Practical Transfusion Medicine

Practical Transfusion Medicine

EDITED BY

Michael F. Murphy, MD, FRCP, FRCPath
Professor of Blood Transfusion Medicine
University of Oxford;
Consultant Haematologist
NHS Blood and Transplant and Department of Haematology
The John Radcliffe Hospital
Oxford, UK

Derwood H. Pamphilon, MD, MRCPCH, FRCP, FRCPath
Consultant Haematologist
NHS Blood and Transplant;
Honorary Clinical Reader
Department of Cellular and Molecular Medicine
University of Bristol
Bristol, UK

FOREWORD BY PROFESSOR DAME MARCELA CONTRERAS

THIRD EDITION

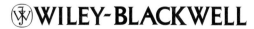

A John Wiley & Sons, Ltd., Publication

This edition first published 2009, © 2001, 2005, 2009 by Blackwell Publishing Ltd

Blackwell Publishing was acquired by John Wiley & Sons in February 2007. Blackwell's publishing program has been merged with Wiley's global Scientific, Technical and Medical business to form Wiley-Blackwell.

Registered office: John Wiley & Sons Ltd, The Atrium, Southern Gate, Chichester, West Sussex, PO19 8SQ, UK

Editorial offices: 9600 Garsington Road, Oxford, OX4 2DQ, UK

The Atrium, Southern Gate, Chichester, West Sussex, PO19 8SQ, UK

111 River Street, Hoboken, NJ 07030-5774, USA

For details of our global editorial offices, for customer services and for information about how to apply for permission to reuse the copyright material in this book please see our website at www.wiley.com/wiley-blackwell

The right of the author to be identified as the author of this work has been asserted in accordance with the Copyright, Designs and Patents Act 1988.

Library of Congress Cataloging-in-Publication Data

Practical transfusion medicine / edited by Michael F. Murphy, Derwood H. Pamphilon. 3rd ed.
p. ; cm.
Includes bibliographical references and index.
ISBN 978-1-4051-8196-9
1. Blood–Transfusion.   I. Murphy, Michael F. (Michael Furber)   II. Pamphilon, Derwood H.
[DNLM: 1. Blood Transfusion.   2. Blood Grouping and Crossmatching.   3. Communicable Disease Control.   4. Specimen Handling. WB 356 P8957 2009]
RM171.P727 2009
615′.39–dc22   2008049829

A catalogue record for this book is available from the British Library.

Set in 9/12pt Meridien by Aptara® Inc., New Delhi, India
Printed & bound in Singapore by Utopia Press Pte Ltd

1   2009

Contents

Colour plates can be found facing page 302

List of contributors

Jean-Pierre Allain, MD, PhD, FRCPath, FMedSc
NHS Blood and Transplant – Cambridge;
Division of Transfusion Medicine
Department of Haematology
University of Cambridge
Cambridge, UK

David L. Allen, FIBMS
Clinical Scientist, NHS Blood and Transplant;
Research Scientist, Department of Clinical Laboratory
  Sciences
University of Oxford
John Radcliffe Hospital
Oxford, UK

Susan Armitage, BSc
Assistant Director
Cord Blood Bank
Department of Stem Cell Transplantation and Cell Therapy
The University of Texas MD Anderson Cancer Center
Houston, Texas, USA

James P. AuBuchon, MD, FCAP, FRCP(Edin)
Professor of Medicine (Hematology) and of Laboratory
  Medicine
University of Washington;
President and CEO
Puget Sound Blood Center
Seattle, Washington, USA

John A.J. Barbara, MA, MSc, PhD, FIBiol, FRCPath
Emeritus Microbiology Consultant
NHS Blood and Transplant and Visiting Professor
University of the West of England
Bristol, UK

Imelda Bates, FRCP, FRCPath
Senior Clinical Lecturer in Tropical Haematology
Liverpool School of Tropical Medicine
Liverpool, UK

Morris A. Blajchman, MD, FRCP (C)
Professor Emeritus, Departments of Pathology and Medicine
McMaster University;
Medical Director, Canadian Blood Services
Hamilton, Ontario, Canada

Anneke Brand, MD, PhD
Consultant
Department of Immunohaematology and Blood Transfusion
Leiden University Medical Center and Sanquin Blood Supply
Leiden, The Netherlands

Susan J. Brunskill, MSc
Senior Scientist
NHS Blood and Transplant
John Radcliffe Hospital
Oxford, UK

Lisa Byrne, BSc
Surveillance Officer (Information)
NHSBT/HPA Infection Surveillance Scheme
Elstree Gate
NBS Colindale
London, UK

Rebecca Cardigan, BSc, PhD
Head of Components Development
NHS Blood and Transplant
Cambridge, UK

Mary E. Clay, MS, MT (ASCP)
Department of Laboratory Medicine and Pathology
University of Minnesota Medical School
Minneapolis, Minnesota, USA

Adrian Copplestone, MBBS, FRCP, FRCPath
Consultant Haematologist
Derriford Hospital
Plymouth, UK

Geoff Daniels, PhD, FRCPath
Head of Molecular Diagnostics and Senior Research Fellow
Bristol Institute for Transfusion Sciences
NHS Blood and Transplant
Bristol, UK

Marcos de Lima, MD
Associate Professor
Department of Stem Cell Transplantation and Cell Therapy
The University of Texas MD Anderson Cancer Center
Houston, Texas, USA

Leandro de Padua Silva, MD
Postdoctoral Fellow
Department of Stem Cell Transplantation and Cell Therapy
The University of Texas MD Anderson Cancer Center
Houston, Texas, USA

Roger Y. Dodd, PhD
Vice President, Research and Development
American Red Cross
Jerome H. Holland Laboratory for the Biomedical Sciences
Rockville, Maryland, USA

Carolyn Doree, PhD
Information Scientist
NHS Blood and Transplant
John Radcliffe Hospital
Oxford, UK

Walter H. Dzik, MD
Co-Director
Blood Transfusion Service
Massachusetts General Hospital;
Associate Professor of Pathology
Harvard Medical School
Boston, Massachusetts, USA

M. P. Eccles, FMedSci
The William Leech Professor of Primary Care Research and
    Professor of Clinical Effectiveness
Institute of Health and Society
Newcastle University
Newcastle, UK

Khaled El-Ghariani, MA, FRCP, FRCPath
Consultant in Haematology and Transfusion Medicine
NHS Blood and Transplant and Sheffield Teaching Hospitals
    NHS Trust;
Honorary Senior Lecturer
University of Sheffield
Sheffield, UK

Deirdre Fehily, PhD
Inspector and Technical Consultant, Tissues and Cells
National Transplant Centre
Rome, Italy

Dean Fergusson, MHA, PhD
Senior Scientist
University of Ottawa Center for Transfusion Research
Clinical Epidemiology Program
The Ottawa Health Research Institute
Ottawa, Ontario, Canada

Stephen Field, FCPath (SA), MMed, MBChB
Consultant in Transfusion Medicine
Welsh Blood Service
Pontyclun, Cardiff, Wales

J. J. Francis, PhD
Senior Research Fellow
Health Services Research Unit
University of Aberdeen
Aberdeen, Scotland

Ian M. Franklin, PhD, FRCP, FRCPath
Professor of Transfusion Medicine
University of Glasgow;
Scottish National Blood Transfusion Service
Glasgow, Scotland

Lawrence Tim Goodnough, MD
Professor of Pathology and Medicine
Director, Transfusion Service
Associate Director of Quality
Department of Pathology
Stanford University School of Medicine
Stanford, California, USA

Paul C. Hébert, MD, FRCPC, MHSc (Epid)
Professor
Department of Medicine
University of Ottawa;
University of Ottawa Center for Transfusion Research
Clinical Epidemiology Program
The Ottawa Health Research Institute
Ottawa, Ontario, Canada

Nancy M. Heddle, MSc, FCSMLS (D)
Associate Professor
Department of Medicine
McMaster University;
Adjunct Scientist
Canadian Blood Services
Hamilton, Ontario, Canada

Patricia E. Hewitt, FRCP, FRCPath
Consultant Specialist in Transfusion Microbiology
NHS Blood and Transplant
and University Hospitals Bristol
NHS Foundation Trust Bristol, UK

Christopher D. Hillyer, MD
Director
Center for Transfusion and Cellular Therapies;
Professor
Department of Pathology and Laboratory Medicine
Emory University School of Medicine
Atlanta, Georgia, USA

Beverley J. Hunt, MD, FRCP, FRCPath
Professor of Thrombosis and Haemostasis
Kings College, London;
Consultant
Departments of Haematology, Pathology and Rheumatology
Guy's and St Thomas' NHS Foundation Trust
London, UK

Chris J. Hyde, MD
Consultant in Public Health Medicine
NHS Blood and Transplant
John Radcliffe Hospital
Oxford, UK

Joan Jones, CSci, FIBMS
Manager
Better Blood Transfusion Team
Welsh Blood Service
Cardiff, Wales

Joanne E. Joseph, MD, FRACP, FRCP
Department of Haematology and Stem Cell Transplantation
St Vincent's Hospital
Darlinghurst, New South Wales, Australia

Ram Kakaiya, MD
Medical Director
LifeSource Blood Services
Glenview, Illinois, USA

Alan D. Kitchen, PhD
Head, National Transfusion Microbiology Reference
  Laboratory;
NHS Blood and Transplant – Colindale
London, UK

Steven H. Kleinman, MD
Clinical Professor of Pathology
University of British Columbia
Victoria, British Columbia, Canada

Sue Knowles, BSc, FRCP, FRCPath
Consultant Haematologist
Epsom and St Helier University Hospitals NHS Trust
Surrey, UK

Mark W. Lowdell, MSc, PhD, FRCPath, MICR
Senior Lecturer in Haematology
University College London Medical School
Honorary Consultant Immunologist,
Royal Free Hospital
London, UK

Geoffrey F. Lucas, BSc, PhD, FIBMS, DMS
Principle Clinical Scientist
Histocompatibility and Immunogenetics
NHS Blood and Transplant
Bristol, UK

Samuel J. Machin, MD, FRCP, FRCPath
Professor of Haematology
Haemostasis Research Unit

University College London
Department of Haematology
London, UK

Edwin Massey, MB ChB, FRCP, FRCPath
Consultant Haematologist
NHS Blood and Transplant
Bristol, UK

Brian McClelland, MB ChB, BSc, FRCP, (cedin), FRCPath
Consultant, Scottish National Blood Transfusion Service
Protein Fractionation Centre
Edinburgh, Scotland

Vickie McDonald, MA, MRCP, FRCPath
Clinical Research Fellow in Haematology
Haemostasis Research Unit
University College London
Department of Haematology
London, UK

David H. McKenna Jr, MD
Assistant Professor
University of Minnesota Medical School;
Medical Director
Molecular and Cellular Therapeutics
Minneapolis/Saint Paul, Minnesota, USA

I. Grant McQuaker
Consultant Haematologist
Bone Marrow Transplant Unit
Beatson West of Scotland Cancer Centre
Glasgow, Scotland

Ellen McSweeney, MB, MRCP(UK), FRCPath
Consultant Haematologist
Irish Blood Transfusion Service
National Blood Centre
Dublin, Ireland

Siraj A. Misbah, MSc, FRCP, FRCPath
Consultant Clinical Immunologist
Honorary Senior Clinical Lecturer in Immunology
Oxford Radcliffe Hospitals
University of Oxford
Oxford, UK

Emma Morris, MA, PhD, MRCP, MRCPath
Senior Lecturer in Immunotherapy
Department of Immunology and Molecular
  Pathology
University College London Medical School
Honorary Consultant Haematologist (BMT)
University College London Hospitals NHS Trust
London, UK

Michael F. Murphy, MD, FRCP, FRCPath
Professor of Blood Transfusion Medicine
University of Oxford;
Consultant Haematologist
NHS Blood and Transplant and Department of
   Haematology
John Radcliffe Hospital
Oxford, UK

William Murphy, MD, FRCPEdin, FRCPath
Medical Director
Irish Blood Transfusion Service;
UCD Senior Clinical Lecturer
University College
Dublin, Ireland

Cristina V. Navarrete, PhD, FRCPath
Consultant Clinical Scientist
Department of Histocompatibility Immunogenetics
NHS Blood and Transplant, Colindale, London
Honorary Reader in Immunology
University College London
London, UK

Willem H. Ouwehand, MD, PhD, FRCPath
Reader in Platelet Biology and Genetics
University of Cambridge;
Consultant Haematologist
NHS Blood and Transplant
Cambridge, UK

**Derwood H. Pamphilon, MD, MRCPCH, FRCP,
   FRCPath**
Consultant Haematologist
NHS Blood and Transplant;
Honorary Clinical Reader
Department of Cellular and Molecular Medicine
University of Bristol
Bristol, UK

Geoff Poole, DBMS, MSc, CSci, FIBMS
Director of Service
Welsh Blood Service
Bridgend, Wales

Chris V. Prowse, MA, DPhil, FRCPath
Research Director
National Science Laboratory
Scottish National Blood Transfusion Service
Edinburgh, Scotland

David Rees, MA, FRCP, FRCPath
Senior Lecturer and Honorary Consultant in Paediatric
   Haematology
Department of Haematological Medicine

King's College Hospital
Denmark Hill
London, UK

David J. Roberts, DPhil, MRCP, FRCPath
Professor of Haematology
University of Oxford;
Consultant Haematologist
NHS Blood and Transplant and Department of Haematology
John Radcliffe Hospital
Oxford, UK

Irene Roberts, MD, FRCP, FRCPath, FRCPCH, DRCOG
Professor of Paediatric Haematology
Honorary Consultant Paediatric Haematologist
Departments of Haematology and Paediatrics
Imperial College London
London, UK

J. Kim Ryland, BSc, MRCP, DipRCPath
Clinical Research Fellow
Haemostasis Research Unit
University College London
Department of Haematology
London, UK

Marion Scott, BSc, PhD
National Research and Development Manager
NHS Blood and Transplant
Bristol, UK

Aryeh Shander, MD, FCCM, FCCP
Chief, Department of Anesthesiology, Critical Care and
Hyperbaric Medicine
Englewood Hospital and Medical Center
Englewood;
Clinical Professor of Anesthesiology, Medicine and Surgery
Mount Sinai School of Medicine
New Jersey, USA

Beth H. Shaz, MD
Director, Blood Bank
Grady Memorial Hospital;
Assistant Professor
Department of Pathology and Laboratory Medicine
Emory University School of Medicine
Atlanta, Georgia, USA

Elizabeth J. Shpall, MD
Professor and Director
Cord Blood Bank
Department of Stem Cell Transplantation and
   Cell Therapy
The University of Texas MD Anderson Cancer Center
Houston, Texas, USA

Simon J. Stanworth, MA, MRCP (Paeds), D. Phil, FRCPath
Consultant Haematologist
NHS Blood and Transplant and Department of Haematology
John Radcliffe Hospital
Oxford, UK

Zbigniew M. Szczepiorkowski, MD, PhD
Consultant Haematologist
Dartmouth-Hitchcock Medical Center
Lebanon
New Hampshire, USA

Dafydd Thomas, MB, ChB, FRCA
Consultant in Intensive Care and Anaesthesia
Welsh Blood Implementation Group
Morriston Hospital
Swansea, Wales

John Thompson, MS, FRCSEd, FRCS
Consultant Surgeon
Royal Devon and Exeter Hospitals
Exeter, UK

Alan T. Tinmouth, MD, MSc (Clin Epi), FRCPC
Associate Professor
Department of Medicine and Pathology and Laboratory
  Medicine
University of Ottawa;
University of Ottawa Centre for Transfusion Research
Clinical Epidemiology Program
Ottawa Health Research Institute
Ottawa, Ontario, Canada

Marc L. Turner, MB, ChB, MBA, PhD, FRCP, FRCPath
Professor of Cellular Therapy
Clinical Director, Edinburgh Blood Transfusion Centre
Royal Infirmary of Edinburgh
Edinburgh, Scotland

Eleftherios C. Vamvakas, MD, PhD
Professor of Pathology
Vice-Chair and Director, Clinical Pathology
Department of Pathology and Laboratory Medicine
Cedars-Sinai Medical Center
Los Angeles, California, USA

Timothy Wallington, BA, MB, BChir, FRCP, FRCPath
Consultant Immunologist
NHS Blood and Transplant
Bristol, UK

Tim Walsh, BSc (Hms), MBChB (Hms), FRCP, FRCA, MD, MRes (PHS)
Department of Anaesthetics
and Intensive care
Royal Infirmary
Edinburgh, Scotland

Ruth M. Warwick, MB, ChB, FRCP, FRCPath
Consultant Specialist in Tissue Services
NHS Blood and Transplant
Edgware, Middlesex, UK

Kathryn E. Webert, MD, FRCP (C)
Department of Medicine
and Department of Pathology and Molecular
  Medicine
McMaster University;
Canadian Blood Services
Hamilton, Ontario, Canada

David Wenham, FIBMS
PTI Manager
NHS Blood and Transplant
Colindale, London, UK

Lorna M. Williamson, BSc, MD, FRCP, FRCPath
Reader in Transfusion Medicine, University of
  Cambridge;
Medical Director
NHS Blood and Transplant
Cambridge, UK

Cynthia Wu, MD, FRCPC
Fellow
Department of Medicine
McMaster University
Hamilton, Ontario, Canada

Foreword

I welcome the third edition of *Practical Transfusion Medicine* coming just under five years after the second edition. It is a pleasure to read this very useful book, written by hand-picked contributors of worldwide renown. As Professor Weatherall notes in his foreword to the second edition, *Transfusion Medicine* spans a large range of subjects and the range has grown wider in this new edition. The reader will not fail to note the extraordinary amplitude of the speciality. Indeed, clinical advances in many areas and particularly in haemato-oncology, cell therapy, solid organ transplantation, and cardiac surgery have been critically dependent on blood component therapy in its many forms and this is evident to the readership of this updated edition.

In its first decades, blood transfusion was largely confined to the treatment of anaemia and massive haemorrhage. The book shows that this is not the case anymore. The speed of advance of transfusion and cellular therapies as well as research in the allied sciences increases year on year. Transfusion medicine is no longer the restricted domain of a few haematologists and biomedical scientists; it is an indispensable tool for many clinical disciplines, i.e. it has become a clinical speciality in itself.

The result of these developments and expansion of the speciality, as well as the interest of the media and the lay public, is that increasing numbers of health care professionals are seeking guidance to particular aspects of the subject or to a rounded view. The book fulfils this role, as it has a wealth of information and guidance on the practicalities of transfusion and transplantation therapy for the specialist as well as for the uninitiated who has hitherto not had the opportunity to explore this interesting topic.

The book is divided into 49 chapters, written in a friendly, accessible, concise and easy style. It has now been expanded from five to seven parts – all very much needed to get a comprehensive view of all aspects of transfusion medicine and allied fields. The chapters are written, with the authority that grows from experience, by practising clinicians, researchers and health care professionals who procure, produce and test blood components, cells and tissues and by those who use them and have to trace them to their final destination. It should enable the reader to obtain a rounded view of what transfusion medicine consists of in the twenty-first century. It also allocates space to different areas according to their relevance in current practice; for example there are full chapters on TRALI, haemovigilance and bacterial contamination. It is recommended for those already involved in blood services and transfusion medicine as well as for those entering the field and who have to make important decisions about patient care. In most cases, the only exposure of health care professionals to transfusion medicine has been a brief session during their undergraduate training; this book will wet their appetite for this very interesting field of medicine. Indeed, *Practical Transfusion Medicine* provides a strong background in those subjects and principles which are so important to anybody involved in the fields of transfusion and transplantation.

Many textbooks devoted to blood transfusion therapy have been published, although surprisingly few deal sufficiently with practical concepts and objectives whilst at the same time dealing with the scientific basis of the many topics embraced. Most books have too much theory and science, neglecting what is important to the clinician and everyday health care practitioner, i.e. 'how to do it' and 'why we are doing it'. This book gives you the answers.

Transfusion Medicine interacts with many other areas of science and medicine and this is clearly shown in the book. The editors have achieved what few books on the subject have done in the past – they have managed to transmit excitement and interest about this growing and fascinating multidisciplinary speciality.

The book is a testimony of the significant progress experienced by transfusion medicine in recent years. Although there is a great deal that we still need to know about clinical transfusion medicine, as is evident after reading the book, a great deal of progress has been made in the last 5 years, including recent discoveries, clinical trials, systematic reviews and progress in quality management and the regulatory environment. I recommend that both specialists and non-specialists read the book from cover to cover and then keep it at hand, as a source of advice and consultation.

Professor Dame Marcela Contreras
Professor of Transfusion Medicine
Chairman, Blood Transfusion International
London, UK
2009

Preface to the third edition

Since the second edition of *Practical Transfusion Medicine* was published in 2005, a number of important developments have taken place in the field of transfusion medicine and the pace of change seems likely to increase further as we embrace new scientific and technological developments.

The primary aim of the third edition remains the same – to provide a comprehensive guide to transfusion medicine. The book includes information in more depth than contained within handbooks of transfusion medicine, and is presented in a more concise and 'user-friendly' manner than standard reference texts. The feedback we received on the previous editions from reviews and colleagues was that this objective has been achieved, and that we have provided a consistent style and format throughout the book which we have attempted to maintain in the third edition. The feedback has also provided many helpful comments that have been taken into account in shaping this edition. We believe that it will continue to provide a text that will be useful to the many clinical and scientific staff, both established practitioners and trainees, who are involved in some aspect of transfusion medicine and who require an accessible text.

The book has been expanded and now has 49 chapters including many new contributions. It is now divided into seven sections which systematically take the reader through the principles of transfusion medicine, the complications of transfusion, the practice of transfusion in blood centres and hospitals, clinical transfusion practice, alternatives to transfusion, cellular and tissue therapy and organ transplantation and development of the evidence base for transfusion. Many chapters such as stem cell processing and the use of recombinant proteins that were included as 'potential advances' now have a secure place in the repertoire of transfusion medicine and are included in the appropriate sections. Once again, a visionary chapter on future advances in the field and written by Walter H. Dzik concludes the book.

The authorship has been expanded and is now more 'international' than in the previous two editions. We are very grateful to the colleagues who have contributed to this book at a time of continuing change and to Jane Graham and Emma Saville for secretarial support. Once again, we have received excellent support from our publishers, particularly Jenny Seward and Maria Khan.

Michael Murphy
Derwood Pamphilon
2009

Preface to the first edition

Blood transfusion continues to enjoy an ever-increasing public profile. This has occurred in part because of the emergence of new pathogens which have posed a significant threat to the safety of the blood supply, and also due to major scientific developments. In the new millennium, advances in technology have facilitated the provision of high-quality blood components and a range of sophisticated diagnostic and specialist services within modern blood centres. There has been enormous progress in transfusion medicine which has developed into a specialist area of its own in the last decade. It now encompasses many important areas of medicine including haematology, immunology, transplantation science, microbiology, epidemiology, clinical practice and research and development.

In this book, we have aimed to provide a comprehensive guide to transfusion medicine. This includes information in more depth than contained within handbooks of transfusion medicine, but at the same time presented in a more concise and 'user-friendly' manner than standard reference texts. Ably assisted by many expert colleagues, we have compiled a text which should prove invaluable to haematologists in training as well as consultants in established practice. We have also aimed to provide useful information to oncologists, surgeons, anaesthetists and other clinicians, nursing staff in general and specialist units and scientific and technical staff in haematology and blood transfusion.

We have endeavoured to provide information that defines practical approaches to the problems that are encountered in transfusion medicine. To this end we have used a consistent format to make access to information easy, irrespective of whether the book is read cover to cover by haematologists updating or revising for exams, or used as a reference book by clinical or laboratory staff faced with specific problems. To facilitate this approach, the book is divided into five sections which systematically take the reader through the principles of transfusion medicine, the use of transfusion in specific clinical areas, its practical aspects in blood centres and hospitals, the complications of transfusion and potential advances, some of which are already with us and some of which will continue to impact significantly on transfusion services in the future.

We are grateful to the colleagues who have contributed to this book at a time of rapid development and considerable organisational change in health care as a whole but specifically within blood services in the UK. We are indebted to Bridget Hunt and Susan Sugden for their patience and forbearance; without their invaluable assistance in compiling the text, this book would not have been possible. We have received enormous support from our publishers, particularly Andrew Robinson, who gave us considerable assistance at a time when this book was at its early conceptual stages, and Marcela Holmes, whose wisdom and expertise have been invaluable in its completion.

Michael Murphy
Derwood Pamphilon
2001

CHAPTER 1

Introduction: recent evolution of transfusion medicine

Ian M. Franklin

Scottish National Blood Transfusion Service, University of Glasgow, Glasgow, Scotland

In the previous introductions to the two earlier editions of *Practical Transfusion Medicine*, an attempt was made to cover a broad sweep of issues of importance in the field. Much of what was included remains relevant, but in this new third edition, a few contemporary issues will be covered to highlight areas of potential development that will have an impact before a fourth edition is published.

As before, blood safety takes centre stage, although there has been some shift in emphasis. In 2004, concerns were over SARS and West Nile virus, the second of which remains important although the impact, at least in North America, appears to be waning as the population develops greater immunity. The wide acceptance by all governments of global warming driven by human activity has been accompanied by the recognition that many infectious diseases previously considered to be tropical are encroaching on temperate countries. The outbreaks of Chikungunya infection in Italy and dengue in the southern US are good examples and are leading to greater concerns over maintaining blood safety. These effects are often made worse by a reduced emphasis on public health systems, by increased international travel and reduced mosquito eradication programmes. These issues are explored in detail in Chapter 16.

Practical Transfusion Medicine, 3rd edition. Edited by Michael F. Murphy and Derwood H. Pamphilon. © 2009 Blackwell Publishing, ISBN: 978-1-4051-8196-9.

Concerns over emerging infections have brought pathogen reduction systems back into the spotlight after a period of decline following the formation of red cell-directed antibodies in recipients of two products in phase 1 trials. An alternative approach to the prevention of transfusion-transmitted infections would be wider testing, ideally perhaps using a generic flavivirus nucleic acid testing (NAT) to detect dengue and Chikungunya viruses. Other expensive interventions, including the introduction of prion reduction filters, are under active consideration and/or development, particularly in the UK and Republic of Ireland, where bovine spongiform encephalopathy (BSE) and then variant Creutzfeldt–Jakob disease (vCJD) have been most prevalent. Happily, the number of new cases of vCJD has fallen to five in each of the past 3 years, and none in the first half of 2008. But concerns remain about a possible later wave of cases in donors who have the less susceptible genotype. What is certain is that vCJD is a transfusion-transmissible agent, albeit very rarely, which has a high degree of probability of disease transmission when transfused shortly before the donor develops evidence of symptoms. So far, all four transmissions of vCJD have occurred prior to the introduction of universal leucocyte reduction in the UK, and the small number of new clinical cases means that the number of persons known to be at risk has not increased recently. This is good news, but not sufficient for complacency. Therefore, trials of prion reduction filters are progressing and some tough decisions will need to be taken soon regarding implementation, assuming that the trials of prion-filtered blood go according to plan. Disadvantages are the cost and also that red cells are lost in the process. The former seems the most difficult issue. At least there will be no perceived problem for donors, which would not be the case for a prion disease test. Though still appearing to be a little way off, the obstacles to successful implementation of a vCJD test will be significant, as described in Chapter 15.

In terms of cost, testing for hepatitis C by NAT continues despite a very high cost indeed per case avoided. Given that the legacy of perceived problems with past blood safety remains with us 15–25 years on – a public inquiry is about to commence in Scotland on this very issue – it appears unlikely that ceasing to perform such a test would be desirable or even politically possible. It will be particularly important to evaluate and assess new safety interventions or tests thoroughly prior to full implementation since ceasing to do any measure that contributes to blood safety appears all but impossible once established.

The high cost of new blood safety initiatives introduced over the past 10 years has been the subject of much discussion within the extended blood transfusion community, particularly as measures against prion transmission are approaching the point at which decisions must be made. Typically, new blood safety interventions cost in excess of US$1,000,000 per quality-adjusted life year (QALY) versus an accepted cost per therapeutic QALY of US$50–100,000 and UK£30,000. More recently, it has been acknowledged that, while high, these costs are not disproportionate to other blood safety procedures introduced in the past. A rational framework for making decisions about which new blood safety measures should be introduced would be most welcome.

Early in 2008, an influential paper was published suggesting, in a retrospective observational study of a large number of patients, that receiving blood older than 14 days post-collection led to an adverse outcome compared with patients receiving younger, fresher red cell transfusions. This

followed on from data from the same group at the Cleveland Clinic and a study from Bristol, UK, amongst other studies, which suggested that receiving a blood transfusion was an independent adverse effect for survival following cardiac surgery.

No one doubts that blood transfusion has a major role in saving life in traumatic and obstetric emergencies, and it is essential to have blood and other blood components available to support major surgery and bone marrow failure. Over the past decades, anxieties about blood safety have tended to be attached to the risks of transfusion-transmitted infections, although these are now extremely rare, or to the more common hazards of a transfusion administration error or transfusion-related acute lung injury. What is emerging now as a more important issue is that transfusion may be an independent risk factor for reduced survival after certain serious events. These include admission to a critical care unit and coronary artery bypass surgery, but may not be confined to these areas of practice.

The first and still the most influential report to question the advisability of a liberal transfusion policy was the transfusion requirements in critical care (TRICC) study. This was well designed and organised, adequately powered and delivered a clear conclusion. A hard end-point – improved survival – was associated with a more restrictive transfusion regime. In neonates, more red cell transfusions conferred no benefit and a recent study in acute lung injury/adult respiratory distress syndrome showed an adverse impact of red cell transfusion. Quite why less transfusion should be as good or better than more is not clear, but these data do fit with a considerable literature from the past decades of often weakly powered studies that have suggested, but never proven, that transfusion is associated with more postoperative infections or recurrent cancer. These transfusion studies are difficult to perform and to analyse, especially as there would appear to be an obvious correlation between the amount of blood required to support a patient and the complexity and risk of the procedure, and how ill the patient is. However, by concentrating on one standard surgical intervention, which has traditionally been associated with a high rate of transfusion, many of these confounding variables have been controlled in recent studies. Coronary artery bypass graft surgery is a common, relatively serious procedure that requires considerable transfusion support to be available – even if many patients do not need blood. Three large retrospective studies have shown that receiving a perioperative blood transfusion is an independent risk factor for short- and long-term survival following cardiac surgery. The differences are not trivial, and avoiding a transfusion could offer at least a 5% improved survival. Although two of the major studies were in the US, where leucocyte reduction of red cell transfusions is not universal, it does not appear to be due simply to an adverse impact of passenger white cells in the transfusions. In the absence of appropriate randomised controlled trials, a potent potential negative impact of transfusion now places the burden of proof on those who use a permissive transfusion regime.

Avoiding a transfusion should not be taken to extremes, however, since pre- and intraoperative anaemia correlates with postoperative renal failure and cerebral dysfunction. Preoperative anaemia, at least for elective surgery, can usually be treated adequately, so transfusion should be avoidable in most cases. Intraoperative anaemia should be amenable to surgical and anaesthetic technique. As with most areas of medicine and life, common sense and a sense of perspective are essential.

Certainly in the UK, the consistent application of known methods to reduce or avoid transfusion has not happened – despite successive initiatives by the chief medical officers in the UK to deliver *better blood transfusion*. Gardner (see Further Reading) also implies that in the US, the peak of enthusiasm for transfusion alternatives may have passed. This state of affairs cannot be allowed to continue. The evidence appears compelling that for elective cardiac surgery – at least – a comprehensive transfusion management programme should be developed for each patient. Preoperative correction of anaemia, peri- and intraoperative blood avoidance interventions and a scrupulous attention to bloodless surgical technique must become the standard of care.

It is likely that such a programme should be developed for all patients about to undergo surgery which has a high probability of needing a transfusion, and particularly for those with cancer. One problem, which the recent study of older blood versus younger blood highlights, is the lack of similar studies in conditions other than heart disease. It is therefore premature to divert supplies of younger red cells to cardiac cases at the expense of other patient groups who may benefit equally. It would seem better to redouble efforts to safely avoid transfusion altogether which would improve supplies of younger transfusions for everybody who really needs blood.

How is this to be delivered? Probably not through further 'top-down' initiatives on blood transfusion practice, although educational and awareness programmes delivered through hospital transfusion teams remain important. One important stakeholder in all this is the patient, and it is currently unlikely that their opinion will be sought, since there is no requirement for formal consent for transfusion in the UK. This can no longer be left up on the 'too difficult' shelf, looked at occasionally by anxious transfusion medicine specialists. Outcome differences with or without transfusion of upwards of 5% surely must be shared with the patient, who should be informed of the mechanisms by which blood transfusion will be avoided and provided, if necessary. None of the methods by which transfusion may be safely avoided are obscure, or difficult. Some may cost money, but if outcomes improve, the total cost should be modest indeed.

Previous debates – mainly within the transfusion community – about consent for transfusion have foundered on concerns about what represents 'consent', when is consent 'informed', is a signature necessary, what about incapable/unconscious patients, or whether there is time in the day to do it – the 'can't be bothered' argument. However, other countries have found no such difficulties, although the recall of patients about what they have been told is often poor. While these niceties are being debated, people – your family member and mine – are being denied their opportunity to share in their care, unless they happen to be a Jehovah's Witness or have an aversion to blood not based on scripture.

Current Scottish guidelines (see further reading) state that 'The decision to transfuse is made following consideration of the potential risks and benefits of, and the alternatives to, transfusion. Where possible, this is discussed between the clinician and patient (or their legal guardian) in advance of transfusion'. It seems unlikely that this will be delivered without a formal requirement to obtain consent prior to transfusion.

At present, the search for perfection is obstructing a sensible, pragmatic attempt to engage patients by seeking their consent to transfusion. In many hospitals, written consent is obtained for bone marrow biopsies and removal of indwelling venous catheters, for example, but not for blood transfusion. Even the most basic system for consent to transfuse would empower those who wish to engage in that aspect of their care. Such a process would also require physicians and surgeons who obtain the consent to be aware of transfusion hazards and alternatives and to ensure that their own practice is current with respect to this area. Certainly, the body of evidence is increasingly supportive of the proposition that the safest transfusion is the one safely avoided.

Further reading

Brunkard JM, Cifuentes E & Rothenberg SJ. Assessing the roles of temperature, precipitation, and enso in dengue re-emergence on the Texas–Mexico border region. *Salud Publica Mex* 2008;50:227–234.

Engoren MC, Habib RH, Zacharias A, Schwann TA, Riordan CJ & Durham SJ. Effect of blood transfusion on long-term survival after cardiac operation. *Ann Thorac Surg* 2002;74:1180–1186.

Gardner TJ. To transfuse or not to transfuse. *Circulation* 2007;116:458–460.

Hebert PC, Wells G, Blajchman MA *et al.*, for Transfusion Requirements in Critical Care Investigators, Canadian Critical Care Trials Group. A multicenter, randomized, controlled clinical trial of transfusion requirements in critical care. *N Engl J Med* 1999;340:409–417.

Jackson B, Busch M, Stramer S & AuBuchon J. The cost-effectiveness of NAT for HIV, HCV, and HBV in whole-blood donations. *Transfusion* 2003;43:721–729.

Kirpalani H, Whyte RK, Andersen C *et al.* The premature infants in need of transfusion (PINT) study: a randomized, controlled trial of a restrictive (low) versus liberal (high) transfusion threshold for extremely low birth weight infants. *J Pediatr* 2006;149:301–307.

Koch CG, Li L, Duncan AI *et al.* Transfusion in coronary artery bypass grafting is associated with reduced long-term survival. *Ann Thorac Surg* 2006;81:1650–1657.

Koch CG, Li L, Sessler DI *et al.* Duration of red-cell storage and complications after cardiac surgery. *N Engl J Med* 2008;358:1229–1239.

Murphy GJ, Reeves BC, Rogers CA, Rizvi SI, Culliford L & Angelini GD. Increased mortality, postoperative morbidity, and cost after red blood cell transfusion in patients having cardiac surgery. *Circulation* 2007;116:2544–2552.

Netzer G, Shah CV, Iwashyna TJ *et al.* Association of RBC transfusion with mortality in patients with acute lung injury. *Chest* 2007;132:1116–1123.

QIS_Scotland. *Clinical Standards – September 2006. Blood Transfusion*. Edinburgh: NHS Quality Improvement Scotland, 2006, p. 40.

Rezza G, Nicoletti L, Angelini R *et al.* Infection with Chikungunya virus in Italy: an outbreak in a temperate region. *Lancet* 2007;370:1840–1846.

PART 1
Basic principles of immunohaematology

CHAPTER 2

Essential immunology for transfusion medicine

Timothy Wallington
NHS Blood and Transplant, Bristol, UK

The immune system is a sophisticated and multi-layered defence against infection. It is based on the recognition of non-self in any potential pathogen. Since donor organs are not-self, their transplantation from one individual to another is only possible if the obstacles inherent in the recipient's immune system can be overcome. The transfer of blood components (either as therapy or during the course of pregnancy) is a form of transplantation. This discussion concentrates on the immunobiology of clinical problems that are encountered as a result. There are excellent texts which discuss human immunobiology in detail (see Further Reading).

The immune system has evolved distinct mechanisms for coping with extracellular pathogens, such as bacteria, based on the production of antibody and intracellular pathogens, such as viruses, based on the activity of effector T cells. Two essential layers of defence are utilised:
• innate immunity which is primitive in evolution and not specific to single pathogens (e.g. mannan-binding protein which binds microbial cell-wall saccharides and Toll-like receptors which can be directly involved in macrophage activation); and
• adaptive immunity in higher animals, which working with innate mechanisms, brings specificity

and memory to immune responses (e.g. antibody formation in defence against bacteria).

Most problems encountered in transfusion medicine are antibody-based – the humoral immune response – and this will be considered in greater detail below.

Cellular basis of the immune response

The key effector cells are T cells, B cells and natural killer (NK) cells. The progenitors of T cells, B cells and NK cells are derived from the same haemopoietic stem cells (HSCs) that give rise to other types of blood cells. Cells of the monocyte–macrophage series, including Langerhans' cells and dendritic cells, process and present antigen to both T and B cells. Progenitor cells migrate from the circulation into the epithelial thymus to become T cells. There they interact with the stromal cells and their soluble products to undergo cell division, clonal selection and maturation. In addition, they acquire their antigen receptor (T-cell receptor or TCR) and other surface molecules which will determine their function, CD8 on cytotoxic T cells, CD4 on helper T cells and the major population of regulatory T cells. Immature T cells initially express both CD4 and CD8 molecules, which interact, respectively, with major histocompatibility complex (MHC) class II or I molecules on thymic stromal

Practical Transfusion Medicine, 3rd edition. Edited by Michael F. Murphy and Derwood H. Pamphilon. © 2009 Blackwell Publishing, ISBN: 978-1-4051-8196-9.

cells to influence their maturation into CD4 or CD8 T cells. Through this process, self-reactive T cells are removed. Later, when they migrate to the periphery, T cells may undergo selective clonal activation triggered by antigen, which leads to proliferation and maturation.

B-cell development is a multifocal process which is concentrated in the fetal liver before bone marrow becomes the major haemopoietic organ. Progenitor cells receiving signals from local stromal cells begin to divide and begin the process that will provide an antigen receptor, in this case surface immunoglobulin (SIg). Like T cells, immature B cells are easily tolerised or killed by premature stimulation via their antigen receptors to prevent damage to self. After migrating from the bone marrow, B cells mature, express SIg antigen receptors, and respond to antigens together with T-cell help from CD4 cells by undergoing proliferation and plasma cell differentiation.

NK cells are non-T, non-B lymphoid cells capable of killing virus-infected cells either specifically targeted by the presence of antibody on their surface (antibody-dependent cell-mediated cytotoxicity – ADCC) or through the recognition of changes in the infected cell surfaces which allow NK cell attack. This mechanism is greatly enhanced by the cytokine interferon-γ, secreted by T cells, illustrating the fact that these key effector cells usually act in concert in the defence against infection.

Humoral immune response

Antibody

Antibody is the specific effector molecule which is secreted into the extracellular space from plasma cells. It is a unique tetramer made up of two identical heavy and two identical light chains (Figure 2.1). These combine variability of amino acid sequence and thus variability of tertiary structure (Fab) with a constant region (Fc), which allows the molecule to bind target antigen via Fab and trigger effector functions through the Fc portion. These molecules are more generally called immunoglobulins. They also serve as antigen receptors on B cells.

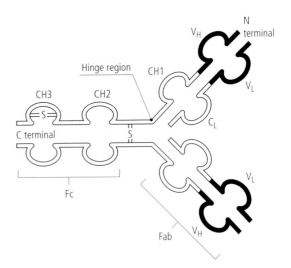

Figure 2.1 Basic structure of an immunoglobulin molecule. Domains are held in shape by disulphide bonds, though only one is shown. CH1–3, constant domain of an H chain; C_L, constant domain of a light chain; V_H, variable domain of an H chain; V_L, variable domain of a light chain.

Antibody effector functions

The constant regions of the heavy (H) chain of immunoglobulins are responsible for the triggering of an effector pathway. This occurs either:
• by binding to appropriate Fc receptors on effector cells, such as leucocytes and mast cells; or
• by activation of the complement cascade.

There are five immunoglobulin isotypes based on different genes for the C domains of the H chain (Table 2.1). Immunoglobulin G (IgG) and IgA have four and two subclasses, respectively. The immunoglobulin isotypes and subtypes differ significantly in their ability to recruit effector functions (Table 2.1). This is of clinical significance in transfusion as the ability of antibodies to bring about erythrocyte or platelet destruction varies according to their isotype and IgG subclass.

Basis of antibody variability

The molecular biology of antibody variability is complex. The genes for the five heavy chains and κ and λ light chains are found on separate chromosomes, at 14q32, 22q11 and 2p11, respectively. Each chain is separately synthesised before being

Table 2.1 Immunoglobulin classes and their functions.

Isotype	Structure			Function		
	Heavy chain	Light chain	Configuration*	Complement fixation†	Cells reacting with FcR	Placental passage
IgM	μ	κ, λ	Pentamer	+++	L	−
IgG1	γ 1	κ, λ	Monomer	+++	M, N, P, L, E	++
IgG2	γ 2	κ, λ	Monomer	+	P, L	+/−
IgG3	γ 3	κ, λ	Monomer	+++	M, N, P, L, E	++
IgG4	γ 4	κ, λ	Monomer	−	N, L, P	+
IgA1	α1	κ, λ	Monomer	−	—	−
IgA2	α2	κ, λ	Dimer in secretion	—	—	−
IgD	δ	κ, λ	Monomer	−	—	−
IgE	ε	κ, λ	Monomer	−	B, E, L	−

* Five basic tetrameric units? pentamer (in vitro good agglutination). Two basic units, dimer. One basic unit, monomer (two or more basic units are held together by a J chain).
† Classical pathway.
B, basophils/mast cells; E, eosinophils; L, lymphocytes; M, macrophages; N, neutrophils; P, platelets.

assembled into an antibody molecule. On chromosome 14, which carries the H chain genes, there are three clusters: 200 variable (V) region genes, which encode the first 95 amino acids of the V portion, 12 diversity (D) region genes and four joining (J) region genes. Together these genes encode for H chain V regions. Like letters of the alphabet, they can be joined at random into three-letter 'words' thus providing much variability in the receptor portion of the H chain. Similarly, 22q11 and 2p11 have two clusters of genes for the V and J portions of the κ and λ light chains, respectively, which can recombine in this way. The incredible diversity of antibody specificity which is found even at the level of the germline is the result of these events, coming together in the tertiary structure of the Fab portions of the immunoglobulin molecule (Figure 2.2). The variability of the receptor for antigen on T lymphocytes (TCR) is the product of similar mechanisms.

Somatic mutation

Antibody function is further refined in the sequential production of immunoglobulin isotypes as the adaptive immune response matures, as follows:

• there is switching in the immunoglobulin isotype mix to molecules that are more effective in neutralising the wide variety of pathogen types that may be encountered; this process is controlled and driven by helper T lymphocytes; and
• mutation at hotspots where the V, D and J genes join and similarly within the V portion of light chains, which refine the shape of the receptor area and thus the specificity of the antibodies produced.

Blood cell antibodies illustrating the above principles

These mechanisms at work are illustrated by the behaviour of commonly found blood cell antibodies. In a typical T-cell-dependent antiprotein (e.g. anti-D) immune response, the switching of the immunoglobulin isotype from IgM to IgG is associated with an increase in the affinity and specificity of the antibody. In the early phase of the response, the V region is encoded by genes from the germline and antibody affinity is low. As a result, in the early phase of an anti-D response, a panreactive antibody, reactive with several blood groups, might

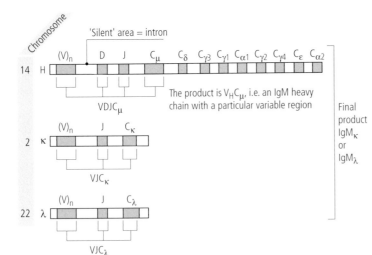

Figure 2.2 Genes encoding IgM antibodies (see the text for explanation).

be detected. This reaction is most likely caused by low-affinity IgM antibodies which, although responding to RhD, are able, particularly at 4°C (which enables low-affinity reactions), to react with other blood groups. Maturation of the response with the selection of B and T cells with greater specificity for RhD results in improved antibody affinity and the disappearance of cross-reactivity. This is the consequence of somatic mutation of the rearranged V gene. In high-affinity anti-D antibodies up to 20 of the 90 codons encoding the V region have changed from germline.

Temperature dependency of antibody–erythrocyte interactions is an indication of antibody affinity.

• Low-affinity antibodies generally do not bind sufficiently strongly at 37°C to be detected by agglutination but they do at lower temperatures. They are also generally of no clinical significance.

• Antibodies of intermediate and high affinity do remain bound and are detected in the antiglobulin test.

Pretreatment of red cells with proteases is also an effective method to reveal the presence of low-affinity antibodies against, for example, RhD as this reduces the strength of interaction between antibody and cell required for agglutination. Some of the isotypes able to activate complement can be detected in haemolysin tests if the antibody is present in excess and the activation of complement is facilitated by lowering the pH of the reaction medium.

Antigen in the adaptive humoral immune response

The immune response is driven by antigens which select the lymphocytes that are able to participate. Therefore, selective use of V genes in antibody production against a certain antigen might be expected. Studies on the V-gene use of blood cell antibodies support this and have thrown light on certain serological anomalies. Most evidence has been acquired by studies on the molecular structure of the V domains of monoclonal antibodies against the carbohydrate antigen I and the protein antigen RhD on the red cell membrane. These studies suggest that:

• there is preferential, but not exclusive use of certain V genes in the generation of these specificities;

• there is a significant overlap in the amino acid sequence of the V domains of cold agglutinins against the lactosylceramide I and anti-D antibodies;

• pathological anti-I cold agglutinins, as observed in the majority of patients with cold haemagglutinin disease, uniquely use the VH gene segment DP63 (V-4.34);

• postinfectious, polyclonal anti-I antibodies seem to make use of the same VH gene segment, whilst cold agglutinins with other specificities do not; and
• in over 50% of monoclonal IgM anti-D antibodies, the VH domain is encoded by the DP63 VH gene, the same as that encountered in pathological anti-I cold agglutinins.

It is attractive to speculate that RhD-specific B cells evolve from B cells with anti-I specificity. This suggests that in the germline these cells provide an SIg receptor which is best fit at that stage in the immune response for the tertiary structure presented by D. In this scenario, the drift in antibody specificity from anticarbohydrate (anti-I) to antiprotein (anti-D) is best explained by minor changes in the amino acid sequence of the V domains of anti-I antibodies brought about by somatic mutation. Ultimately, the low-affinity binding for I is lost. This is also influenced by the switch from IgM to IgG. In serology, these structural observations are supported by the functional observations on low-affinity interactions mentioned earlier and by the fact that certain IgM monoclonal antibodies used for D typing show reactivity at 4°C with protease-treated RhD-negative red cells.

The isotype and subclass of blood cell antibodies are at least, in part, determined by the chemical nature of the antigen which had stimulated their production.
• Blood cell antibodies against carbohydrate antigens are generally IgM or IgG2 and IgG4 or a combination of these.
• Antibodies against protein blood group antigens are typically of the IgG class with predominantly IgG1 and IgG3, although autoantibodies can be IgA. This suggests a direct involvement of the antigen. The source of antigen might not be red cells if the same structure is shared, so-called cross-reactivity. An increase in the titre of anti-I antibodies occurs after infection with *Mycoplasma pneumoniae*. Some preparations of the vaccine TAB (typhoid, paratyphoid A and paratyphoid B) stimulate anti-A and anti-B and cause not only a rise in agglutinin titre but also a change in antibody isotype. Many of the low-affinity reactions seen in red cell serology reflect part of the response to bacterial antigens, usually carbohydrate. When the affinity and concentration of such antibodies increases above certain thresholds, complement-mediated haemolysis can occur and this is clearly of clinical significance.

T-cell-independent antibody formation

As we have seen, the formation of antibodies by B cells is dependent on interaction with helper T cells. However, some antigens can stimulate a subset of B cells (B1 cells) directly, independent of T help. These cells provide an early response to bacteria by producing antibody specific to bacterial polysaccharide. This is also important in the response to certain gylcosylation-based red cell antigens. The presence of naturally occurring IgM antibodies against A and B is an excellent example of T-cell-independent antibody formation. Isoagglutinins to the missing A or B antigens are always present, although there has been no exposure to red cells carrying these antigens. The response is essentially limited to IgM because T cells are not involved and not available to trigger isotype switching, although some switching does occur in the absence of T cells. The repetitive carbohydrate structures (epitopes) presented by the A- and B-determining portions of the relevant blood groups are structurally the same as bacterial polysaccharide and indeed it is antigens from gastrointestinal bacteria that trigger isoagglutinin production. These isoagglutinins are present from the first months of life.

T-cell-dependent antibody formation

Unlike glycolipids and glycoproteins, the formation of antibodies against blood cell membrane proteins is always dependent on interaction with T-helper cells. The immune response to RhD is an example.
• RhD is the most immunogenic red cell membrane protein antigen. RhD is a 30-kDa non-glycosylated membrane protein.
• Analysis suggests that only short peptide loops, part of the molecule, are displayed on the cell surface.
• Ample evidence indicates that anti-D antibodies recognise discontinuous amino acid sequences derived from several of the extracellular RhD loops.

• These discontinuous residues come together in the tertiary structure of the RhD protein. Therefore, isolation of RhD from the membrane disrupts the majority of B-cell epitopes and reactivity with anti-D antibodies.

This is not a repetitive structure as with ABO and the B-cell response requires T-cell help. The response of T-helper cells, like B cells, is antigen-specific but triggered in a totally different way. T-helper cells recognise short linear segments of amino acids derived by intracellular digestion from the RhD protein and presented to the helper T cell by the HLA class II molecule. This is achieved most effectively by professional antigen-presenting cells (APCs). APCs belong to a family of cells with diverse anatomical locations and of diverse ontogeny:

• Langerhans' cells in the skin;
• interdigitating, follicular and germinal centre dendritic cells in lymph nodes and spleen; and
• B cells and macrophages.

The antibody response to a red cell antigen like RhD involves the interaction of at least three cell types and of antigen in two forms, both intact and digested. This is the basis of two important features of the immune response:

• an efficient mechanism for tolerance to self-antigens preventing failure to discriminate self from non-self that is the basis of autoimmunity; and
• the maturation of the antibody response, through isotype switching, that is driven by the T cell.

This is illustrated in detail by the specific example from transfusion medicine described below.

Human platelet antigen-1a presentation via the HLA class II route

If a human platelet antigen (HPA-1a)-negative mother is carrying an HPA-1a-positive fetus, platelets may enter the maternal circulation and immunise her against HPA-1a. This is the end result of quite complex events and can have disastrous consequences for the fetus (see Chapters 5 and 26). Fetal HPA-1a are ingested by maternal APCs and digested by endosomal enzymes like cathepsin G. Short fragments of 12–15 amino acids will be produced in endosomes, which in the *trans*-Golgi network fuse with HLA class II-containing vesicles. The fusion results in a downwards pH shift, which results in the removal of the invariant chain from the HLA class II molecule (this chain prevents the premature loading of the cleft in the molecule which is used for presentation of the digested antigen). Many peptides will be bound in the HLA class II groove, of which some will have been derived from the fetal GPIIIa. Once migrated to the surface of the APC, specific helper T cells recognise the change in the HLA class II molecule produced by the peptides to which they are specific and proliferate. Cytokines produced by these T-helper cells will drive the expansion of HPA-1a-specific B cells responding to intact HPA-1. With time the process of antigen take-up, processing and presentation will pass from the classical APCs to HPA-1a-specific B cells. This helps to bring together the complex interaction of cells needed for a mature antibody response as both the surface molecules needed for antigen presentation to the helper T cells and for interaction with intact HPA-1 are present on the same cell set.

HLA class II restriction of antibody response

We have seen that there must be a genetic element to an individual's immune response in that the first encounter with antigen is dependent on the germline V region genes, which show differences between individuals. Whether or not processed peptide from a particular alloantigen can interact with a particular HLA class II molecule to trigger a T cell is also dependent on genetic variability. In the immune response this is important to the immunogenicity of antigens in individuals. Sometimes the peptide is presented exclusively by a certain HLA class II molecule and a linkage between HLA class II type and antibody response can be observed. The HLA DRB3*0101 restricted response against HPA-1a (GPIIIa–leucine 33) is a good example of an HLA class II-restricted response in humans. The very much lower immunogenicity of the antithetical antigen HPA-1b (HPA-1b–proline 33) is most likely explained by a less good fit of the peptide-containing proline at position 33 when compared with the one containing leucine at that position.

T regulatory cells

Brief mention was made earlier in this chapter of regulatory T cells. The observation that a key function of T cells is to downregulate immune responses is not novel. The so-called suppressor T cells were first observed in 1970 and there is clearly not a single species of T cells with this general function but through the characterisation of both intracellular and cell membrane molecules a subset of T cells has been characterised comprising between 5 and 10% of T cells found in peripheral blood and with expression of CD4 and CD25 on their surface and Foxp3 in their cytoplasm. These are natural T regulatory cells (nTregs) which once activated are able to non-specifically suppress both helper and cytotoxic T cell activity and thus downregulate a wide range of immune responses. They play a major role in maintaining peripheral tolerance and the prevention of autoimmunity. These cells have clear potential for use in treatment and are the subject of much promising research.

Antibody-mediated blood cell destruction

Most red blood cell allo- and autoantibodies of the IgG isotype bring about lysis via the interaction of the IgG constant domain with Fcγ receptors on cells of the mononuclear phagocytic system. Several receptor types are described.

- FcγRI is the most important to blood cell destruction. This is a high-affinity receptor found predominantly on monocytes. The consequence of adherence of IgG-coated red cells to FcγRI-positive cells is phagocytosis and lysis. This is usually extravascular and takes place in the spleen. The lysis can be demonstrated in vitro as antibody-dependent cell cytotoxicity (ADCC).
- FcγRII is a lower affinity receptor found on monocytes, neutrophils, eosinophils, platelets and B cells.
- FcγRIII is also of relatively low affinity and found on macrophages, neutrophils, eosinophils and NK cells. It is responsible for the ADCC demonstrable in vitro with NK cells.

- There is also an FcRn (neonatal) on the placenta and other tissues of a different molecular family which mediates the transfer of IgG into the fetus and is involved in the control of IgG concentrations. The severity of haemolysis by IgG antibodies is determined by the concentration of antibody, its affinity for the antigen, antigen density and the IgG subclass. IgG2 and IgG4 antibodies generally do not reduce red cell survival, whilst IgG1 and IgG3 do. There is ample evidence in patients with warm-type autoimmune haemolytic anaemia that IgG1 and IgG3 are more effective in causing red cell destruction than IgG2 and IgG4. The level of IgG1 coating of red cells needs to exceed a threshold of approximately 1000 molecules per red cell to cause cell destruction. For a long time, it has been speculated that polymorphisms in the genes of the family of FcγRs might be significant in causing differences of severity of blood cell destruction observed between patients with apparently similar levels of IgG coating. So far, firm evidence for such polymorphisms has been lacking, although a single amino acid polymorphism of the FcγRIIa receptor dramatically alters the affinity for human IgG2 and additional polymorphisms might have an effect on the interaction with IgG1 and IgG3.

Complement system

The complement system, either working alone or in concert with antibody, is important to effective immunity to many extracellular pathogens. It also often plays an important part in immune red cell destruction and can be the reason for important systemic complications of haemolysis. Naturally occurring IgM antibodies against the A and B antigens are often of low affinity and do not bind to red cells at 37°C. However, when ABO blood group antibodies do bind at 37°C, there will be rapid complement-mediated destruction of incompatible red cells where there is a major A to O or B to O mismatch. This may result from a transfusion error and remains an important cause of transfusion-related mortality and morbidity

Blood cell antibodies which can activate complement are more effective in achieving haemolysis

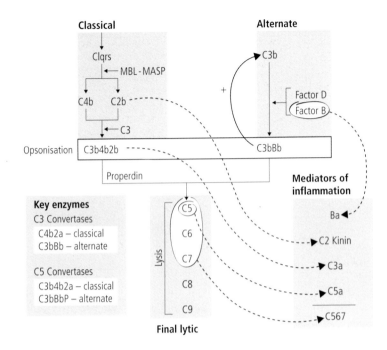

Figure 2.3 The different pathways for complement activation. MBL, mannan-binding lectin; MASP, MBL-associated serine protease.

than non-complement-activating antibodies. In contrast to extravascular FcγR-mediated destruction, complement-mediated lysis occurs in the intravascular compartment. The ensuing release of anaphylatoxins such as C3a and C5a contributes to the acute systemic effects that occur. IgM, IgG1 and IgG3 antibodies are the most effective in binding C1q and initiating activation of the complement cascade via the classical pathway. However, they are dependent on aggregation for a high enough antibody density to trigger C1q and overcome the regulators of complement activation that are present. The concentration of antibody may be too low to achieve the density necessary. The antigen topography (e.g. of RhD) can prevent the binding and activation of the C1q molecule.

Complement is a system of plasma proteins, both part of innate immunity and vital to the effector functions of complement-fixing immunoglobulin isotypes. Central to complement's function is the activation of C3 as this leads to the opsonisation of bacteria (Figure 2.3). C3 can be activated by three routes:
- the classical pathway;

- the alternate pathway; and
- lectin binding.

Lysis is dependent on activation, downstream from C3, of components of the membrane attack pathway.

The classical complement pathway consists of:
- four numbered components (C1–C4); and
- two regulatory proteins (C1 inhibitor, C4-binding protein).

The first component (C1) comprises three subcomponents, C1q, C1r and C1s. It is the interaction between C1q and aggregated IgG or IgM bound to antigen that initiates activation of the classical complement sequence. The fixation of C1q activates C1r and C1s. C1s cleaves C4 and C2, whose active fragments C4b and C2a form the classical pathway C3 convertase.

The alternative pathway to C3 activation consists of:
- C3b, factor B and factor D; and
- the regulatory proteins, properdin, factors H and I.

Factor B binds to a cleavage fragment of C3, C3b, to form C3bB. Factor D cleaves the bound factor B to form the alternative pathway C3 convertase (C3bBb). It activates C3 in a fashion similar to the C3 convertase of the classical pathway, C4b2a. Properdin acts to stabilise this alternative pathway C3 convertase, as do carbohydrate-rich cell surfaces, by partially shielding the convertase from inhibitors. Activation via the alternative pathway would otherwise be unchecked if it were not inhibited, as it requires no specific stimulus.

The lectin pathway is initiated by mannan-binding lectin: This is structurally related to C1q and binds avidly to carbohydrate on the surface of microorganisms. It activates C4 through a serine protease, which is similar to C1r and C1s with the same outcome.

The attack pathway is dependent on the formation of the trimolecular complex of C4b2a3b or C5 convertase, which cleaves C5 to two fragments C5a and C5b. The former is a potent anaphylatoxin. C5b forms a complex with C6, C7 and C8, which facilitates the insertion of a number of C9 molecules in the membrane. The C5b-8 and the multimeric C9 molecules form the membrane attack complex (MAC), creating a lytic pore in the membrane and lysing the target cell. Cells not involved in the process but close to it can also be lysed by excess MAC transferred to them – so-called bystander lysis.

Blood cells coated with C3b will bind to cells carrying receptors for C3b (CR1 or CD35). This adherence can lead to extravascular cell destruction mainly in the liver, but if the bound C3b degrades to its inactive components iC3b and C3dg before the cell is lysed then the cell is protected from lysis. Membrane-bound molecules such as decay accelerating factor (DAF) and membrane inhibitor of reactive lysis (MIRL) protect red cells from lysis in this way. They are of clinical importance as:

• DAF (CD55) and MIRL (CD59) are linked to the blood cell membrane via a glycosylphosphatidylinositol (GPI) anchor;

• patients with paroxysmal nocturnal haemoglobinuria (PNH) have an acquired mutation in the PIG-A gene in a subset of their HSC which prevents synthesis of the anchor;

• progeny from the affected stem cells lack GPI-linked membrane proteins; and

• the absence of DAF and MIRL from red cells increases the sensitivity for complement-mediated lysis which occurs when the pH is marginally lowered during sleep; this results in intravascular lysis and haemoglobinuria. In vitro acidification is used in the Ham's acid test to reveal the presence of a population of erythrocytes with increased sensitivity for complement-mediated lysis. Flow cytometric analysis looking for the absence of GPI-linked proteins on a subset of leucocytes derived from mutated stem cells is an alternative test for the diagnosis of PNH.

Cell-mediated immunity

Antigen-specific cell-mediated responses are carried out by T cells. They provide the immune system's main defence against intracellular microorganisms and can lyse cells expressing specific antigens – cytotoxicity. In addition, they release cytokines which can trigger inflammation and are responsible for delayed hypersensitivity and symptoms usually associated with infection such as fever, myalgia and fatigue.

Cytotoxic T cells
Cytotoxicity is the job of cytotoxic T cells, which are distinguished by the presence of CD8 on the cell surface. This facilitates their interaction with HLA class I on the surface of cells altered by the presence of antigen, usually as the result of virus infection. Cytotoxic T cells are the main means of protection against virus infection. They are also important mediators of allograft rejection. Like the B-cell response, the cytotoxic T-cell response requires help from helper T cells.

Delayed hypersensitivity
Delayed hypersensitivity is an example of another crucial role for helper T cells. It is dependent on the secretion of the cytokines interleukin (IL)-1, IL-2, tumour necrosis factor (TNF) and interferon (IFN)-γ – so-called proinflammatory or Th1-type cytokines. These recruit inflammatory cells, in particular macrophages, to sites of infection and arm them to kill certain bacteria, e.g. *Mycobacterium*

tuberculosis, which normally proliferate inside cells and are resistant to killing after phagocytosis. Helper T cells also function in a Th2 manner, releasing cytokines which promote antibody formation including production of IgE, which is important in protection against parasites. The core Th2 cytokine profile is IL-4, IL-5, IL-10 and IL-13.

Cell-mediated immunity in transfusion medicine

Cell-mediated immunity is of much less importance to the transfusion of blood cells than humoral immunity. It is important to the defence against blood-borne virus (as discussed below). Th1-type cytokines released from leucocytes in stored blood are the main cause of non-allergic febrile transfusion reactions in susceptible individuals.

As we have seen, virally infected target cells are marked for recognition by cytotoxic T cells by the presence of oligopeptides derived from viral proteins in the cleft of the HLA class I molecule. This is a process analogous to that which occurs for antigen presentation on class II HLA by APCs. The cytotoxic T-cell response to this antigen is very intense. Studies with cytomegalovirus (CMV)-derived peptides captured in HLA class I tetramers have revealed that up to 8% of CD8-positive T cells are CMV-specific during CMV infection and similar results have been obtained with peptides derived from other viruses. Biologically, the antibody response can afford to lag behind this response and usually does. This is of importance to transfusion practice.

Prevention of the transmission of hepatitis B, hepatitis C, human immunodeficiency virus (HIV) type 1 and 2 and CMV by blood transfusion is one of the major challenges of transfusion medicine. Counselling of donors, together with the detection of viral antigens and antibodies, and the development of tests for virally-derived nucleic acid, is the bedrock for the prevention of viral transmission. Antibody-based immunoassays are the mainstay but after a first encounter with a virus the formation of viral antibodies will require time; they are not the first line of defence or even the means to recovery from infection for many of the pathogens concerned but the basis of immunity against subsequent infection. There is a critical window, which may be several months, in which the donor carries the virus but is still antibody-negative.

The sequence of immunodominant oligopeptides which appear in the HLA class I molecule for all four main blood-borne viruses and several others of clinical significance has been defined and applied to treatment. Such short oligopeptides can be used to load APCs for in vitro education and proliferation of virus-specific cytotoxic T cells. These educated T cells can be used for the treatment of viral infection in immunosuppressed transplant patients.

• Adoptive immunotherapy for prevention of post-transplant Epstein–Barr virus (EBV)-associated lymphomas by infusion of virus-specific cytotoxic T lymphocytes (CTLs) has been successfully applied in allogeneic bone marrow transplantation in children.

• Preliminary data suggest that CMV infection in allogeneic bone marrow transplant patients can be prevented in a similar way.

Blood services, as they are adept at handling cells in vitro, are increasingly supporting the clinical development of these novel cellular therapies, which are a direct application of the underlying immunobiology.

Antigen presentation and its clinical implications

The interaction between APCs and helper T cells is complex (Figure 2.4). We now understand which of the many interactions are critical in turning on T-cell activity. This knowledge provides a means to specific manipulation of immune responses.

The requirement is for concurrent signalling over two independent pathways, one antigen-specific via the TCR and HLA/peptide and the other non-specific via the CD28/CD80 pathway. This interaction also provides control to prevent inappropriate T-cell proliferation. Initial triggering via CD28 results in T-cell proliferation and IL-2 production, which in turn induces the expression of CTLA-4 on the expanding T-cell clone. CTLA-4 is a competitive inhibitor of proliferation and competes with CD28 for binding with CD80.

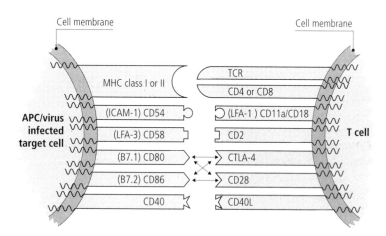

Figure 2.4 Adhesion molecules and signalling pathways in T-cell activation.

This molecular competition in the control of T-cell proliferation results in a balanced expansion of antigen-specific T-cell clones. The absence of initial signalling through CD80 from the APC when antigen is appropriately presented leads to apoptosis of the helper T cell. This can be exploited in the modulation of immune responses through molecules which block the interaction. The following are examples which are of relevance to transfusion medicine.

• Clinical studies in HSC transplantation suggest that donor lymphocytes can be tolerised for incompatible HLA alloantigens on host cells by ex vivo exposure to them in the presence of a recombinant CTLA-4–IgG fusion protein (abatacept) which blocks CD80.

• In platelet transfusion, alloimmunisation to HLA antigens with subsequent failure to increment after further platelet transfusions is a clinical problem. This may be reduced by leucocyte-depleting blood components, thus removing APCs along with other white cells. A similar effect is obtained by treatment which modifies cell membranes and particularly the CD80 signal, such as ultraviolet irradiation.

Conversely, immune responses can be deliberately induced by priming separated dendritic cells with immunogenic peptide derived from the relevant antigen. This approach is under investigation in cancer therapy and again blood services are involved due to their familiarity with the safe handling of such cells under conditions of good manufacturing practice (GMP).

Similar molecular switches and controls influence the B-cell response to antigen. In B–T-helper cell interaction, the CD40/CD154 (CD40-ligand) pathway exercises control over B-cell isotype switching and subsequent maturation of the antibody response. This pathway is also important to certain aspects of effector T-cell function. Again there is the potential for clinical exploitation. Anti-CD40 antibodies might be powerful therapeutic reagents in kidney transplantation. HLA-incompatible transplants can be achieved successfully in monkeys if pretreated with anti-CD40 antibodies. The ability of anti-CD40 antibodies to control autoreactive B cells in treatment-refractory autoimmune thrombocytopenia has promised. Such designer therapeutic biologics look likely to replace less-specific therapies such as with polyvalent intravenous immunoglobulin.

The amount of antigen required to activate B cells is reduced if C3d is covalently bound to antigen as this leads to the concurrent signalling of CD21 (the complement receptor type 2 on B cells) as well as SIg by antigen. This is also a pathway that is open to manipulation.

Key points

1 The immune system has evolved to deal with infection and is able to distinguish microbes

from self and destroy them. Transplants are non-self.

2 Immunological matching of a transplant donor to the recipient allows the transplant, whether of blood cells or a solid organ, to be treated as self (or close to it) and reduces the likelihood of rejection.

3 Most immunological problems encountered in transfusion medicine are antibody-based.

4 The ability of antibodies to bring about erythrocyte or platelet destruction varies according to their isotype and temperature of reaction. This determines clinical significance.

5 The source of the antigen that causes the production of blood group antibodies may not be blood cells. Cross-reactivity with intestinal bacteria means antibodies to groups A and B are triggered independent of transfusion and present from infancy. This makes ABO matching especially critical.

6 Blood cell destruction by antibodies is either mediated through Fcγ receptor-mediated phagocytosis with extravascular haemolysis or complement when haemolysis is predominantly intravascular and the clinical symptoms more acute and serious.

7 Mismatch within the ABO blood group system leads to intravascular haemolysis and remains an important cause of transfusion-related mortality and morbidity.

8 The clinical use of blood cell immunotherapies based on growing knowledge of immunology is a growing area of transfusion medicine practice.

Further reading

Murphy KM, Travers P & Walport M. *Immuno Biology. The Immune System in Health and Disease*, 7th edn. London: Garland Science Textbooks, 2008.

CHAPTER 3

Human blood group systems

Geoff Daniels

Bristol Institute for Transfusion Sciences, NHS Blood and Transplant, Bristol, UK

A blood group may be defined as an inherited character of the red cell surface detected by a specific alloantibody. This definition would not receive universal acceptance as cell surface antigens on platelets and leucocytes might also be considered blood groups, as might uninherited characters on red cells defined by autoantibodies or xenoantibodies. The definition is suitable, however, for the purposes of this chapter.

Most blood groups are organised into blood group systems. Each system represents a single gene or a cluster of two or more closely linked homologous genes. Of the 308 blood group specificities recognised by the International Society for Blood Transfusion, 270 belong to one of 30 systems (Table 3.1). All these systems represent a single gene, apart from Rh, Xg and Chido/Rodgers, which have two closely-linked homologous genes, and MNS with three genes.

Most blood group antigens are proteins or glycoproteins, with the blood group specificity determined primarily by the amino acid sequence, and most of the blood group polymorphisms result from single amino acid substitutions, though there are many exceptions. The four types of red cell surface glycoproteins, based on their integration into the red cell membrane, are shown in Figure 3.1. Some blood group antigens, including those of the ABO, P, Lewis, H and I systems, are carbohydrate structures on glycoproteins and glycolipids. These antigens are not produced directly by the genes controlling their polymorphisms, but by genes encoding transferase enzymes that catalyse the final biosynthetic stage of an oligosaccharide chain.

The two most important blood group systems from the clinical point of view are ABO and Rh. They also provide good models for contrasting carbohydrate and protein-based blood group systems.

The ABO system

ABO is often referred to as a histo-blood group system because, in addition to being expressed on red cells, ABO antigens are present on most tissues and in soluble form in secretions. At its most basic level, the ABO system consists of two antigens, A and B, indirectly encoded by two alleles, *A* and *B*, of the *ABO* gene. A third allele, *O*, produces neither A nor B. These three alleles combine to effect four phenotypes: A, B, AB and O (Table 3.2).

Clinical significance

Two key factors make ABO the most important blood group system in transfusion medicine. Firstly, almost without exception, the blood of adults contains antibodies to those ABO antigens lacking from their red cells (Table 3.2). In addition to anti-A and anti-B, group O individuals have anti-A,B, an antibody to a determinant common to A and B. Secondly, ABO antibodies are IgM, though they

Practical Transfusion Medicine, 3rd edition. Edited by Michael F. Murphy and Derwood H. Pamphilon. © 2009 Blackwell Publishing, ISBN: 978-1-4051-8196-9.

Table 3.1 Human blood group systems.

No.	Name	Symbol	Number of antigens	Gene symbol(s)	Chromosome
001	ABO	ABO	4	*ABO*	9
002	MNS	MNS	46	*GYPA, GYPB, GYPE*	4
003	P	P1	1	*P1*	22
004	Rh	RH	50	*RHD, RHCE*	1
005	Lutheran	LU	19	*BCAM*	19
006	Kell	KEL	31	*KEL*	7
007	Lewis	LE	6	*FUT3*	19
008	Duffy	FY	6	*DARC*	1
009	Kidd	JK	3	*SLC14A1*	18
010	Diego	DI	21	*SLC4A1*	17
011	Yt	YT	2	*ACHE*	7
012	Xg	XG	2	*XG, CD99*	X/Y
013	Scianna	SC	7	*ERMAP*	1
014	Dombrock	DO	6	*ART4*	12
015	Colton	CO	3	*AQP1*	7
016	Landsteiner-Wiener	LW	3	*ICAM4*	19
017	Chido/Rodgers	CH/RG	9	*C4A, C4B*	6
018	H	H	1	*FUT1*	19
019	Kx	XK	1	*XK*	X
020	Gerbich	GE	8	*GYPC*	2
021	Cromer	CROM	15	*CD55*	1
022	Knops	KN	9	*CR1*	1
023	Indian	IN	4	*CD44*	11
024	Ok	OK	1	*BSG*	19
025	Raph	RAPH	1	*CD151*	11
026	John Milton Hagen	JMH	5	*SEMA7A*	15
027	I	I	1	*GCNT2*	6
028	Globoside	GLOB	1	*B3GALT3*	3
029	Gill	GIL	1	*AQP3*	9
030	RHAG	RHAG	3	*RHAG*	6

may also have an IgG component, activate complement, and cause immediate intravascular red cell destruction, which can give rise to severe and often fatal haemolytic transfusion reactions (HTRs) (see Chapter 7). Major ABO incompatibility (i.e. donor red cells with an ABO antigen not possessed by the recipient) must be avoided in transfusion and, ideally, ABO-matched blood (i.e. of the same ABO group) should be provided.

ABO antibodies seldom cause haemolytic disease of the fetus and newborn (HDFN) and when they do it is usually mild. The prime reasons for this are (1) that IgM antibodies do not cross the placenta, (2) IgG ABO antibodies are often IgG2, which do not activate complement or facilitate phagocytosis

and (3) ABO antigens are present on many fetal tissues and even in body fluids, so the haemolytic potential of the antibody is greatly reduced.

A and B subgroups

The A (and AB) phenotype can be subdivided into A_1 and A_2 (and A_1B and A_2B). In a European population, about 80% of group A individuals are A_1 and 20% A_2 (Table 3.2). A_1 and A_2 differ quantitatively and qualitatively. A_1 red cells react more strongly with anti-A than A_2 cells. In addition, A_2 red cells lack a component of the A antigen present on A_1 cells and some individuals with the A_2 or A_2B phenotype produce anti-A_1, an antibody that agglutinates A_1 and A_1B cells, but not A_2 or A_2B

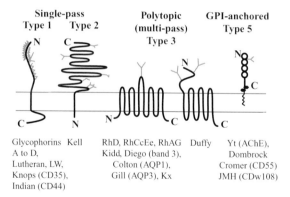

Figure 3.1 Diagrammatic representation of the four types of glycoproteins of the red cell surface membrane, with examples of blood group antigens expressed on those types of glycoproteins.

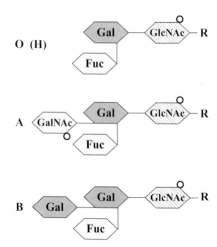

Figure 3.2 Diagram of the tetrasaccharides representing A and B antigens, and their biosynthetic precursor (H), which is abundant in group O. R, remainder of molecule.

cells. Anti-A_1 is seldom reactive at 37°C and generally considered clinically insignificant.

There are numerous other ABO variants, involving weakened expression of A or B antigens (A_3, A_x, A_m, A_{el}, B_3, B_x, B_m, B_{el}), but all are rare. At least 60 subgroups of A and 30 subgroups of B have been recognised by molecular genetical methods, but the symbols A_x, A_{el}, etc., represent phenotypic characteristics and not single genetic entities.

Biosynthesis and molecular genetics

Red cell A and B antigens are expressed predominantly on oligosaccharide structures on integral membrane glycoproteins, mainly the anion transporter band 3 and the glucose transporter GLUT1, but are also on glycosphingolipids embedded in the membrane. The tetrasaccharides that represent the predominant form of A and B antigens on red cells are shown in Figure 3.2, together with their biosynthetic precursor, the H antigen, which is abundant on group O red cells. The product of the A allele is a glycosyltransferase that catalyses the transfer of N-acetylgalactosamine (GalNAc) from a nucleotide donor substrate, UDP-GalNAc, to the fucosylated galactose (Gal) residue of the H antigen, the acceptor substrate. The product of the B allele catalyses

Table 3.2 The ABO system.

| Phenotype | Genotypes | Frequency | | | Antibodies present |
		Europeans*	Africans†	Indians‡	
O	O/O	43%	51%	31%	anti-A, -B, -A,B
A_1	A^1/A^1, A^1/O, A^1/A^2	35%	18%	26%	anti-B
A_2	A^2/A^2, A^2/O	10%	5%	3%	sometimes anti-A_1
B	B/B, B/O	9%	21%	30%	anti-A
A_1B	A^1/B	3%	2%	9%	none
A_2B	A^2/B	1%	1%	1%	sometimes anti-A_1

* English people.
† Donors from Kinshasa, Congo.
‡ Makar from Mumbai.

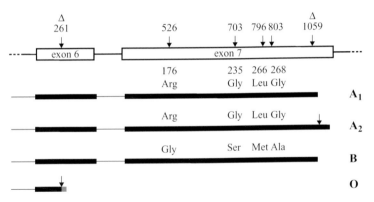

Figure 3.3 Diagrammatic representation of exons 6 and 7 of the *ABO* gene, showing the position of the nucleotide deletions (Δ) responsible for the common form of O (exon 6) and for A_2 (exon 7), and the positions of the four nucleotide changes in exon 7 responsible for the amino acid residues that are characteristic of A- and B-transferases. Below are representations of the encoded transferases.

the transfer of Gal from UDP-Gal to the fucosylated Gal residue of the H antigen. GalNAc and Gal are the immunodominant sugars of A and B antigens, respectively. The *O* allele produces no transferase, so the H antigen remains unmodified.

The *ABO* gene on chromosome 9 consists of seven exons. The A^1 and *B* alleles differ by seven nucleotides in exons 6 and 7, which encode a total of four amino acid substitutions at positions 176, 235, 266 and 268 of their glycosyltransferase products (Figure 3.3). It is primarily the amino acids at positions 266 and 268 that determine whether the gene product is a GalNAc-transferase (A) or Gal-transferase (B). The most common *O* allele (O^1) has an identical sequence to A^1, apart from a single nucleotide deletion in exon 6, which shifts the reading frame and introduces a translation stop codon before the region of the catalytic site, so that any protein produced would be truncated and have no enzyme activity. Another common *O* allele, called O^{1v}, differs from O^1 by at least nine nucleotides, but has the same single nucleotide deletion as that in O^1 and so cannot produce any functional enzyme. O^2, which represents about 3% of *O* alleles in a European population, does not have the nucleotide deletion characteristic of most *O* alleles and encodes a complete protein product, but with a charged arginine residue instead of a neutral glycine (A) or alanine (B) at position 268. This amino acid change at a vital position inactivates the enzyme activity. The A^2 allele has a sequence almost identical to A^1, but has a single nucleotide deletion immediately before the translation stop codon. The resultant frame shift abolishes the stop codon, so the protein product has an extra 21 amino acids at its C-terminus, which reduces the efficiency of its GalNAc-transferase activity and might alter its acceptor substrate specificity.

Biochemically related blood group systems – H, Lewis and I

H antigen is the biochemical precursor of A and B (Figure 3.2). It is synthesised by an α1,2-fucosyltransferase, which catalyses the transfer of fucose from its donor substrate to the terminal Gal residue of its acceptor substrate. Without this fucosylation neither A nor B antigens can be made. Two genes, active in different tissues, produce α1,2-fucosyltransferases: *FUT1*, active in mesodermally derived tissues and responsible for H on red cells, and *FUT2*, active in endodermally derived tissues and responsible for H in many other tissues and in secretions. Homozygosity for inactivating mutations in *FUT1* leads to an absence of H from red cells and, therefore, an absence of red cell A or B, regardless of *ABO* genotype. Such mutations are rare, as are red cell H-deficient phenotypes. In contrast, inactivating mutations in *FUT2* are relatively common and about 20% of White Europeans (non-secretors) lack H, A, and B from body secretions despite expressing those antigens on their red cells. Very rare individuals who have H-deficient red cells and are also H non-secretors (Bombay phenotype)

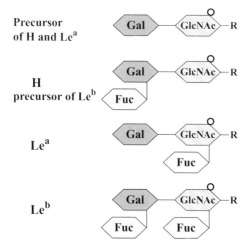

Figure 3.4 Diagram of oligosaccharide structures representing Le^a and Le^b expression and their biosynthetic precursors. R, remainder of molecule.

produce anti-H together with anti-A and -B and can cause a severe transfusion problem.

Antigens of the Lewis system are not produced by erythroid cells, but become incorporated into the red cell membrane from the plasma. Their corresponding antibodies are not usually active at 37°C and are not generally considered clinically significant. Le^a and Le^b are not the products of alleles. The Lewis gene (*FUT3*) product is an α1,3/4-fucosyltransferases that transfers fucose to the GlcNAc residue of the secreted precursor of H in non-secretors to produce Le^a and to secreted H in secretors to produce Le^b (Figure 3.4). Consequently, H secretors are Le(a−b+) or Le(a+b+), H non-secretors are Le(a+b−), and individuals homozygous for *FUT3* inactivating mutations (secretors or non-secretors) are Le(a−b−).

I antigen represents branched *N*-acetyl-lactosamine (Galβ1–4GlcNAc) structures in the complex carbohydrates that also express H, A and B antigens. The I gene (*GCNT2*) encodes a branching enzyme, which only becomes active during the first months of life. Consequently, red cells of neonates are I-negative. Rare individuals are homozygous for inactivating mutations in *GCNT2* and never form I on their red cells. This phenotype, called adult i, is associated with production of anti-I,

which is usually only active below 37°C, but may occasionally be haemolytic at body temperature.

The Rh system

Rh is the most complex of the blood group systems, with 50 specificities. The most important of these is D (RH1).

Rh genes and proteins
The antigens of the Rh system are encoded by two genes, *RHD* and *RHCE*, which produce D and CcEe antigens, respectively. The genes are highly homologous, each consisting of 10 exons. They are closely linked, but in opposite orientation, on chromosome 1 (Figure 3.5). Each gene encodes a 417 amino acid polypeptide that differs by only 31–35 amino acids, according to Rh genotype. The Rh proteins are palmitoylated, but not glycosylated, and span the red cell membrane 12 times, with both termini inside the cytosol and with six external loops, the potential sites of antigenic activity (Figure 3.5).

D antigen
The most significant Rh antigen from the clinical point of view is D. About 85% of White people are

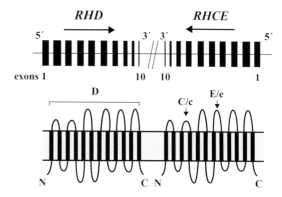

Figure 3.5 Diagrammatic representation of the Rh genes, *RHD* and *RHCE*, shown in opposite orientation as they appear on the chromosome, and of the two Rh proteins in their probable membrane conformation, with 12 membrane-spanning domains and 6 extracellular loops expressing D, C/c and E/e antigens.

D+ (Rh-positive) and 15% are D− (Rh-negative). In Africans, only about 3–5% are D− and in the Far East D− is rare.

The D− phenotype is usually associated with absence of the whole D protein from the red cell membrane. This explains why D is so immunogenic, as the D antigen comprises numerous epitopes on the external domains of the D protein. In White people, the D− phenotype almost always results from homozygosity for a complete deletion of *RHD*. D-positives are either homozygous or heterozygous for the presence of *RHD*. In Africans, in addition to the deletion of *RHD*, D− often results from an inactive *RHD* (called *RHD*Ψ) containing translation stop codons within the reading frame. Other genes containing inactivating mutations are also found in D− Africans and Asians.

Numerous variants of D are known, though most are rare. They are often split into two types, partial D and weak D, though this dichotomy is not adequately defined and of little value for making clinical decisions. Partial D antigens lack some or most of the D epitopes. If an individual with a partial D phenotype is immunised by red cells with a complete D antigen, they might make antibodies to those epitopes they lack. The D epitopes comprising partial D may be expressed weakly, or may be of normal or even enhanced strength. Weak D antigens (previously known as D^u) appear to express all epitopes of D, but at a lower site density than normal D. D variants result from amino acid substitutions in the D protein occurring either as a result of one or more missense mutations in *RHD* or from one or more exons of *RHD* being exchanged for the equivalent exons of *RHCE* in a process called gene conversion.

Anti-D

Anti-D is almost never produced in D− individuals without immunisation by D+ red cells. However, D is highly immunogenic and at least 30% of D− recipients of transfused D+ red cells make anti-D. Anti-D can cause severe immediate or delayed HTRs and D+ blood must never be transfused to a patient with anti-D.

Anti-D is the most common cause of severe HDFN. The effects of HDFN caused by anti-D are, at its most severe, fetal death at about the seventeenth week of pregnancy. If the infant is born alive, the disease can result in hydrops and jaundice. If the jaundice leads to kernicterus, this usually results in infant death or permanent cerebral damage. The prevalence of HDFN resulting from anti-D has been substantially reduced by anti-D immunoglobulin prophylaxis. In 1970, at the beginning of the anti-D prophylaxis programme, there were 1.2 deaths per thousand births in England and Wales due to HDFN caused by anti-D; by 1989, this figure had been reduced to 0.02.

Prediction of fetal Rh genotype by molecular methods

Knowledge of the molecular bases for D− phenotypes has made it possible to devise tests for predicting fetal D type from fetal DNA. This is a valuable tool in assessing whether the fetus of a woman with anti-D is at risk from HDFN. Most methods involve PCR tests that detect the presence or absence of *RHD*. It is important that the tests are devised so that *RHD*Ψ and other variant *RHD* genes do not give false phenotype predictions. Initially, the usual source of fetal DNA was amniocytes obtained by amniocentesis, which has an inherent risk of fetal loss and of feto-maternal haemorrhage. A far superior source of fetal DNA, avoiding invasive procedures, is the small quantity of free fetal DNA present in maternal plasma. This non-invasive form of fetal D typing is now provided as a reference service in some countries for alloimmunised D− women. In the near future it is likely that non-invasive fetal *RHD* genotyping will be offered to all D− pregnant women, so that only those with a D+ fetus will receive routine antenatal anti-D prophylaxis (see Chapter 26).

C and c, E and e

C/c and E/e are two pairs of allelic antigens produced by *RHCE*. The fundamental difference between C and c is a serine-proline substitution at position 103 in the second external loop of the CcEe protein (Figure 3.5), though the

Table 3.3 Rh phenotypes and the genotypes that produce them (presented in DCE and shorthand terminology).

Phenotype					Frequency (%)			Genotypes	
D	C	c	E	e	Europeans*	Africans[†]	Asians[‡]		
+	+	−	−	+	18.5	0.7	56.0	*DCe/Dce*	*R¹/R¹*
								DCe/dCe	*R¹r′*
+	−	+	+	−	2.3	1.3	3.5	*DcE/DcE*	*R²R²*
								DcE/dcE	*R²r″*
+	−	+	−	+	2.1	58.9	0.2	*Dce/dce*	*R°r*
								Dce/Dce	*R°R°*
+	+	−	+	−	rare	rare	rare	*DCE/DCE*	*RᶻRᶻ*
								DCE/dCE	*Rᶻrʸ*
+	+	+	−	+	34.9	13.2	8.4	*DCe/dce*	*R¹r*
								DCe/Dce	*R¹R°*
								Dce/dCe	*R°r′*
+	−	+	+	+	11.8	18.3	2.1	*DcE/dce*	*R²r*
								DcE/Dce	*R²R°*
								Dce/dcE	*R°r″*
+	+	−	+	+	0.2	rare	1.1	*DCe/DCE*	*R¹Rᶻ*
								DCE/dCe	*Rᶻr′*
								DCe/dCE	*R¹rʸ*
+	+	+	+	−	0.1	rare	0.3	*DcE/DCE*	*R²Rᶻ*
								DCE/dcE	*Rᶻr″*
								DcE/dCE	*R²rʸ*
+	+	+	+	+	13.4	2.1	28.1	*DCe/DcE*	*R¹R²*
								DCe/dcE	*R¹r″*
								DcE/dCe	*R²r′*
								DCE/dce	*Rᶻr*
								Dce/DCE	*R°Rᶻ*
								Dce/dCE	*R°rʸ*
−	+	−	−	+	rare	0.1	rare	*dCe/dCe*	*r′r′*
−	−	+	+	−	rare	rare	rare	*dcE/dcE*	*r″r″*
−	−	+	−	+	15.1	4.1	0.1	*dce/dce*	*rr*
−	+	−	+	−	rare	rare	rare	*dCE/dCE*	*rʸrʸ*
−	+	+	−	+	0.1	1.3	0.1	*dCe/dce*	*r′r*
−	−	+	+	+	0.1	rare	rare	*dcE/dce*	*r″r*
−	+	−	+	+	rare	rare	rare	*dCe/dCE*	*r′rʸ*
−	+	+	+	−	rare	rare	rare	*dcE/dCE*	*r″rʸ*
−	+	+	+	+	rare	rare	rare	*dcE/dCe*	*r″r′*
								dCE/dce	*rʸr*

* English donors.
[†] Yoruba of Nigeria.
[‡] Cantonese of Hong Kong.

situation is more complex than that. E and e represent a proline-alanine substitution at position 226 in the fourth external loop. Taking into account the presence and absence of D, and of the C/c and E/e polymorphisms, eight different haplotypes can be recognised. The frequencies of these haplotypes and the shorthand symbols often used to describe them are shown in Table 3.3.

Anti-c is clinically the most important Rh antigen after anti-D and may cause severe HDFN. On the other hand, anti-C, -E and -e rarely cause HDN and when they do the disease is generally mild, though all have the potential to cause severe disease.

Other Rh antigens

Of the 50 Rh antigens, 20 are polymorphic, that is have a frequency between 1 and 99% in at least one major ethnic group, 21 are rare antigens and 9 are very common antigens. Antibodies to many of these antigens have proved to be clinically important and it is prudent to treat all Rh antibodies as being potentially clinically significant.

Other blood group systems

Of the remaining blood group systems (Table 3.1), the most important clinically are Kell, Duffy, Kidd, Diego and MNS, and these are described below.

The Kell system

The original Kell antigen, K (KEL1) (Met193), has a frequency of about 9% in Caucasians, but is rare in other ethnic groups. Its allelic antigen, k (KEL2) (Thr193), is common in all populations. The remainder of the Kell system consists of one triplet and four pairs of allelic antigens – Kp^a, Kp^b and Kp^c; Js^a and Js^b; K11 and K17; K14 and K24; VLAN and VONG – plus 12 high-frequency and 3 low-frequency antigens. Almost all represent single amino acid substitutions in the Kell glycoprotein.

Anti-K can cause severe HTRs and HDFN. About 10% of K− patients who are given one unit of K+ blood produce anti-K, making K the next most immunogenic antigen after D. About 0.1% of all cases of HDFN are caused by anti-K; most of the mothers will have had previous blood transfusions. HDFN caused by anti-K differs from Rh HDFN in that anti-K appears to cause fetal anaemia by suppression or erythropoiesis, rather than immune destruction of mature fetal erythrocytes. Anti-k is a very rare antibody. It is always immune and has been incriminated in some cases of mild HDFN. Most other Kell-system antibodies are rare and best detected by an antiglobulin test.

The Kell antigens are located on a large glycoprotein, which crosses the cell membrane once and has a glycosylated, C-terminal extracellular domain, maintained in a folded conformation by multiple disulphide bonds. The Kell glycoprotein belongs to a family of endopeptidases, which process biologically important peptides, and is able to cleave the biologically inactive peptide big endothelin-3 to produce endothelin-3, an active vasoconstrictor.

The Duffy system

Fy^a and Fy^b represent a single amino acid substitution (Gly42Asp) in the extracellular N-terminal domain of the Duffy glycoprotein. Their incidence in Caucasians is Fy^a 68%, Fy^b 80%. About 70% of African Americans and close to 100% of West Africans are Fy(a−b−) (Table 3.4). They are homozygous for an Fy^b allele containing a mutation in a binding site for the erythroid-specific GATA-1 transcription factor, which means that Duffy glycoprotein is not expressed in red cells, though it is present in other tissues (Table 3.5). The Duffy glycoprotein is the receptor exploited by *Plasmodium vivax* merozoites for penetration of erythroid cells. Consequently, the Fy(a−b−) phenotype confers resistance to *P. vivax* malaria. The Duffy glycoprotein (also called Duffy-Antigen Chemokine Receptor, DARC) is a red cell receptor for a variety of chemokines, including interleukin-8.

Anti-Fy^a is not infrequent and is found in previously transfused patients who have usually already made other antibodies. Anti-Fy^b is very rare. Both may cause acute or delayed HTRs and HDFN varying from mild to severe.

Table 3.4 The Duffy system: phenotypes and genotypes.

Phenotype	Genotype	Frequency (%)	
		Europeans	Africans
Fy(a+b−)	*Fy^a/Fy^a* or *Fy^a/Fy*	20	10
Fy(a+b+)	*Fy^a/Fy^b*	48	3
Fy(a−b+)	*Fy^b/Fy^b* or *Fy^b/Fy*	32	20
Fy(a−b−)	*Fy/Fy*	0	67

Table 3.5 Nucleotide polymorphisms in the promoter region and in exon 2 of the three common alleles of the Duffy gene.

Allele	GATA box sequence −64 to −69 (promoter)	Codon 42 (exon 2)	Antigen
Fy^a	TT**AT**CT	G**GT** (Gly)	Fy^a
Fy^b	TT**AT**CT	G**AT** (Asp)	Fy^b
Fy	TT**AC**CT	G**AT** (Asp)	Red cells – none Other tissues – probably Fy^b

The Kidd system

Kidd has two common alleles, *Jk*^{a} and *Jk*^{b}, which represent a single amino acid change (Asp280Asn) in the Kidd glycoprotein. Both Jk^a and Jk^b antigens have frequencies of about 75% in Caucasian populations. A Kidd-null phenotype, Jk(a−b−), results from homozygosity for inactivating mutations in the Kidd gene, *SLC14A1*. It is very rare in most populations, but reaches an incidence of greater than 1% in Polynesians. The Kidd glycoprotein is a urea transporter in red cells and in renal endothelial cells.

Anti-Jk^a is uncommon and anti-Jk^b is very rare, but they both cause severe transfusion reactions and, to a lesser extent, HDFN. Kidd antibodies have often been implicated in delayed HTRs. They are often difficult to detect serologically and tend to disappear rapidly after stimulation.

The Diego system

Diego is a large system of 21 antigens: two pairs of allelic antigens – Di^a and Di^b (Leu854Pro), Wr^a and Wr^b (Lys658Glu) – plus 17 antigens of very low frequency. All represent single amino acid substitutions in band 3, the red cell anion exchanger. The original Diego antigen, Di^a, is very rare in Caucasians and Black people, but relatively common in Mongoloid people, with frequencies varying between 1% in Japanese and 50% in some native South Americans. Anti-Di^a and -Di^b are immune and rare, and can cause severe HDFN.

Wr^a has a frequency of about 0.1%. Its high frequency allelic antigen, Wr^b, is dependent on an interaction of band 3 with glycophorin A for its expression. Naturally occurring anti-Wr^a is present in approximately 1% of blood donors and can cause severe transfusion reactions. Very rarely, anti-Wr^a causes HDFN. Autoanti-Wr^b is a relatively common autoantibody and may be implicated in autoimmune haemolytic anaemia.

The MNS system

MNS, with a total of 46 antigens, is second only to Rh in complexity. These antigens are present on one or both of two red cell membrane glycoproteins, glycophorin A (GPA) and glycophorin B (GPB). They are encoded by two homologous genes, *GYPA* and *GYPB*, on chromosome 4.

The M and N antigens, both with frequencies of about 75%, differ by amino acids at positions 1 and 5 of the external N-terminus of GPA (Ser1Leu, Gly5Glu). S and s have frequencies of about 55% and 90%, respectively, in a Caucasian population, and represent an amino acid substitution in GPB (Met29Thr). About 2% of Black West Africans and 1.5% of African Americans are S− s−, a phenotype virtually unknown in other ethnic groups, and most of these lack the U antigen, which is present when either S or s is expressed. The numerous MNS variants mostly result from amino acid substitutions in GPA or GPB and from the formation of hybrid GPA-GPB molecules, formed by intergenic recombination between *GYPA* and *GYPB*. The phenotypes resulting from these hybrid proteins are rare in Europeans and Africans, but the GP.Mur (previously Mi.III) phenotype occurs in up to 10% of Southeast Asians. GPA and GPB are exploited as receptors by the malaria parasite *Plasmodium falciparum*.

Anti-M and -N are not generally clinically significant, though anti-M is occasionally haemolytic. Anti-S, the rarer anti-s, and anti-U can cause HDFN and have been implicated in HTRs. Although rare elsewhere, anti-Mur, which detects red cells of the GP.Mur phenotype, is common in Southeast Asia and causes severe HTRs and HDFN.

The biological significance of blood group antigens

The functions of several red cell membrane protein structures bearing blood group antigenic determinants are known, or can be deduced from their structure. Some are membrane transporters, facilitating the transport of biologically important molecules through the lipid bilayer: band 3 membrane glycoprotein, the Diego antigen, provides an anion exchange channel for HCO_3^- and Cl^- ions; the Kidd glycoprotein is a urea transporter; the Colton glycoprotein is aquaporin 1, a water channel; the GIL antigen is aquaporin 3, a glycerol transporter. The Lutheran, LW, and Indian (CD44) glycoproteins are adhesion molecules, possibly serving their primary functions during erythropoiesis. The MER2 antigen is located on the tetraspanin CD151, which associates with integrins within basement membranes, but its function on red cells is not known. The Duffy glycoprotein is a chemokine receptor and could function as a 'sink' or scavenger for unwanted chemokines. The Cromer and Knops antigens are markers for decay accelerating factor (CD55) and complement receptor 1 (CD35), respectively, which protect the cells from destruction by autologous complement. Some blood group glycoproteins appear to be enzymes, though their functions on red cells are not known: the Yt antigen is acetylcholinesterase, the Kell antigen is an endopeptidase, and the sequence of the Dombrock glycoprotein suggests that it belongs to a family of adenosine diphosphate (ADP)-ribosyltransferases. The C-terminal domains of the Gerbich antigens, GPC and GPD, and the N-terminal domain of the Diego glycoprotein, band 3, are attached to components of the cytoskeleton and function to anchor it to the external membrane. The carbohydrate moieties of the membrane glycoproteins and glycolipids, especially those of the most abundant glycoproteins, band 3 and GPA, constitute the glycocalyx, an extracellular coat that protects the cell from mechanical damage and microbial attack.

The Rh proteins are associated with the glycoprotein RhAG in the red cell membrane, and these proteins are part of a macrocomplex of red cell surface proteins which include band 3, LW, GPA, GPB and CD47. The function of the Rh proteins and RhAG are not known, but it has been proposed that RhAG might form an oxygen and carbon dioxide channel, or possibly an ammonia channel or ammonium transporter.

The structural differences between allelic red cell antigens (e.g. A and B, K and k, Fy^a and Fy^b) are small, often being just one monosaccharide or one amino acid. The biological importance of these differences is unknown and there is little evidence to suggest that the product of one allele confers any significant advantage over the other. Some blood group antigens are exploited by pathological microorganisms as receptors for attaching and entering cells, so in some cases absence or changes in these antigens could be beneficial. It is likely that interaction between cell surface molecules and pathological microorganisms has been a major factor in the evolution of blood group polymorphism.

Key points

1 The International Society of Blood Transfusion recognises 308 blood group specificities, 270 of which belong to one of 30 blood group systems.
2 The most important blood group systems clinically are ABO, Rh, Kell, Duffy, Kidd and MNS.
3 ABO antibodies are almost always present in adults lacking the corresponding antigens and can cause fatal intravascular HTRs.
4 ABO antigens are carbohydrate structures on glycoproteins and glycosphingolipids.
5 Anti-RhD is the most common cause of HDFN.
6 Red cell surface proteins serve a variety of functions, though many of their functions are still not known.

Further reading

Avent ND & Reid ME. The Rh blood group system: a review. *Blood* 2000;95:375–387.
Chester AM & Olsson ML. The ABO blood group gene: a locus of considerable genetic diversity. *Transfus Med Rev* 2001;15:177–200.
Daniels G. *Human Blood Groups*, 2nd edn. Oxford: Blackwell Science, 2002.

Daniels G. Functions of red cell surface proteins. *Vox Sang* 2007;93:331–340.

Daniels G & Bromilow I. *Essential Guide to Blood Groups.* Oxford: Blackwell Publishing, 2006.

Daniels GL, Fletcher A, Garratty G *et al.* Blood group terminology 2004. From the ISBT Committee on Terminology for Red Cell Surface Antigens. *Vox Sang* 2004;87:304–316.

Hillyer C, Shaz BH, Winkler AM & Reid M. Integrating molecular technologies for red blood cell typing and compatibility testing into blood centers and transfusion services. *Transfus Med Rev* 2008;22:117–132.

Mohandas N & Gallagher PG. Red cell membrane: past, present, and future. *Blood* 2008;112:3939–3948.

Poole J & Daniels G. Blood group antibodies and their significance in transfusion medicine. *Transfus Med Rev* 2007;21:58–71.

Reid ME & Lomas-Francis C. *The Blood Group Antigen Facts Book,* 2nd edn. New York: Academic Press, 2004.

Storry JR & Olsson ML. Genetic basis of blood group diversity. *Br J Haemat* 2004;126:759–771.

Watkins WM. (ed) Commemoration of the centenary of the discovery of the ABO blood group system. *Transfus Med* 2001;11:239–351.

CHAPTER 4
Human leucocyte antigens

Cristina V. Navarrete
NHS Blood and Transplant, Colindale, University College, London, UK

Introduction

The genes coding for the human leucocyte antigens (HLAs) are located on the short arm of chromosome 6 spanning a distance of approximately 4 Mb. This genomic region is divided into three subregions.

- Class I subregion contains genes coding for the heavy (α) chain of the classical (HLA-A, -B and -C) and non-classical (HLA-E, -F and -G) class I molecules. The non-classical major histocompatibility complex class I chain-related gene A and gene B (*MICA* and *MICB*) have also been mapped to this subregion, centromeric to the HLA-B gene (Figure 4.1).
- Class II subregion contains the classical HLA-DR, -DQ and -DP genes and the non-classical HLA-*DMA*, -*DMB*, -*DOA* and -*DOB* genes. The low-molecular-mass polypeptide genes *LMP2* and *LMP7*, *TAP1* and *TAP2* transporters and the Tapasin (Tpn) genes involved in the processing, transport and loading of HLA class I antigenic peptides are also located in this subregion (see Figure 4.1).
- Class III subregion lies between the other two subregions and contains genes coding for a diverse group of proteins, including complement components (C4Bf), tumour necrosis factor (TNF) and heat-shock proteins (HSPs).

The non-classical class I-like gene *HFE* has been mapped to a locus located 4 Mb telomeric to HLA-F.

Practical Transfusion Medicine, 3rd edition. Edited by Michael F. Murphy and Derwood H. Pamphilon. © 2009 Blackwell Publishing. ISBN: 978-1-4051-8196-9.

Mutations in this gene are involved in the development of hereditary haemochromatosis (HH).

HLA class I genes

The HLA class I genes are classified according to their structure, expression and function as classical (HLA-A, -B and -C) and non-classical (HLA-E, -F and -G). Both classical and non-classical HLA class I genes code for a heavy (α) chain, of approximately 43 kDa, non-covalently linked to a non-polymorphic light chain, the β_2-microglobulin of 12 kDa, which is coded for by a gene on chromosome 15. The extracellular portion of the heavy chain has three domains (α1, α2 and α3) of approximately 90 amino acids long. These domains are encoded by exons 2, 3 and 4 of the class I gene, respectively. The α1 and α2 domains are the most polymorphic domains of the molecule and they form a peptide-binding groove that can accommodate antigenic peptides approximately eight to nine amino acids long.

The exon/intron organisation of the non-classical HLA class I genes (E, F and G) is very similar to the classical class I genes, but they have a more restricted polymorphism. The MICA and MICB gene products, however, do not bind β_2-microglobulin and do not present antigenic peptides.

A schematic representation of the classical HLA class I gene and molecule is shown in Figure 4.2.

HLA class II genes

The classical HLA class II DR, DQ and DP A and B genes code for heterodimers formed by

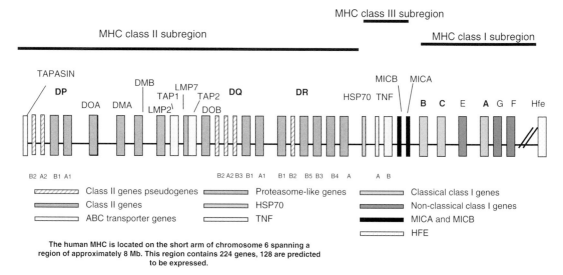

Figure 4.1 Map of the human leucocyte antigen complex. HSP, heat-shock protein; TNF, tumour necrosis factor. (Adapted from Trowsdale and Campbell, 1997.)

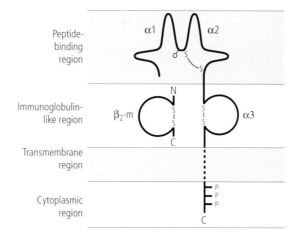

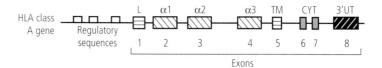

Figure 4.2 HLA class I molecule. β_2-m, β_2-microglobulin.

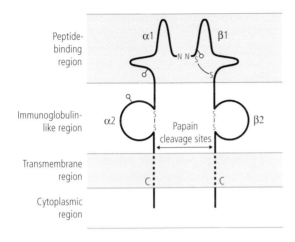

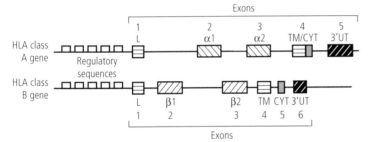

Figure 4.3 HLA class II molecule.

non-covalently associated α and β chains of approximately 34 and 28 kDa, respectively. The expressed α and β chains consist of two extracellular domains and a transmembrane and cytoplasmic domains. The α1/β1 and α2/β2 domains are encoded by exon 2 and exon 3 of the class II gene, respectively. The majority of the polymorphism is located in the β1 domain of the DR molecules and in the α1 and β1 domains of the DQ and DP molecules. Similarly to the class I molecules, these domains also form a peptide-binding groove. However, in the case of the class II molecules (DR), the groove is open at both sides and it can accommodate antigenic peptides of varying size, although most of them are approximately 13–25 amino acids long. A schematic representation of the HLA class II gene and molecule is shown in Figure 4.3.

The non-classical HLA class I *DMA*, *DMB*, *DOA* and *DOB* genes have a similar structure to the classical class II genes, but show limited polymorphism.

Genetic organisation and expression of HLA class II genes

There is one *DRA* gene of limited polymorphism and nine *DRB* genes, of which B1, B3, B4 and B5 are highly polymorphic and B2, B6 and B9 are pseudogenes. The main serologically defined DR specificities (DR1–DR18) are determined by the polymorphic *DRB1** gene. The number of *DRB* genes expressed in each individual varies according to the DRB1 allele expressed (Figure 4.4). There are a few exceptions to this pattern of gene expression, e.g. a *DRB5* gene has been found to be expressed with some DR1 alleles. Some non-expressed or null *DRB5* and *DRB4* genes have also been identified. In contrast to the *DRB* genes, there are two *DQA* and three *DQB* genes, but only the *DQA1* and *DQB1* are expressed and both are polymorphic. Similarly, there are two *DPA* and two *DPB* genes, and only the *DPA1* and *DPB1* are expressed and both are polymorphic.

Specifications

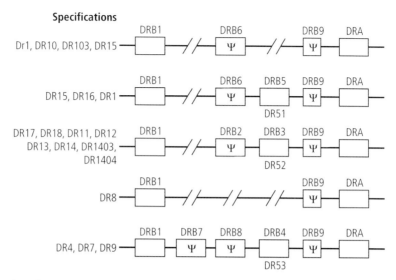

Figure 4.4 Expression of HLA-DRB genes.

Expression of HLA molecules

The classical HLA class I molecules (A, B, C) are expressed on the majority of tissues and blood cells, including T and B lymphocytes, granulocytes and platelets. Low levels of expression have been detected in endocrine tissue, skeletal muscle and cells of the central nervous system. HLA-E and -F are also expressed on most tissues tested, but HLA-G shows a more restricted tissue distribution and to date HLA-G products have only been found on extravillous cytotrophoblasts of the placenta and mononuclear phagocytes. MICA and MICB molecules are expressed on fibroblasts, endothelial, intestinal and tumour epithelial cells.

The HLA class II molecules are constitutively expressed on B lymphocytes, monocytes and dendritic cells, but can also be detected on activated T lymphocytes and activated granulocytes. It is not clear whether they are also present on activated platelets. HLA class II expression can be induced on a number of cells such as fibroblasts and endothelial cells as the result of activation and/or the effect of certain inflammatory cytokines, such as interferon (IFN)-γ, TNF and interleukin (IL)-10.

Both classical and non-classical HLA molecules can also be found in soluble forms and it has been suggested that they may play a role in the induction of peripheral tolerance.

Genetics

HLA genes are codominantly expressed and are inherited in a mendelian fashion. One of the main features of the HLA genes is their high degree of polymorphism and the strong linkage disequilibrium (LD) in which they segregate. LD is a phenomenon where the observed frequency of alleles of different loci segregating together is greater than the frequency expected by random association. Whereas some of the polymorphism and the patterns of LD are expressed with similar frequencies in all populations, others are unique to some population groups. For example, HLA-A2 is expressed at a relatively high frequency in most population groups studied so far, whereas B53 is found predominantly in Black people.

The genetic region containing all HLA genes on each chromosome is termed the haplotype. Some HLA haplotypes are also found across different ethnic groups, e.g. HLA-B44-DR7, whereas others are unique to a particular population, e.g. HLA-B42-DR18 in Black Africans. This characteristic is particularly relevant for the selection of HLA-compatible family donors for patients requiring solid organ or haemopoietic stem cell (HSC) transplantation.

Function of HLA molecules

The main function of HLA molecules is to present antigenic peptides to T cells and this requires a fine interaction between the HLA molecules, the antigenic peptide and the T-cell receptor. A number of costimulatory molecules (e.g. CD80 and CD86) and adhesion molecules such ICAM-1 (CD54) and LFA-3 (CD58) also contribute to these interactions.

The HLA class I molecules are primarily, but not exclusively, involved in the presentation of endogenous antigenic peptides to CD8 cytotoxic T cells. Both the classical and non-classical HLA class I molecules also interact with a new family of receptors present on natural killer (NK) cells. Some of these receptors, which are polymorphic and differentially expressed, have an inhibitory role whereas others are activating. The killer-activating and killer-inhibitory receptors belong to two distinct families: the immunoglobulin superfamily called killer immunglobulin receptors (KIRs) and the C-type lectin superfamily CD94-NKG2. The interaction between the inhibitory receptors and the relevant HLA ligand results in the prevention of NK lysis of the target cell. Thus, NK cells from any given individual will be alloreactive towards cells lacking their corresponding inhibitory KIR ligands, e.g. tumour or allogeneic cells. In contrast, NK cells will be tolerant to cells from individuals who express the corresponding KIR ligands. The *MICA* molecules, which are induced by stress, also interact with the NK activatory receptor NKG2D and with γδT cells.

The *LMP2* and *LMP7* are thought to improve the capacity of the proteosomes to generate peptides of the appropriate size and specificity to associate with the class I molecules whereas *TAP1* and *TAP2* are primarily involved in the transport of the proteosome-generated peptides to the endoplasmic reticulum, where they associate with the class I molecules.

Classical HLA class II molecules are mostly involved in the presentation of exogenous antigenic peptides to CD4 helper T cells. Once activated, these CD4 cells can initiate and regulate a variety of processes leading to the maturation and differentiation of cellular (CD8 cytotoxic T cells) and humoral effectors (such as antibody production by plasma cells). Activated effectors also secrete proinflammatory cytokines (IL-2, IFN-γ, TNF-α) and regulatory cytokines (IL-4, IL-10 and transforming growth factor-β).

The main function of HLA-DM molecules is to facilitate the release of the class II-associated invariant chain (Ii) peptide from the peptide-binding groove of the HLA-DR molecules so that the groove can be loaded with the relevant antigenic peptide and this function is modulated by the DO molecules.

Identification of HLA gene polymorphism

The HLA polymorphisms were initially defined using serological and cellular techniques. With the development of gene cloning and DNA sequencing, it is now possible to perform a detailed analysis of these genes at the single nucleotide level. This analysis has shown the existence of certain locus-specific nucleotide sequences in both coding (exons) and non-coding (introns) regions of the genes and also the existence of regions of nucleotide sequences that are common to several alleles of the same and/or different loci. The DNA sequencing of a number of HLA alleles of various loci has also demonstrated that the majority of the variation is located in the α1 and α2 domain of the class I molecules and in the α1 and β1 domain of the class II molecules. These are called hypervariable regions.

Based on this information, a number of techniques have been developed to characterise these polymorphisms. Most of the described techniques make use of the polymerase chain reaction (PCR) to amplify the specific genes or region to be analysed. These techniques include PCR-SSP (PCR-sequence-specific priming), PCR-SSOP

Table 4.1 Number of recognised HLA antigens/alleles.

	Alleles	Antigens
HLA class I		
HLA-A	349	24
HLA-B	627	50
HLA-C	182	9
HLA-E	5	
HLA-F	2	
HLA-G	15	
HLA class II		
HLA-DRB1	394	17
HLA-DRA1	3	—
HLA-DRB3	41	1
HLA-DRB4	13	1
HLA-DRB5	18	1
HLA-DQB1	61	6
HLA-DQA1	28	—
HLA-DPB1	116	6*
HLA-DPA1	22	—

*Cellularly defined.
Adapted from Marsh *et al.* (2004).

(PCR-sequence-specific oligonucleotide probing) and DNA sequencing-based typing (SBT).

The number of recognised serologically defined antigens and DNA-identified HLA alleles is shown in Table 4.1.

PCR-sequence-specific priming

This technique involves the use of primers designed to anneal with DNA sequences unique to each allele and locus. The detection of the PCR-amplified product is then carried out by running the amplified product on an agarose gel. This technique allows the rapid identification of the HLA alleles in individual samples since the readout of this method is the presence or absence of the product for which specific primers were used. However, although this is a very rapid procedure, many PCR reactions have to be set up per sample in order to detect most of the defined alleles, e.g. at least 24 reactions for low-resolution DR typing. Furthermore, for PCR-SSP typing the DNA sequence of the alleles must be known since novel unknown sequences may not always be detected.

PCR-sequence-specific oligonucleotide probing

In this technique, the gene of interest is amplified using primers designed to anneal with DNA sequences common to all alleles of the loci of interest. The amplified PCR product is then immobilised onto support (e.g. nylon) membranes and the specificity of the products analysed by reacting the membranes with labelled allele-specific oligonucleotides. By scoring the probes that bind to specific regions, it is possible to assign the HLA type.

A modification of this technique, called reverse blot, involves the binding of the PCR-amplified product to labelled probes immobilised on membranes (strips) or plates. More recently, Luminex analysers are used to read the binding of the DNA to beads coated with oligonucleotide probe. Reverse SSOP is useful when large numbers of samples need to be HLA-typed, e.g. bone marrow or cord blood donors.

DNA sequencing-based typing

DNA sequencing involves the denaturation of the DNA to be analysed to provide a single-strand template. Sequencing primers, exon- or locus-specific, are then added and the DNA extension is performed by the addition of Taq polymerase in the presence of excess nucleotides. The sequencing mixture is divided into four tubes, each of which contains specific dideoxyribonucleoside triphosphate (ddATP). When these are incorporated into the DNA synthesis, elongation is interrupted with chain-terminating inhibitors. In each reaction, there is random incorporation of the chain terminators and therefore products of all sizes are generated. The sequencing products are detected by labelling the nucleotide chain inhibitors with radioisotopes and, more recently, with fluorescent dyes. The products of the four reactions are then analysed by electrophoresis in parallel lanes of a polyacrylamide–urea gel and the sequence is read by combining the results of each lane using an automated DNA sequencer. In HLA SBT, some ambiguous results can be obtained with heterozygous samples and these may need to be retested by using PCR-SSP or reverse PCR-SSOP.

Table 4.2 Advantages and disadvantages of DNA-based techniques.

Technique	Advantages	Disadvantages
Sequence-specific oligonucleotide probing (SSOP)	Needs only one pair of genetic primers, fewer reactions to set up Larger number of samples can be processed simultaneously Requires small amount of DNA cheap	Different temperatures required for each probe Probes can cross-react with different alleles Large numbers of probes required to identify specificity Difficult to interpret pattern of reactions
Sequence-specific priming (SSP)	Provides rapid typing with higher resolution than SSOP All PCR amplifications are carried out at same time, temperature and conditions Fast and simple to read and interpret	Too many sets of primers are needed to fully HLA type Requires a two-stage amplification to provide HR typing
Reference strand conformational analysis (RSCA)	Easy to perform Provides higher resolution than SSOP and SSP	Requires expensive equipment Requires established data on viability value of each allele studied
Sequencing-based typing (SBT)	Provides the highest level of resolution Able to identify new alleles Does not require previous sequence data to identify new allele	Not easy to perform Requires expensive reagents and equipments Difficult to interpret Requires DNA sequence data to compare results Slower than SSOP (reverse blot), SSP and RSCA

SBT permits high-resolution HLA typing, which is known to be important in the selection of HLA-matched HSC unrelated donors.

A major advantage of all DNA-based techniques is that no viable cells are required to perform HLA class I and II typing. Furthermore, since all the probes and primers are synthesised to order, there is a consistency of reagents used, allowing the comparison of HLA types from different laboratories. However, although serological typing is being rapidly replaced by DNA-based typing techniques, serological reagents may still be required for antigen expression studies.

The advantages and disadvantages of the various techniques described above are given in Table 4.2.

Formation of HLA antibodies

HLA-specific antibodies are induced by pregnancy, transplantation, blood transfusions and planned immunisations. The affinity, avidity and class of the antibodies produced depend on various factors, including the route of immunisation, the persistence and type of immunological challenge and the immune status of the host. Cytotoxic HLA antibodies can be identified in approximately 20% of human pregnancies. The antibodies produced are normally multi-specific, high titre, high affinity and of the IgG class. Although these HLA IgG antibodies can cross the placenta, they are not harmful to the fetus. Antibodies produced following transplantation are mostly IgG, although rarely HLA IgM antibodies have been identified. In contrast, the majority of HLA antibodies found in multitransfused patients are multi-specific IgM and IgG and are mostly directed at public epitopes. The introduction of leucocyte-depleted blood components (see Chapter 21) may lead to a reduction in alloimmunisation in naive recipients, but it may not be very effective in preventing alloimmunisation in already sensitised recipients, i.e. women who have become immunised as a result of pregnancy.

The deliberate immunisation of healthy individuals to produce HLA-specific reagents is nowadays difficult to justify ethically. However, planned HLA immunisation is still carried out in some centres to treat women with a history of recurrent miscarriages. These women are immunised with white cells from their partners or a third party to attempt to induce an immunomodulatory response that results in the maintenance of the pregnancy.

Detection of HLA antibodies

A number of techniques to detect HLA antibodies have been developed. These include the complement-dependent lymphocytotoxicity (LCT) test, enzyme-linked immunosorbent assay (ELISA) and flow cytometry and more recently, a Luminex-based technique.

Complement-dependent cytotoxicity test

The complement-dependent cytotoxicity (CDC) test, developed by Terasaki and McClelland (1964), involves mixing equal volumes of serum and cells to allow the binding of the specific antibody to the target cell followed by the addition of rabbit complement. Complement-fixing antibodies reacting with the HLA antigen present on the cell surface lead to the activation of complement via the classical pathway and result in the disruption of the cell membrane. The lysed cells are then detected by adding ethidium bromide (EB) and the live cells are identified by adding acridine orange (AO) at the end of the incubation period. Live cells stained with AO when exposed to ultraviolet (UV) light, appear green, whereas lysed cells allow the entry of EB,

which binds to DNA, and they appear red under UV light. The reactions are scored by estimation of the percentage of dead cells in each well after establishing baseline values in the negative and positive as follows: 0–10% (1 background cell death, negative); 11–20% (2 doubtful negative); 21–50% (4 weak positive); 51–80% (6 positive); 81–100% (8 strong positive).

The CDC assay, however, does not discriminate between HLA and non-HLA cytotoxic lymphocyte-reactive antibodies including autoantibodies. However, the majority of lymphocytotoxic autoantibodies are IgM and can be identified by screening the serum with and without dithiothreitol (DTT). The addition of DTT to the serum results in the breakdown of the intersubunit disulphide bonds in the IgM molecule, leading to the loss of cytotoxicity due to IgM. Prolonged exposure or excess DTT can lead to the breakdown of intramolecular disulphide bonds in the IgG molecules and also inactivate complement, but this can be inhibited by the addition of cystine.

The presence of lymphocytotoxic autoreactive antibodies in itself is not thought to be of clinical significance in solid organ transplant recipients or in patients immunologically refractory to random donor platelet transfusions.

Since the CDC test only detects cytotoxic HLA-specific antibodies, other techniques such as the ELISA or flow cytometry are needed to detect non-cytotoxic HLA-specific antibodies.

Enzyme-linked immunosorbent assay

ELISA-based methods have often been the technique of choice for antibody detection particularly where there has been a requirement for testing large numbers of samples. In this technique, a pool of purified HLA antigens is immobilised on a microwell plate, directly or via an antibody directed against a non-polymorphic region of the HLA antigen or against the β2-microglobulin. Antibodies directed against the non-polymorphic region of the HLA class I molecule, i.e. the α3 domain, are used to immobilise the specific HLA antigen to the microwell, ensuring that the more polymorphic α1 and α2 domains are available for antibody binding. HLA-specific antibodies bound to the immobilised antigens are then detected with an enzyme-linked secondary antibody which, upon addition of specific substrate, catalyses a colour change reaction that is detected in an ELISA reader.

In order to detect HLA specificity, each specific HLA antigen is isolated from an individual cell or cell line. Large panels of cells are cell lines used to purify these antigens in order to cover all the major HLA specificities at least once. A number of commercial kits are now available to screen for HLA antibodies and to define their specificities.

One of the main advantages of this ELISA technique is that they detect HLA-specific antibodies since it relies on the binding of the antibodies to wells coated with pools of solubilised or purified HLA antigens.

Flow cytometry

In this technique, cells and serum are incubated to allow the binding of the antibody to the target antigen. The bound antibody is then detected by using an antibody against human immunoglobulin labelled with a fluorescent marker such as fluorescein isothiocyanate or R-phycoerythrin. At the end of the incubation period, the cells are passed through the laser beam of the flow cytometer to identify the different cell populations based on their morphology/granularity and on the fluorescence. Normally, test sera with median fluorescence values greater than the mean $+$ 3SD of the negative controls are considered positive, but each laboratory needs to establish its own positive and negative cut-off point values. By using a second antibody against cell-specific markers such as CD3 or CD19, it is possible to identify T or B cell reactivity.

The main advantages of flow cytometric techniques are the increased sensitivity when compared with LCT- and ELISA-based techniques and the detection of non-complement-fixing antibodies, allowing early detection of sensitisation. However, one of the disadvantages is that it also detects non-HLA lymphocyte-reactive antibodies which are of unclear clinical relevance.

The use of flow cytometric techniques was initially investigated as an alternative cross-match technique and was shown to be more sensitive than previously described techniques. The increased

sensitivity may be due to the fact that it detects both cytotoxic and non-cytotoxic antibodies, some of which may be HLA specific.

Luminex

This technique uses fluorochrome-dyed polystyrene beads coated with specific HLA antigens. The precise ratio of these fluorochromes creates 100 distinctly coloured beads, each of them coated with a different antigen. The beads are then incubated with the patient's serum and the reaction is developed using a PE-conjugated antihuman IgG (Fc specific) antibody. The positive or negative reactions are then read using a Luminex analyser which can distinguish between up to 100 different beads sets in a single tube. Luminex is the most sensitive technique currently available for the detection of HLA antibodies. Most recently, this technology has been further improved by the introduction of beads coated with single antigens which improve the identification of antibody specificities that were not previously detected. In this technique, the beads can be coated with either HLA antigens for antibody screening or HLA oligonucleotide probes for HLA typing.

The CDC test and flow cytometry are the two main techniques used to perform antibody cross-matching between the patient's serum and the potential donor's cells in the solid organ transplant setting.

Clinical relevance of HLA antigens and antibodies

Although the main role of the HLA molecules is to present antigenic peptides to T cells, HLA molecules can themselves be recognised as foreign by the host T cells by a mechanism known as allorecognition. Two pathways of allorecognition have been identified, direct and indirect.

In the direct pathway, the host's T cells recognise HLA molecules (primarily class II) expressed on donor tissues, e.g. tissue dendritic cells and endothelial cells. Indirect allorecognition involves the recognition by the host T cells of donor-derived HLA class I and II antigenic peptides presented by the host's own antigen-presenting cells. Because of this mechanism, HLA antigen incompatibility is one of the main barriers to success of solid organ or HSC transplantation and also results in the strong alloimmunisation seen in patients following transplantation or blood transfusion.

Solid organ transplantation

Matching for HLA-A, -B and -DR antigens is an important factor influencing the outcome of solid organ transplantation and particularly renal transplants. The application of the PCR-based techniques has allowed the identification of molecular differences between otherwise serologically identical HLA types of donor and recipient pairs, particularly in the HLA-DRβ1 chain. Correlation of these results with graft survival has shown a higher kidney graft survival rate when recipients and donors are HLA-DR identical by serological and molecular techniques than when they were HLA-DR identical by serological but not molecular methods (87% versus 69%).

The presence of circulating HLA-specific antibodies directed against donor antigens in renal and cardiac recipients has been associated with hyperacute rejection of the graft. It is therefore important that these antibodies are detected and identified as soon as the patient is registered on the transplant waiting list to ensure that incompatible donors are not considered for transplantation.

Antibodies against the MICA and HLA DP antigens also seem to influence graft outcome suggesting the possible need to screen for these antibodies in patients awaiting transplantation.

Furthermore, the appearance of donor-specific antibodies after transplantation has been associated with graft rejection, indicating the importance of post-transplant antibody monitoring for some groups of patients.

HLA and haemopoietic stem cell transplantation

HLA-DR incompatibility is one of the main factors associated with the development of acute graft-versus-host disease (aGVHD) but mismatches at the HLA-A and -B alleles, and to lesser extent HLA-C alleles, are also independent risk factors particularly

when using matched unrelated donors. Although HSC transplantation between HLA-identical siblings ensures matching for all HLA-A, -B, -C, -DR and -DQ genes, acute GVHD still develops in about 20–30% of these patients. This is probably due to the effect of untested HLA antigens, such as DP, or minor histocompatibility antigens in the activation of donor T cells. However, patients receiving grafts from HLA-matched unrelated donors have a higher risk of developing GVHD than those transplanted using an HLA-identical sibling.

The use of DNA-based methods has provided a unique opportunity to improve the HLA matching of patients and unrelated donors and to reduce the development of GVHD. However, it has been shown that the increased GVHD seen as a result of HLA mismatch is also associated with lower relapse rates, probably due to a graft-versus-leukaemia (GVL) response associated with the graft-versus-host response. On the other hand, the use of T-cell-depleted marrow, which has successfully decreased the incidence of GVHD, has resulted in an increased incidence of leukaemia relapse. Thus, it appears that mature T cells in the marrow, which may be responsible for GVHD, may also be involved in the elimination of residual leukaemic cells. Conversely, the rate of graft rejection is significantly higher in recipients of an HLA-mismatched transplant than in those receiving a transplant from an HLA-identical sibling (12.3% versus 2.0%).

HSC transplantation using cord blood from HLA-matched and HLA-mismatched donors has now been associated with a reduced risk and severity of GVHD and with no increase in relapse rates. It is possible that the immaturity of the immunological effectors present in cord blood may contribute to the reduced GVHD without impairment of the GVL effect.

Graft failure, which is thought to be mediated by residual recipient T and/or NK cells reacting with major or minor histocompatibility antigens present in the donor marrow cells, has been shown to be associated also with antibodies reacting with donor's HLA antigens. Thus, rejection is particularly high in HLA-alloimmunised patients. However, in spite of these reports, HLA antibodies are more relevant in the post-transplant period, where highly immunised patients can develop immunological refractoriness to random platelet transfusions due to the presence of HLA antibodies. These patients require transfusions of HLA-matched platelets (see Chapter 27).

Blood transfusion

White cells and platelets present in transfused products express antigens which, if not identical to those present in the recipient, are able to activate T cells and lead to the development of antibodies and/or effector cells responsible for some of the serious complications of blood transfusion. Also, antibodies (and T cells) present in the transfused product may react directly with the relevant antigens in the recipient and lead to the development of a transfusion reaction. Amongst the transfusion reactions due to the presence of antibodies in the recipient are febrile non-haemolytic transfusion reaction (FNHTR) and immunological refractoriness to random platelet transfusions.

Although the occurrence of FNHTR has been commonly associated with the presence of HLA (and to a lesser extent HPA (human platelet antigen) or HNA (human neutrophil antigen)) antibodies in the recipient reacting with white blood cells or platelets present in the transfused product, it has recently been described that FNHTR may also be triggered by the direct action of cytokines such as IL-1β, TNF-α, IL-6 and/or by chemokines such as IL-8 which are found in transfused products.

Immunological refractoriness to random platelet transfusions is primarily due to the presence of HLA and, to a lesser extent, HPA and high-titre ABO alloantibodies in the patient and reacting with the transfused incompatible platelets leading to the lack of platelet increments after the transfusion. Following the introduction of universal leucodepletion, the proportion of multitransfused patients with HLA antibodies seems to have decreased to approximately 10–20% and these patients are in general, previously sensitised the transplanted or transfused recipients and multiparous women.

The development of transfusion-related acute lung injury (TRALI) has been associated with the transfusion of blood components containing HLA and HNA antibodies able to recognise the relevant antigen(s) on recipient white cells and triggering an immunological reaction leading to the accumulation of neutrophils in the lungs and oedema. TRALI has sometimes been associated with the presence of HLA or HNA antibodies in recipients reacting with transfused leucocytes and/or to inter-donor antigen–antibody reactions in pooled platelets.

Transfusion-associated (TA)-GVHD which is a rare but often severe and fatal transfusion reaction is the result of immunocompetent HLA-matched T lymphocytes present in blood or blood products reacting with HLA and/or minor histocompatibility antigens present on the recipient cells. TA-GVHD occurs primarily in immunosuppressed individuals, although it can also occur in immunocompetent recipients. The diagnosis of TA-GVHD depends on finding evidence of donor-derived cells, chromosomes or DNA in the blood and/or affected tissues of the recipient.

HLA and disease

HLA genes are known to be associated with a number of autoimmune and infectious diseases, and different mechanisms to explain these associations have been postulated, including linkage disequilibrium with the relevant disease susceptibility gene, the preferential presentation of the pathogenic peptide by certain HLA molecules and molecular mimicry between certain pathogenic peptides and host-derived peptides. A number of diseases associated with both HLA class I and II have been described in Table 4.3.

Hereditary haemochromatosis

HH is a clinical condition of iron overload caused by an inherited disorder in the genes involved in the metabolism of iron. HH is a common genetic disorder in Northern Europe, where between 1 in 200 and 1 in 400 individuals suffer from the disease, with an estimated carrier frequency of between 1 in 8 and 1 in 10. Clinical manifestations of HH include cirrhosis of the liver, diabetes and cardiomyopathy. Detection of asymptomatic iron

Table 4.3 HLA-associated diseases.

HLA class I genes
Birdshot chorioretinopathy: HLA-A29
Behçet's disease: HLA-B51
Ankylosing spondylitis: HLA-B27
Psoriasis: HLA-Cw6
Malaria: HLA-B53

HLA class II genes
Rheumatoid arthritis
   HLA-DRB1*0401
   HLA-DRB1*0404
   HLA-DRB1*0405
   HLA-DRB1*0408
   HLA-DRB1*0101/0102
   HLA-DRB1*1402
   HLA-DRB1*1001
Narcolepsy: HLA-DQB1*0602/DQA1*0102
Coeliac disease: HLA-DQB1*0201/DQA1*0501
Neonatal alloimmune thrombocytopenia: HLA-DRB3*0101
Malaria: HLA-DRB1*1302/DQB1*0501
Insulin-dependent diabetes mellitus:
   HLA-DQB1*0302/DQA1*0301

HLA-linked diseases
Haemochromatosis: (HLA-A3) HFE gene C282Y, H63D and
   S65C
21-OH deficiency: (HLA-B47) 21-OH gene

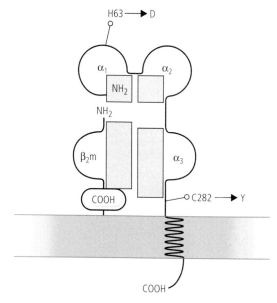

Figure 4.5 HFE molecule. β_2-m, β_2-microglobulin.

overload is important since removal of excess iron by phlebotomy can prevent organ damage.

HH was originally described associated to HLA-A3 although this was not very specific since the majority of HLA-A3-positive individuals do not have HH. It was later found that mutations in the HFE gene located 3 Mb telomeric from the HLA-F gene was partly responsible for this condition. A number of mutations have now been identified and clinical data indicate that at least three of these mutations (C282Y, H63D and S65C) may predispose to and affect the clinical outcome of this condition. Over 90% of HH patients in the UK are homozygous for the mutation that replaces a cysteine (C) with a tyrosine (Y) at codon 282 in the *HFE* gene. The second and third mutations (H63D and S65C) are thought to be less important, although it may have an additive effect if inherited with the first mutation (Figure 4.5). Recent studies on blood donors

have shown that approximately 1 in 280 donors is homozygous for the mutations.

A DNA-based technique to detect these three mutations simultaneously has now been developed and provides a simple, rapid and unambiguous definition of these mutations.

Neonatal alloimmune thrombocytopenia

Neonatal alloimmune thrombocytopenia (NAIT) is a serious condition in the newborn and is due to fetomaternal incompatibility for HPAs (see also Chapters 5 and 26). More than 80% of cases occur in women who are homozygous for the HPA-1b allele. Although the majority of cases are associated with the presence of HPA-1a antibodies, about 15% of cases are due to anti-HPA-5b. The production of HPA-1a antibodies is strongly associated with the HLA-DRB3*0101 allele. However, only approximately 35% of HPA-1a-negative, DRB3*0101-positive women develop antibodies upon exposure to the antigen, suggesting that other genes or factors may be involved in the development of alloimmunisation against HPA-1a.

Diseases in which the molecular mimicry mechanism has been postulated include ankylosing spondylitis and *Klebsiella* infection. However, the precise pathogenic mechanisms involved remain unknown. More recently, it has been shown that HLA genes are also involved in the response to certain drugs such as the association of HLAB-57 and abacavir, a drug used in the treatment of HIV.

Key points

1 HLA molecules are crucial in the induction and regulation of immune responses and in the outcome of transplantation using allogeneic-related and -unrelated donors and are also responsible for some of the serious immunological complications of blood transfusion.
2 The main feature of HLA genes is their high degree of polymorphism and linkage disequilibrium and depending on their molecular structure, expression and function, they are classified as classical or non-classical.
3 The detection of HLA polymorphisms is currently performed using DNA-based techniques at various degrees of resolution depending on the clinical needs and relevance.
4 The techniques currently used to screen and define the specificity of HLA antibodies allow the discrimination of HLA and non-HLA cytotoxic and non-cytotoxic antibodies.
5 HLA antibodies produced following transfusion, transplantation or pregnancy are responsible for some of the most serious complications of blood transfusion.
6 HLA matching and cold ischaemia time are the two most important factors influencing the outcome of renal transplantation.
7 In the HSC transplantation setting, HLA matching for HLA class I and II genes is essential to minimise the development of aGVHD.
8 HLA genes are involved in the pathogenesis of a variety of diseases either directly through the presentation of pathogenic peptides or indirectly through their linkage disequilibrium with the relevant disease susceptibility gene(s).

Further reading

Bomford A. Genetics of haemochromatosis. *The Lancet* 2002;360:1673–1681.

Brown C & Navarrete C. HLA antibody screening by LCT, LIFT and ELISA. In: Bidwell J & Navarrete C. (eds), *Histocompatibility Testing*. London: Imperial College Press, 2000, pp. 65–98.

Campbell RD. The human major histocompatibility complex: a 4000-kb segment of the human genome replete with genes. In: Davies KE & Tilghman SM. (eds), *Genome Analysis. Vol. 5: Regional Physical Mapping*. New York: Cold Spring Harbor Laboratory Press, 1993, pp. 1–33.

Dyer PA & Claas FHJ. A future for HLA matching in clinical transplantation. *Eur J Immunogenet* 1997;24:17–28.

Gruen JR & Weissman SM. Evolving views of the major histocompatibility complex. *Blood* 1997;90:4252–4265.

Harrison J & Navarrete C. Selection of platelet donors and provision of HLA matched platelets. In: Bidwell J & Navarrete C. (eds), *Histocompatibility Testing*. London: Imperial College Press, 2000, pp. 379–390.

Horton R, Wilming L, Rand V *et al.* Gene map of the extended human MHC. *Nat Rev* 2004;5:889–899.

Howell M & Navarrete C. The HLA system: an update and relevance to patient–donor matching strategies in clinical transplantation. *Vox Sang* 1996;71:6–12.

Lardy NM, Van Der Hjorst AR, Ten Berge IJM *et al.* Influence of HLA-DRB1* incompatibility on the occurrence of rejection episodes and graft survival in serologically HLA-DR-matched renal transplant combinations. *Transplantation* 1997;64:612–616.

Madrigal JA, Arguello R, Scott I & Avakian H. Molecular histocompatibility typing in unrelated donor bone marrow transplantation. *Blood Rev* 1997;11:105–117.

Madrigal JA, Scott I, Arguello R, Szydlo R, Little A-M & Goldman JM. Factors influencing the outcome of bone marrow transplants using unrelated donors. *Immunol Rev* 1997;157:153–166.

Marsh SG, Albert ED, Bodmer WF *et al.* Nomenclature for factors of the HLA system, 2004. *Int J Immunogenet* 2004;32:107–159.

Mura C, Raguenes O & Ferec C. HFE mutations analysis in 711 haemochromatosis probands: evidence for S65C implication in mild form of hemochromatosis. *Blood* 1999;93:2502–2505.

Opelz G & Döhler B. Effects of human leucocyte antigen compatibility of kidney graft survival: comparative analysis of two decades. *Transplantation* 2007;84:137–143.

Parham P & McQueen KL. Alloreactive killer cells: hindrance and help for haematopoietic transplants. *Nat Rev Immunol* 2003;3:108–121.

Petersdorf EW, Malkki M, Gooley TA *et al.* MHC haplotype matching for unrelated hematopoietic cell transplantation. *PloS Med* 2007;4:59–68.

Suthanthiran M & Strom TB. Renal transplantation. *N Engl Med J* 1994;331:365–376.

Terasaki PL & McClelland JD. Microdroplet assay of human serum cytokines. *Nature* 2000;204:998–1000.

Thorsby E. HLA associated diseases. *Hum Immunol* 1997;53:1–11.

CHAPTER 5

Platelet and neutrophil antigens

David L. Allen[1], Geoffrey F. Lucas[2], Michael F. Murphy[3] & Willem H. Ouwehand[4]

[1]NHS Blood and Transplant; Department of Clinical Laboratory Sciences, University of Oxford, John Radcliffe Hospital, Oxford, UK

[2]NHS Blood and Transplant, Bristol, UK

[3]University of Oxford; NHS Blood and Transplant and Department of Haematology, John Radcliffe Hospital, Oxford, UK

[4]University of Cambridge; NHS Blood and Transplant, Cambridge, UK

Antigens on platelets and granulocytes

Antigens on human platelets and granulocytes can be categorised according to their biochemical nature into:

- carbohydrate antigens on glycolipids and glycoproteins;

  (a) A, B and O

  (b) P and Le on platelets; I on granulocytes

- protein antigens;

  (a) human leucocyte antigen (HLA) class I (A, B and C)

  (b) glycoprotein (GP)IIb/IIIa, GPIa/IIa, GPIb/IX/V, etc. on platelets

  (c) FcγRIIIb (CD16), CD177, etc. on granulocytes

- hapten-induced antigens:

  (a) quinine, quinidine

  (b) some antibiotics, e.g. penicillins and cephalosporins

  (c) heparin.

These antigens can be targeted by some or all of the following types of antibodies:

- autoantibodies;
- alloantibodies;
- isoantibodies; and
- drug-dependent antibodies.

Many platelet and granulocyte antigens are shared with other cells, e.g. ABO and HLA class I (Table 5.1); other platelet and granulocyte antigens, however, are restricted to these lineages. This chapter therefore is divided into two sections: the first focuses on proteins expressed predominantly on platelets (although several of these are also present on some other blood cells), and in particular the alloantigens on these proteins commonly referred to as platelet-specific alloantigens or human platelet antigens (HPAs), whilst the second section focuses on the equivalent protein alloantigens expressed predominantly on granulocytes (human neutrophil antigens, HNAs).

Human platelet antigens

Seventeen polymorphisms have been described (Table 5.2); most were first discovered during the investigation of cases of neonatal alloimmune thrombocytopenia (NAIT). The majority of these antigens are located on the β3 subunit of the αIIbβ3 integrin (GPIIb/IIIa, CD41/CD61) which is present at high density on the platelet membrane. Others are located on the αIIb subunit of αIIbβ3, on α2β1 (GPIa/IIa, CD49b), GPIb/IX/V and CD109.

These receptor complexes are critical to platelet function and are responsible for the stepwise

Practical Transfusion Medicine, 3rd edition. Edited by Michael F. Murphy and Derwood H. Pamphilon. © 2009 Blackwell Publishing, ISBN: 978-1-4051-8196-9.

Table 5.1 Antigen expression on peripheral blood cells.

Antigens	Erythrocytes	Platelets	Neutrophils	B lymphocytes	T lymphocytes	Monocytes
A, B, H	+++	++/(+)	−	−	−	−
I	+++	++	++	−	−	−
Rh*	+++	−	−	−	−	−
K	+++	−	−	−	−	−
HLA class I	−/(+)	+++	+++	+++	+++	+++
HLA class II	−	−	−/+++[†]	+++	−/+++[†]	+++
GPIIb/IIIa	−	+++	(+)[‡]	−	−	−
GPIa/IIa	−	+++	−	−	++	−
GPIb/IX/V	−	+++	−	−	−	−
CD109	−	(+)/++[†]	−	−	−/++[†]	(+)

* Non-glycosylated.
[†] On activated cells.
[‡] GPIIIa(β_3) in association with an alternative α chain (α_v).

process of platelet attachment to the damaged vessel wall. GPIb/IX/V is the receptor for von Willebrand Factor (vWF) and is implicated in the initial tethering of platelets to damaged endothelium and the GPIbα-bound vWF interacts with collagen facilitating the interaction of collagen with its signalling (GPVI) and attachment receptors (GPIa/IIa). Outside-in signalling via GPVI leads to a change in the platelet integrins αIIbβ3 (GPIIb/IIIa) and α2β1 (GPIa/IIa) from the 'locked' to 'open' configurations, exposing the high-affinity binding sites for collagen and fibrinogen, respectively. GPIIb/IIIa is the main platelet receptor for fibrinogen and is critical to the final phase of platelet aggregation, but it also binds fibronectin, vitronectin and vWF. The function of CD109 has not been fully elucidated although recent studies suggest a role in the regulation of TGFβ-mediated signalling. Glanzmanns' thrombasthenia and Bernard-Soulier syndrome are rare and severe, autosomal recessive, platelet bleeding disorders caused by mutations in the genes encoding GPIIb and GPIIIa, or GPIbα, GPIbβ and GPIX, respectively.

Inheritance and nomenclature

Most of the HPAs reported to date have been shown to be biallelic, with each allele being codom-

inant. Historically, platelet-specific antigens were named by the authors first reporting the antigen, usually using an abbreviation of the name of the propositus in whom the alloantibody was first detected. Some systems were published simultaneously by different investigators and several names were assigned, e.g. Zw and Pl^A and Zav, Br and Hc, and only later were they found to be the same polymorphism. In 1990, a working party for platelet immunology of the International Society of Blood Transfusion (ISBT) agreed a new nomenclature for platelet-specific alloantigens, the HPA nomenclature, and subsequently the International Platelet Nomenclature Committee has published guidelines for the naming of newly discovered platelet-specific alloantigens. In this nomenclature, each system is numbered consecutively (HPA-1, -2, -3 and so on) (Table 5.2) according to its date of discovery, with the major allele in each system being designated 'a' and the minor allele 'b'. Antigens are only included in a system if antibodies against the alloantigen encoded by both the major and minor alleles have been reported; if an antibody against only one allele has been reported, a 'w' (for workshop) is added after the antigen name, e.g. HPA-10bw.

With the advent of techniques such as immunoprecipitation of radioactive-labelled platelet membrane proteins, the monoclonal antibody-specific immobilisation of platelet antigen (MAIPA) assay (Figure 5.1) and the polymerase chain reaction

Table 5.2 HPA systems.

HPA system	Antigen	Alternative names	Phenotype frequency[*] (%)	Glycoprotein	SNP	SNP rs number	Amino acid change
1	1a	Zw^a, Pl^{A1}	97.9	GPIIIa	T^{196}	rs5918	Leucine[33]
	1b	Zw^b, Pl^{A2}	28.8		C^{196}		Proline[33]
2	2a	Ko^b	>99.9	GPIbα	C^{524}	rs6065	Threonine[145]
	2b	Ko^a, Sib^a	13.2		T^{524}		Methionine[145]
3	3a	Bak^a, Lek^a	80.95	GPIIb	T^{2622}	rs5911	Isoleucine[843]
	3b	Bak^b	69.8		G^{2622}		Serine[843]
4	4a	Yuk^b, Pen^a	>99.9	GPIIIa	G^{526}	rs5917	Arginine[143]
	4b	Yuk^a, Pen^b	<0.1		A^{526}		Glutamine[143]
5	5a	Br^b, Zav^b	99.0	GPIa	G^{1648}	rs10471371	Glutamic acid[505]
	5b	Br^a, Zav^a, Hc^a	19.7		A^{1648}		Lysine[505]
6				GPIIIa	G^{1564}	rs13306487	Arginine[489]
	6bw	Ca^a, Tu^a	0.7		A^{1564}		Glutamine[489]
7				GPIIIa	C^{1267}		Proline[407]
	7bw	Mo^a	0.2		G^{1267}		Alanine[407]
8				GPIIIa	T^{2004}		Arginine[636]
	8bw	Sr^a	<0.01		C^{2004}		Cysteine[636]
9				GPIIb	G^{2603}		Valine[837]
	9bw	Max^a	0.6		A^{2603}		Methionine[837]
10				GPIIIa	G^{281}		Arginine[62]
	10bw	La^a	<1.6		A^{281}		Glutamine[62]
11				GPIIIa	G^{1996}		Arginine[633]
	11bw	Gro^a	<0.25		A^{1996}		Histidine[633]
12				GPIbβ	G^{141}		Glycine[15]
	12bw	Iy^a	0.4		A^{141}		Glutamic acid[15]
13				GPIa	C^{2531}		Threonine[799]
	13bw	Sit^a	0.25		T^{2531}		Methionine[799]
14				GPIIIa	Δ AAG$^{1929-1931}$		Δ Lysine[611]
	14bw	Oe^a	<0.17				
15	15a	Gov^b	74	CD109	C^{2108}	rs10455097	Serine[703]
	15b	Gov^a	81		A^{2108}		Tyrosine[703]
16				GPIIIa	C^{517}		Threonine[140]
	16bw	Duv^a	<1		T^{517}		Isoleucine [140]
17				GPIIIa	C^{622}		Threonine[195]
	17bw	Va^a	<0.4		T^{622}		Methionine[195]

[*] Frequencies based on studies in Caucasians.
SNP, single nucleotide polymorphism; rs, the international SNP reference number in the dbSNP database.

(PCR), the genetic and molecular basis of all HPAs has been elucidated (Figure 5.2 and Table 5.2). For all but one of the 17 HPAs, the difference between the two alleles is a single nucleotide polymorphism (SNP) which changes the amino acid in the corresponding protein (Figure 5.2). Twelve of the HPAs are grouped into six HPA systems (HPA-1 to -5 and HPA-15) and for all of these, except HPA-3 and HPA-15, the minor allele frequency is ≤0.2; homozygosity for the minor allele is therefore relatively rare. This places significant demands on blood services in providing compatible blood products for patients with alloantibodies against the high-frequency allele. Some SNPs are population-specific, for example the SNP rs5918, at the basis of the HPA-1a system, is absent in

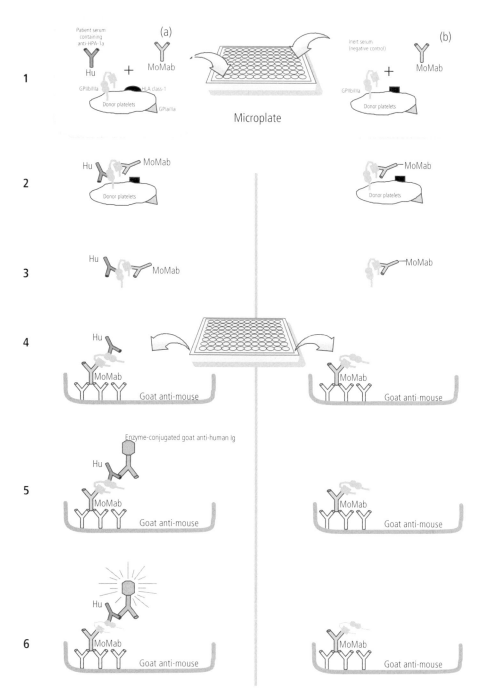

Figure 5.1 Monoclonal antibody-specific immobilisation of platelet antigens. (1) A cocktail of target platelets, murine monoclonal antibody (MoMab) directed against the glycoprotein being studied, e.g. GPIIb/IIIa and human serum is prepared; in (a) the test serum contains anti-HPA-1a and (b) no platelet antibodies are present. (2) After incubation a trimeric (a) or dimeric (b) complex is formed. Excess serum antibody and MoMab is removed by washing. (3) The platelet membrane is solubilised in a non-ionic detergent releasing the complexes into the fluid phase and particulate matter is removed by centrifugation. (4) The lysates containing the glycoprotein/antibody complexes are added to the wells of a microtitre plate previously coated with goat anti-mouse antibody. (5) Unbound lysate is removed by washing and an enzyme-conjugated goat anti-human antibody added. (6) Excess conjugate is removed by washing and a substrate solution added. Cleavage of the substrate, i.e. a colour reaction indicates binding of human antibody to the target platelets.

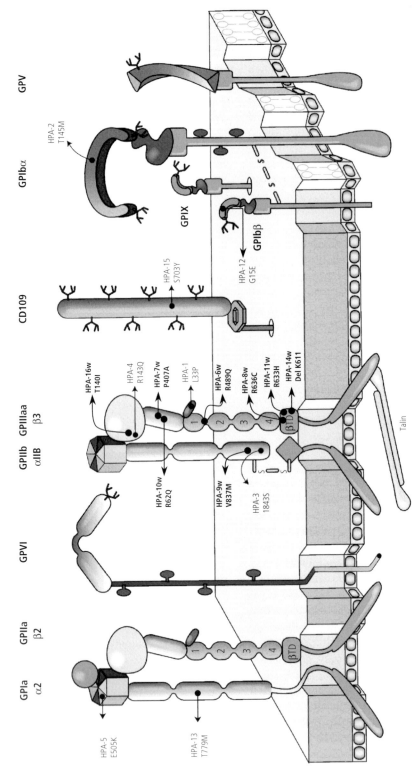

Figure 5.2 Representation of the platelet membrane and the glycoproteins (GP) on which the human platelet antigens (HPA) are localised. From left to right are depicted GPIa/IIa (α2β1), GPIIb/IIIa (αIIbβ3), CD109 and GPIbα/Ibβ/IX/V. The molecular basis of the HPAs are indicated by black dots, with the amino acid change in single-letter code and by residue number in the mature protein.

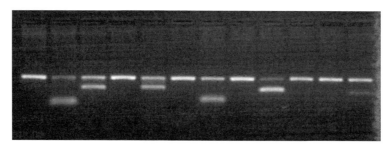

Figure 5.3 PCR-SSP determination of HPA-1, -2, -3, -4, -5 and -15 genotypes. The upper band present in all lanes is the 429-bp product of human growth hormone. The lower bands are the products of sequence-specific primers. The results are read from left to right, i.e. lane 1 HPA-1a, lane 2 HPA-1b, etc. The HPA genotype in this case is 1b/1b, 2a/2a, 3a/3a, 4a/4a, 5a/5a, 15b/15b. (Courtesy of Dr Paul Metcalfe (NIBSC).

populations of the Far East; conversely, the HPA-4 SNP (rs5917) is not present in Caucasians but is present in Far Eastern populations. It is therefore important to take ethnicity into account when investigating clinical cases of suspected HPA alloimmunisation.

Typing for HPAs

Until the early 1990s, HPA typing was performed by serological assays ('phenotyping'). These required the use of monospecific antisera, which were relatively uncommon as the majority of immunised individuals produced HLA class I antibodies in addition to the HPA antibodies. The development of more advanced assays, such as the MAIPA assays (Figure 5.1) that were able to elucidate complex mixtures of antibodies against different GPs, permitted more extensive phenotyping, but some antisera were simply not available.

Many DNA-based typing techniques have been developed; these have largely overcome the earlier problems in platelet typing and have replaced phenotyping in the majority of platelet laboratories. One such assay is the PCR using sequence-specific primers (PCR-SSP). This is a fast and reliable technique with minimal post-PCR handling and it has become one of the cornerstone techniques in HPA genotyping (see Figure 5.3). High-throughput HPA SNP typing techniques with automated readout, such as Taqman assays, are now

also in routine use and allow typing at reduced cost. With the ongoing genomics revolution, novel techniques for the simultaneous detection of numerous SNPs are emerging and these will become the routine method for typing in blood centres.

Genotyping of fetal DNA from amniocytes or from chorion villous biopsy samples is of clinical value in cases of HPA alloimmunisation in pregnancies where there is a history of severe NAIT and the father is heterozygous for the implicated HPA SNP. Non-invasive HPA genotyping assays based on the presence of trace amounts of fetal DNA in maternal plasma are currently under development and these will reduce the risk to the fetus from invasive sampling procedures.

Platelet isoantigens, autoantigens and hapten-induced antigens

GPIV is absent from the platelet membrane in 4% of African Blacks and 3–10% of Japanese. If these individuals are exposed to normal, GPIV-positive blood through pregnancy or transfusion, they may produce GPIV isoantibodies. These antibodies may cause NAIT or platelet refractoriness and may be responsible for non-haemolytic febrile transfusion reactions in multi-transfused recipients. Similarly, formation of isoantibodies can complicate the transfusion support of patients with Glanzmanns' thrombasthenia or Bernard-Soulier syndrome.

The GPs carrying the HPAs are the target of autoantibodies in autoimmune thrombocytopenia (AITP). Such autoantibodies bind to the platelets of all individuals, regardless of their HPA type. Platelet autoimmunity is frequently associated with B-cell malignancies and in the post-haemopoietic stem cell transplantation period during immune cell re-engraftment. In both situations, the presence of autoantibodies may contribute to the refractoriness to donor platelets.

Some drugs too small to elicit an immune response in their own right may bind to platelet GPs in vivo and act as a hapten. In some patients, the haptenised platelet GP can trigger the formation of antibodies that only bind to the GP in the presence of hapten; a classic example is quinine and its stereo-isomer quinidine. Typically, quinine-dependent antibodies are against either GPIIb/IIIa and/or GPIb/IX/V although other GPs are sometimes the target. Many other drugs, including several antibiotics, have been associated with hapten-mediated thrombocytopenia. In haemato-oncology patients, who often receive a spectrum of drugs, unravelling the causes of persistent thrombocytopenia or poor responses to platelet transfusions can be complex because of the many possible causes of thrombocytopenia. If the thrombocytopenia is hapten-mediated, withdrawal of the drug will result in rapid recovery of the platelet count.

Another form of drug-dependent thrombocytopenia may be observed in coronary artery disease patients treated with ReoPro (Abciximab). This function-blocking chimeric human–mouse F(Ab) fragment against GPIIb/IIIa causes precipitous thrombocytopenia in approximately 1% of patients due to the presence of pre-existing antibodies against ReoPro-induced neoepitopes.

The interaction of heparin with platelet factor 4 induces epitope formation that can cause antibody production and lead to a drug-dependent thrombocytopenia, but the reduction in platelet count is less profound than in the classic examples of hapten-mediated immune thrombocytopenia. The risk of thrombotic complications is the main concern in patients who show a mild but significant reduction in their platelet count after heparin administration.

Detection of HPA alloantibodies

Over the last five decades, techniques for the detection of HPA antibodies have evolved from being non-specific and insensitive, e.g. the platelet agglutination test, to become more sensitive, e.g. the platelet immunofluorescence test (PIFT), which is still non-specific as it is unable to distinguish between HPA and HLA class I antibodies, and on to assays that use purified or captured GPs such as the MAIPA assay and solid-phase ELISA assays. Despite this limitation, the PIFT remains a widely used assay and, when results are analysed by a flow cytometer, is one of the most sensitive assays available. The principles of the PIFT are shown in Plate 5.1. However, assays based on the use of purified or captured GPs have become the cornerstone for the detection and identification of HPA antibodies. The MAIPA assay, which is widely used, captures specific GPs using monoclonal antibodies and can be used to analyse complex mixtures of platelet antibodies in patient sera. The principle of this assay is shown in Figure 5.1. However, the MAIPA assay requires considerable operator expertise in order to ensure maximum sensitivity and specificity. The selection of appropriate screening cells is critical, i.e. use of platelets heterozygous for the relevant antigen or from donors who have a low expression of particular antigens, e.g. HPA-15, may result in the failure to detect clinically significant alloantibodies. A further disadvantage of assays that use purified rather than captured GPs as in the MAIPA assay GPs is that not all clinically important GPs are available, e.g. CD109.

Clinical significance of HPA alloantibodies

HPA alloantibodies are responsible for the following clinical conditions:
• NAIT: this condition is described in detail below (but also see Chapter 26);
• refractoriness to platelet transfusions (described in detail in Chapter 27); and
• post-transfusion purpura (PTP) (described in detail in Chapter 12).

Neonatal alloimmune thrombocytopenia

History

The first case of NAIT was described by van Loghem in 1959. The existence of the platelet equivalent of haemolytic disease of the newborn (HDN) had long been suspected, but laboratory confirmation was delayed because the detection of platelet antibodies was more technically demanding than that of red cell antibodies.

NAIT is now a well-recognised clinical entity with an estimated incidence of severe thrombocytopenia due to maternal HPA antibodies of between 1 in 1000 and 1200 live births. Unlike HDN, about 30% of cases of NAIT occur in first pregnancies.

Definition and pathophysiology

NAIT is due to maternal HPA alloimmunisation caused by fetomaternal incompatibility for a fetal HPA inherited from the father and which is absent in the mother. Maternal IgG alloantibodies against the fetal HPA cross the placenta and bind to fetal platelets and, dependent on the quantity, affinity and subclass of the IgG antibodies, the density of the target antigen and as yet other undefined factors, platelet survival is reduced. Severe thrombocytopenia in the term neonate, accompanied by haemorrhage, is generally caused by HPA-1a antibodies if the mother is Caucasian or Black African. Antibodies against antigens in the HPA-2 and HPA-4 systems are generally implicated in cases of Far Eastern ethnicity. In the latter and in Black Africans, GPIV deficiency should also be considered. Anti-HPA-5b tends to cause mild thrombocytopenia, although on rare occasions intracranial cerebral haemorrhage (ICH) has been reported.

NAIT due to alloantibodies against the other HPAs is infrequent and HLA class I antibodies, present in 15–25% of multiparous women, are not thought to be responsible for fetal thrombocytopenia.

Destruction of IgG-coated fetal platelets is assumed to take place in the spleen through interaction with mononuclear cells bearing receptors for the constant domain of IgG, the so-called Fcγ receptors.

HPA-1a is known to be expressed on fetal platelets from 16 weeks' gestation, and placental transfer of IgG antibodies can occur from 14 weeks, so thrombocytopenia can occur early in pregnancy and ICH has been reported as early as 16 weeks' gestation.

Incidence

Prospective screening of pregnant Caucasian women has shown that about 1 in 1200 neonates has severe thrombocytopenia ($<50 \times 10^9/L$) because of alloimmunisation against HPA-1a. However, the authors' experience and other studies, where prospective screening was not carried out, indicate that the number of samples referred for investigation of suspected NAIT is considerably less than this suggesting that many cases are undiagnosed. HPA-5b antibodies are frequently found in pregnant women, but they cause clinically significant platelet destruction much less frequently than anti-HPA-1a, possibly due to the low copy number of the GPIa/IIa complex (1–2000 compared to approximately 50,000 for GPIIb/IIIa).

Clinical features

A typical case of NAIT presents as skin bleeding (purpura, petechiae and/or ecchymoses) or more serious haemorrhage such as ICH, in a full-term and otherwise healthy newborn with a normal coagulation screen and isolated thrombocytopenia. There are less common presentations in utero, including ventriculomegaly, cerebral cysts and hydrocephalus, which may be discovered by routine ultrasound. Although rare, hydrops fetalis has been reported in association with NAIT and this diagnosis should be considered if there are no other obvious reasons for the hydrops.

The precise incidence of ICH due to NAIT is unknown, but conservative estimates suggest that it is as low as 1 in 20,000 live births, which equates to approximately 35 cases per annum in the UK. Nearly 50% of severe ICHs occur in utero, usually between 30 and 35 weeks' gestation, but sometimes even before 20 weeks. At the other end of the clinical spectrum, NAIT can be discovered incidentally when a blood count is performed for other reasons.

Severe NAIT (platelet count $<30 \times 10^9$/L) in a neonate is a serious condition and requires correction of the platelet count. Appropriate management (see below) is essential to prevent ICH and the possibility of lifelong disability.

Differential diagnosis

Other causes of neonatal thrombocytopenia are infection, prematurity, intrauterine growth retardation, inherited chromosomal abnormalities (particularly trisomy 21), maternal AITP and, very rarely, inherited forms of inadequate megakaryopoiesis, e.g. those caused by mutations in the gene encoding the receptor for thrombopoietin.

Precise figures on the incidence of neonatal thrombocytopenia caused by viral infection are not available. Maternal platelet autoimmunity is rarely associated with severe thrombocytopenia in the neonate, but should be considered in women with a history of AITP.

Platelet-type von Willebrand's disease, in which mutations in the *GPIbα* gene are associated with a propensity for in vitro platelet aggregation, can lead to falsely low platelet counts.

Laboratory investigations

Only alloantibodies against HPAs or isoantibodies against GPIIb/IIIa, GPIb/IX and GPIV are thought to cause immune thrombocytopenia in the fetus and neonate.

For appropriate clinical management, the cause of severe thrombocytopenia in an otherwise healthy neonate should be determined with urgency. Detection of maternal HPA antibodies must be carried out by techniques with appropriate sensitivity and specificity. The combination of two techniques such as the indirect PIFT and the MAIPA assay, using a panel of HPA-typed platelets, remains the preferred option in many reference laboratories.

HPA antibodies are detected in approximately 15% of referrals of suspected NAIT. The most frequently detected specificities are anti-HPA-1a and anti-HPA-5b which are implicated in about 85% and 10% of clinically diagnosed cases of NAIT, respectively. The ability of an HPA-1a-negative

mother to form anti-HPA-1a is partly controlled by the HLA DRB3*0101 allele. This allele is present in approximately 30% of Caucasoid women and the chance of HPA-1a antibody formation is greatly enhanced in HPA-1a-negative women who are HLA DRB3*0101-positive, with an odds ratio of 140 when compared to DRB3*0101-negative women. Such an explicit linkage between an HLA class II type and the formation of alloantibodies against a blood group antigen is exceptional and has not been observed for any of the other blood group antigens on platelets, red cells or leucocytes. Although the negative predictive value of the absence of HLA-DRB3*0101 for HPA-1a alloimmunisation in HPA-1a-negative women is >90%, its positive predictive value is only 35%, limiting its potential usefulness as part of an antenatal screening programme. However, it remains of clinical use when counselling female siblings from index cases who have formed HPA-1a antibodies in pregnancy. About 15% of HPA-1a-negative pregnant women develop anti-HPA-1a in pregnancy, and about 30% of these will deliver a neonate with a platelet count $<50 \times 10^9$/L. The HPA-15 system was described a decade ago, but its clinical relevance has only recently been demonstrated, with a number of studies having shown that it is the third most commonly encountered HPA antibody specificity and that the effects may be as severe as in anti-HPA-1a-mediated NAIT .

Molecular typing of the parents and neonate for HPA-1, -2, -3, -5 and HPA-15 should be performed because the results will be informative when interpreting the results of the antibody investigations. For patients from the Far East, HPA-4 must also be included and the platelets should be investigated for GPIV expression status.

Alloimmunisation against low-frequency HPAs, e.g. HPA6-bw can be an explanation for some of the NAIT referrals that have a negative antibody screen for the common HPA antibody specificities. Screening all NAIT referrals for antibodies against low-frequency HPAs is prohibitively expensive and a recent study of more than 1000 paternal DNA samples from NAIT referrals showed the presence of HPA-bw alleles in less than 10 paternal samples. Investigations for alloimmunisation against rare

HPA-bw alleles should therefore be reserved for clinically severe cases of NAIT where there is no alternative clinical diagnosis. Genotyping of the paternal DNA sample for the 11 HPA-bw SNPs seems to be the most cost-effective approach in this clinical setting.

Neonatal management

A cord platelet count of $<100 \times 10^9$/L should be confirmed on a venous sample, and a blood film examined. A careful examination of the neonate for skin or mucosal bleeding is indicated if a low platelet count is confirmed. If the platelet count is $<30 \times 10^9$/L or if there are signs of bleeding with a low count, it is strongly recommended that the neonate is transfused with donor platelets that are preferably HPA-1a and -5b-negative, as these will be compatible with the maternal HPA alloantibody in over 95% of NAIT cases. The authors have shown that the transfusion of platelets that are HPA-1a- and HPA-5b-negative in NAIT caused by HPA-1a or HPA-5b antibodies results in a higher increment and more prolonged platelet survival than transfusion of random donor (HPA-1a positive) platelets. However, if HPA-1a- and -5b-negative platelets are not immediately available and there is an urgent clinical need for transfusion then random, ABO and RhD compatible, donor platelets should be used in the first instance. Following the transfusion of platelets, a platelet count should be performed approximately 1 hour after the transfusion is completed, and subsequently at least daily until the platelet count has been demonstrated not to be falling. Furthermore, the results of the laboratory investigations should not delay immediate platelet transfusion, as full investigation may be time-consuming and the risk of cerebral bleeds is highest in the first 48 hours post-delivery. In a typical case, the platelet count should recover to normal within a week, although a more protracted recovery can occur. Intravenous immunoglobulin (IvIgG) is not recommended as first-line treatment as it is only effective in about 75% of cases and there is a delay of 24–48 hours before a satisfactory count is achieved; this is in contrast to the immediate effect of the transfusion of HPA-compatible donor platelets. A cerebral ultrasound scan of the baby within the first week of life should be considered if the platelet count is $<50 \times 10^9$/L, and is recommended when the platelet count is 30×10^9/L.

Antenatal management

In a subsequent pregnancy of a mother with a previously affected pregnancy with NAIT, a decision needs to be taken on the mother's care plan in partnership with a team that is experienced in the management of this type of high-risk pregnancy. Treatment during the subsequent pregnancy is based on the history of haemorrhage and fetal/neonatal thrombocytopenia in previous pregnancies.

In all cases, the mother should be advised to avoid any non-steroidal anti-inflammatory drugs as well as aspirin. There are two main treatment options: high-dose IvIgG to the mother, or in utero platelet transfusion. Over the last decade, it has become increasingly clear that the former is the safest and most effective intervention to reduce the risk of ICH in the fetus. The dose is 1 g/kg body weight at weekly intervals, usually from 20 weeks' gestation onwards; some fetal medicine specialists use a lower dose (0.5 g/kg/week) and may start between 12 and 20 weeks' gestation depending on the history of NAIT in previous pregnancies. Early commencement of treatment is indicated in those cases where there is a history of antenatal ICH in previous pregnancies, because the earliest reports of ICH are at 16 weeks. A beneficial effect of IvIgG on the fetal platelet count occurs in approximately 70% of cases. There is debate about the need to perform fetal blood sampling (FBS) to ascertain the platelet count and many centres do this at 28 weeks (usually after 8 weeks' treatment with IvIgG). If FBS reveals IvIgG to be ineffective in achieving a safe fetal platelet count doubling the dose of IvIgG and/or adding corticosteroids (prednisolone, 0.5 mg/kg body weight) should be considered. If the increased intensity of treatment is ineffective, it may be necessary to switch to weekly fetal platelet transfusions. In utero platelet transfusions, carried out with FBS, carry a significant risk of fetal morbidity and mortality and should not be chosen as first-line treatment but as a rescue therapy or in the management of pregnancies with a history of treatment failure on IvIgG. The transfusion

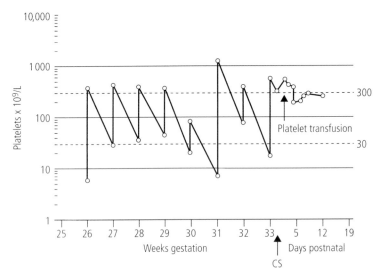

Figure 5.4 Seventh pregnancy of a patient who has had five miscarriages. The last of these was shown to have hydrops and hydrocephalus and a platelet count of only $17 \times 10^9/L$, and the serological findings supported a diagnosis of NAIT due to anti-HPA-1a. The fetal platelet count was $<10 \times 10^9/L$ at 25 weeks' gestation in the sixth pregnancy, and a cord haematoma developed during FBS resulting in fetal death. In the seventh pregnancy, prednisolone 20 mg/day and IvIgG immunoglobulin 1 g/kg/week were administered to the mother from 16 weeks until delivery. The figure shows pre- and post-transfusion platelet counts following serial FBS and platelet transfusions. The fetal platelet count was $<10 \times 10^9/L$ at 26 weeks. The aim was to maintain the fetal platelet count above $30 \times 10^9/L$ by raising the immediate post-transfusion platelet count to above 300 $\times 10^9/L$ after each transfusion. The fetal platelet count fell below $10 \times 10^9/L$ on one occasion when there were problems in preparing the fetal platelet concentrate and the dose of platelets was inadequate. CS, caesarean section.

of platelets has more complications compared to red cell transfusions for HDN, e.g. bradycardia, post-needle withdrawal cord bleeds. Once commenced, the technically demanding procedure of in utero platelet transfusions is generally repeated at weekly intervals (Figure 5.4).

The delivery also needs careful planning between obstetric, paediatric and haematology teams in close consultation with the consultant haematologist to ensure the appropriate mode of delivery and timely provision of HPA-compatible platelets for the neonate. For neonates that have been transfused in utero, irradiation of cellular blood products is recommended.

Counselling

Counselling of couples with an index case about the risks of severe fetal/neonatal thrombocytopenia in a subsequent pregnancy needs to be based on the severity of disease in the infant(s) and the outcome of immunological investigations. The following should be taken into account:
• thrombocytopenia in subsequent cases is as severe or, generally, more severe;
• the best predictors of severe fetal thrombocytopenia in a future pregnancy are the occurrence of antenatal ICH and severe thrombocytopenia (platelet count $<30 \times 10^9/L$) in a previous pregnancy;
• antibody specificity, titre or bioactivity does not reliably correlate with the severity of NAIT, and are probably of no value in informing clinical management; and
• the HPA zygosity of the partner.

HPA-typed donor panels

Establishing donor panels for fetal and neonatal platelet transfusion requires a major commitment from blood services and identification of suitable donors requires the use of high-throughput typing techniques that are now available. Although the frequency of HPA-1a-negative individuals amongst Caucasians is 2.5%, potential donors for fetal/neonatal transfusions must also be negative for the mandatory microbiological tests, negative for antibodies against red cells, platelets and leucocytes, and be cytomegalovirus (CMV) seronegative. Thus, in order to recruit one HPA-1a-negative donor who is able to meet all of the above criteria, approximately 1500–2000 donors will have to be typed for HPA-1a. In addition, therapeutic platelets should be RhD matched, as small amounts of red cells present in platelet concentrates may immunise RhD-negative recipients and be negative for high titre anti-A and anti-B antibodies. In order to recruit a single O RhD-negative HPA-1a-negative donor whose platelets will be suitable for a first fetal or neonatal platelet transfusion, where the fetal/neonatal blood group is unknown, approximately 15,000–20,000 donors need to be typed.

Human neutrophil antigens

The antigens on the membrane of human neutrophils can, as with platelets, be divided into different categories. There are common antigens which have a wider distribution on other blood cells and tissues, e.g. I and P blood group systems and HLA class I. There are 'shared' antigens which have a limited distribution amongst other cell types, e.g. HNA-4a and HNA-5a polymorphisms associated with CD11/18. There are also a limited number of truly granulocyte-specific antigens, e.g. HNA-1a, HNA-1b, HNA-1c polymorphisms on FcγRIII or CD16. The current nomenclature for the HNA systems includes polymorphisms that are both cell-specific and 'shared' (see Table 5.3).

HNA-1 system
The most immunogenic polymorphisms, the tri-allelic HNA-1 system, are localised on neutrophil FcγRIIIb (CD16), one of two low-affinity receptors (R) for the constant domain (Fc) of human IgG(γ) found on granulocytes. Four amino acid differences with arginine/serine, asparagine/serine, aspartic acid/asparagine and valine/isoleucine substitutions at positions 36, 65, 82 and 106, respectively, define the difference between HNA-1a and -1b, while a single amino acid substitution alanine/asparagine at position 78 defines the HNA-1c polymorphism (see Figure 5.5). The expression of HNA-1c is frequently associated with the presence of an additional FcγRIIIb gene and increased expression of FcγRIIIb.

Two other FcγRIIIb-associated high-frequency alloantigens, the LAN and SAR antigens, have been reported. The FcγRIIIb 'null' phenotype is rare and is based on a double deletion of the FcγRIIIb gene and is, in some cases, associated with a deletion of the FcγRIIc gene. The deficiency for the most abundant FcγR on neutrophils can cause immune neutropenia in the newborn due to maternal anti-FcγRIIIb isoantibodies.

PCR-SSP can be used to determine the HNA-1a, -1b, -1c, -4a, -4b, -5a, -5b and FcγRIIIb null genotypes and transfected cells expressing the FcγRIIIb HNA-1a, -1b and -1c allotypes have been used for alloantibody detection.

HNA-2 system
HNA-2a, formerly known as NB1, is localised on a 58–64. kDa glycoprotein (CD177) expressed as a glycosylphosphatidylinositol-anchored membrane GP found both on the neutrophil surface membrane and on secondary granules. The percentage of neutrophils expressing HNA-2a varies between individuals and HNA-2a alloantibodies typically give a bimodal fluorescence profile with granulocytes from HNA-2a-positive donors. The HNA-2a status can be determined by phenotyping with polyclonal or monoclonal antibodies. The HNA-2a-negative phenotype is associated with particular sequence haplotypes from which non-productive HNA-2a transcripts are generated, resulting in the HNA-2a null phenotype. There is no antithetical antigen to HNA-2a; an anti-NB2 antiserum was originally thought to define the antithetical antigen to HNA-2a (NB1), but this serum may instead contain antibodies against human monocyte antigen 1.

Table 5.3 HNA systems.

HNA system	Antigen	Original acronym for antigen	Phenotype frequency* (%)	Glycoprotein	Nucleotide change	Amino acid change
1	1a	NA1	46	FcγRIIIb	G^{108}	Arginine[36]
					C^{114}	None
					A^{197}	Asparagine[65]
					G^{247}	Aspartic acid[82]
					G^{319}	Valine[106]
	1b	NA2	88	FcγRIIIb	C^{108}	Serine[36]
					T^{114}	None
					G^{197}	Serine[65]
					A^{247}	Asparagine[82]
					A^{319}	Isoleucine[106]
	1c	SH+	5	FcγRIIIb	A^{266}	Aspartic acid[78]
		SH−			C^{266}	Alanine[78]
2	2a	NB1	97	CD177	nk	nk
—		NB2	32	nk	nk	nk
—	ND	ND1	98.5	nk	nk	nk
—	NE	NE1	23	nk	nk	nk
—	LAN	LAN[a]	>99	FcγRIIIb	nk	nk
—	SAR	SAR[a]	>99	FcγRIIIb	nk	nk
—	Five	5a	—	nk	nk	nk
3a	Five	5b	—	70–95 kDa	nk	nk
4a	Mart	Mart[a](+)	99.1	CD11b	G^{302}	Arginine[61]
		Mart[a](−)		CD11b	A^{302}	Histidine[61]
5a	Ond	Ond[a](+)	>99	CD11a	G^{2466}	Arginine[766]
		Ond[a](−)		CD11a	C^{2466}	Threonine[766]

* Frequencies based on studies in Caucasians.
nk, not known.

HNA-3 system

HNA-3a (previously known as 5[b]) was originally described using antisera obtained from women immunised during pregnancy and was reported as being present on granulocytes, platelets, lymphocytes, kidney, spleen and lymph node tissue. Some evidence suggests that HNA-3a may be granulocyte-specific and that the previously reported wider antigen distribution was caused by the presence of HLA antibodies. The HNA-3a antigen has been localised on a granulocyte glycoprotein with a molecular weight of 70–95 kDa. The gene frequency of HNA-3a has been variously estimated as 0.66 and 0.82. Antisera to 5[a] (the proposed antithetical antigen to 5[b]) were described many years ago. The clinical significance and molecular localisation of the 5[a] antigen remain unknown, and 5[a] is not recognised as the antithetical antigen to HNA-3a within the HNA nomenclature.

Alloantigens on CD11a and CD11b

The genes encoding the α_M and α_L subunits of the β_2 integrin or CD11b and CD11a are polymorphic and are associated with HNA-4a and HNA-5a, respectively. Alloantibody formation against these two polymorphisms has been observed in transfusion recipients, and recently a case of neonatal neutropenia due to HNA-4a alloantibodies has been described. The low incidence of neonatal neutropenia associated with these antibodies is probably

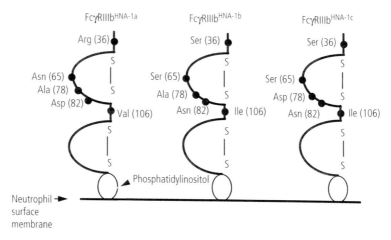

Figure 5.5 Representation of the amino acid substitutions resulting in the HNA-1a, -1b, -1c forms of FcγRIIIb. The positions of the amino acid substitutions arising from the allelic variation of the FcγRIIIb gene are depicted by black dots. Amino acids are given in three-letter acronyms. The intra-chain disulphide bonds create two domains which are closely related to the C-terminal heavy chain domains of IgG.

explained by the wide distribution of these proteins on granulocytes, monocytes and lymphocytes.

Detection of neutrophil antibodies

The reliable detection and identification of neutrophil antibodies can be technically difficult. The main problems are the abundant expression of the two low-affinity receptors (FcγRII and FcγRIIIb) for the constant domain of human IgG, which results in increased binding of circulating immunoglobulins in normal sera and the requirement for fresh and typed donor neutrophils as panel cells, since the neutrophils cannot be stored. The incidence of antibody-mediated neutropenias is comparatively rare and, therefore, the best strategy for investigation of clinical cases is in a single national laboratory so that adequate technical expertise and the required reagents are available.

Many techniques for neutrophil/granulocyte antibody detection have been evaluated over the years. Early assays such as the granulocyte cytotoxicity and agglutination tests had a very low specificity. The granulocyte immunofluorescence and granulocyte chemiluminescence tests have the advantage of good sensitivity but are not spe-

cific, i.e. they cannot readily distinguish between granulocyte-specific and HLA class I antibodies without further investigations. For some HNA systems, e.g. antigens expressed on CD16, CD177 and C11/18, assays comparable with the MAIPA assay can be applied but, otherwise, immunoprecipitation of surface radioactive-labelled neutrophils remains the only reliable technique to determine the nature of the antigen. The principles of the granulocyte immunofluorescence test and the monoclonal antibody immobilisation of granulocyte antigen (MAIGA) assays are analogous to the equivalent platelet tests described in Plate 5.1 and Figure 5.1, respectively. Increased understanding of the molecular nature of HNA has opened the potential to develop recombinant HNA and these have the potential to transform the serological investigation of granulocyte antibodies.

Typing for HNAs is generally based on the use of monospecific alloantisera derived from immunised patients. However, for some HNAs, for example HNA-1a, -1b and -2a, murine monoclonal antibodies with allele-specific reactivity are now available. Furthermore, for some of the HNA systems (HNA-1a, -1b, -1c, -4a, -4b, 5a and -5b) the molecular basis has been determined and PCR-based genotyping can be used.

Clinical significance of HNA antibodies

Neutrophil-specific antibodies are implicated in:
- neonatal alloimmune neutropenia;
- non-haemolytic febrile transfusion reactions (NHFTR) (see Chapter 8);
- transfusion-related acute lung injury (TRALI) (see Chapter 9);
- transfusion-related alloimmune neutropenia (TRAIN);
- autoimmune neutropenia; and
- persistent post-bone marrow transplant neutropenia.

Neonatal alloimmune neutropenia

Maternal alloimmunisation against neutrophil-specific alloantigens on fetal/neonatal neutrophils is rare as a clinically significant entity. The incidence of the disorder is estimated at 0.1–0.2% of live births but there are no reliable prevalence figures. Clinical presentation is mainly one of bacterial infections with a selective neutropenia on a whole blood count. Severe but reversible neutropenia in the newborn may require treatment with antibiotics and/or GCSF to control bacterial infections and hasten recovery to a normal neutrophil count. Left untreated, the neutropenia in some cases caused by HNA-1a and -1b antibodies has been reported to extend up to 28 weeks. HNA-1a and -2a are the most commonly implicated antibody specificities.

FNHTRs and TRALI (see Chapters 8 and 9)

Non-haemolytic, febrile transfusion reactions (NHFTRs) are usually caused by bacterially contaminated blood products, particularly platelet concentrates, but can occasionally be associated with the presence of leucocyte (HLA and HNA) alloantibodies in the recipient. In the UK, where there is universal leucocyte depletion of blood products, investigations for other causes of high fever associated with transfusion are carried out, e.g. tests for bacterial contamination and IgA-deficiency. The clinical management of NHFTRs, if pre-medication with corticosteroids is not effective,

is to alter product specification by using red cells or platelets with reduced plasma content. Serological investigations for platelet, HLA and granulocyte antibodies are of limited clinical value as the diagnostic specificity of these tests for NHFTRs is low. Nonetheless, testing for HNA antibodies may be required in the rare cases in which a severe NHFTR cannot be otherwise explained and plasma-reduced components have proved ineffective.

TRALI is a severe and sometimes life-threatening transfusion reaction. The majority of cases are caused by donor leucocyte alloantibodies against alloantigens present on the patient's leucocytes, although patient alloantibodies may be involved in some cases. In most TRALI cases, HLA class I- and II-specific antibodies are implicated but HNA antibodies have also been implicated as causal agents with HNA-1a and HNA-3a antibody specificities being found most commonly. TRALI investigations are logistically complex but should include a screen for both HLA and HNA alloantibodies in samples from donors and the patient. In some cases, a crossmatch between the donor's sera and the patient's granulocytes and lymphocytes may be required.

Transfusion-related alloimmune neutropenia

The first case of TRAIN occurred following the infusion of 80 mL of plasma-reduced blood after surgery on a 4-week-old infant. The plasma from the blood donor was found to contain HNA-1b alloantibodies, and resulted in an absolute neutropenia in the infant, who typed as HNA-1a(+), 1b(+). The neutropenia was resolved after 7 days after treating the infant with GCSF. The case is of interest since it demonstrates, that in some circumstances, infused passive HNA antibodies can trigger neutropenia rather than TRALI. This clinical entity has recently been confirmed by an additional report of three cases.

Autoimmune neutropenia

Autoimmune neutropenia is a rare condition which can occur as a transient, self-limiting autoimmunity in young children or in a chronic form in adults. The autoantibodies tend to target the FcγRIIIb (CD16), CD177 or CD11/18 molecules but can also be HNA-specific, typically HNA-1a, especially in children. The most sensitive method for the detection of autoantibodies is to test the patient's neutrophils using the direct immunofluorescence test. However, the combination of severe neutropenia and the requirement for a fresh sample limits the applicability of this test, especially in children. Screening of a patient's serum sample with a panel of typed neutrophils in the indirect granulocyte immunofluorescence and granulocyte chemiluminescence or granulocyte agglutination tests provide a suitable alternative and, in some studies, this approach has been found to be only slightly less sensitive than the direct test.

Persistent post-bone marrow transplant neutropenia

Antibody-mediated neutropenia may be a serious complication of bone marrow transplantation. In this context, the neutrophil antibodies may be autoimmune and/or alloimmune in nature and laboratory investigation requires serological and typing studies to elucidate the nature of the antibodies involved.

Key points

1 Allo-, auto-, iso- and drug-induced antigens may be found on platelets and neutrophils and are implicated in a range of immune cytopenias.
2 Alloantigens on platelets are known as HPAs; alloantigens on neutrophils are known as HNAs.
3 Reliable detection and identification of HPA- and HNA-specific antibodies requires the use of both whole-cell type assays such as the PIFT/GIFT and antigen-capture type assays such as the MAIPA/MAIGA assays.
4 NAIT is a common disorder and HPA-1a or HPA-5b antibodies are responsible for approximately 95% of cases.
5 Optimal postnatal treatment of NAIT is the transfusion of HPA-1a/5b-negative donor platelets.
6 Optimal antenatal treatment is yet to be determined but maternal treatment with IvIgG is the safest initial treatment.

Further reading

Bassler D, Greinacher A, Okascharoen C *et al.* A systematic review and survey of the management of unexpected neonatal alloimmune thrombocytopenia. *Transfusion.* 2008;48:92–98.

Bux J, Behrens G, Jaeger G & Welte K. Diagnosis and clinical course of autoimmune neutropenia in infancy: analysis of 240 cases. *Blood* 1998;91:181–186.

Bux J & Sachs UJH. The pathogenesis of transfusion related acute lung injury (TRALI). *Br J Haematol* 2007;36:788–799.

Ghevaert C, Campbell K, Stafford P. *et al.* HPA-1a antibody potency and bioactivity do not predict severity of fetomaternal alloimmune thrombocytopenia. *Transfusion* 2007;47:1296–1305.

Kjeldsen-Kragh J, Killie MK, Tomter G *et al.* A screening and intervention program aimed to reduce mortality and serious morbidity associated with severe neonatal alloimmune thrombocytopenia. *Blood* 2007;110:833–839.

Lucas GF & Metcalfe P. Platelet and granulocyte polymorphisms. *Transfus Med* 2000;10:157–174.

Metcalfe P, Watkins NA, Ouwehand WH *et al.* Nomenclature of human platelet antigens. *Vox Sang* 2003;85:240–245.

Murphy MF & Bussel JB. Advances in the management of alloimmune thrombocytopenia. *Br J Haematol* 2007;136:366–378.

Ouwehand WH, Stafford P, Ghevaert C *et al.* Platelet immunology, present and future. *ISBT Science Series* 2006;1:96–102.

Shastri KA & Logue GL. Autoimmune neutropenia. *Blood* 1993;81:1984–1995.

Von dem Borne AE, de Haas M, Roos D, Homburg CH & van der Schoot CE. Neutrophil antigens, from bench to bedside. *Immunol Invest* 1995;24:245–272.

Wallis JP, Haynes S, Stark G *et al.* Transfusion related alloimmune neutropenia (TRAIN), a previously undescribed complication of blood transfusion. *Lancet* 2002;360:1073.

Warkentin TE & Smith JW. The alloimmune thrombocytopenic syndromes. *Transfus Med Rev* 1997;11:296–307.

Williamson LM, Hackett G, Rennie J *et al.* The natural history of fetomaternal alloimmunization to the platelet-specific antigen HPA-1a (PlA1, Zwa) as determined by antenatal screening. *Blood* 1998;92:2280–2287.

PART 2
Complications of transfusion

CHAPTER 6

Investigation of acute transfusion reactions

Nancy M. Heddle[1] *& Kathryn E. Webert*[2]

[1]Department of Medicine, McMaster University; Canadian Blood Services, Hamilton, Ontario, Canada
[2]Department of Medicine and Department of Pathology and Molecular Medicine, McMaster University; Canadian Blood Services, Hamilton, Ontario, Canada

The investigation of suspected acute reactions to blood products and plasma derivatives cannot be summarised in a single simple algorithm for several reasons:

• signs and symptoms are not specific for one type of reaction;

• the frequency and type of reactions vary with different blood products, e.g. leucocyte-reduced or not;

• risks are variable with different patient populations;

• the severity and risk of reactions must be taken into account to ensure a balance between the safety, availability and cost of blood.

In this chapter, an algorithmic approach is provided for the clinical management and laboratory investigation of transfusion reactions.

Understanding the clinical presentation and differential diagnosis

Acute reactions can usually be placed into one of eight categories:

• acute haemolysis;
• allergic;
• anaphylactic;
• transfusion-related acute lung injury (TRALI);
• febrile non-haemolytic reactions (FNHTR);
• bacterial contamination;
• hypotension; and
• transfusion-associated circulatory overload (TACO).

Other reactions that may occur acutely but may not always be recognised initially include cytopenias such as transfusion-associated graft-versus-host disease, post-transfusion purpura, alloimmune thrombocytopenia and alloimmune neutropenia. These reactions are discussed in other chapters.

The diagnosis of an acute transfusion reaction can be complicated as signs and symptoms are not specific for each type of reaction as illustrated. The diagnosis becomes more challenging when more than one reaction occurs simultaneously. In Table 6.1, symptoms have been categorised as cutaneous, inflammatory, pain, respiratory, gastrointestinal and cardiovascular. For some reactions, the clinical presentation can be identical (i.e. acute haemolysis and bacterial contamination). To ensure management strategies and investigations that minimise risks to patients, health care professionals need to understand the aetiology and pathophysiology of each type of acute reaction (Table 6.2). It is

Practical Transfusion Medicine, 3rd edition. Edited by Michael F. Murphy and Derwood H. Pamphilon. © 2009 Blackwell Publishing. ISBN: 978-1-4051-8196-9.

Table 6.1 Summary of the signs/symptoms typically observed with different types of acute transfusion reactions.

Reaction type	Common symptoms and signs					Cardiovascular	
	Cutaneous (hives, urticaria)	Inflammatory (fever, chills, rigors)	Pain	Respiratory	Gastrointestinal (nausea and vomiting)	Hypotension	Hypertension
AHTR		✓	✓	✓	✓	✓	
Allergic	✓			✓	✓		
Anaphylactic	✓			✓		✓	✓
TRALI		✓		✓		✓	
FNHTR		✓	✓		✓		
Bacterial contamination		✓	✓	✓	✓	✓	
Hypotensive transfusion reaction	✓			✓	✓	✓	
TACO				✓			✓

AHTR, acute haemolytic transfusion reaction; TRALI, transfusion-related acute lung injury; FNHTR, febrile non-haemolytic transfusion reaction; TACO, transfusion-associated circulatory overload.

also essential to understand the typical clinical presentation for each type of reaction so that a differential diagnosis can be formulated as part of the investigative process. Some considerations to assist in the decision-making process and investigation are summarised below.

Patient history

• The reason for the patient's admission and current diagnosis may give some indication as to the type of reaction. For example, if the patient being transfused because of anaemia but is also in congestive heart failure, TACO could be the cause of the reaction.
• Consider whether the patient has been previously transfused or pregnant as this can lead to alloimmunisation to red cell and leucocyte antibodies which are known to be associated with certain types of reactions (acute haemolytic, FNHTR).
• What blood products have been transfused and what is the transfusion timeline? If plasma-containing products have been recently transfused, consider whether the reaction could be caused by passive infusion of antibody or soluble allergens that may now be reacting with the product being transfused.

• Has the patient had a history of reactions when blood products are transfused? Some patients are prone to developing recurrent FNHTR and/or allergic reactions when transfused.
• Is the patient known to be IgA deficient? Some patients with IgA deficiency develop anti-IgA antibodies which may cause anaphylactic transfusion reactions when an IgA-containing blood product is transfused.

Medications

• Determine what medications the patient is receiving or has received in the time period leading up to the transfusion. Considerations should include:
  ○ the use of premedications given to prevent acute reactions such as allergic (antihistamines) or FNHTR (antipyretics);
  ○ antimicrobial medication;
  ○ pyrogenic agents that are known to cause fever such as amphotericin or monoclonal antibodies;
  ○ ACE inhibitors which have been associated with hypotensive reactions; and,
  ○ pruritogenic agents such as vancomycin, narcotics etc.

Table 6.2 Summary of acute transfusion reactions.

Reaction	Frequency	Mechanism	Clinical presentation	Differential diagnosis	Laboratory investigations	Management
AHTR	1:25,000 (fatal 1:600,000)	Result from the destruction of donor red cells by preformed recipient antibodies. Antibodies fix complement and cause rapid intravascular haemolysis. Usually due to ABO incompatibility which is most often the result of clerical error	Fever, flank pain and red/brown urine. Hypotension, shock, death	FNHTR. Bacterial contamination. TRALI	Positive DAT free haemoglobin in plasma and urine. Positive cross-match	Stop the transfusion immediately. Begin infusion of normal saline. Alert the blood bank, check for clerical error, send entire transfusion setup to blood bank for testing. Obtain bloodwork: DAT, plasma for free haemoglobin, antibody screen. Obtain urine sample: haemoglobinuria
Allergic transfusion reaction	1:100–300 transfusions	Soluble allergenic substances in the plasma of the donated blood product react with pre-existing IgE antibodies in the recipient. Causes mast cells and basophils to release histamine, leasing to hives or urticaria	Hives. Urticaria. Flushing	Anaphylactic transfusion reaction. TRALI. TACO	Rule out anaphylactic reaction	Stop the transfusion until a more serious reaction is ruled out. Antihistamine may improve symptoms. If no evidence of dyspnea or anaphylaxis, the transfusion may be continued with close observation

(Continued)

Table 6.2 *(Continued)*

Reaction	Frequency	Mechanism	Clinical presentation	Differential diagnosis	Laboratory investigations	Management
Anaphylactic transfusion reaction	1:20,000–50,000 transfusions	Usually due to the presence of anti-IgA antibodies in recipients who are IgA deficient	Rapid onset of shock, hypotension, angioedema and respiratory distress (2° to bronchospasm and laryngeal oedema)	Allergic transfusion reaction TRALI TACO	IgA level Testing for anti-IgA (if IgA deficient)	Stop the transfusion Epinephrine Airway maintenance, oxygenation Maintain haemodynamic status (IV fluids, vasopressor medications)
TRALI	2–8 cases per 10,000 allogeneic transfusion (0.014–0.08%) 0.5–2 cases per 1000 patients transfused (0.04–0.16%)	Antibodies or neutrophil-priming agents in the infused blood product likely interact with the recipient's leucocyte antigens Activation of the WBC results in the production of inflammatory mediators that increase vascular permeability Leads to capillary leak and pulmonary tissue damage	Shortness of breath Fever Hypotension or hypertension Acute non-cardiogenic pulmonary oedema (elevated JVP, bilateral lung crackles)	Bacterial contamination TACO Anaphylactic transfusion reaction Cardiogenic pulmonary oedema ARDS Pneumonia	Antigranulocyte or anti-HLA antibodies in the donor CXR (bilateral pulmonary infiltrates) BNP (possible useful).	Stop the transfusion Respiratory support as required (supplemental oxygen, mechanical ventilation) Maintain haemodynamic status (IV fluids, vasopressor medications)
FNHTR	Commonly occur during transfusions of red cells, platelets, or plasma 1:100 RBC transfusions; 1:5 platelet transfusions	Likely caused by cytokines that are generated and accumulate during the storage of blood components	Fever, rigors, chills Other: nausea, vomiting, dyspnea, hypotension Typically occur during the transfusion, but may present up to 6 hours after transfusion	AHTR Bacterial contamination TRALI Co-morbid conditions causing fever (i.e. infection, haematologic malignancies, solid tumour) Drugs causing fever	No specific tests Rule out other transfusion reactions	Stop the transfusion until a more serious reaction is ruled out Antipyretics (i.e. acetaminophen) and meperidine may help patients with severe chills and rigors

Reaction	Incidence	Pathophysiology	Signs/symptoms	Differential diagnosis	Laboratory investigation	Management
Bacterial contamination	1:10,000 (platelets), 1:>1 million (RBC)	Bacteria in the blood product from: donor skin (venipuncture site); donor with bacteremia; contamination during collection/storage	High fevers, rigors, Hypotension	AHTR, FNHTR, Allergic transfusion reaction	Gram stain and culture of remaining blood component; Gram stain and culture of patient's blood	Stop the transfusion, IV fluids, Broad spectrum antibiotics
Hypotensive transfusion reaction	Unknown but thought to be rare	Unknown. May be related to generation of bradykinin and/or its active metabolite. Majority of reactions occur during transfusion of blood components administered through a negatively charged filter or to patients receiving an angiotensin-converting enzyme (ACE) inhibitor	Hypotension, Dyspnea, urticaria, flushing, pruritis, GI symptoms. Most reactions occur within minutes of the beginning of the transfusion and resolve rapidly with cessation of the transfusion and supportive care	AHTR, Bacterial contamination, TRALI, Anaphylactic transfusion reaction, Unrelated to blood transfusion (i.e. due to blood loss)	No specific tests. Rule out other transfusion reactions	Stop the transfusion, Maintain haemodynamic status (IV fluids, vasopressor medications)
TACO	May be as high as 1:100 transfusions	Increase in central venous pressure, increase in pulmonary blood volume, and decrease in pulmonary compliance with resultant secondary congestive heart failure and pulmonary oedema	Elevated JVP, Bilateral crackles on auscultation, Hypertension, Dry cough, Orthopnea, Pedal oedema	TRALI, Anaphylactic transfusion reaction	Chest X-ray, Clinical examination, BNP (possible useful)	Stop the transfusion, Supplemental oxygen, Diuretics

AHTR, acute haemolytic transfusion reaction; FNHTR, febrile non-haemolytic transfusion reaction; TRALI, transfusion-related acute lung injury; DAT, direct antiglobulin test; TACO, transfusion-associated circulatory overload; IV, intravenous; HLA, human leucocyte antigen; CXR, chest X-ray; JVP, jugular venous pressure; ARDS, adult respiratory distress syndrome; GI, gastrointestinal; BNP, brain natriuretic peptide.

Type of blood product being transfused

• Does the product contain significant volumes of plasma? Infusion of plasma is associated with a variety of reactions including allergic, anaphylactic, TRALI and acute haemolysis caused by passive antibody incompatibility with the patient's red cells.

• Does the product contain a significant number of red cells? If greater than 50 mL of red cells are present in the product, acute haemolysis needs to be considered as a possible cause of the adverse reaction.

• Was the product stored at room temperature or in a refrigerator? Platelets have a higher risk of bacterial contamination as they are stored at room temperature. However, products stored at colder temperatures can also be contaminated with bacteria, especially those strains that are known to grow at cold temperatures.

• Is the product leucocyte-reduced and if so was leucocyte reductions performed pre- or post-storage? Non-leucocyte-reduced blood products (especially platelets) are associated with a higher frequency of FNHTR. Post-storage leucocyte reduction also has limited effectiveness in preventing FN-HTR to platelets whereas pre-storage leucocyte reduction is highly effective. In contrast, both post- and pre-storage leucocyte reductions are effective in preventing most FNHTR to red cells.

Was fever present?

• Fever is a common finding in most types of reactions. However, it does not occur in allergic transfusion reactions or with anaphylaxis. Therefore, fever can be useful to help differentiate between severe hypotension caused by bacterial contamination, acute haemolysis or TRALI (fever may be present) versus hypotension caused by anaphylactic shock (fever is absent).

• Was the rise in temperature $\geq 2°C$? Significant temperature increases are typically seen with bacterial contamination especially if the patient has not been premedicated with an antipyretic or is not receiving antibiotic therapy. Increases in temperature greater than $2°C$ are not usually seen with other types of reactions.

Volume of product transfused

The volume of the product transfused can also be an important consideration for a differential diagnosis.

• Some types of reactions are dose dependent; hence, they tend to occur towards the end of the transfusion after most of the product has been given. Such reactions include allergic reactions, FN-HTR and TRALI. This observation becomes less useful when symptoms occur during the transfusion of multiple blood products. In this situation, it is difficult to determine if the reaction is caused by the first unit transfused or the current unit that is being administered.

• Anaphylactic reactions can present after a small amount of product is transfused (1–10 mL).

• Acute haemolytic reactions usually require at least 50–100 mL of red cells to be transfused before symptoms appear.

Other considerations

• Always remember that the patient's clinical comorbidities and therapies could also be causing many of the symptoms typical of acute transfusion reactions. Hence, these always need to be considered as part of the differential diagnosis.

• Although most reactions are relatively infrequent, it is possible for a patient to have more than one type of reaction concurrently. This possibility should always be considered when the patient presents with atypical findings.

• For many reaction types, there is a spectrum of severity, ranging from mild to severe depending on such factors as characteristics of the patient and blood product and amount of blood transfused. For example, bacterial contamination of a blood product may result in an acute septic reaction with high fever and hypotension. Alternately, such a product may cause no or only mild symptoms.

• Consider how well you know the patient and their previous response to blood product transfusions. Less concern may be appropriate for a patient who develops hives every time they are transfused; whereas, action would be appropriate for sudden development of moderate respiratory symptoms in the multi-transfused patient who has previously had no adverse events.

General approach for investigation and treatment of acute transfusion reactions

Using all of the information noted above, the clinician must make a decision whether to stop the administration of the blood product temporarily or discontinue the transfusion and must decide the extent of the investigations to be performed. Stopping and investigating every transfusion reaction is often assumed to provide the highest level of safety for the patient, but in reality may contribute to other morbidities such as bleeding or respiratory/cardiovascular morbidity if an essential transfusion is delayed. Hence, some clinical judgement is required to ensure a balance between risk and benefit. The following approach should be used when there is any concern about patient safety and an investigation is required.

Action to be taken on the clinical unit

• Stop the transfusion immediately. The severity of some reactions is dose dependent. For example, the risk of severe morbidity and mortality with acute haemolysis is generally proportional to the volume of product transfused.
• Keep the line open with saline (or other appropriate IV solution) in the event that a decision is made to continue the transfusion if the patient requires other IV therapy.
• Support the patient's clinical symptoms with appropriate medical therapy.
• Perform a bedside clerical check to ensure that the name on the blood product and requisition matches the patient's armband/identifier.
• Look carefully at the remaining blood product to determine if there is any evidence of haemolysis or particulate matter. A contaminated unit of red cells may have discolouration either in the primary bag or in the first few segments closest to the blood bag.
• Complete a transfusion reaction form and notify the blood transfusion laboratory that a reaction has occurred; it is essential that it is notified whenever a reaction occurs, and that it reports relevant reactions to its country's haemovigilance system (see Chapter 18). These in turn provide cumulative statistics about reactions, and this information may be the first clue of a new emerging threat to the blood supply or a problem with product manufacturing. In many countries, there is also a regulatory requirement to report severe reactions to the supplying blood service to ensure that appropriate action is taken. For example, it is important to exclude blood donors whose blood products have caused TRALI reactions.
• If a decision is made to perform a more extensive investigation to rule out problems with a donor unit (e.g. serological incompatibility causing haemolysis, bacterial contamination, TRALI), the remainder of the blood bag should be returned to the blood transfusion laboratory and/or blood service for further testing. Local policies should be followed for additional patient samples to be collected for specialised testing.

Action to be taken in the laboratory

When a reaction is reported to the blood transfusion laboratory, there should always be a clerical check performed to verify that the paperwork is accurate and that the correct product was issued for transfusion. To rule out haemolysis from the differential diagnosis, the following screening tests should be performed:
• clerical check as mentioned above;
• centrifuge a post-transfusion sample of the patient's blood and observe the plasma for visual evidence of haemolysis; and
• perform a direct antiglobulin test on a post-transfusion EDTA sample taken from the patient.
If the clerical check does not indicate any problems and the two screening tests are negative, acute haemolysis as the cause of the reaction can usually be eliminated. However, if the patient's symptoms are severe and consistent with a haemolytic reaction, a complete serological work-up may be indicated, including repeating the compatibility test on both the pre- and post-transfusion patient samples, and specific tests for haemolysis (i.e. lactate dehydrogenase, haptoglobin, methemalbumin etc.).

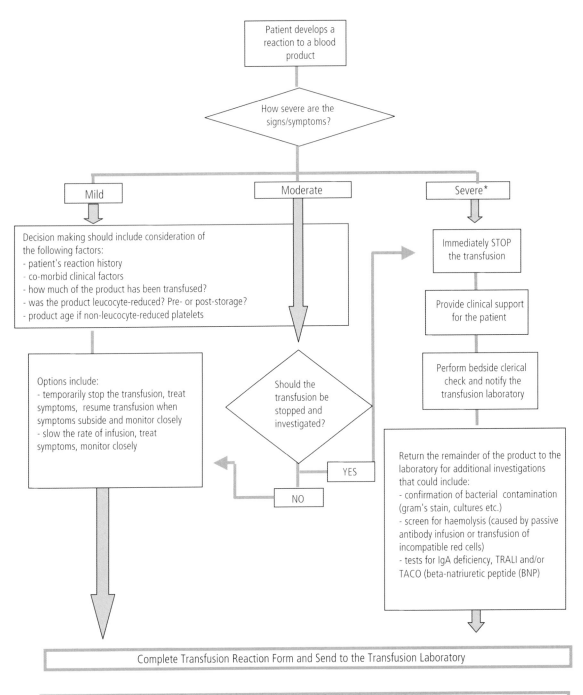

Figure 6.1 Flow diagram illustrating a possible approach for the management and investigation of an acute transfusion reaction.

All blood transfusion laboratories should have specific protocols for the investigation of other types of reactions. The Public Health Agency of Canada has developed guidelines for the investigation of suspected reactions caused by bacterial contamination which can be accessed from the website (http://www.phac-aspc.gc.ca). Investigation of TRALI, anaphylaxis and TACO requires specialised testing which may be available only from a reference centre or specialised laboratory. However, each facility should have policies and procedures in place to direct and facilitate these investigations. Results from these specialised tests are not usually available in a timely manner. Hence, treatment and prevention strategies must be made based on clinical findings and test results available on site.

Algorithm (Figure 6.1)

As mentioned previously, some clinical judgement is required when deciding what reactions to investigate more fully and the management strategies required. Aggressive investigation of mild reactions can burden resources within the health care setting and may cause unnecessary delays in transfusion therapy for a patient in critical need of blood products. In contrast, patient safety should always be paramount. The following algorithm can be used as a guide to develop a safe but logical approach to managing acute transfusion reactions.

Key points

1 Decisions related to the investigation of acute transfusion reactions require some clinical judgement based on the severity of the reactions (Figure 6.1).

2 Effective management decision-making requires that health care professionals understand the types of acute transfusion reactions that can occur and their pathophysiology (Table 6.2).

3 Patient factors to consider when formulating the differential diagnosis include history of transfusion, pregnancy, medications, previous reactions, types of symptoms (Table 6.1) and diagnosis and clinical morbidities.

4 Product factors to consider when formulating the differential diagnosis include type of product, leucocyte reduction status, volume transfused and product age.

5 Each institution must have policies and procedures for the investigation of acute reactions.

Further reading

Bakdash S & Yazer MH. What every physician should know about transfusion reactions. *CMAJ* 2007;177:141–147.

Callum JL & Pinkerton PH. *Bloody Easy 2, Blood Transfusions, Blood Alternatives and Transfusion Reactions: A Guide to Transfusion Medicine*, 2nd edn. 2005. Available at https://secure.shopsunnybrook.ca.

Eder AF & Chambers LA. Noninfectious complications of blood transfusion. *Arch Pathol Lab Med* 2007;131(5):708–718.

Guidelines for the Investigation of Suspected Transfusion Transmitted Bacterial Contamination, Public Health Agency of Canada. Available at http://www.phac-aspc.gc.ca/hcai-iamss/tti-it.

Sandler SG. How I manage patients suspected of having had an IgA anaphylactic transfusion reaction. *Transfusion* 2006;46(1):10–13.

Stroncek DF, Fadeyi E & Adams S. Leucocyte antigen and antibody detection assays: tools for assessing and preventing pulmonary transfusion reactions. *Transfus Med Rev* 2007;21(4):273–286.

Vassallo RR. Review: IgA anaphylactic transfusion reactions. Part I. Laboratory diagnosis, incidence, and supply of IgA-deficient products. *Immunohematology* 2004;20(4):226–233.

CHAPTER 7

Haemolytic transfusion reactions

Edwin Massey[1] & *Geoff Poole*[2]

[1]NHS Blood and Transplant, Bristol, UK
[2]Welsh Blood Service, Bridgend, Wales

A haemolytic transfusion reaction (HTR) is the occurrence of lysis or accelerated clearance of red cells in a transfusion recipient. With few exceptions, these reactions are caused by immunological incompatibility between the blood donor and the recipient.

HTRs can be classified either with respect to the time of their occurrence following the transfusion or to the predominant site of red cell destruction:
- acute HTRs (AHTRs) occur during or within 24 hours of the transfusion;
- delayed HTRs (DHTRs) occur more than 24 hours after a transfusion, typically 5–7 days later;
- haemolysis can be predominantly intravascular, when it is characterised by gross haemoglobinaemia and haemoglobinuria, or predominantly extravascular, when the only feature may be the fall in haemoglobin (Hb); and
- in general, intravascular haemolysis is seen in AHTRs and extravascular haemolysis in DHTRs.

Pathophysiology of HTRs

There are three phases involved (Figure 7.1):
- antibody binding to red cell antigens, which may involve complement activation;

Practical Transfusion Medicine, 3rd edition. Edited by Michael F. Murphy and Derwood H. Pamphilon. © 2009 Blackwell Publishing, ISBN: 978-1-4051-8196-9.

- these opsonised red cells interacting with and activating phagocytes; and
- production of inflammatory mediators.

Antigen–antibody interactions

Where an immunological incompatibility is responsible, the course of the reaction depends upon:
- the class and the subclass (in the case of IgG) of the antibody;
- the blood group specificity of the antibody;
- the thermal range of the antibody;
- the number, density and special arrangement of the red cell antigen sites;
- the ability of the antibody to activate complement;
- the concentration of antibody in the plasma; and
- the amount of red cells transfused.

The characteristics of the antibody and antigen

The characteristics of the antibody (such as immunoglobulin class, specificity and thermal range) and those of the antigen sites against which antibody activity is directed (such as site density and special arrangement) are inter-related. Antibodies of a certain specificity, from different individuals, are often found only within a particular immunoglobulin class and have similar thermal characteristics; and red cells of a certain blood group phenotype, from different individuals, tend to be relatively homogenous regarding the attributes of the relevant antigen. It is for this reason that a

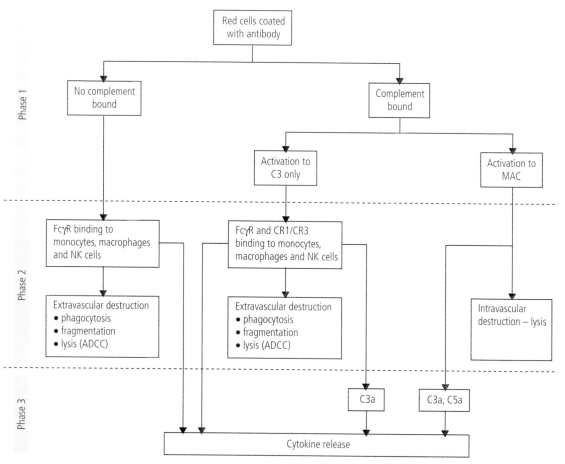

Figure 7.1 Pathophysiology of haemolytic transfusion reaction (HTR). ADCC, antibody-dependent cell-mediated cytotoxicity; MAC, membrane attack complex; NK, natural killer.

knowledge of the specificity of an antibody can be highly informative in predicting its clinical significance. Three examples illustrate this:

• Anti-A, anti-B and anti-A,B antibodies are regularly present in moderate to high titre in the plasma of group O persons. These antibodies are often both IgM and IgG, having a broad thermal range up to 37°C, and are often strongly complement-binding. The A and B antigens are often present in large site numbers (e.g. up to 1.2×10^6 A_1 antigen sites per cell) and are strongly *immunogenic* (provoking an immune response in an individual lacking the antigen). Anti-A, anti-B and/or anti-A,B are frequently implicated in AHTRs.

• Anti-Jk^a antibodies may be produced following immunisation of a Jk(a−) person. They are usually IgG (but may also have an IgM component), are active at 37°C and may be complement-binding. In Jk(a+b−) persons, there are about 1.4×10^4 Jk^a antigen sites per cell. Jk^a antigens are not particularly immunogenic. However, the antibody is sometimes difficult to detect in pre-transfusion testing (because of the low titre of antibody); consequently, Jk(a+) blood may be inadvertently transfused to patients with pre-existing anti-Jk^a. These antibodies are frequently implicated in DHTRs.

• Anti-Lu^a antibodies may be produced following the immunisation of a Lu(a−) person, or may be 'naturally occurring'. They are usually IgM (but often have IgA and IgG components), are only sometimes reactive at 37°C, and are not usually complement-binding. The Lu^a antigens show variable distribution on the red cells of an individual and are poorly immunogenic. The antibody may not be detected in pre-transfusion testing, because screening cells usually do not possess the Lu^a antigen, and because antibody levels fall after immunisation. Anti-Lu^a antibodies have not been implicated in AHTRs and only rarely in (mild) DHTRs.

Complement activation

Antibody-mediated intravascular haemolysis is caused by sequential binding of complement components (C1–C9). IgM alloantibodies are more efficient activators of C1 than IgG, since the latter must be sufficiently close together on the red cell surface to be bridged by C1q in order to activate complement. Activation to the C5 stage leads to release of C5a into the plasma and assembly of the remaining components of the membrane attack complex (MAC) on the red cell surface, leading to lysis.

Extravascular haemolysis is caused by non-complement-binding IgG antibodies or those which bind sublytic amounts of complement. IgG subclasses differ in their ability to bind complement, with the following order of reactivity: IgG3>IgG1>IgG2>IgG4.

Activation of the C3 stage leads to C3b and iC3b deposition on red cells, promoting binding to two complement receptors, CR1 and CR3, which are both expressed on macrophages and monocytes, and to the release of C3a into the plasma. Hence, C3b and iC3b augment macrophage-mediated clearance of IgG-coated cells, and antibodies binding sublytic amounts of complement (e.g. Duffy and Kidd antibodies) often cause more rapid red cell clearance and more marked symptoms than non-complement-binding antibodies (e.g. Rh antibodies).

C3a and C5a are anaphylatoxins with potent proinflammatory effects including oxygen radical production, granule enzyme release from mast cells and granulocytes, nitric oxide production and cytokine production.

Fc receptor interactions

IgG alloantibodies bound to red cell antigens interact with phagocytes through Fc receptors. The affinity of Fc receptors for IgG subclasses varies, with most efficient binding to IgG1 and IgG3. After attachment to phagocytes, the red cells are either engulfed, or lysed external to the monocyte membrane by lysosomal enzymes excreted by the monocyte, i.e. antibody-dependent cell-mediated cytotoxicity (ADCC).

Cytokines

Cytokines are generated during an HTR as a consequence of both anaphylotoxin generation (C3a, C5a) and monocyte FcγRI interaction with red cell-bound IgG. Some biological actions of cytokines implicated in HTRs are given in Table 7.1.

ABO incompatibility stimulates the release of high levels of tumour necrosis factor (TNF)-α into the plasma, within 2 hours, followed by interleukin (IL)-8 and monocyte chemotactic protein (MCP)-1. In IgG-mediated haemolysis, TNF-α is produced at a lower level together with IL-1β and IL-6. IL-8 production follows a similar time course to that in ABO incompatibility.

IgG-mediated haemolysis, as opposed to ABO incompatibility, also results in the production of the IL-1 receptor antagonist, IL-1ra. The relative balance of IL-1 and IL-1ra may also, at least in part, account for some of the clinical differences between intravascular and extravascular haemolysis.

Antibody specificities associated with HTRs

These are given, together with the site of red cell destruction, in Table 7.2.

Acute HTRs

Aetiology and incidence

These reactions arise as a result of existing antibodies, in either the recipient or donor plasma, which are directed against red cell antigens of the other party. The majority of AHTRs are due to the transfusion of ABO-incompatible transfusions, predominantly red cells, but can also be due to the

Table 7.1 Cytokines implicated in haemolytic transfusion reactions.

Terminology	Biological activity
Proinflammatory cytokines	
TNF, IL-1	Fever
	Hypotension, shock, death
	Mobilisation of leucocytes from marrow
	Activation of T and B cells
	Induction of cytokines (IL-1, IL-6, IL-8, TNF-α, MCP)
	Induction of adhesion molecules
IL-6	Fever
	Acute-phase protein response
	B-cell antibody production
	T-cell activation
Chemokines	
IL-8	Chemotaxis of neutrophils
	Chemotaxis of lymphocytes
	Neutrophil activation
	Basophil histamine release
MCP-1	Chemotaxis of monocytes
	Induction of respiratory burst
	Induction of adhesion molecules
	Induction of IL-1
Anti-inflammatory cytokines	
IL-1ra	Competitive inhibition of IL-1 type I and II receptors

Table 7.2 Antibody specificities associated with haemolytic transfusion reactions.

Blood group system	Intravascular haemolysis	Extravascular haemolysis
ABO, H	A, B, H	
Rh		All
Kell	K	K, k, Kp^a, Kp^b, Js^a, Js^b
Kidd	Jka	Jk^a, Jk^b, Jk^3
Duffy		Fy^a, Fy^b
MNS		M, S, s, U
Lutheran		Lu^b
Lewis	Le^a	
Cartwright		Yt^a
Vel	Vel	Vel
Colton		Co^a, Co^b
Dombrock		Do^a, Do^b

Table 7.3   Errors resulting in 'wrong blood' incidents.

Prescription, sampling and request
Failure to identify correct recipient at sampling
Correct patient identity at sampling but incorrectly labelled sample
Selection of incompatible products in an emergency
Transfusion laboratory
Took a correctly identified sample and aliquoted it into an improperly labelled test tube for testing
Took a wrongly identified sample through testing
Tested the correct sample but misinterpreted the results
Tested the correct sample but recorded the results on the wrong record
Correctly tested the sample but labelled the wrong unit of blood as compatible for the patient
Incorrect serological reasoning, e.g. O-positive FFP to non-O-positive recipient
Collection of unit
Failure to check recipient identity with unit identity
Bedside administration error
Recipient identity checked through case notes or prescription chart, and not wristband
Wristband absent or incorrect

administration of plasma containing high titres of ABO haemolysins. ABO-incompatible transfusions are the result of the 'wrong' blood being given to the 'wrong' patient because of clerical or administrative errors, occurring at any stage during the transfusion process.

The serious hazards of transfusion (SHOT) confidential reporting scheme has shown that in cases where the patient was transfused with a blood component or plasma product that did not meet the appropriate requirements or that was intended for another patient, clinical areas were the site of primary error in 65% of cases, and hospital laboratories were the site of primary error in 34% of cases. The reports have also highlighted that multiple errors contribute to incorrect blood component transfusion (IBCT). Examples of reported errors from several series are given in Table 7.3. Estimates of ABO-incompatible transfusions vary and may be underestimates, since some may be unrecognised or not reported, but two recent surveys have found a frequency of 1 in approximately 30,000 transfusions.

Table 7.4   Fatal acute haemolytic transfusion reactions reported to the FDA between 1976 and 1985.

Incompatibility	Number of deaths
O recipient and A red cells	80
O recipient and B/AB red cells	26
B recipient and A/AB red cells	12
A recipient and B red cells	6
O plasma to A/AB recipient	6
B plasma to AB recipient	1
Total ABO incompatibilities	131
Anti-K	5
Anti-EKP$_1$	1
Anti-Jk^b	1
Anti-Jk^{a}Jk^{b}Jk^3	1
Anti-Fy^a	1
Total non-ABO incompatibilities	9

Not all ABO-incompatible transfusions cause morbidity and mortality; mortality is dependent on the amount of incompatible red cells transfused and is reported to be 25% in recipients receiving 1–2 units of blood and reaches 44% with more than 2 units. However, as little as 30 mL group A cells given to a group O recipient can be fatal. Less frequently, Kell, Kidd and Duffy antibodies can be responsible and the acute reaction is due to a failure to detect, or take account of, the red cell alloantibody in either the antibody screen or cross-match.

Details of the incompatibilities resulting in deaths reported to the Food and Drug Administration between 1976 and 1985 are provided in Table 7.4. In the UK, with voluntary reporting to the SHOT scheme, HTR has accounted for 6.4% and IBCT 75.3% of reported errors. Nearly all deaths as a result of IBCT are due to ABO incompatible transfusions and there have been 7 deaths definitely attributable to IBCT, with 4 further probable deaths and 13 possible deaths attributable to IBCT, between 1996 and 2006. Over the same period there have been 99 cases of major morbidity due to IBCT and 29 others attributable to acute and delayed HTR.

On a positive note, in 2006, the number of incidents of the 'wrong blood' being given to the 'wrong patient' fell for the first time since reporting

commenced in the UK. This fall was greater than would be expected to result from the reduction in the number of red cell units transfused. There was also a fall in the number of ABO incompatible transfusions reported and no deaths as a result of ABO incompatibility. This progress is probably due to a number of initiatives to improve hospital transfusion practice, including providing better training of the large number of staff involved at some stage of the transfusion process (see Chapter 23).

Symptoms and signs

These may become apparent within receiving as little as 20 mL of ABO-incompatible red cells. Initial clinical presentations include the following:

• fever, chills or both;
• pain at the infusion site, or localised to the loins, abdomen, chest or head (the aetiology is unclear, but may be related to rapid complement activation at the site of infusion, and the generation of bradykinin following complement activation);
• hypotension, tachycardia or both;
• agitation, distress and confusion, particularly in the elderly;
• nausea or vomiting;
• dyspnoea;
• flushing; and
• haemoglobinuria.

In anaesthetised patients, the only signs may be uncontrollable hypotension or excessive bleeding from the operative site, as a result of disseminated intravascular coagulation (DIC).

These symptoms and signs can also be features of a reaction to bacterial contamination of the unit.

Complications

Renal failure develops in up to 36% of patients as a result of acute tubular necrosis induced by both hypotension and DIC. Thrombus formation in renal arterioles may also cause cortical infarcts.

DIC develops in up to 10% of patients. TNF-α can induce tissue factor expression by endothelial cells and together with IL-1 can reduce the endothelial expression of thrombomodulin. Thromboplastic material is also liberated from leucocytes during the course of complement activation.

Table 7.5 Immediate medical management of an acute transfusion reaction.

Symptoms/signs	Likely diagnosis	Actions
Isolated fever or fever and shivering, stable observations, correct unit given	Febrile non-haemolytic transfusion reaction (FNHTR)	Paracetamol 1 g po, continue transfusion slowly observations of P, BP and T every 15 min for 1 h, then hourly. If no improvement then call haematology medical staff
Fever with pruritus, urticaria	Allergic transfusion reaction	Chlorpheniramine 10 mg IV and other actions as for suspected FNHTR
Any other symptoms/signs, hypotension, or incorrect unit	Assume to be an acute haemolytic transfusion reaction in first instance	Discontinue transfusion, normal/saline to maintain urine output >1 mL/kg/h. Full and continuous monitoring of vital signs. Call haematology medical and transfusion laboratory staff immediately for further advice/action. Send discontinued unit of blood with attached giving set and other empty packs, after clamping securely, to the transfusion laboratory

Immediate management of suspected AHTR (see Chapter 6)

Actions for nursing staff
In the presence of a fever of more than 1.5°C above the patient's pre-transfusion temperature, and/or any symptoms or signs mentioned above, the nursing staff should:
- stop the transfusion, leaving the giving set attached;
- use a new giving set and keep the intravenous infusion running with normal saline;
- call a member of the medical staff;
- check that the patient identity as provided on the wristband corresponds with that given on the label on the blood pack and on the compatibility form;
- save any urine the patient passes for later examination for haemoglobinuria; and
- monitor the pulse (P), blood pressure (BP) and temperature (T) at 15-minute intervals.

Actions for medical staff
The immediate actions depend upon the presenting symptoms and signs, and are summarised in Table 7.5.

Investigation of suspected AHTR
Blood samples should be taken from a site other than the infusion site for the investigations listed in Table 7.6.

Other reactions characterised by haemolysis
In patients with autoimmune haemolytic anaemia, transfusion may exacerbate the haemolysis and be associated with haemoglobinuria.

Donor units of red cells may also be haemolysed as a result of:
- bacterial contamination;
- excessive warming;
- erroneous freezing;
- addition of drugs or intravenous fluids;
- trauma from extracorporeal devices; or
- red cell enzyme deficiency.

Management of a confirmed AHTR
- Maintain adequate renal perfusion by:
  a maintenance of circulating volume with crystalloid and/or colloid infusions and
  b if necessary, inotropic support.

Table 7.6   Laboratory investigation of suspected acute haemolytic transfusion reaction.

Blood test	Rationale/findings
Full blood count	Baseline parameters, red cell agglutinates on film
Plasma/urinary haemoglobin	Evidence of intravascular haemolysis
Haptoglobin, bilirubin, LDH	Evidence of intravascular or extravascular haemolysis
Blood group	Comparison of post-transfusion and retested pre-transfusion samples, to detect ABO error not apparent at bedside. Unexpected ABO antibodies post-transfusion may result from transfused incompatible plasma. The donor ABO group should be confirmed
Direct antiglobin test (DAT)	Positive in majority, pre-transfusion sample should be tested for comparison. May be negative if all incompatible cells destroyed
Compatibility testing	An IAT antibody screen and IAT cross-match using the pre- and post-transfusion sample provide evidence for the presence of alloantibody. Elution of antibody from post-transfusion red cells may aid identification of antibody, or confirm specificities identified in serum in cases of non-ABO incompatibility. Red cell phenotype should also be performed on recipient pre-transfusion sample and unit in cases of non-ABO incompatibility, to confirm absence in patient and presence in unit of corresponding antigen
Urea/creatinine and electrolytes	Baseline renal function
Coagulation screen	Detection of incipient DIC
Blood cultures	In event of septic reaction caused by bacterial contamination of unit, which may be suspected from inspection of pack for lysis, altered colour or clots

- Transfer to a high dependency area where continuous monitoring can take place.
- Repeat coagulation and biochemistry screens 2- to 4-hourly.
- If urinary output cannot be maintained at 1 mL/kg/h, seek expert renal advice.
- Haemofiltration or dialysis may be required for the acute tubular necrosis.
- In the event of the development of DIC, blood component therapy may be required.
- Having ascertained the nature of the incompatibility causing the AHTR, transfusion of compatible blood may be required for life-threatening anaemia.

Prevention of AHTRs

Prevention of 'wrong blood' incidents
- Prevention of the multiplicity of errors which can contribute to the transfusion of ABO-incompatible red cells must depend upon the creation of an effective quality system for the entire process, which will involve:

   (a) adherence to national guidelines and standards;

   (b) local procedures which are agreed, documented and validated;

   (c) training and retraining of key staff;

   (d) regular error analysis and review;

   (e) reporting to local Risk Management/Assurance Committee; and

   (f) reporting to regulatory bodies such as the Medicines and Healthcare products Regulatory Agency (MHRA) in the UK, the Food and Drug Administration in the US, and to national haemovigilance schemes to contribute to the understanding of the extent and underlying causes. These aspects are specifically covered in Chapter 23.
- Since the majority of errors leading to an ABO-incompatible transfusion are due to misidentification of the patient or patient's sample, due attention must be paid to the comprehensive use of unique patient identifiers throughout the hospital and automation within the laboratory.
- Access to previous transfusion records containing historical ABO groups should be available at all times.

• It is desirable that computerised systems are used to verify at the bedside the matches between the patient and the sample taken for compatibility testing, and at the time of transfusion between the patient and the unit of blood.

Prevention of non-ABO AHTRs

• In the case of recurrently transfused patients, due attention should be paid to the interval between sampling and transfusion, to optimise the detection of newly developing antibodies. For patients transfused within the previous 72 hours, the pretransfusion sample should not be taken more than 24 hours before the next transfusion; for patients transfused within the previous 14 days, the pretransfusion sample should not be taken more than 3 days before the next transfusion.

• In the presence of multiple red cell alloantibodies, when it is not feasible to obtain compatible red cells in an emergency, intravenous immunoglobulin (1 g/kg/day for 3 days) and/or steroids (hydrocortisone 100 mg 6-hourly or methylprednisolone 1 g daily for 3 days) have been used with anecdotal reports of ameliorating a potential haemolytic or 'hyperhaemolytic' episode (see below).

Delayed HTRs

Aetiology and incidence

With few exceptions, DHTRs are due to secondary immune responses following re-exposure to a given red cell antigen. The recipient has been primarily sensitised to the antigen in pregnancy or as a result of a previous blood transfusion and a few days after a subsequent transfusion there is a rapid increase in the antibody concentration, resulting in the destruction of red cells.

• The antibodies most commonly implicated and reported to SHOT between 1996 and 2006 were those from the Kidd blood group system followed by those from the Rh, Duffy and Kell systems. One analysis showed that in approximately 10% reported cases, more than one alloantibody was found in the serum.

• Frequently, there are no clinical signs of red cell destruction, but subsequent patient investigations reveal a positive direct antiglobulin test (DAT) and the emergence of a red cell antibody. This situation has been termed a delayed serological transfusion reaction (DSTR).

• Kidd and Duffy antibodies are more likely to cause symptoms and be associated with a DHTR rather than a DSTR.

• Estimates of the frequency of DHTR and DSTR vary, but in a series reported from the Mayo Clinic, the frequency of DHTR was 1 in 5405 units and of DSTR was 1 in 2990 units, giving a combined frequency of 1 in 1900 units transfused.

• DHTRs are in themselves rarely fatal, although in association with the underlying disease can lead to mortality.

• Ten per cent of transfusion fatalities reported to the American Food and Drug Administration (FDA) between 1976 and 1985 were due to DHTR; in 75% of cases, more than one alloantibody was present in the serum, and the same proportion involved non-Rh antibodies.

• Six deaths reported to SHOT between 1996 and 2006 have been due to DHTRs. Tragically in some instances, there were delays in diagnosis, investigation and provision of compatible units which led to marked anaemia and contributed to mortality.

Signs and symptoms

These usually appear within 5–10 days following the transfusion, but intervals as short as 24 hours and as late as 21 days have been recorded. The exact onset may be difficult to define since haemolysis can be initially insidious and may only be appreciated from results of post-transfusion samples. The commonest features are:
• fever;
• fall in haemoglobin concentration; and
• jaundice and haemoglobinuria.
Hypotension and renal failure are uncommon (6% of cases). In the postoperative period in particular, the diagnosis may be overlooked and the symptoms and signs incorrectly attributed to continuing haemorrhage or sepsis.

Management

The majority of DHTRs require no treatment because red cell destruction occurs gradually as antibody synthesis increases. However, particularly in a bleeding patient, haemolysis will contribute to the development of life-threatening anaemia and urgent investigations are required to ensure the timely provision of antigen-negative units.

Expert medical advice may be required for treatment of the hypotension and renal failure. When accompanied by circulatory instability and renal insufficiency, a red cell exchange transfusion with antigen-negative units can curtail the haemolytic process. Future transfusions of red cells should also be negative for the antigen in question.

Investigation of suspected DHTR
(see Chapter 6)
• The peripheral blood film is likely to show spherocytosis.
• Other evidence of haemolysis – namely, hyperbilirubinaemia, reduced serum haptoglobin, haemoglobinaemia, haemoglobinuria and haemosiderinuria – is useful to confirm the nature of the reaction and to monitor progress.
• The DAT usually becomes positive within a few days of the transfusion until the incompatible cells have been eliminated.
• Further serological testing on pre- and post-transfusion samples should be undertaken in accordance with the schedule provided for AHTR.
• The antibody may not be initially apparent in the post-transfusion serum but can be eluted from the red cells. If the red cell eluate is inconclusive, then a repeat sample should be taken after 7–10 days, to allow for an increase in antibody titre. However, additional, more sensitive techniques may have to be employed to detect the antibody and it is advisable to seek the help of a reference laboratory.
• Since a significant proportion of cases have more than one alloantibody in the serum, it is important that the panels used for antibody identification have sufficient cells of appropriate phenotypes to exclude additional specificities.

Prevention

Access to previous transfusion records may disclose the presence of antibodies undetectable at the time of cross-matching, and all patients should be questioned regarding previous transfusions and pregnancies. Patients found to have developed a clinically significant red cell alloantibody should be provided with an antibody card. When the care of patients requiring transfusion support is shared between hospitals, there must be adequate communication between laboratories and clinical teams.

Laboratories should ensure that their antibody screen is effective in detecting weak red cell alloantibodies and that screening cells are taken from homozygotes where the corresponding antibodies show a dosage effect (i.e. they are less easy to detect when red cells with heterozygous expression of the relevant antigen are used rather than cells with homozygous expression).

Haemopoietic stem cell transplants
(see Chapter 27)
Most patients transplanted with minor ABO-incompatible marrow develop a positive DAT, but only 10–15% of patients develop clinically significant haemolysis.

Haemolysis in minor ABO incompatibility is short-lived and exchange transfusion is rarely required. Red cells and plasma-containing components (platelets, FFP and cryoprecipitate) should be compatible with both recipient and donor.

It has been suggested that the use of peripheral blood stem cells may increase the risk of significant haemolysis since the number of lymphocytes infused with the graft is increased, and three deaths due to an AHTR were reported between 1997 and 1999 in minor ABO-incompatible transplants. Several cases due to anti-D have been described, and antibody production has persisted for up to 1 year.

Solid organ transplants (see Chapter 45)
In ABO-unmatched organs, the frequency of occurrence of donor-derived antibodies and haemolysis increases with the lymphoid content of the graft, from kidney to liver to heart–lung transplants. The figures for haemolysis are 9%, 29% and 70%,

respectively. The frequency of haemolysis increases with an O donor and A recipient. The ABO antibodies, which appear 7–10 days after transplant, last for approximately 1 month. Haemolysis is usually mild, although several cases of renal failure and one death have been reported. It can be prevented by switching to group O cells, either at the end of surgery or postoperatively if the DAT becomes positive.

Rh antibodies have been described following kidney, liver and heart–lung transplants. They can cause haemolysis for up to 6 months, which can be sufficiently severe to merit therapy.

Delayed haemolysis following organ transplantation (passenger lymphocyte syndrome)

Donor-derived B lymphocytes within the transplanted organ may mount an anamnestic response against the recipient's red cell antigens. Donor-derived antibodies are usually directed against antigens within the ABO and Rh systems.

Haemolysis occurs 7–10 days after transplantation, with an unpredictable and abrupt onset.

In minor ABO-incompatible transplants (O donors and recipients of other groups), pre-transplant isohaemagglutinin titres do not appear to predict the incidence or severity of haemolysis. In both haemopoietic stem cell and solid organ transplants, the haemolytic syndrome is almost exclusively associated with the use of cyclosporin and tacrolimus. The ex vivo removal of T cells has a similar enhancing effect on the function of transplanted donor memory B lymphocytes.

Haemolytic transfusion reactions in sickle-cell disease

The frequency of alloimmunisation in sickle-cell anaemia is dependent upon the nature and success of the extended red cell antigen matching policy employed. Approximately, 40% of patients who are alloimmunised have experienced or will experience a DHTR.

Although DHTRs are characteristically mild in other groups of recipients, they can be responsible for major morbidity in sickle-cell disease. The term 'sickle-cell haemolytic transfusion reaction (SCHTR) syndrome' has been suggested to capture some of the distinctive features which can be seen to accompany a reaction. A similar syndrome has been described in other transfusion-dependent patients so the term 'hyperhaemolytic transfusion reaction (HHTR)' may be more appropriate. These features are as follows:

• symptoms suggestive of a sickle-cell pain crisis that develop or are intensified during the HTR;
• marked reticulocytopenia (for the patient);
• development of a more severe anaemia after transfusion than was present before: this may be due to the suppression of erythropoiesis as a result of the transfusion but hyperhaemolysis of autologous red cells (bystander immune haemolysis) has also been suggested. There have been reports that bone marrow aspirates performed on patients suffering from this complication have shown evidence of active erythropoiesis during the reticulocytopenic phase and haemophagocytosis. This has led to the suggestion that erythroid precursors and reticulocytes are removed by adhesion to monocytes via other mechanisms, in addition to IgG and Fc receptors, such as the integrins $\alpha 4\beta 1$ and VCAM-1;
• subsequent transfusions may further exacerbate the anaemia and it may become fatal; and
• patients often have multiple red blood cell alloantibodies and may also have autoantibodies, which make it difficult or impossible to find compatible units of red blood cells.

However, in other patients the DAT may be negative, no alloantibodies are identified, and serological studies may not provide an explanation for the HTR: even red cells which are phenotypically matched with multiple patient antigens may be haemolysed.

Management involves withholding further transfusion and treating with corticosteroids (hydrocortisone 100 mg 6-hourly or methylprednisolone 1 g daily for 3 days); IVIG (1 g/kg/day) may have been beneficial in some cases.

It is recommended that patients with sickle-cell disease are phenotyped prior to transfusion and that blood is selected for Rh and K (see Chapter 28).

Key points

1 HTRs are the second commonest cause in the UK and the US of immediate morbidity and mortality following a transfusion (the most common cause is transfusion-related acute lung injury (TRALI)).

2 The clinical presentations are diverse and they can be unrecognised or misdiagnosed.

3 Most fatal AHTRs are due to the transfusion of ABO-incompatible red cells.

4 The transfusion of ABO-incompatible red cells is the result of an error occurring at any stage in the transfusion process.

5 Devising and successfully implementing measures to overcome these preventable and fatal errors is a challenge but should be a priority for those involved in hospital transfusion.

Further reading

Beauregard P & Blajchman MA. Haemolytic and pseudo-haemolytic transfusion reactions: an overview of the haemolytic transfusion reactions and the clinical conditions that mimic them. *Transfus Med Rev* 1994;8:184–199.

British Committee for Standards in Haematology. Guidelines for compatibility procedures in blood transfusion laboratories. *Transfus Med* 2004;14:59–73.

Davenport RD. Haemolytic transfusion reactions. In: Popovsky MA. (ed), *Transfusion Reactions.* Bethesda: AABB Press, 1996, pp. 1–44.

Klein H & Anstee D. Haemolytic transfusion reactions. In: Klein HG & Anstee D (eds), *Mollison's Blood Transfusion in Clinical Medicine.* Oxford: Backwell Science, 2006.

Linden JV & Kaplan HS. Transfusion errors: causes and effects. *Transfus Med Rev* 1994;8:169–183.

National Patient Safety Agency. *Right Patient, Right Blood.* Safer Practice Notice No. 14. London: NPSA, 2006. Available at www.npsa.nhs.uk.

National Patient Safety Agency. *Standardising Patient Wristbands Improves Patient Safety.* Safer Practice Notice No. 24. London: NPSA, 2007. Available at www.npsa.nhs.uk.

Petz LD, Calhoun L, Shulman IA, Johnson C & Herron RM. The sickle cell haemolytic transfusion reaction syndrome. *Transfusion* 1997;37:382–392.

Ramsey G. Red cell antibodies arising from solid organ transplants. *Transfusion* 1991;31:76–86.

Sazama K. Reports of 355 transfusion-associated deaths: 1976 through 1985. *Transfusion* 1990;30:583–590.

Serious Hazards of Transfusion. *Annual Report 2006.* Manchester: SHOT Office. Available at www.shotuk.org.

Vamvakas EC, Pineda AA, Reisner R, Santrach PJ & Moore SB. The differentiation of delayed haemolytic and delayed serologic transfusion reactions: incidence and predictors of haemolysis. *Transfusion* 1995;35:26–32.

CHAPTER 8

Febrile and allergic transfusion reactions

Cynthia Wu[1] & Nancy M. Heddle[1,2]
[1]Department of Medicine, McMaster University, Hamilton, Ontario, Canada
[2]Canadian Blood Services, Hamilton, Ontario, Canada

Febrile and allergic reactions frequently occur during or following the transfusion of blood products. Interpretation of the signs and symptoms of the reaction to establish the cause, clinical relevance and management strategy can be challenging for the physician as the clinical findings are not necessarily specific to one type of reaction. In this chapter, two of the more common adverse events are described: febrile non-haemolytic transfusion reactions (FN-HTRs) and both mild and severe forms of allergic reactions.

Febrile non-haemolytic transfusion reactions

Clinical presentation

In the classical FNHTR, the patient will present with fever (usually defined as $\geq 1\,^{\circ}C$ rise in temperature) during or within 2 hours of completing the transfusion, along with other typical symptoms that include a cold feeling, chills and a generalised feeling of discomfort. Less frequently headache, nausea and vomiting may also occur. Rigors also occur in the severest reactions. Although this is the classical

definition, in practice only 15% of patients develop a fever but typically present with the other symptoms described above.

Differential diagnosis

Unfortunately, these symptoms are not specific for a FNHTR; hence, the challenge for the transfusing physician is to consider the other possibilities and develop a systematic approach for excluding other causes to establish a definitive diagnosis. When a patient presents with fever, the differential diagnosis should include:
- FNHTR;
- acute haemolytic reactions;
- delayed haemolytic reactions;
- bacterial contamination;
- transfusion-related acute lung injury (TRALI);
- co-morbid conditions; and
- medications.

It is especially important to rule out acute haemolysis, bacterial contamination and TRALI as these conditions can be associated with frequent morbidity and mortality unless rapidly recognised and treated. In contrast, FNHTRs cause discomfort and distress for the patient and consume additional health care resources to treat and investigate; however, long-term morbidity or mortality does not occur.

To further complicate the investigative process in patient populations where transfusion-associated

Practical Transfusion Medicine, 3rd edition. Edited by Michael F. Murphy and Derwood H. Pamphilon. © 2009 Blackwell Publishing, ISBN: 978-1-4051-8196-9.

fever occurs frequently, clinical judgement has to be incorporated into the decision-making process.

Frequency

The frequency of reactions varies with the:
- patient population;
- type of blood product being transfused; and
- age of the blood product.

Reactions to platelets are more common than reactions to red cells. In a general hospital population, red cell reactions occur with 0.04–0.44% of transfusions, while the frequency of platelet reactions is higher, ranging from 0.06 to 2.2% of transfusions. In specific patient populations such as haematology/oncology patients, reactions to platelets are more common occurring in up to 37% of transfusions if non-leucocyte-reduced blood products are used. When pre-storage leucocyte-reduced blood platelets are transfused, the frequency of acute reactions decreases dramatically (<2% of transfusions). FNHTRs to products other than red cells and platelets are rare and there are limited data to estimate the frequency.

Pathogenesis

The pathogenesis of FNHTRs is multifactorial and varies for red cells and platelets. Our current understanding of why FNHTRs occur with red cells and platelets is summarised below.
- *Antibody mechanism*: The patient's serum contains a leucocyte antibody that reacts with leucocytes present in the blood product. An antigen–antibody reaction occurs resulting in the release of endogenous pyrogens by the donor leucocytes. These pyrogens act on the hypothalamus to cause fever. This antigen–antibody hypothesis is believed to be the primary mechanism causing FNHTRs to red cells.
- *Leucocyte/platelet-derived biological response modifiers*: During storage of the blood product, proinflammatory cytokines (interleukin 1, interleukin 6 and tumour necrosis factor α) are released from leucocytes present in blood products stored at room temperature (platelets). These cytokines accumulate to high levels by the end of the product storage period and, when infused, cause fever by stimulation of the hypothalamus. This is the primary mechanism responsible for FNHTRs to

platelets. Platelets are stored at room temperature for a maximum of 5 days and have high cytokine concentrations at the end of the storage period. This mechanism is unlikely to contribute to red cell reactions as the red cells are stored in the cold preventing significant levels of cytokines from accumulating. Platelet-derived cytokines also accumulate in stored platelet products and may play a role in some reactions. There are over 15 different cytokines that have been shown to accumulate in platelets during storage.
- *Other biological response modifiers (BRMs)*: Other BRMs such as complement and/or neutrophil priming lipids have been detected in some stored blood products and it is hypothetically possible that they may cause or contribute to fever in some patients. However, there are no clinical data linking these substances to an increased risk of FNHTRs.

Management of FNHTRs

The management of FNHTRs includes the exclusion of other causes of fever. However, the strategy requires some clinical judgement and must balance benefit versus risk. The following questions should be considered as part of the decision-making process about the management approach. The rationale for considering these questions is also presented.
- *Is the blood product being transfused leucocyte-reduced?* The risk of an FNHTR in a setting where all blood products are universally leucocyte-reduced is low occurring in less than 1% of red cell transfusions and approximately 2% of platelet transfusions. In contrast, if leucocyte-reduced blood products are not being transfused then reactions will be very common: 6–8% of red cells and up to 37% of platelets transfused, respectively. In this latter situation, stopping the transfusion and investigating every reaction not only consumes significant health care resources but may put patients at risk as they may not receive the required product in a timely manner.
- *Does the patient have a history of FNHTRs?* Some patients are susceptible to repeated FNHTRs when blood products are transfused, e.g. because of the presence of leucocyte antibodies.

• *If a temperature increase occurred, was it greater than or equal to 2°C?* It is very uncommon for the temperature to rise more than 2°C with an FNHTR. In this situation, bacterial contamination should be suspected, the blood product should be stopped immediately and appropriate investigations initiated.

• *Would you describe the patient's signs and symptoms as mild, moderate or severe?* If the symptoms are mild, a less aggressive management approach may be initiated but careful observation of the patient is essential. If the symptoms are severe, the product should be stopped immediately and supportive care given to the patient. If the clinical findings are categorised as moderate, the points above need to be considered and clinical judgement is required as to how patient management should proceed.

Finally, the management strategy for red cells should include an approach to rule out an acute haemolytic transfusion reaction. Haemolysis following platelet transfusion is rare but can occur when the plasma of the platelet product contains a high titre ABO antibody that reacts with the patient's red cells.

The management approach should also alleviate the signs and symptoms associated with an FNHTR. This may involve temporary discontinuation of the transfusion while antipyretic medication is administered to the patient. Medications should never be injected into the blood product. In most cases, the transfusion can be resumed once the signs and symptoms subside. There is some evidence that pethidine (or meperidine in North America) is effective treatment for alleviating rigors associated with transfusions.

A conservative strategy for minimising the risk to patients while investigating reactions would include the following steps:

• temporarily stop the transfusion but keep the line open with saline;

• perform a bedside clerical check between the blood and the patient to ensure that the right blood has been transfused;

• observe the blood product to determine if there is discolouration or particulate matter present; and

• notify the blood transfusion laboratory and send appropriate samples if laboratory investigations are deemed necessary to rule out other causes of acute reactions with fever.

Prevention of FNHTRs

As the pathogenesis of FNHTRs is different for red cells and platelets, the strategy for prevention of these reactions also varies depending on the blood product being transfused.

Red cells

Since most reactions are caused by the leucocyte antigen–antibody mechanism, the primary way to prevent these reactions is to remove some of the leucocytes from the red cell product. Prevention can be accomplished for most patients by removing approximately one log of leucocytes from the red cell product to a level of approximately 10^8 leucocytes/product. This can be achieved by post-storage filtration, centrifugation with buffy coat removal (either during the manufacturing process or post-storage) or pre-storage filtration during the component preparation phase. Filtration (pre- or post-storage) using current leucocyte reduction filters results in red cell products with less than 10^6 leucocytes which is well below the threshold needed to prevent most red cell reactions. If a patient still reacts to a leucocyte-reduced product, other options for preventing future reactions include washing the product prior to transfusion and/or selecting fresher blood for transfusion.

Platelets

Most platelet reactions (90%) are caused by leucocyte-derived cytokine accumulation during storage. Hence, post-storage leucocyte reduction is not an effective strategy for preventing most FNHTR to platelets. FNHTRs to platelets can be prevented by pre-storage leucocyte reduction by either filtration or centrifugation (buffy coat method of platelet preparation). If pre-storage leucocyte-reduced products are not available, the plasma supernatant on the stored platelets can be removed and replaced with a compatible solution, the product can be washed to remove the cytokine-rich plasma, or fresher platelets (≤3 days of storage) can be transfused.

Premedication of the patient with an antipyretic drug, paracetamol in the UK and acetaminophen in North America, has become standard practice to prevent FNHTRs. Aspirin should not be used as a premedication in any patient requiring platelet transfusions as it affects platelet function. In some centres, it is routine practice to premedicate all patients prior to transfusion. However, there are no clinical data to justify this universal approach and when using leucocyte-reduced blood products such a practice is not warranted. However, patients with recurrent FNHTRs can be treated with an antipyretic approximately 30 minutes prior to starting the transfusion, which should help to alleviate or prevent symptoms.

Allergic transfusion reactions

Generally, an allergic transfusion reaction is defined as a type I hypersensitivity response mediated by IgE antibodies binding to a soluble allergen and resulting in the activation of mast cells. In these reactions, the allergen is often not known and the actual mechanism continues to remain largely speculative. In contrast, severe reactions that involve anaphylaxis which are not mediated by IgE antibodies but involve IgG anti-IgA are classified as type III reactions. These reactions result in complement activation with subsequent amplified release of anaphylotoxins C3a and C5a leading to anaphylaxis. When the aetiology of an allergic reaction is identified, it usually falls into one of the following categories:
• recipient pre-existing antibodies to plasma proteins in the blood product;
• recipient antibodies against a substance in the blood product that either is lacking or has a distinctly different allelic expression in the recipient (i.e. IgA, haptoglobulin, C_4); and
• extraneous substances in the product (i.e. passively transmitted donor IgE antibodies, drugs, other allergens).

Incidence
It is estimated that about 1% of transfusions are adversely affected by allergic reactions and that aller-

gic reactions comprise 13–33% of all transfusion reactions. Rates of allergic transfusion reactions vary widely between the studies depending on product type and preparation. In a review of the studies done between 1990 and 2005:
• allergic transfusion reactions to packed red blood cell (RBC) were reported to range from 0.03 to 0.61% with a median of 0.15% (1 reaction per 667 transfusions);
• allergic transfusion reactions to platelet occurred at a higher rate, ranging from 0.09 to 21% with a median of 3.7% (1 reaction per 27 transfusions); and,
• the frequency of allergic transfusion reactions to plasma is lower than platelets but more common than reactions to red cells.

True anaphylaxis is a systemic reaction caused by antigen-specific cross-linking of IgE molecules on the surface of tissue mast cells and peripheral blood basophils, with immediate release of potent mediators. In contrast, immediate systemic reactions that mimic anaphylaxis but are not caused by an IgE-mediated immune response are termed anaphylactoid reactions. Both anaphylactic or anaphylactoid reactions are severe and life-threatening, but fortunately they are rare and comprise only about 1.3% of all transfusion reactions, affecting 1/20,000–1/47,000 transfusions.

Clinical presentation
Allergic transfusion reactions can be either non-systemic/localised or systemic/generalised and are classified as mild, moderate or severe.
• Non-systemic reactions are usually mild, consisting of urticaria and occasionally focal angioedema. These are benign and self-limiting though still cause symptoms that are distressing to the patient.
• Systemic reactions range from moderate (generalised urticaria) to severe and life-threatening. Although urticaria is considered a pathognomonic finding for an allergic reaction, 9.5% of allergic transfusion reactions lack all skin findings.
• Anaphylactic and anaphylactoid reactions behave identically clinically and are managed the same. These reactions should be considered a medical emergency as failure to initiate prompt treatment can have fatal consequences. Anaphylaxis

usually begins 1–45 minutes after starting the transfusion and, in addition to an urticarial rash, presents with hypotension/shock, upper or lower airway obstruction (hoarseness, wheezing, chest pain, stridor, dyspnoea, anxiety, feeling of impending doom), gastrointestinal symptoms and rarely death.

To ensure that appropriate treatment is administered in a timely fashion, patients presenting with systemic symptoms should also be promptly evaluated for:

• other causes of respiratory distress including circulatory overload, TRALI or any other co-morbid condition such as pulmonary embolism and exacerbations of chronic lung disease; and,

• other causes of shock such as acute haemolytic transfusion reactions, sepsis and other co-morbid clinical conditions that can be associated with shock.

Management

When there is a suspicion for any transfusion reaction, a general principle of treatment is to discontinue the transfusion immediately and until the patient is clinically assessed.

• Mild non-systemic allergic transfusion reactions are usually treated with an antihistamine, commonly diphenhydramine 25–50 mg IM or IV in North America and chlorphenamine (Piriton) 10–20 mg IM or IV in the UK. The transfusion can often be restarted at a slower rate once symptoms are medicated.

• Moderate reactions can additionally be treated with a dose of corticosteroids and the transfusion is usually discontinued indefinitely.

• In severe reactions, the transfusion is never restarted. Anaphylaxis is treated as with any other anaphylactic reaction.

However, the management strategy differs for adults and paediatric patients. For adults/adolescents, immediate administration of epinephrine (adrenaline in Europe) 500 µg (0.5 mL of 1:1000 solution) IM is key. Aggressive volume expansion with IV normal saline, oxygen supplementation and antihistamines are also required. If the hypotension is intractable, adrenaline

500 µg (5 mL 1:10000 solution) IV can be given every 5–10 minutes and preparations should be made to transfer the patient to an intensive care unit where an IV drip of inotropic therapy can be maintained. Intubation may be necessary if the airway becomes compromised.

For paediatric patients, the treatment of anaphylaxis should include: epinephrine/adrenaline 10 µg/kg 1:1000 concentration IM (e.g. under 6 months: 50 µg or 0.05 mL of adrenaline 1 in 1000; 6 months to 6 years: 120 µg or 0.12 mL; 6–12 years, 250 µg or 0.25 mL) that can be repeated every 5 minutes (maximum dose 500 µg). A µg/kg dose should be used rather than a mL/kg dose as there are different concentrations of epinephrine/adrenaline. Administration of diphenhydramine 1 mg/kg IV/IM (or chlorphenamine 250 µg/kg IV for children 1 month to less than 1 year of age; 2.5–5 mg for 1–5 years; 5–10 mg for 6–12 years; 10 mg for over 12 years) and ranitidine 1 mg/kg IV (maximum dose 50 mg) are also effective for supportive management.

While the above drugs are being prepared, the focus should be on resuscitation, including oxygen therapy, suctioning and positioning of patient to open the airway, maintenance of the circulation, oxygen saturation monitoring, establishing an IV if possible and administering a fluid bolus with 20 mL/kg sodium chloride 0.9% if venous access is established. If signs and symptoms persist despite a single dose IM of epinephrine/adrenaline then a paediatric intensive care specialist should be consulted to provide airway and further haemodynamic support.

Prevention

Premedication with antipyretics and/or antihistamines

It has been reported that 50–80% of transfusions in Canada and the US are premedicated. Interestingly, the only prospective, randomised trial assessing the efficacy of premedication in non-haemolytic transfusion reactions (NHTRs) found a 15.2% rate of NHTR in the placebo arm versus a 15.4% rate in the acetaminophen plus diphenhydramine pretreated arm (51 adult oncology patients, 98 transfusions). A retrospective review of 7900 transfusions in 385 paediatric oncology patients also found no statistically significant difference in allergic transfusion reactions between those who received premedication and those who did not. This study also found that there was no difference in allergic reactions with or without premedication even in those with a previous history of two or more allergic reactions and that these were not more common in those with a history of two or more allergic transfusion reactions. Although premedication does not appear to affect the incidence of allergic reactions, there have been no studies to date that have evaluated if premedication has an effect on the severity of such reactions.

Leucocyte reduction

Unlike FNHTRs, there is no significant reduction in allergic transfusion reactions with the use of leucocyte-reduced blood products.

Washed products/plasma-reduced products

Washing a cellular blood product may decrease allergic transfusion reactions particularly in patients with recurrent, moderate to severe reactions but there is a paucity of data to confirm this beneficial effect.

IgA-deficient blood products

IgA deficiency is the most common primary immunodeficiency in the Western world, affecting up to 1 in 20 people. Severe IgA deficiency, defined as IgA <0.05 mg/L, can be associated with anaphylactic reactions to blood products containing IgA. Patients with anaphylactic transfusion reactions should have further testing to quantify their serum IgA level as well as anti-IgA antibody titres. If allergic transfusion reactions secondary to IgA antibodies due to IgA deficiency is confirmed, IgA-deficient products should be given in any future transfusions. Since anaphylactic transfusion reactions are rare and often not due to IgA deficiency, while transfusions are common and often urgent, it is both impractical and not cost-effective to widely screen for IgA deficiency in the pre-transfused population.

Key points

1 Allergic and FNHTRs are the most common transfusion reactions. Anaphylaxis is rare.
2 Mild allergic reactions usually only require antihistamine treatment and the transfusion can be continued unless systemic symptoms develop.
3 Mild FNHTRs usually respond to the administration of an antipyretic.
4 If a moderate to severe transfusion reaction is suspected, the transfusion must be stopped until the patient is assessed and possible causes of the reaction are investigated.
5 Systemic symptoms warrant prompt clinical assessment as treatment can vary widely between diagnoses and, in particular, failure to administer epinephrine (adrenaline) in anaphylactic reactions can be fatal.

Further reading

Domen RE & Hoeltge GA. Allergic transfusion reactions. An evaluation of 273 consecutive patients. *Arch Pathol Lab Med* 2003;127:316–320.

Geiger TL & Howard SC. Acetaminophen and diphenhydramine premedication for allergic and febrile nonhemolytic transfusion reactions: good prophylaxis or bad practice? *Transfus Med Rev* 2007;21:1–12.

Heddle NM. Febrile non hemolytic transfusion reactions. In: Popovsky MA. (ed), *Transfusion Reactions*, 3rd edn. Bethesda, MD: AABB Press, 2007, pp. 57–103.

Paglino JC, Pomper GJ, Fisch GS, Champion MH & Snyder EL. Reduction of febrile but not allergic reactions to RBCs and platelets after conversion to universal prestorage leukoreduction. *Transfusion* 2004;44:16–24.

Sanders SG & Zantek ND. Review: IgA anaphylactic transfusion reactions. Part II. Clinical diagnosis and bedside management. *Immunohematology* 2004;20:234–239.

Sandler SG. How I manage patients suspected of having had an IgA anaphylactic transfusion reaction. *Transfusion* 2006;46:10–13.

Tobian AA, King KE & Ness PM. Transfusion premedications: a growing practice not based on evidence *Transfusion* 2007;47:1089–1096.

Vamvakas E & Pineda AA. Allergic and anaphylactic reactions. In: Popovsky MA. (ed), *Transfusion Reactions*, 3rd edn. Bethesda, MD: AABB Press, 2007, pp. 105–156.

Vassallo RR. Review: IgA anaphylactic transfusion reactions. Part I. Laboratory diagnosis, incidence, and supply of IgA-deficient products. *Immunohematology* 2004;20:226–233.

Wang SE, Lara PN Jr, Lee-Ow A *et al.* Acetaminophen and diphendydramine as premedication for platelet transfusions: a prospective randomized double-blind placebo-controlled trial. *Am J Hematol* 2002;70:191–194.

CHAPTER 9
Transfusion-related acute lung injury

Steven H. Kleinman[1] & Ram Kakaiya[2]
[1]University of British Columbia, Victoria, British Columbia, Canada
[2]Life Source Blood Services, Glenview, Illinois, USA

Definition

The clinical syndrome of transfusion-related acute lung injury (TRALI) is characterised by acute onset of respiratory distress during or within 6 hours of transfusion, associated with oxygen desaturation (hypoxemia) and bilateral lung infiltrates, without evidence for left atrial hypertension or circulatory overload. No specific treatment for TRALI exists; in 90% of the cases, the patient recovers completely within 96 hours; the remaining 10% of the cases are fatal.

Incidence

Haemovigilance data establish that TRALI is the number one cause of acute mortality from transfusion. In the US, reports of transfusion-related fatalities to the Food and Drug Administration (FDA) indicate that TRALI has been the number one cause of fatalities from 2003 to 2006 and in the UK, the 2005 Serious Hazards of Transfusion (SHOT) report lists TRALI as the leading cause of transfusion-related mortality.

There is a consensus that TRALI is both under-recognised and underreported; thus, the precise in-

cidence of fatal plus non-fatal TRALI is unknown. An overall risk of approximately 1:5000 transfused units in the general hospital population was reported in 1985 and this incidence number is frequently cited in the literature. The risk of TRALI may be higher for certain patient groups. An incidence of 1:1300 has been observed in patients in critical care units when careful monitoring has been performed. Data are less clear for other predisposing patient conditions, with occasional reports indicating higher risk for surgical patients (see pathogenesis), patients with haematologic malignancies, and patients receiving large amounts of plasma during plasma exchange.

Pulmonary dysfunction that is not severe enough to meet the definition of TRALI may also occur following transfusion. In one randomised crossover trial, patients in the intensive care unit were transfused with a fresh frozen plasma (FFP) unit from a multiparous donor, preceded or followed by a unit from a donor without a history of transfusion or pregnancy. Five patients from a total of 100 developed oxygen desaturation; four cases followed transfusion of plasma from multiparous donors, and one case followed the transfusion of control plasma.

Clinical manifestations

Males and females are equally affected. Most cases occur in adults. Previous transfusion history is

Practical Transfusion Medicine, 3rd edition. Edited by Michael F. Murphy and Derwood H. Pamphilon. © 2009 Blackwell Publishing. ISBN: 978-1-4051-8196-9.

unremarkable and recurrent TRALI is extremely rare. At least one case of TRALI from an autologous transfusion has been recorded. A few cases have occurred in children. Directed donations from mother to child can cause TRALI due to maternal leucocyte antibodies against the child's leucocyte antigens.

The onset of TRALI is often quite dramatic, with symptoms occurring either during the transfusion or usually within 2 hours (but this can be up to 6 hours) of its completion. The syndrome manifests as acute respiratory distress syndrome (ARDS) or as non-cardiogenic pulmonary oedema, and is characterised by acute onset of respiratory distress with dyspnoea, tachypnea and oxygen desaturation. The patient may appear cyanotic and may develop hypotension or hypertension. Oxygen desaturation is often severe, requiring mechanical ventilation in 70% of cases. Mild cases of respiratory distress that are unaccompanied by hypoxia, do not require any oxygen administration, or resolve quickly do not fit the diagnostic criteria for TRALI. Some patients with TRALI experience a low-grade fever for several hours. Symptoms and signs may be muted in patients under general anaesthesia and the first indication of TRALI might be the appearance of copious amounts of yellow frothy sputum from the endotracheal tube.

Auscultation of the lungs will detect the presence of bilateral rales or crackles. Hypoxia, defined as PaO_2/FiO_2 <300, and the development of new bilateral lung infiltrates on chest X-ray are essential in making a diagnosis. Hypoxia may also manifest as cyanosis or oxygen saturation of <90% on room air by pulse oximetry.

New acute lung injury (ALI) is defined by the development of new bilateral lung infiltrates on the chest X-ray. The chest X-ray may show 'white out', a radiographic finding in which both lungs show uniform white opacities throughout. More commonly, pulmonary infiltrates are located peripherally, especially in both lower lung fields (Figure 9.1). Because some patients with TRALI have acute transient leucopenia (neutropenia) around the time of symptom onset, a complete blood count with white cell count differential can be a useful adjunct test.

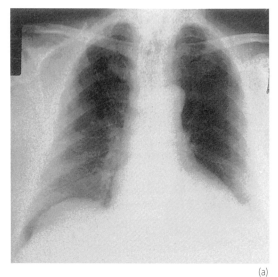

(a)

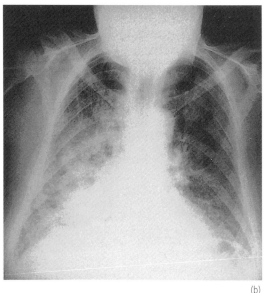

(b)

Figure 9.1 Chest X-rays of a patient with transfusion-related acute lung injury: (a) 1 day before a platelet transfusion and (b) shortly after transfusion showing diffuse bilateral shadowing of the lungs and a normal-sized heart. (From Virchis *et al.*, 1997, with permission.)

Types of blood components that can cause TRALI

TRALI has been caused by all types of blood components, including red cell concentrates, FFP, platelet concentrates, platelets collected by apheresis, cryoprecipitate and rarely intravenous immunoglobulin. Plasma-rich components, namely FFP, platelet concentrates collected by the buffy coat method, and platelets collected by apheresis pose a greater per-unit risk than plasma-poor components (e.g. red cell concentrates). Plasma that has been treated by the solvent-detergent (SD) method that is currently in use in Europe, manufactured by pooling a large number of plasma units thus diluting the leucocyte antibodies contained in donor blood, has not been shown to cause TRALI.

Pathogenesis

Two different mechanisms – antibody-mediated and non-antibody-mediated – have been postulated as causes of TRALI. It appears that cases caused by the antibody mechanism are of greater clinical severity and more often require mechanical ventilation.

• Leucocyte antibodies may bind to the recipient's neutrophils that possess the corresponding cognate antigen/s, causing them to aggregate in the pulmonary vasculature, or may bind to endothelial cells, leading to neutrophil adherence and neutrophil activation. Activated neutrophils subsequently release cytotoxic enzymes, which leads to increased vascular permeability and intra-alveolar oedema. Antigen–antibody complex formation may also lead to increased vascular permeability through complement activation.

• Non-antibody-mediated TRALI results from transfusion of bioactive substances, which accumulate in cellular blood components during their storage. These bioactive substances include lipids (lysophosphatidylcholines), cytokines (IL-6 and IL-8), secretory phopholipase2 (sPLA2) and soluble CD40 ligand. This mechanism of TRALI has been termed the two-hit hypothesis. The first hit is a patient stressor (e.g. surgery or sepsis) that causes the expression of endothelial cell adhesion molecules, leading to neutrophil adherence and activation in the pulmonary microvasculature. The second hit, consisting of passive administration of bioactive substances in stored blood components, leads to intravascular release of neutrophil enzymes, causing increased vascular permeability and resultant intra-alveolar oedema. Laboratory tests to measure bioactive substances are not widely available.

It is unclear what percentage of TRALI cases are due to each of these mechanisms. Most (but not all) series report that the large majority of TRALI cases are caused by the antibody mechanism, with 80–85% of these due to donor leucocyte antibodies directed at HLA or neutrophil-specific antigens present on the recipient's cells. The remainder are due to recipient antibody reactions with leucocytes in the transfused unit; this phenomenon was probably more common prior to the widespread use of leucocyte-reduced blood components. Implicated antibodies include HLA class I antibodies directed against A and B locus antigens, HLA class II antibodies directed mostly against DR antigens, and neutrophil antibodies directed against human neutrophil antigens (HNAs). Involved donors can have multiple types of antibodies. The presence of a cognate antigen in the recipient that corresponds to the antibody specificity in the involved donor, or a positive cross-match between the donor's serum and the recipient's leucocytes provide strong support for the diagnosis of antibody-mediated TRALI. HNA-3a(5b) antibodies are rare but are important to detect as these have been associated with several fatal cases of TRALI. Currently, neutrophil antibody detection assays are not widely available and are not automated. It has been reported that anti-HNA-3a may be missed unless a leucoaggultination assay or an enhanced immunofluorescense assay is used.

Lung histology

Fatal cases of TRALI show massive alveolar oedema on histological examination (Figure 9.2). Alveolar–capillary membrane disruption is widespread with

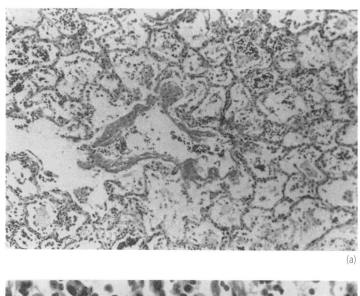

(a)

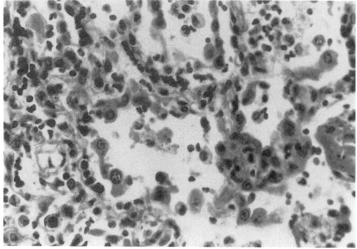

Figure 9.2 Thin sections of fixed lung from a patient with transfusion-related acute lung injury. There is acute diffuse alveolar damage with intra-alveolar oedema and haemorrhage. There was no histological evidence of infection, and all postmortem cultures (bacterial, viral and fungal) were negative. Magnification: (a) x40;(b) x440. (From Silliman *et al.*, 1997 with permission.)

(b)

hyaline membrane formation. Interstitium and alveoli are infiltrated with inflammatory cells consisting of neutrophils and macrophages. The diffuse alveolar damage resembles findings seen in ARDS from other causes.

Differential diagnosis

Diagnosis of TRALI remains difficult because patients who experience severe respiratory distress during or after transfusion are often quite ill, have multiple other morbidities, may have cardiac or pulmonary compromise, and could be suffering from conditions that are known to cause ALI or ARDS. Clinical evaluation should include investigation of other causes of ALI, which include sepsis syndrome (with or without septic shock), trauma, aspiration, smoke inhalation, near drowning, pneumonia, systemic inflammatory response syndrome, pancreatitis, post-cardiopulmonary bypass and drug overdose. In any given patient, the presence of one or more of these other causes of ALI makes the diagnosis of TRALI quite difficult. A recent Consensus Conference has recommended that ALI occurring within 6 hours of transfusion in a patient with other ALI risk factors be designated as possible TRALI, as it is often extremely difficult to determine whether it was the transfusion or the alternate risk factor that caused the ALI. The diagnosis of TRALI is difficult, if not impossible, to make in patients with pre-existing ALI.

The lack of certain clinical findings helps in the differential diagnosis between TRALI and transfusion associated circulatory overload (TACO). This latter syndrome consists of cardiogenic pulmonary oedema, which may show one or more of the following features:

- positive fluid balance, weight gain, orthopnoea or paroxysmal nocturnal dyspnoea;
- peripheral oedema;
- hepatomegaly;
- hepatojugular reflux, heart murmur;
- new onset cardiac gallop rhythm (S3 and S4);
- an increased jugular venous pressure;
- elevated pulmonary artery wedge pressure (≥ 18 mm Hg) in invasively monitored patients;
- an enlarged heart with or without pleural effusion on the chest X-ray;
- radiographic appearance of pulmonary infiltrates that are more central with or without Kerley septal lines;
- some TRALI patients experience low-grade fever and acute onset of leucopenia and these features, if present, suggest TRALI rather than TACO;
- a 50% elevation of B-type natriuretic peptide (BNP) in a post- versus a pre-transfusion sample supports TACO whereas a BNP level of <250 pg/mL measured immediately after the onset of acute pulmonary oedema supports the diagnosis of TRALI.

In addition to TACO, other conditions that can mimic TRALI include anaphylactic transfusion reactions and sepsis from transfusion of bacterially contaminated blood components. Respiratory stridor, localised or generalised skin rash, hypotension and/or shock favour a diagnosis of anaphylactic reaction. High fever, chills, rigor, shock, disseminated intravascular coagulation, a positive gram stain and culture from the transfused blood component and positive blood cultures from the recipient support a diagnosis of transfusion-transmitted bacterial sepsis. Finally, a low-grade fever seen in TRALI must be differentiated from a haemolytic transfusion reaction. A clerical check of the transfusion episode showing the lack of any error, plus an absence of visual haemolysis in the serum or plasma and a negative direct antiglobulin test, suggest that a haemolytic transfusion reaction is unlikely.

More recently, the new term 'transfusion-associated dyspnoea' (TAD) has been coined for those cases of dyspnoea following transfusion that do not fit into any of the known transfusion reaction categories.

Clinical information helpful in the differential diagnosis of TRALI is listed in Table 9.1.

Management

Patient management is supportive. Virtually all patients will require some sort of oxygen support with many requiring mechanical ventilation with or without intubation. There is no evidence to support the use of corticosteroids. Fluid management may include the use of intravenous fluids to correct profound hypotension. Diuretics may be indicated if blood pressure is stable and if an element of congestive heart failure or circulatory overload is present or cannot be excluded.

Clinicians should obtain a chest X-ray, HLA phenotype, leucocyte antibody identification, and pre- and post-transfusion BNP levels in all suspected cases of TRALI. Patients with leucocyte antibodies may benefit from transfusion of leucocyte-reduced blood components. Further transfusions, if needed, do not require any other special precautions since recurrent TRALI is extremely rare. The use of platelets that are stored for less than 4 days and red cell units less than 14 days have been advocated by some authors, but there are no clinical data to support the need for such products.

Outcome and morbidity

TRALI is often quite severe and patients require mechanical ventilation for adequate oxygenation

Table 9.1 Clinical information that may assist in differential diagnosis of pulmonary transfusion reactions.

Clinical parameter	Interpretation
History	Underlying cardiac dysfunction and positive fluid balance may suggest TACO. Sepsis or aspiration in the previous 24 h suggest ALI and the designation of 'possible TRALI'. IgA deficiency may suggest allergic reaction
Physical examination	Sudden elevation of blood pressure, jugular venous distension and wheezing suggest TACO. Hypotension suggests TRALI. Stridor, wheezing and urticaria suggest allergic reaction. Fever suggests febrile reaction, sepsis/bacterial contamination
Chest X-ray	Bilateral infiltrates indicate pulmonary oedema (TACO or TRALI). Cardiomegaly (cardiothoracic ratio > 0.55) and increased vascular pedicle width (>65 mm) suggest TACO
Arterial blood gas analysis, arterial oxygen saturation (pulse oximetry)	$PaO_2/FIO_2 < 300$ (or O_2 saturation < 90% on room air) meets the Consensus Conference definition of ALI (TRALI or possible TRALI)
Haemodynamic monitoring: central venous and pulmonary artery pressures	Increase in central venous (>12–15 mm Hg) or pulmonary artery wedge pressure (>18–20 mm Hg) at the time of reaction suggest TACO
Echocardiography	Systolic (ejection fraction < 45%) or diastolic dysfunction suggest TACO or other cause of cardiogenic oedema
Pulmonary oedema fluid	The ratio of pulmonary oedema albumin over plasma albumin of >0.55 suggest ALI rather than hydrostatic (TACO) oedema
Beta-natriuretic peptide (BNP)	Low values of BNP (<250 pg/mL) suggest TRALI. Increase in BNP >1.5 of pre-transfusion values may suggest TACO
Leucocyte and neutrophil count before and after the implicated transfusion	Sudden, transient drop in neutrophil or leucocyte count after the transfusion suggests TRALI
Response to diuretic therapy	Rapid (minutes to hours) resolution of pulmonary oedema after diuresis may suggest TACO
Timing of the reaction in relation to transfusion and other potential risk factors	Sudden onset during or shortly after the transfusion is suggestive of a transfusion reaction rather than a pulmonary complication related to another risk factor

in two thirds or more of the cases. The remaining cases require oxygen therapy by non-mechanical modalities. Pulmonary infiltrates resolve in the vast majority of patients (≥80%) in 96 hours. Slow recovery of pulmonary functions occur in 10%. Mortality is approximately 6–10%. Recurrence is extremely rare. Those who recover do not have any chronic sequelae.

Prevention

For non-antibody-mediated TRALI, no preventive steps have been recommended or undertaken. For antibody-mediated TRALI, there is general agree-

ment that a donor who is clearly 'implicated' in a case of TRALI should be deferred. An 'implicated donor' is defined as one who is shown to possess leucocyte antibodies that correspond to the recipient's antigen/s, or a donor whose serum is reactive against the recipient's leucocytes in a cross-match test. It remains uncertain if the donor should be deferred if he or she has leucocyte antibodies but cognate antigens are not present in the recipient or if the cross-match test is negative.

In the UK, steps were taken in late 2003 to reduce transfusing FFP units collected from female donors. With this intervention, the number of TRALI cases from FFP transfusion decreased from 14 cases in 2003 to 6 cases in 2004 to 1 case in

2005. In view of these and other data, in late 2006, the AABB (formerly, American Association of Blood Banks) recommended that plasma for transfusions be prepared from donors who are less likely to be alloimmunised. Therefore, plasma units for transfusion are now increasingly prepared predominantly from male donors. In some European countries, SD plasma has been used as an alternative product to reduce the incidence of TRALI, but this option is not currently available in the US.

There are probably sufficient male donor plasma units available for blood groups O and A such that transfusion needs can be met almost exclusively by transfusion of male-only plasma. For blood groups B and AB plasma, some plasma from female donors may be necessary to meet the transfusion demand. In this regard, plasma from nulliparous female donors would be preferred to plasma from multiparous donors. Prevention approaches for platelets will likely require different measures as there are an insufficient number of male platelet apheresis donors to achieve a practice similar to the one described for plasma transfusion. Alternatively, deferral of females who have been pregnant at least once would still result in the loss of 40–60% of female donors, and such a donor loss would likely create a critical shortage. Because of these considerations, screening blood donors, especially female donors with a history of pregnancy, for HLA antibodies and then deferring those who have them from plateletpheresis donations is currently under intense study. At present, techniques for neutrophil antibody identification are cumbersome and cannot be applied for screening a large number of donors.

Key points

1 TRALI is a leading cause of death from transfusion.
2 It manifests as ARDS or non-cardiogenic pulmonary oedema during or within 6 hours of transfusion.

3 Leucocyte antibodies (HLA and neutrophil-specific) and neutrophil priming agents in blood components are responsible for the syndrome.
4 Treatment is supportive, but fatality occurs in 10% of diagnosed cases.
5 Those who recover show no long-term lung injury.
6 Preventive measures include exclusion of blood donors implicated in TRALI cases.
7 Other steps being implemented include reducing the number of transfusions of plasma-containing blood components from donors who are likely to possess leucocyte antibodies.

Further reading

Bux J. Transfusion-related acute lung injury (TRALI): a serious adverse event of blood transfusion. *Vax Sang* 2005;89:1–10.

Bux J & Sachs UJH. The pathogenesis of transfusion-related acute lung injury (TRALI). *Br J Haematol* 2007;136:788–799.

Eder AF, Herron R, Strupp A *et al.* Transfusion-related acute lung injury surveillance (2003–2005) and the potential impact of the selective use of plasma from male donors in the American Red Cross. *Transfusion* 2007;47:599–607.

Gajic O, Gropper MA & Hubmayr RD. Pulmonary edema after transfusion: how to differentiate transfusion-associated circulatory overload from transfusion-related acute lung injury. *Crit Care Med* 2006;34:S109–S113.

Goldman M, Webert KE, Arnold DM, Freedman J, Hannon J & Blajchman MA. Proceedings of a consensus conference: towards an understanding of TRALI. *Transfus Med Rev* 2005;19:2–31.

Kleinman S, Caufield T, Chan P *et al.* Toward an understanding of transfusion-related acute lung injury: statement of a consensus panel. *Transfusion* 2004;44:1774–1789.

Moore SB. Transfusion-related acute lung injury (TRALI); clinical presentation, treatment, and prognosis. *Crit Care Med* 2006;34(Suppl):S114–S117.

Popovsky MA & Moore SB. Diagnostic and pathogenetic considerations in transfusion-related acute lung injury. *Transfusion* 1985;25:573–577.

Rana R, Fernandez-Perez ER, Khan SA *et al.* Transfusion-related acute lung injury and pulmonary edema in critically ill patients: a retrospective study. *Transfusion* 2006;46:1478–1483.

Silliman CC, Ambruso DR & Boskov LK. Transfusion-related acute lung injury. *Blood* 2005;105:2266–2273.

Silliman CC, Paterson AJ, Dickey W *et al.* The association of biologically active lipids with the development of

transfusion-related acute lung injury. *Transfusion* 1997;37:719–726.

Stroncek DF. Pulmonary transfusion reactions. *Semin Hematol* 2007;44:2–14.

Virchis AE, Patel RK, Contreras M *et al.* Acute non-cardiogenic lung oedema after platelet transfusion. *Br Med J* 1997;314:880–882.

CHAPTER 10

Transfusion-related immunomodulation

Morris A. Blajchman[1] *& Eleftherios C. Vamvakas*[2]

[1]Departments of Pathology and Medicine, McMaster University; Canadian Blood Services, Hamilton, Ontario, Canada
[2]Department of Pathology and Laboratory Medicine, Cedars-Sinai Medical Center, Los Angeles, California, USA

As knowledge about immune tolerance evolves, and as more tools to measure immune alterations appear, more immunologic consequences of allogeneic blood transfusion (ABT) are detected. ABT causes a decrease in the helper/suppressor lymphocyte ratio, a decrease in natural killer (NK) cell function, defective antigen presentation, suppression of lymphocyte blastogenesis and a reduction in delayed-type hypersensitivity. The lingering question has been whether these observations are mere laboratory curiosities or reflect some clinically relevant alteration in the immune function of the transfusion recipient.

Transfusion-related immunomodulation (TRIM) encompasses the documented laboratory immune alterations that follow ABT, as well as any established or purported, beneficial or deleterious, clinical effects that may be ascribed to immunosuppression resulting from ABT, which include:

• enhanced survival of renal allografts;
• increased risk of recurrence of resected malignancies and of postoperative bacterial infections;
• increased short-term (up to 3-month post-transfusion) mortality from all causes; and
• activation of endogenous CMV or HIV infection in transfused compared with untransfused patients.

Practical Transfusion Medicine, 3rd edition. Edited by Michael F. Murphy and Derwood H. Pamphilon. © 2009 Blackwell Publishing, ISBN: 978-1-4051-8196-9.

Any ABT-related increase in short-term post-transfusion mortality (perhaps secondary to an increased risk of multiple organ failure [MOF]) would likely be mediated by 'pro-inflammatory' rather than 'immunomodulatory' mechanisms; however, the term TRIM has recently been used more broadly, to encompass transfusion complications mediated via either immunomodulatory or pro-inflammatory pathways.

The only *established* clinical TRIM effect is beneficial, not deleterious: it is the enhanced survival of renal allografts after pre-transplant ABT. This effect has been confirmed by animal data and clinical experience worldwide. Before the advent of cyclosporine and potent immunosuppressive drugs, this ABT effect was exploited clinically, through the deliberate exposure of patients awaiting renal transplantation to transfusion of non-white blood cell (WBC)-reduced red blood cells (RBCs). The benefit from ABT is small in the current era, but a randomised controlled trial (RCT) documented that it is still evident. Importantly, compared with transfusions of non-WBC-reduced RBCs, patients receiving WBC-reduced, washed, or frozen-thawed-deglycerolised RBCs (i.e. RBCs depleted of allogeneic WBCs by various methods) derive less benefit from pre-transplant ABT. Thus, whether pre-transplant ABT continues to confer a benefit in countries that have converted to universal WBC reduction remains to be determined.

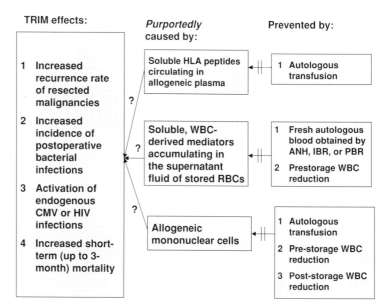

Figure 10.1 TRIM effects, postulated mediators of TRIM, and preventive strategies that could be effective if the TRIM effects were mediated by each corresponding mediator. ANH, acute normordemic hemodilution; IBR, intraoperative blood recovery; PBR, postoperative blood recovery (Modified with permission from *Am J Clin Pathol* 2006;126(Suppl 1):S71–S85.)

The existence of deleterious clinically relevant TRIM effects has not yet been established; neither do we know the mechanism(s) of TRIM nor the specific blood constituent(s) that mediate(s) TRIM. TRIM may be mediated by one (or more) of the following (Figure 10.1):

• allogeneic mononuclear cells (AMCs) present in RBC units stored for less than 2 weeks;

• pro-inflammatory soluble mediators released from WBC granules or membranes and accumulating progressively in the supernatant of RBCs during storage; and/or

• soluble, class I HLA molecules circulating in allogeneic plasma.

Clinical studies of adverse TRIM effects

Some 200 observational studies and 22 RCTs have reported on adverse TRIM effects in humans. Sixteen RCTs assumed that the TRIM effect is mediated by allogeneic WBCs and compared recipients of non-WBC-reduced versus WBC-reduced allogeneic RBCs or whole blood. Six RCTs assumed that the TRIM effect is mediated by either allo-geneic WBCs or allogeneic plasma and compared recipients of non-WBC-reduced allogeneic versus autologous blood.

Thus, the available RCTs differ in ways that determine the conclusions to be drawn about mechanisms of TRIM. Patients randomised to receive non-WBC-reduced allogeneic RBCs received units that were either buffy-coat-reduced (in Europe) or buffy-coat-rich (in the US). Buffy-coat-reduced RBCs are units from which approximately two-thirds of WBCs are removed, without filtration, by the method used to separate blood into components. If WBCs do indeed mediate TRIM, buffy-coat-rich RBCs should have more of a TRIM effect than buffy-coat-reduced RBCs.

Patients randomised to receive autologous or WBC-reduced allogeneic RBCs received units that were either replete with or devoid of WBC-derived soluble mediators. During storage of a non-WBC-reduced RBC unit, WBCs deteriorate over 2 weeks, progressively releasing soluble mediators. RBCs WBC-reduced by filtration after storage are full of WBC-derived mediators, because such mediators (as well as apoptotic or necrotic WBCs) are not retained by WBC reduction filters. RBCs WBC-reduced by filtration before storage are free of WBC-derived mediators, because their WBCs are removed before they can release mediators into the supernatant fluid. Stored autologous blood, obtained by preoperative donation, is full of mediators, because autologous WBCs also deteriorate during storage, releasing mediators. Fresh autologous blood, obtained by acute normovolemic haemodilution (ANH), intraoperative blood recovery (IBR), or postoperative blood recovery (PBR), and transfused within hours of collection and processing, is free of WBC-derived soluble mediators.

WBC reduction, performed either before or after storage, can prevent TRIM effects mediated by AMCs, but it cannot prevent TRIM effects mediated by soluble molecules circulating in allogeneic plasma (Figure 10.1). Only pre-storage, as opposed to post-storage, WBC reduction can prevent TRIM effects mediated by WBC-derived, soluble mediators. Autologous transfusion can prevent TRIM effects mediated by AMCs as well as by molecules circulating in allogeneic plasma. Only fresh, as opposed to stored, autologous blood can prevent TRIM effects mediated by WBC-derived, soluble mediators.

TRIM effects mediated by AMCs

The best argument that the adverse TRIM effects are mediated by AMCs is that the established beneficial TRIM effect in renal transplantation requires viable WBCs. Also, immune suppression has been induced in mice receiving allogeneic WBCs free of plasma and platelets.

A recent theory attributes TRIM to donor myeloid dendritic cells that have both CD11c and CD200 on their surface. The receptor for CD200 is found on some T cells in the recipient. The interaction between the donor CD200 and its receptor in the recipient produces a tolerance signal that suppresses T-cell immune responses and induces proliferation of $\gamma\delta$-suppressor T cells that release cytokines, especially transforming growth factor (TGF)-β that promotes tumour growth. Thus, in an experimental animal model of tumour growth, mice injected intravenously with syngeneic fi-

brosarcoma cells have shown a dose–response relationship between the volume of transfused allogeneic blood and the number of pulmonary tumour nodules, along with proliferation of suppressor TGF-β-positive cells in the spleen. The growth promoting effect could be blocked by antibodies to either CD11c or CD200, implicating the subset of donor dendritic cells that have both CD11c and CD200 on their surface in the pathogenesis of TRIM.

Accordingly, fresh donor blood (containing functional dendritic cells) should provoke growth of tumours stimulated by TGF-β (i.e. sarcomas); and tumours for which the immune response plays a major role (i.e. skin tumours and virally induced tumours). However, no RCT of ABT and cancer recurrence has transfused fresh RBCs to patients randomised to receive non-WBC-reduced RBCs, to study the effects of AMCs. Also, instead of enrolling patients with sarcomas, skin tumours, or virally induced tumours, the three available RCTs enrolled patients with colorectal cancer (i.e. a tumour that is not sufficiently antigenic to render the immune response to the tumour important in controlling its growth). Thus, when the results of these three RCTs were integrated by a meta-analysis, no association was observed between non-WBC-reduced ABT and colorectal cancer recurrence.

The only RCT to study the effect of AMCs has been the Viral Activation Transfusion Study, which studied transfusion-induced activation of endogenous CMV or HIV infection. All RBCs transfused in this study had been stored for less than 2 weeks. There was no difference between the arms of the RCT in any end-point studied. Median survival was 13.0 months in recipients of pre-storage filtered, WBC-reduced allogeneic RBCs, as compared with 20.5 months in recipients of buffy-coat-rich, non-WBC-reduced allogeneic RBCs ($p = 0.12$).

TRIM effects mediated by WBC-derived soluble mediators

Histamine, eosinophil cationic protein and eosinophil protein X, which may inhibit neutrophil function, increase 3- to 25-fold in the supernatant of RBCs during storage. These mediators are contained in intracellular WBC granules and are released as the WBCs deteriorate. Fas ligand is similarly released from WBC membranes during storage. The infusion of soluble Fas ligand may impair the function of NK and cytotoxic T cells of the recipient, because the infused Fas ligand binds to the Fas molecule on NK and cytotoxic T cells, thereby preventing the binding of the Fas molecule on these immune cells to the Fas ligand on virus-infected cells. Apoptotic WBCs may also have TRIM effects, and the importance of pre-storage (as compared with post-storage) WBC reduction for removing such soluble WBC-derived mediators (thereby preventing the tumour growth promoting effect of ABT) has been documented in an animal model.

In this model, New Zealand White rabbits with established tumours were blood recipients and California Black rabbits were allogeneic donors; and siblings of the recipients were syngeneic donors. Infusion of epithelial tumour cells was followed by non-WBC-reduced allogeneic, post-storage WBC-reduced allogeneic, pre-storage WBC-reduced allogeneic, or syngeneic transfusion. When the pulmonary tumour nodules were counted, there was no difference between non-WBC-reduced versus post-storage WBC-reduced ABT, or between pre-storage WBC-reduced allogeneic versus syngeneic transfusion, but the difference between the former two and the latter two groups was statistically significant.

With regard to infections, a recent theory attributes the purported susceptibility of transfused patients to infection to a sustained inhibition of neutrophil chemotaxis caused by TGF-β. Both exogenous TGF-β, contained in the supernatant of stored RBCs, and endogenous TGF-β, produced by the recipient's neutrophils in response to soluble Fas ligand and soluble HLA molecules contained in the transfused supernatant have been implicated. Pre-storage WBC reduction has abrogated this ABT effect.

However, the 12 RCTs that compared the risk of postoperative infection between patients randomised to receive non-WBC-reduced versus WBC-reduced ABT (in the event that they needed perioperative transfusion) have not supported the theory that attributes TRIM to WBC-derived soluble mediators. These RCTs are medically heterogeneous, having been conducted at various settings, having transfused various blood products, and having diagnosed infection based on varying criteria. Thus, not all 12 RCTs targeted a TRIM effect that was *biologically* similar in all cases, making it inappropriate to combine the results of all 12 RCTs in a meta-analysis. However, if we were to integrate these findings despite the extreme heterogeneity of the studies, we would find no association between non-WBC-reduced ABT and an increased risk of infection across all the available RCTs, whether we relied on 'intention-to-treat' analyses (that retain all randomised subjects, whether transfused or not) or on 'as-treated' analyses (that remove the untransfused subjects).

What has medical relevance, however, is the integration of medically homogeneous studies. Integration of such subsets of homogeneous studies produced results antithetical from those expected from theory. Across nine RCTs transfusing allogeneic RBCs filtered before storage to the WBC-reduced arm, and enrolling approximately 5000 subjects, no TRIM effect was detected. If WBC-derived, soluble mediators did cause TRIM, pre-storage filtration should abrogate any increased infection risk associated with non-WBC-reduced ABT. Thus, a deleterious TRIM effect would be expected in this analysis, but no such effect was found (summary odds ratio [OR] = 1.06; 95% confidence interval [CI], 0.91–1.24; $p > 0.05$) (Figure 10.2a).

In contrast, across the four RCTs transfusing allogeneic RBCs or whole blood filtered after storage to the non-WBC-reduced arm, there was a 2.25-fold increase in the risk of infection in association with non-WBC-reduced ABT (summary OR = 2.25; 95% CI, 1.12–4.25; $p < 0.05$) (Figure 10.2b). Thus, the TRIM effect appeared to be prevented by post-storage filtration, contradicting the theory that attributes TRIM to WBC-derived, soluble mediators. Such mediators would have been present equally in both the non-WBC-reduced and WBC-reduced RBCs, because they would not have been removed by post-storage filtration.

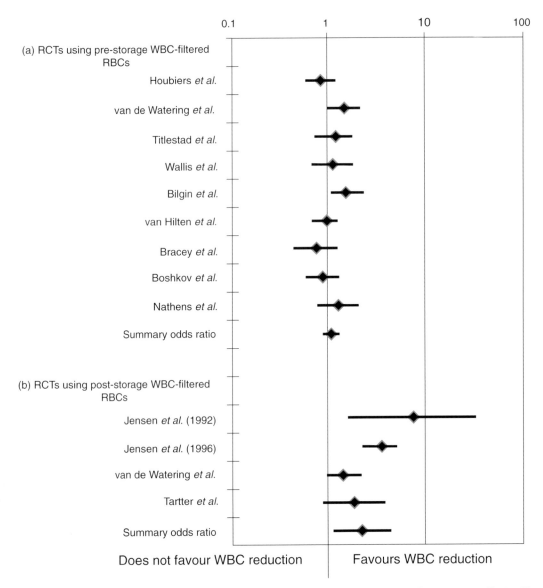

Figure 10.2   RCTs of ABT and postoperative infection administering pre-storage WBC filtered (a) or post-storage WBC filtered (b) allogeneic RBCs to the WBC-reduced arm. The figure shows the OR of postoperative infection, as calculated from an intention-to-treat analysis of each study; and the summary OR across the depicted RCTs, as calculated from a meta-analysis. A deleterious ABT effect (and thus a benefit from WBC reduction) is demonstrated by an OR > 1, provided that the effect is statistically significant ($p < 0.05$; i.e. provided that the associated 95% CI does not include the null value of 1). The RCT of van de Watering et al. included recipients of both pre-storage filtered and post-storage filtered RBCs and found no difference between these two arms. For the references to the listed studies, see Further Reading, Vamvakas & Blajchman (2007)

TRIM effects mediated by soluble molecules circulating in allogeneic plasma

Only one RCT has been specifically designed to study the effects of soluble HLA molecules circulating in allogeneic plasma as mediators of TRIM. Wallis randomised patients undergoing open-heart surgery to receive plasma-reduced, buffy-coat-reduced, or WBC-reduced RBCs. The highest risk of infection was observed in the plasma-reduced arm, although the difference between the three arms was not significant. This finding suggested that plasma removal does not prevent TRIM; or, by extension, that allogeneic plasma does not mediate TRIM. Similarly, integration of the five RCTs that compared recipients of allogeneic versus autologous blood demonstrated no increased risk of infection in association with ABT.

Association between non-WBC-reduced ABT and short-term mortality

The association of non-WBC-reduced ABT with short-term mortality from all causes started out as a data-derived hypothesis to account for an unexpected transfusion effect. The RCT of van de Watering et al. (Figure 10.2) had been designed to investigate differences in postoperative infection between recipients of non-WBC-reduced versus WBC-reduced allogeneic RBCs. However, it detected, instead, differences in 60-day mortality between the arms (Figure 10.3). The authors suggested that non-WBC-reduced ABT may predispose to MOF, which, in turn, may predispose to mortality.

Tissue injury is mediated by reactive oxygen species and by proteolytic enzymes released from activated neutrophils. Transfusion of stored, non-WBC-reduced blood may have a neutrophil-priming effect, mediated by bioactive lipids that accumulate during storage. Deteriorating WBCs may release enzymes that act on RBC membranes to produce bioactive lipids responsible for neu-

trophil priming and endothelial cell activation. Supernatant from stored RBCs primes neutrophils for superoxide production and enhanced cytotoxicity and also activates pulmonary endothelial cells, showing a dose–response relationship with the length of RBC storage. Pre-storage WBC reduction abrogates this ABT effect.

If 11 medically heterogeneous RCTs comparing recipients on non-WBC-reduced versus WBC-reduced ABT and reporting on short-term mortality were to be combined, there would be no increase in mortality in association with non-WBC-reduced ABT. These studies transfused to the non-WBC-reduced arm either buffy-coat-rich or buffy-coat-reduced allogeneic RBCs; as already discussed, the former should have more of an effect than the latter. However, this theoretical prediction is the opposite of what the analysis actually showed. Across six RCTs transfusing buffy-coat-reduced RBCs to the non-WBC-reduced arm, and pre-storage filtered RBCs to the WBC-reduced arm, there was a 60% increase in mortality in association with non-WBC-reduced ABT (summary OR = 1.60; 95% CI, 1.14–2.24; $p < 0.05$) (Figure 10.3a). In this analysis, pre-storage filtration appeared to abrogate an increased mortality risk, but the benefit from pre-storage filtration was not seen where more of an ABT effect would have been expected. Across the RCTs that transfused buffy-coat-rich RBCs to the non-WBC-reduced arm, no ABT effect was detected, although some 4500 subjects had been enrolled in these studies.

Perhaps, the benefit observed in the analysis of studies transfusing buffy-coat-reduced versus pre-storage filtered RBCs (Figure 10.3a) was due to over-representation in that analysis of the cardiac surgery studies: three of the six RCTs included in that analysis (i.e. the studies by van de Watering et al., Bilgin et al. and Wallis et al.) had been conducted in open-heart surgery. Across all five RCTs conducted in cardiac surgery (Figure 10.3b), there was a 72% increase in mortality in association with non-WBC-reduced ABT (summary OR = 1.72; 95% CI, 1.05–2.81; $p < 0.05$). In contrast, across the six RCTs conducted in other surgical settings, there was no ABT effect (summary OR = 0.99; 95% CI, 0.73–1.33; $p > 0.05$).

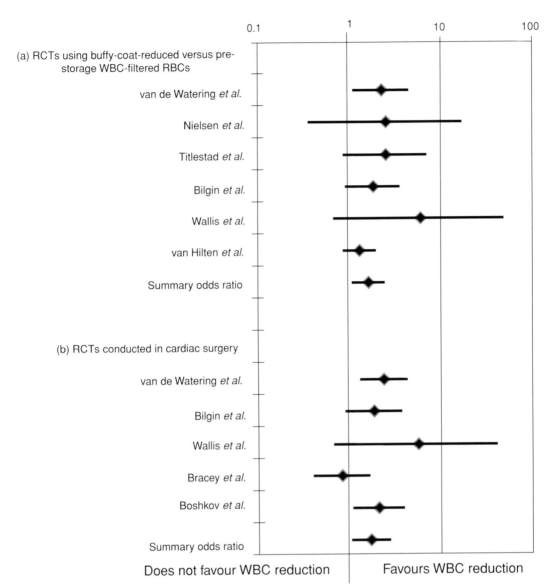

Figure 10.3   RCTs investigating the association of non-WBC-reduced ABT with short-term (up to 3-month post-transfusion), all-cause mortality and transfusing buffy-coat-reduced versus pre-storage filtered allogeneic RBCs (a) or conducted in cardiac surgery (b). For each RCT, the figure shows the OR of short-term mortality, as calculated from an intention-to-treat analysis; and the summary OR across the depicted RCTs, as calculated from a meta-analysis. A deleterious ABT effect (and thus a benefit from WBC reduction) is demonstrated by an OR > 1, provided that the effect is statistically significant ($p < 0.05$; i.e. provided that the associated 95% CI does not include the null value of 1). For the references to the listed studies, see Further Reading, Vamvakas & Blajchman (2007).

Thus, the ABT-related mortality risk, which is not seen in any other setting, may relate to another effect present in patients undergoing cardiac surgery. Bioactive lipids that accumulate during storage and/or AMCs may act as a second inflammatory insult, compounding the diffuse inflammatory response related to exposure to the extracorporeal circuit, and predisposing to MOF and mortality. Thus, the effect seen in cardiac surgery may be pro-inflammatory rather than immunomodulatory. However, this explanation is speculative as, hitherto, no cardiac surgery RCT has reported an association between non-WBC-reduced (versus WBC-reduced) ABT and MOF.

Conclusions

TRIM appears to be a real biologic phenomenon resulting in at least one established beneficial clinical effect in humans, the enhanced survival of renal allografts in patients receiving pre-transplant ABT, but the existence of deleterious clinical TRIM effects manifest across other clinical settings has not yet been confirmed by adequately powered RCTs. Except for cardiac surgery, there is no setting where the results of the RCTs of deleterious TRIM effects have been consistent. In cardiac surgery patients, the use of non-WBC-reduced ABT has been consistently associated with increased mortality, but, even in this setting, the reasons for the excess deaths remain elusive.

The other TRIM effects shown in Figures 10.2b and 10.3a, the one on postoperative infection prevented by post-storage filtration, and the one on short-term mortality mediated by non-WBC-reduced ABT of buffy-coat-reduced RBCs, appear to contradict current theories about TRIM pathogenesis, because they are not accompanied by similar (or larger) ABT effects prevented by pre-storage filtration or mediated by buffy-coat-rich RBCs. The effect prevented by post-storage filtration may be due to the inclusion in that analysis of two early studies by Jensen *et al.* that transfused blood products no longer used today (non-WBC-reduced versus WBC-reduced allogeneic whole blood or post-storage filtered, WBC-reduced allogeneic RBCs).

These studies reported extraordinarily large adverse TRIM effects (Figure 10.2b). No TRIM effect is detected if these studies are excluded from the meta-analysis.

The effect on mortality mediated by buffy-coat-reduced RBCs may be due to over-representation in that analysis of the cardiac surgery RCTs. Thus, the only adverse TRIM effect of non-WBC-reduced ABT that has been clinically documented in humans is increased mortality in cardiac surgery. Until further studies are conducted to pinpoint the mechanisms for these excess deaths (or to refute this association), we believe that all cellular blood components transfused in cardiac surgery should be WBC-reduced products. At this time, however, the totality of the evidence from RCTs does not support a policy of universal WBC reduction introduced specifically to prevent TRIM, although universal WBC reduction can be justified based on other clinical benefits of WBC reduction.

The evidence for such a policy decision based on TRIM data may not be available, because the requisite adequately powered studies have not been conducted. The design of the available RCTs has not been based on specific hypotheses about the mechanisms of TRIM formulated in the preclinical studies. For example, animal models of ABT and tumour growth have convincingly documented that allogeneic blood containing functional dendritic cells can facilitate the growth of selected tumours. However, none of the available RCTs has transfused fresh, non-WBC-reduced RBCs to test this theory, or has enrolled patients with tumours whose growth could be augmented by ABT.

Moreover, it is possible that much of the voluminous literature on adverse TRIM effects may have been focusing on the 'wrong' outcomes: searching for impairments in immunity rather than for organ dysfunction. In the Canadian 'before-and-after' study of premature infants, there was no difference in deaths or in infections between infants transfused with non-WBC-reduced RBCs before implementation of WBC reduction and infants transfused with WBC-reduced RBCs after implementation of universal WBC reduction. However, there was a difference in several secondary outcomes involving several organ systems (e.g. bronchopulmonary dysplasia, retinopathy of prematurity, necrotising enterocolitis), an observation consistent with a diffuse pro-inflammatory microvascular effect of allogeneic WBCs or their products. Although this explanation is a data-derived hypothesis offered by the authors to account for their findings, it is indicative of a shift that is currently occurring in this area of investigation (from purported deleterious 'immunomodulatory' effects towards postulated adverse 'pro-inflammatory' effects). Whether such 'pro-inflammatory' ABT effects will be documented by future research remains to be seen.

Key points

1 TRIM is a real biologic phenomenon, resulting in at least one established beneficial clinical effect in humans (enhancement of renal-allograft survival).

2 The existence of deleterious clinical TRIM effects has not yet been confirmed by adequately powered RCTs.

3 In cardiac surgery, transfusion of WBC-reduced (compared with non-WBC-reduced) allogeneic RBCs appears to reduce short-term (up to 3 months post-transfusion) all-cause mortality, but the reasons for the observed excess deaths remain elusive.

4 Based on the available data, WBC reduction of all cellular blood components – introduced specifically for the prevention of adverse TRIM effects – is indicated in cardiac surgery.

Further reading

Blajchman MA & Bordin JO. Mechanisms of transfusion-associated immunosuppression. *Curr Opin Hematol* 1994;1:457–461.

Bordin JO, Bardossy L & Blajchman MA. Growth enhancement of established tumors by allogeneic blood transfusion in experimental animals and its amelioration by leukodepletion: the importance of timing of the leukodepletion. *Blood* 1994;84:344–348.

Fergusson D, Hébert PC, Lee SK *et al.* Clinical outcomes following institution of universal leukoreduction of blood transfusions for premature infants. *JAMA* 2003;289:1950–1956.

Ghio M, Contini P, Mazzei C *et al.* Soluble HLA Class I, HLA Class II, and Fas ligand in blood components: a possible key to explain the immunomodulatory effects of allogeneic blood transfusion. *Blood* 1999;93:1770–1777.

Hébert PC, Fergusson D, Blajchman MA *et al.* Clinical outcomes following institution of the Canadian universal leukoreduction program for red blood cell transfusions. *JAMA* 2003;289:1941–1949.

Opelz G, Sengar DP, Mickey MR *et al.* Effect of blood transfusions on subsequent kidney transplants. *Transplant Proc* 1973;5:253–259.

Vamvakas E & Blajchman MA. Universal white-cell reduction: the case for and against. *Transfusion* 2001;41:691–712.

Vamvakas EC & Blajchman MA (eds). *Immunomodulatory Effects of Blood Transfusion*. Bethesda, MD: AABB Press, 1999, 295 pp.

Vamvakas EC & Blajchman MA. Deleterious clinical effects of transfusion-associated immunomodulation: fact or fiction? *Blood* 2001;97:1180–1195.

Vamvakas EC & Blajchman MA. Transfusion-related immunomodulation (TRIM): an update. *Blood Rev* 2007; 21:327–348.

CHAPTER 11

Transfusion-associated graft-versus-host disease and microchimerism

Beth H. Shaz & Christopher D. Hillyer
Center for Transfusion and Cellular Therapies; Department of Pathology and Laboratory Medicine,
Emory University School of Medicine, Atlanta, Georgia, USA

Transfusion-associated graft-versus-host disease

Transfusion-associated graft-versus-host disease (TA-GVHD) is an uncommon yet highly fatal complication of cellular blood product transfusion (red blood cells (RBC), platelets and granulocytes). TA-GVHD is defined by the UK haemovigilance system Serious Hazards of Transfusion (SHOT) as fever, rash, liver dysfunction, diarrhoea, and pancytopenia occurring 1–6 weeks after transfusion, without other apparent cause. The development of GVHD requires that the product must contain immunologically competent lymphocytes and the recipient must express tissue antigens absent in the donor and must be incapable of mounting an effective immune response to destroy the foreign lymphocytes. Cellular blood products contain viable lymphocytes that can proliferate and result in TA-GVHD. Inactivation of these lymphocytes, usually through irradiation, prevents TA-GVHD. The identification of individuals at high risk for TA-GVHD, such as immune-impaired patients or those receiving products from relatives, and the subsequent requirement that these individuals receive irradiated products, reduces the incidence of TA-GVHD, but its elimination requires universal irradiation or lymphocyte inactivation of all cellular blood products.

Pathogenesis

TA-GVHD results from the engraftment of transfused donor T-lymphocytes in a recipient whose immune system is unable to reject them. The mechanism of TA-GVHD is similar to that of acute GVHD after haemopoietic progenitor cell (HPC) transplantation. Donor lymphocytes recognise recipient HLA antigens as foreign, resulting in activation and proliferation of the lymphocytes, which leads to host cell death and tissue destruction.

Clinical features

TA-GVHD is an acute illness characterised by fever, rash, pancytopenia, diarrhoea and liver dysfunction which begins 4–30 days (median 8–10 days) after transfusion and results in death within 3 weeks from symptom onset in over 90% of the cases. In neonates the clinical manifestations are similar,

Practical Transfusion Medicine, 3rd edition. Edited by Michael F. Murphy and Derwood H. Pamphilon. © 2009 Blackwell Publishing, ISBN: 978-1-4051-8196-9.

yet the interval between transfusion and onset is longer; the median time of onset of fever is 28 days, rash 30 days, and death 51 days. Fever is usually the presenting symptom followed by an erythematous maculopapular rash, which begins on the face and trunk and spreads to the extremities. The liver dysfunction usually manifests as an obstructive jaundice or an acute hepatitis. Gastrointestinal complications include nausea, anorexia or massive diarrhoea. Leucopenia and pancytopenia develop later and progressively become more severe, which is the primary reason for death resulting from sepsis, candidiasis and multiorgan failure.

Diagnosis

The diagnosis of TA-GVHD is usually based on the characteristic clinical manifestations, pathologic findings on tissue biopsy, and if possible evidence of donor-derived lymphocytes in the recipient's blood or affected tissues. Laboratory data demonstrate pancytopenia and abnormal liver function tests. Skin biopsy changes include epidermal basal cell vacuolisation and mononuclear cell infiltration. Liver biopsy findings include degeneration of the small bile ducts, periportal mononuclear infiltrates and cholestasis. The bone marrow is usually hypocellular or aplastic, which is the primary contrast between TA-GVHD and GVHD occurring after HPC transplantation. The discovery of donor lymphocytes or DNA in the patient's peripheral blood or tissue biopsy with the appropriate clinical picture confirms the diagnosis. Donor-derived DNA is usually detected using polymerase chain reaction (PCR)-based HLA typing, but other methods include the use of restriction fragment length polymorphisms, variable-number tandem repeat analysis, microsatellite markers and cytogenetics.

Treatment

Most treatments of TA-GVHD are largely ineffective though corticosteroids, antithymocyte globulin and ciclosporin are often employed after treatment with growth factors. However, there are reports of spontaneous resolution and successful treatment with a combination of ciclosporin, steroids and OKT3 (anti-CD3 monoclonal antibody) or antithymocyte globulin. Transient improvement has been seen with nafmostat mesilate, a serine protease inhibitor that inhibits cytotoxic T lymphocytes. There are case reports of successful treatment with autologous or allogeneic HPC transplantation.

Prevention

Since treatment options for TA-GVHD are mostly unsuccessful, patients at increased risk must be identified and transfused with lymphocyte inactivated products, usually through gamma-irradiation or pathogen inactivation methods. Gamma-radiation is derived from decay of radioactive isotopes, such as caesium-137 or cobalt-60. Properly installed and maintained radioisotope instruments are safe, but their use requires radiation safety protocols and training. Some pathogen reduction technologies have been shown in human clinical trials, mouse models and other lymphocyte proliferation assays to inactivate T-lymphocytes (Table 11.1). Gamma-irradiation is the most common method used to prevent TA-GVHD, but in

Table 11.1 Potential methods for leucocyte inactivation.

Method	Leucocyte inactivation
Ultraviolet B	Inhibits TA-GVHD in dog transfusion model
8-Methoxypsoralen	Inhibits activation and proliferation
Aminomethyl trimethylpsoralen	Inhibits activation and proliferation
Amotosalen (S-59)	Inhibits activation and proliferation
	Inhibits TA-GVHD in murine transfusion model
Methylene blue	Does not inactivate leucocytes
Dimethylmethylene blue	Inactivates leucocytes
Riboflavin	Inhibits activation and proliferation
Inactine – PEN 110	Inhibits TA-GVHD in murine transfusion model
	Inhibits activation and proliferation
Thionine – Two-step process with UVB	Inhibits activation and proliferation

(Adapted by permission from Macmillan Publishers Ltd: *Bone Marrow Transplant* 2004,33(1):1–7, copyright 2004.)

Europe the use of pathogen inactivation platelets is growing.

Source and dose of ionising radiation

Both gamma-rays and X-rays inactivate T-lymphocytes and can be used to irradiate blood products. Usually gamma-rays originate from caesium-137 or cobalt-60 while X-rays are generated from linear accelerators. Quality assurance measures should be performed, including dose mapping, adjustment of irradiation time to correct for isotopic decay, assurance of no radiation leakage, timer accuracy, turntable operation, preventive maintenance, and qualitative indicator label to confirm that blood products have been properly irradiated.

The dose of irradiation must be sufficient to inhibit lymphocyte proliferation but not significantly damage RBCs, platelets, and granulocytes or their function. Assays to assess the effect of irradiation on T-lymphocyte proliferation include the mixed lymphocyte culture (MLC) assay and the limiting dilution analysis (LDA). Recommended dose varies between 15 and 50 Gy (Table 11.2). Of note, there have been three patients transfused with irradiated blood products, two at doses of 20 Gy and one at 15 Gy, who developed TA-GVHD, but it is unknown if there was a process or dose failure.

Adverse effects of irradiation

At recommended doses, radiation causes some oxidation and damage to lipid components of membranes over time. Products irradiated immediately prior to transfusion appear to be unaffected and have virtually normal function. In stored products, radiation harms RBCs, but does not appear to significantly affect platelet and granulocyte function in the clinically utilised doses. The effects on RBC products include increase in extracellular potassium and decrease in post-transfusion RBC survival. The increase in extracellular potassium is usually not of clinical significance because of post-transfusion dilution of the potassium. However, there may be certain patients who may be sensitive to the increased potassium, such as premature infants, infants receiving large RBC volumes, and those receiving intrauterine transfusions

(IUT), neonatal exchange transfusions, or intracardiac transfusions via central line catheters. The potassium increase can be prevented by either irradiating the RBC product shortly (usually within 24 hours) or washing the RBC product prior to transfusion. The in vivo viability of irradiated RBCs evaluated at 24-hour recovery is reduced by 3–10% compared to non-irradiated RBCs. As a consequence, RBC product outdate is variably shortened to 14–28 days after irradiation (Table 11.2).

Blood product factors

Age of blood

Fresh blood increases the risk of TA-GVHD. A Japanese series of cases of TA-GVHD in immunocompotent patients found that 62% of patients had received blood less than 72 hours old and a US series found about 90% of cases received blood less than 4 days old. A possible reason is with storage time lymphocytes undergo apoptosis and fail to stimulate an MLC response. Therefore, older blood may be less likely to cause TA-GVHD.

Leucocyte dose

Leucocyte reduction of blood products may decrease the risk of TA-GVHD, but it does not eliminate it. The SHOT data reported a decrease in the number of TA-GVHD cases following universal leucocyte reduction of blood components in the UK in 1999.

Blood products

All cellular blood products, including RBCs, platelets, granulocytes, whole blood, and fresh plasma (not fresh frozen plasma), contain viable T-lymphocytes that are capable of causing TA-GVHD (Table 11.2). Granulocyte transfusions are the highest risk product because they are given fresh, have a high lymphocyte count and are administered to neutropenic and immunosuppressed patients. Therefore, it is recommended that all granulocyte transfusions undergo irradiation prior to transfusion and the remaining cellular blood products be irradiated for patients at increased risk.

Table 11.2 Comparison of irradiation guidelines, including dose and indications.

	UK	United States	Japan
Techniques	Gamma-irradiation	Gamma-irradiation	Gamma-irradiation
Dose	Minimum 2500 cGy No part >5000 cGy	2500 cGy at centre of product Minimum 1500 cGy at any point Maximum 5000 cGy	Between 1500 and 5000 cGy
Type of product	All cellular products: Whole blood RBCs Platelets Granulocytes	All cellular products: Whole blood RBCs Platelets Granulocytes	All cellular products: Whole blood RBCs Platelets Granulocytes Fresh plasma
Age of product	RBCs <14 days after collection Platelets – anytime during 5 day storage For exchange or intrauterine transfusion (IUT): <24 h	RBCs – any time Platelets Granulocytes	RBCs: ≤ 3 days – regardless of recipient ≤ 14 days – if clinically indicated At any time – if patient immunocompromised
Expiration	RBCs stored for 14 days after irradiation	RBCs stored for up to 28 days after irradiation or original outdate, whichever is sooner	Irradiated RBCs – up to 3 weeks after collection
General	All blood from relatives All HLA-selected products All granulocytes	All blood from relatives All HLA-selected products	All blood from relatives All HLA-selected products
Neonates	Intrauterine transfusions Exchange transfusions in IUT babies	IUT	All
Congenital immunodeficiency	All	All	All
Allogeneic HPC transplantation	All – at least 6 mo post BMT; longer in selected patients	All	All
Autologous HPC transplantation	All – at least 3 mo post BMT; 6 mo if TBI used		
Leukaemia	No	*	Yes
Hodgkin's disease	All stages	*	All
Purine analogues (fludarabine)	All	*	
Non-Hodgkin's lymphoma	Not necessary – under review	*	
Solid tumours	No	*	All
Solid organ transplants	No	*	All
Cardiovascular surgery	No	No	Yes
AIDS	No	No	Yes

*According to policies and procedures developed by the blood bank or transfusion service.
(Modified with permission from Schroeder ML 2002).

Table 11.3 Indications for irradiated cellular blood products to prevent TA-GVHD.

Clear indications
Congenital immunodeficiency syndromes (suspected or known)
Allogeneic and autologous haemopoietic progenitor cell transplantation
Transfusions from blood relatives
HLA-matched or partially HLA-matched products (platelet transfusions)
Granulocyte transfusions
Hodgkin's disease
Treatment with purine analogue drugs (fludarabine, cladribine and deoxycoformycin)
Treatment with Campath (anti-CD52) and other drugs/antibodies that affect T-lymphocyte number or function
Intrauterine transfusions

Indications deemed appropriate by most authorities
Neonatal exchange transfusions
Pre-term infants/low birth-weight infants
Infant/child with congenital heart disease (secondary to possible DiGeorge syndrome)
Acute leukaemia
Non-Hodgkin's lymphoma and other haematologic malignancies
Aplastic anaemia
Solid tumours receiving intensive chemotherapy and/or radiotherapy
Recipient and donor pair from a genetically homogeneous population

Indications unwarranted by most authorities
Solid organ transplantation
Healthy newborns/term infants
HIV/AIDS

Patients at increased risk

Patient populations have varying risks for developing TA-GVHD (Table 11.3). It is difficult to quantify any of these risks because the number of these patients, number who are transfused, or number of transfusions or type of products received is unknown. The risk is therefore derived from case reports or haemovigilance data, which is biased by underrecognition, misdiagnosis, and under- and passive reporting.

Congenital immunodeficiency patients

The first reported cases of TA-GVHD occurred in the 1960s in children with T-lymphocyte congenital immunodeficiency syndromes. Children with severe congenital immunodeficiency syndromes (SCID) and with variable immunodeficiency syndromes, such as Wiskott–Aldrich and DiGeorge syndromes, have developed TA-GVHD. These children may be transfused prior to the recognition of these syndromes. This appears true for at least two cases in young infants in Canada. Because of the possibility of the patient not being known to be immunodeficient, it may be prudent to irradiate all blood components for children under a certain age. This is particularly true with infants undergoing cardiac surgery who may have unrecognised DiGeorge syndrome. In three reported cases of TA-GVHD in SCID patients, allogeneic HPC transplantation was successful in treating the disease. It is recommended that all patients with suspected or confirmed congenital immunodeficiency receive irradiated products.

Allogeneic and autologous HPC recipients

Both allogeneic and autologous HPC transplant recipients are at increased risk of TA-GVHD. Patients who undergo allogeneic HPC transplantation have received irradiated blood products routinely for over 40 years. Multiple organisations, including The European School of Haematology (ESH), European Group for Blood and Marrow Transplantation (EMBT), and Foundation for the Accreditation of Cellular Therapy (FACT), recommend irradiated blood products for allogeneic and autologous HPC recipients, but it is unclear for how long before and after transplantation these patients require irradiated blood products.

Leukaemia and lymphoma patients

Patients with haematologic malignancies are at increased risk for TA-GVHD, especially patients with Hodgkin's disease (HD). Twenty cases were reported in patients with malignant lymphoma, 13 in association with HD and 7 with NHL, and all undergoing therapy for active disease at the time. Five of thirteen cases reported to SHOT were associated with haematologic malignancies (Table 11.4).

Table 11.4 Cases of TA-GVHD reported to SHOT 1996 through 2001*.

Year	Number of cases	Case	Diagnosis and/or possible risk factor	RBCs and/or platelets leukodeple-tion	Donor-recipient HLA haplotype share
1996–1997	4	1	Immunodeficient neonate, not diagnosed at time of transfusion	No	Reported as haplotype share; no other details provided
		2	Epistaxis, age 88	No	NK
		3	B-cell NHL	No	NK
		4	B-cell NHL	No	NK
1997–1998	4	5	Waldenstom's macroglobulinaemia	No	Donor reported as homozygous; no other details provided; patient's HLA type not determined
		6	B-cell NHL	No	Yes; donor homozygous: A1; B8; DR17 Patient: A1, A31; B7, B8, Bw6; Cw7; DR17; DQ2
		7	CABG, RBCs less than 3 days old	No	Yes; donor homozygous: A*01; B*0801; DRB1*0301
		8	ITP, treated with prednisolone	No	NK
1998–1999	4	9	Myeloma, 6 units of RBCs, all less than 7 days old	Yes	NK
		10	Male, age 53; uncharacterised immunodeficiency; HIV-negative	No	NK; 100% XX cells in marrow
		11	CABG, also received platelets	No	NK (32 donors)
		12	CABG	No	Donor homozygous: A*01; B*0801; Cw*0701/06/07; DRB1*0301; DQB1*0201/02 Patient: A*01, A*3301/03; B*0801, B*14202/03; Cw*0701/06/07; Cw*0802; DRB1*0301, DRB1*0701/03; DQB1*03032/06, DQB1*0201/02
1999–2000	0				
2000–2001	1	13	Relapsed ALL on UKALL R2. Died despite 'rescue' HPC allograft	Yes	NK; chimerism shown by variable-number tandem repeat analysis but no donor HLA typing performed
Total	**13**				

*No cases were reported from 2002 through 2005.
CABG, coronary artery bypass grafting; ITP, immune thrombocytopenia; NHL, non-Hodgkin's lymphoma; NKs, not known.
(Reprinted with permission from Williamson *et al.*, 2007).

In the 1970s and 1980s, cases of TA-GVHD occurred in patients with acute leukaemia undergoing chemotherapy; the majority of these patients had received granulocyte transfusions. It is recommended that patients with haematologic malignancies receive irradiated products; however, it is less clear if this requirement should be only during active treatment.

Recipients of fludarabine and other purine analogues as well as other drugs/antibodies that affect T-lymphocyte number or function

TA-GVHD was initially reported in patients with CLL receiving fludarabine, which is a purine analogue and results in profound lymphopenia. There are nine cases of TA-GVHD in CLL, AML, and NHL patients who received fludarabine up to 11 months prior to transfusion. In addition, TA-GVHD occurred in a patient who received fludarabine for autoimmune disease. Other purine analogues, including deoxycoformycin (pentostatin) and chlorodeoxyadenosine (cladribine), have been associated with the development of TA-GVHD. It is recommended that all patients who have received fludarabine or other purine analogues as well as Campath (anti-CD52) or other drugs/antibodies that affect T-lymphocyte function or number be transfused with irradiated products; however, it is unclear if this requirement should only be for at least a year and until recovery from the resulting lymphopenia following the administration of these drugs.

Fetus and neonate

Fetuses and neonates have immature immune systems and may be at increased risk of TA-GVHD. In neonates, most cases of TA-GVHD reported are in those with congenital immunodeficiency or that received products from related donors. At least ten cases were reported after neonatal exchange transfusions; four occurred in infants who had previously received IUT. Seven cases were in preterm infants (excluding those who received a product from a relative). A single case report involved a full-term infant receiving extracorporeal membrane oxygenation (ECMO). The use of irradiated products for fetal and neonatal transfusions is recommended

for exchange transfusions and IUT, preterm infants, infants with congenital immunodeficiency, and those receiving products from relatives; its need is less clear for other neonatal transfusions.

Aplastic anaemia patients

Since patients with aplastic anaemia are usually treated with intensive chemotherapy regimens and possible HPC transplantation, some authorities recommend they receive irradiated products, especially during myelosuppressive therapy.

Patients receiving chemotherapy and immunotherapy

TA-GVHD has occurred in patients with solid tumours, including neuroblastoma, rhabdomyosarcoma, and bladder and small cell lung cancer, during intensive myeloablative therapy. Therefore, it is recommended that patients with solid tumours receive irradiated products, especially during myelosuppressive therapy.

Solid organ transplantation recipients

GVHD is a rare complication of solid organ transplantation, which usually results from the passenger lymphocytes contained within the solid organ and not from transfusion, even though these individuals are highly immunosuppressed and transfused. There have been four cases of TA-GVHD in solid organ transplant recipients; one was a liver transplant recipient with pre-existing pancytopenia, one a heart transplant recipient, and two were inconclusive cases in kidney recipients. The risk of TA-GVHD in solid organ transplant recipients appears low and the use of irradiated products is generally considered to be unwarranted.

Human immunodeficiency virus (HIV) and acquired immunodeficiency syndrome (AIDS) patients

HIV/AIDS is not considered a risk factor for TA-GVHD as there is only a single case report of a child with AIDS developing transient TA-GVHD. It is postulated that HIV infects the transfused T-lymphocytes. The use of irradiated blood products in HIV/AIDS patients is not warranted, but approximately a quarter of institutions in the US choose to take this precaution likely because of the immunosuppresive nature HIV/AIDS and the high degree of fatality of TA-GVHD.

Cardiovascular surgery patients

Prior to the Japanese changing their irradiation policies, their reported incidence of TA-GVHD following cardiovascular surgery was 0.15–0.47%. Fifty-six of the 122 cases of TA-GVHD reported in Japan from 1985 to 1993 were patients after cardiovascular surgery; 28% used blood from a relative and 72% used blood less than 72 hours old. They also reported a lower risk for women than men possibly secondary to women having previous exposure to leucocytes during pregnancy and childbirth. There are 5 cases reported in the US and the UK (Table 11.4). Possible reasons for the increased risk are that the RBC products are usually less than 72 hours old and cardiac surgery may result in reduced cell-mediated immunity. The recommendation for irradiated products is warranted in Japan but not in the US or UK at this time.

Immunocompetent patients

TA-GVHD has been reported in immunocompetent patients, especially those who received transfusions of blood products donated by close relatives. The majority of cases reported in immunocompetent patients occurred with the use of fresh whole blood from a close relative. In a review of 122 cases of TA-GVHD in immunocompetent Japanese patients, 67% had not received products from a related donor, and of the 66 non-cardiovascular surgery patients, 39 had solid tumours and 27 had other conditions. The risk of receiving a blood product from a homozygous donor is greatest in populations with limited HLA haplotype polymorphisms, such as Japan (Table 11.5). The frequency of reported cases is substantially lower than these estimates, which may be a result of unrecognised and/or unreported cases, lymphocytes in blood products that are either non-viable or insufficient to cause disease, and/or recipients may be able to destroy the donor lymphocytes based on minor HLA differences between donor and recipient. Irradiation of products from close relatives and HLA matched products is recommended, but the risk is minimal for other immunocompetent patients.

Table 11.5 Frequency of homozygous HLA donors in various populations.

Frequency of transfusion from homozygous donors to potential heterozygous recipients		
Population	Parent/child	Sibling	Unrelated
US whites	1:475	1:902	1:7174
Japan	1:102	1:193	1:874
Canada whites	1:154	1:294	1:1664
Germany	1:220	1:424	1:3144
Korea	1:183	1:356	1:3220
Spain	1:226	1:438	1:3552
South African blacks	1:286	1:558	1:5519
Italy	1:434	1:854	1:12870
France	1:762	1:2685	1:16835

Guidelines and requirements for irradiated products

In 1989, AABB institutional members were surveyed about their blood product irradiation practice. Approximately 10.1% of the products transfused were irradiated, which has remained fairly constant. The indications included patients with allogeneic HPC transplantation (88%), autologous HPC transplantation (81.4%), congenital immunodeficiency syndrome (62.4%), premature newborn (53.9%), leukaemia (51.4%), organ transplantation (40.5%), HD (34.0%), NHL (32.0%), HLA matched product (31.0%), AIDS (24.5%), term newborn (24.0%), and solid tumour (20.0%). This survey highlighted the need for guidelines. In 1996, the UK published guidelines for the use of gamma-irradiation to prevent TA-GVHD (Table 11.2) as well as the American Society for Clinical Pathology. Japan has elected to irradiate all blood products.

Only 2 of the 13 TA-GVHD cases reported to SHOT fulfilled the current UK guideline criteria as requiring irradiated blood products, which highlights the need to continually monitor and revise the definition of high-risk individuals.

Universal irradiation

As case reports cited above indicate, TA-GVHD can occur in immunocompetent patients and in individuals where degree of immunocompromise was not known or properly identified prior to transfusion. Given that TA-GVHD is fatal in almost all cases and the risk of radiation of a product includes only minimal cost and effect on product potency, many authorities consider that the cost: benefit ratio is weighted in favour of universal irradiation. Consideration of universal irradiation should be undertaken on a local, regional, or national basis, as appropriate.

Haemovigilance

Some countries have begun comprehensive tracking systems for adverse events of blood transfusion (Chapter 18). SHOT data from 1996 to 2005 revealed 11 cases of TA-GVHD occurred with the use of non-leucocyte-reduced and only 2 cases with leucocyte-reduced products (Table 11.4). In addition there were 405 reports where irradiated products were indicated and were not used due to error. From 1992 to 2000, 2 cases of TA-GVHD have been reported to Health Canada with the addition of 1–2 cases that were presented but not reported. Irradiated blood products were used in Canada for highly immunocompromised patients and patients receiving directed donation from close relatives. With this information, it is estimated that the risk of TA-GVHD in Canada is less than 1 per million products transfused. The continued occurrence of TA-GVHD is likely from lack of agreement on the level of immunodeficiency that results in increased risk and patients with immunocompromised conditions who receive non-irradiated products either secondary to not being identified prior to transfusion or the product not being irradiated by error. On the other hand, the low incidence reported may be secondary to underreporting and/or under-recognition, the fact that lymphocytes are no longer capable of proliferating because the blood is older by the time of transfusion, the risk is decreased by leucocyte reduction of blood products, and the multiracial nature of Canadians.

Transfusion-associated microchimerism

Chimerism is defined as the presence of two genetically distinct cell lines in a single organism. Haemopoietic chimerism refers to the persistence of allogeneic donor lymphocytes in a recipient. Microchimerism (MC) occurs when these donor cells represent a small population (less than 5%) and can be a consequence of pregnancy, organ transplantation, or transfusion. With increased sensitivity of methods, MC can be detected not infrequently after transfusion, but the conditions that facilitate and consequences of this phenomenon are unknown.

Normal clearance of transfused lymphocytes

In a study investigating the clearance of lymphocytes in immunocompetent recipients, three phases were found: first, 99.9% of the lymphocytes were cleared over the first 2 days, second, there was a 1-log increase in the number of circulating donor lymphocytes on days 3–5, and lastly there was a secondary clearance. It was postulated that this transient increase in donor lymphocytes represents one arm of an in vivo mixed lymphocyte reaction with activated donor T-lymphocytes proliferating in reaction to HLA-incompatible recipient cells.

Clinical data

TA-MC has been reported most extensively in trauma patients, but has also been reported in sickle cell disease and thalassemia patients. HIV-positive individuals do not have sustained TA-MC. Irradiation of products prevents TA-MC. Leucocyte reduction of blood products does not decrease the incidence of TA-MC. In addition, TA-MC can be sustained for decades after transfusion. Age, sex, injury severity score, splenectomy and number of units transfused did not correlate with the establishment of TA-MC in trauma patients. When patients were evaluated for symptoms suggestive of chronic GVHD several months after transfusion, TA-MC did not correlate with these symptoms. One study reported decrease in donor-specific lymphocyte response in TA-MC trauma patients versus non-TA-MC patients. TA-MC may occur, especially in trauma patients, but its conditions and consequences are unknown.

Testing for TA-MC

Detection of TA-MC requires the ability to detect small amounts of minor population DNA among large amounts of host DNA and selection of optimal genetic differences. One technique is to use real-time PCR. Initially this technique was to look for the Y chromosome in women who received blood transfusions from at least one male donor. This has been expanded to a panel of 12 HLA-DR polymorphisms. A third improvement was the addition of a panel of 12 insertion/deletion (InDel) polymorphisms.

Testing limitations

The ability to detect TA-MC is limited by sample volume and sampling error. Large sample volume will create too much DNA and result in difficulties in testing. Sampling error is likely when an extremely low level of TA-MC exists. Techniques that look for Y chromosome in women transfused with male blood products are limited, because this can result from the previous carrying of a male fetus.

Clinical consequences

To date, no clear relationship of TA-MC to clinical outcomes has been elucidated. To determine the association between TA-MC and autoimmune or other diseases, important confounding factors would need to be accounted for, and long follow-up would be needed as these diseases can take years to develop and may result in vague symptoms. Currently, the conditions that facilitate TA-MC and its consequences remain to be established.

Key points

1 TA-GVHD is a rare yet highly fatal complication of cellular blood product transfusion.
2 TA-GVHD can be prevented by using irradiated or leucocyte-inactivated blood products.

3 Patients at increased risk for TA-GVHD include those who are immune impaired and those receiving blood products donated from relatives.
4 Leucocyte dose and age of the blood product, HLA matching between the donor and the recipient, and the immune state of the recipient contribute to the likelihood of developing TA-GVHD.
5 With increased sensitivity of methods to detect chimerism, microchimerism can be detected not infrequently after transfusion, but the conditions that facilitate it and its consequences are unknown.

Further reading

Corash L & Lin L. Novel processes for inactivation of leukocytes to prevent transfusion-associated graft-versus-host disease. *Bone Marrow Transplant* 2004;33(1):1–7.

BCSH Blood Transfusion Task Force. Guidelines on gamma irradiation of blood components for the prevention of transfusion-associated graft-versus-host disease. *Transfus Med* 1996;6(3):261–271.

Hume HA & Preiksaitis JB. Transfusion associated graft-versus-host disease, cytomegalovirus infection and HLA alloimmunization in neonatal and pediatric patients. *Transfus Sci* 1999;21(1):73–95.

Moroff G & Luban NLC. The irradiation of blood and blood components to prevent graft-versus-host disease: technical issues and guidelines. *Transfus Med Rev* 1997;11(1):15–26.

Schroeder ML. Transfusion-associated graft-versus-host disease. *Br J Haematol* 2002;117(2):275–287.

Utter GH, Reed WF, Lee TH & Busch MP. Transfusion-associated microchimerism. *Vox Sang* 2007;93(3):188–195.

Williamson LM, Stainsby D, Jones H *et al.* The impact of universal leukodepletion of the blood supply on hemovigilance reports of posttransfusion purpura and transfusion-associated graft-versus-host disease. *Transfusion* 2007;47(8):1455–1467.

CHAPTER 12
Post-transfusion purpura

Michael F. Murphy

University of Oxford; NHS Blood and Transplant and Department of Haematology, John Radcliffe Hospital, Oxford, UK

In 1959, van Loghem and colleagues described a 51-year-old woman who developed severe thrombocytopenia 7 days after elective surgery. The thrombocytopenia did not respond to transfusion of fresh blood, but there was a spontaneous recovery after 3 weeks. The patient's serum contained a strong platelet alloantibody, which enabled the description of the first human platelet antigen (HPA) (Zw, see Chapter 5). However, the relationship of platelet alloimmunisation to post-transfusion thrombocytopenia was not recognised until 2 years later when Shulman and colleagues studied a similar case, naming the antibody anti-Pl[A1] (later shown to be the same as anti-Zw), and coined the term post-transfusion purpura (PTP).

Definition

PTP is an acute episode of severe thrombocytopenia occurring about a week after a blood transfusion. It usually affects HPA-1a-negative women who have previously been alloimmunised by pregnancy. The transfusion precipitating PTP causes a secondary immune response, boosting the HPA-1a antibodies, although the mechanism of destruction of the patient's own HPA-1a-negative platelets remains uncertain.

Practical Transfusion Medicine, 3rd edition. Edited by Michael F. Murphy and Derwood H. Pamphilon. © 2009 Blackwell Publishing, ISBN: 978-1-4051-8196-9.

Incidence

PTP is considered to be a rare complication of transfusion. Over 200 cases had been reported in the literature till 1991. However, this may not reflect the true incidence of PTP, which is not known. Forty-three cases were reported in the first 6 years of the Serious Hazards of Transfusion (SHOT) scheme during which approximately 20 million blood components were transfused, giving an approximate incidence of 1 case in 465,000 transfusions. Since the introduction of universal leucocyte reduction of blood components in the UK in 1999, there has been a reduction in the number of reported cases from about 10 per year in the late 1990s to just 2 in 2005, and none in 2006.

The low incidence of PTP relative to the 2.5% of the population who are HPA-1a negative and at risk of the condition raises the question of individual susceptibility. As in neonatal alloimmune thrombocytopenia (NAIT), the antibody response to HPA-1a is strongly associated with a certain HLA class II type (HLA-DR3*0101) (Chapter 5).

Clinical features

PTP typically occurs in middle-aged or elderly women (mean 57 years, range 21–80), although it has also been reported in a small number of males. All patients, apart from rare exceptions, have had previous exposure to platelet antigens through pregnancy and/or transfusion. The interval

117

between pregnancy and/or transfusion and PTP is variable: the shortest being 3 years and the longest 52 years. The initial maternal sensitisation to platelet antigens during pregnancy in females subsequently developing PTP is rarely of sufficient degree to cause NAIT.

Blood components implicated in causing PTP are:
- whole blood;
- packed red cells; and
- red cell concentrates.

There are two reports of PTP following the transfusion of plasma.

Severe thrombocytopenia and bleeding usually occur about 5–12 days after transfusion; shorter or longer intervals are rare. The onset is usually rapid, with the platelet count falling from normal to $<10 \times 10^9$/L within 12–24 hours. Haemorrhage is very common and sometimes severe. There is typically widespread purpura and bleeding from mucous membranes and the gastrointestinal and urinary tracts. In many cases the precipitating transfusion has been associated with a febrile non-haemolytic transfusion reaction, probably due to the presence of HLA antibodies stimulated by previous pregnancy and/or transfusion.

Megakaryocytes are present in normal or increased numbers in the bone marrow and coagulation screening tests are normal in uncomplicated PTP.

In untreated cases the thrombocytopenia usually lasts between 7 and 28 days although it occasionally persists for longer.

Differential diagnosis

The rapid onset of severe thrombocytopenia in a middle-aged or elderly woman should arouse suspicion of PTP and a history of recent blood transfusion should be sought. The differential diagnosis includes other causes of acute immune thrombocytopenia such as:
- autoimmune thrombocytopenia;
- drug-induced thrombocytopenia, e.g. heparin-induced thrombocytopenia (HIT);
- non-immune platelet consumption, e.g. disseminated intravascular coagulation (DIC) and thrombotic thrombocytopenic purpura (TTP);

- a less likely possibility is passively transfused platelet-specific alloantibodies from an immunised blood donor when thrombocytopenia occurs within the first 48 hours after the transfusion; and
- pseudothrombocytopenia due to ethylenediamine tetra-acetic acid (EDTA)-dependent antibodies should be excluded in any patient with unexplained thrombocytopenia by examination of the blood film.

Laboratory investigations

A preliminary diagnosis of PTP on clinical grounds needs to be confirmed by the detection of platelet-specific alloantibodies. The majority (80–90%) of cases of PTP are associated with the development of HPA-1a antibodies in HPA-1a-negative patients. Antibodies against HPA-1b, HPA-3a, HPA-3b, HPA-4a, HPA-5a, HPA-5b, HPA-15b and Nak[a] have been associated with PTP, and occasionally multiple antibodies are present, e.g. anti-HPA-1a, anti-HPA-2b and anti-HPA-3a were found in one case.

HLA antibodies are often present in patients with PTP. There is no evidence that they are involved in causing PTP but their presence complicates the detection of platelet-specific antibodies. Modern platelet serological techniques such as the monoclonal antibody immobilisation of platelet antigens (MAIPA) assay are useful for resolving mixtures of antibodies in patients with PTP (Chapter 5).

Pathophysiology

The time course of events in PTP is shown in Figure 12.1. A blood transfusion triggers a rapid secondary antibody response against HPA-1a, and there is acute thrombocytopenia about a week after the transfusion. It is difficult to understand why the patient's own HPA-1a-negative platelets are destroyed. There remains no generally accepted mechanism to explain this although a number of suggestions have been made as follows:
- Transfused HPA-1a-positive platelets release HPA-1a antigen, which is adsorbed on to the patient's HPA-1a-negative platelets, making them a target for anti-HPA-1a. Support for this hypothesis

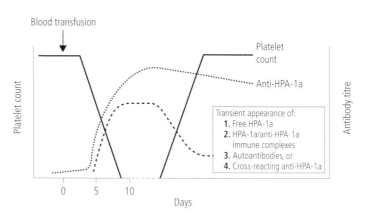

Figure 12.1 A typical time course of post-transfusion purpura. Purpura and severe thrombocytopenia occurred 5–10 days after a blood transfusion. The figure indicates the secondary antibody response of anti-HPA-1a, and the postulated transient appearance of free HPA-1a antigen in the plasma, which binds to HPA-1a-negative platelets, HPA-1a/anti-HPA-1a immune complexes, platelet autoantibodies or cross-reacting HPA-1a antibodies.

comes from observations such as the elution of anti-HPA-1a from HPA-1a-negative platelets in some cases of PTP, and the demonstration of the adsorption of HPA-1a antigen on to HPA-1a-negative platelets after incubation with plasma from HPA-1a-positive stored blood.

• The released HPA-1a antigen forms immune complexes with anti-HPA-1a in the plasma, and the immune complexes become bound to the patient's platelets, causing their destruction.

• The transfusion stimulates the production of platelet autoantibodies as well as anti-HPA-1a. Evidence in favour of this mechanism is the detection of positive reactions of some PTP patients' sera from the acute thrombocytopenic phase with autologous platelets.

• In the early phase of the secondary antibody response, anti-HPA-1a may be produced which has the ability to cross-react with autologous as well as allogeneic platelets.

Management

Immediate treatment is essential as the risk of fatal haemorrhage is greatest early in the course of PTP. In a review of 71 cases of PTP, five died within the first 10 days because of intracranial haemorrhage. The main aim of treatment is to prevent severe haemorrhage by shortening the duration of severe thrombocytopenia.

No randomised controlled trials of treatment for PTP have been carried out. Comparison of various therapeutic measures is complicated because it may be difficult to differentiate a response to treatment from a spontaneous remission in individual cases.

High-dose intravenous immunoglobulin (IVIgG) (2 g/kg given over 2 or 5 days) is the current treatment of choice, with responses in about 85% of cases; there is often a rapid and prompt increase in the platelet count (Figure 12.2). Steroids and plasma exchange were the preferred treatments before the availability of IVIgG, and plasma exchange, in particular, appeared to be effective in some but not all cases.

Platelet transfusions are usually ineffective in raising the platelet count but may be needed in large doses to control severe bleeding in the acute phase, particularly in patients who have recently undergone surgery before there has been a response to high-dose IVIgG. There is no evidence that platelet concentrates from HPA-1a-negative platelets are more effective than those from random donors in the acute thrombocytopenic phase; the dose of platelets may be more important than the platelet type of the donor platelets. There is no evidence to suggest that further transfusions in the acute phase prolong the duration or severity of thrombocytopenia.

Platelet transfusions have been reported to cause severe febrile and occasionally pulmonary reactions in patients with PTP; these were probably due to HLA antibodies reacting against leucocytes in non-leucocyte-reduced platelet concentrates.

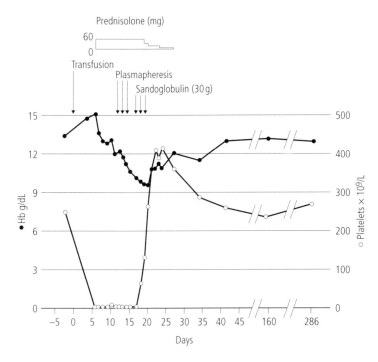

Figure 12.2 Haematological course of a patient with post-transfusion purpura showing the onset of profound thrombocytopenia 6 days after a blood transfusion. Initial treatment with random platelet concentrates caused rigors and bronchospasm, and there was no platelet increment. There was no response to prednisolone (60 mg/day) or plasma exchange (2.5 L/day for 3 days), but there was a prompt remission following high-dose IVIgG (30 g/day for 3 days). (Redrawn with permission from Berney et al., 1985.)

Prevention of recurrence of PTP

Recurrence of PTP has been reported. However, it is unpredictable and has usually occurred following a delay of 3 years or more after the first episode. The patient should be issued with a card to indicate that he/she has previously had PTP and 'special' blood is required for future transfusions.

Future transfusion policy should be to use red cell and platelet concentrates from HPA-compatible donors or autologous transfusion. If these are not available, leucocyte-depleted blood components are considered to be safe. There have been occasional reports of recurrence of PTP with leucocyte-reduced red cell concentrates, but the implicated components would not have complied with current standards for leucocyte reduction.

Key points

1 Post-transfusion purpura (PTP) is characterised by an acute episode of severe thrombocytopenia occurring about a week after a transfusion.

2 The pathophysiology remains uncertain.

3 PTP typically occurs in HPA-1a-negative women who have been alloimmunised by pregnancy.

4 Haemorrhage is common and sometimes severe, although the thrombocytopenia resolves spontaneously within a few weeks.

5 High-dose intravenous immunoglobulin (IVIgG) (2 g/kg given over 2 or 5 days) is the current treatment of choice to shorten the duration of thrombocytopenia, with responses in about 85% of cases.

6 Universal leucocyte reduction of blood components in the UK has resulted in a marked reduction in the number of reported cases.

Further reading

Becker T, Panzer S, Maas D et al. High-dose intravenous immunoglobulin for post-transfusion purpura. Br J Haematol 1985;61:149–155.

Berney SI, Metcalfe P, Wathen NC & Waters AH. Post-transfusion purpura responding to high-dose intravenous IgG: further observations on pathogenesis. Br J Haematol 1985;61:627–632.

Kr von dem Borne AEG & van derPlas-van Dalen CM. Further observations on post-transfusion purpura. *Br J Haematol* 1986;62:374–375.

Kickler TS, Ness PM, Herman JH & Bell WR. Studies on the pathophysiology of post-transfusion purpura. *Blood* 1986;68:347–350.

Loghem JJ van, Dorfmeijer H, Hart M van der & Schreuder F. Serological and genetical studies on a platelet antigen (Zw). *Vox Sang* 1959;4:161–169.

Mueller-Eckhardt C. Post-transfusion purpura. *Br J Haematol* 1986;64:419–424.

Shulman NR. Post-transfusion purpura: clinical features and the mechanism of platelet destruction. In: Nance SJ. (ed.), *Clinical and Basic Science Aspects of Immunohaematology*. Arlington, VA: American Association of Blood Banks, 1991, pp. 137–154.

Shulman NR, Aster RH, Leitner A & Hiller MC. Immunoreactions involving platelets. V. Post-transfusion purpura due to a complement-fixing antibody against a genetically controlled platelet antigen. A proposed mechanism for thrombocytopenia and its relevance in 'autoimmunity'. *J Clin Invest* 1961;40:1597–1620.

Waters AH. Post-transfusion purpura. *Blood Rev* 1989;3:83–87.

CHAPTER 13

Transfusion-transmitted infections

Alan D. Kitchen[1] *& John A.J. Barbara*[2]

[1]National Transfusion Microbiology Reference Laboratory; NHS Blood and Transplant, Colindale, London, UK
[2]NHS Blood and Transplant; University of the West of England, Bristol, UK

This chapter considers the subject of transfusion-transmitted infection (TTI) by describing the range of infectious agents, including their biology and epidemiology, currently known to be transmissible by blood transfusion, transfusion-transmissible infectious agents (TIAs), and by considering the options available for their detection and the general effectiveness of screening in ensuring the microbial safety of donated blood and blood products. Although not a focus of this section, in general, the same considerations in terms of transmissible infections and screening approaches can be applied to tissue and stem cell donations. Emerging infections are considered in detail in Chapter 16.

It is only over the last 25 years that the true significance of the potential of blood transfusion as a vehicle for the transmission of infectious agents has been recognised widely. While transmission of syphilis and hepatitis B virus (HBV) has been recognised for many years, it was the identification of human immunodeficiency virus (HIV) and hepatitis C virus (HCV) that opened many eyes not only to the potential of transfusion as a route of infection, but also to its startling efficiency in the transmission of a whole range of infectious agents.

Viruses, bacteria and protozoa have been clearly demonstrated to be transmitted by transfusion of blood or blood products. More recently, the potential for the transfusion transmission of protein-based agents, prions, has been highlighted and it is in the area of these and emerging or re-emerging viruses that much current interest is focussed.

The detection of TIAs, although described in Chapter 20, merits a brief mention here in the context of understanding the roles of donor selection and laboratory screening, and the strengths and limitations of each in relation to specific TIAs.

- The process of identifying donors potentially carrying TIAs begins with donor selection.
- The identification and deferral of donors considered to be 'high risk', by activity or association, is central to donor selection, which aims to minimise any risk of TTI from donations which may have been collected from donors in the 'window period' of an infection (infectious but not at that time detectable by the screening tests performed).
- The brief assessment of donors prior to donation, even when performed thoroughly, can only be an initial filtering process to identify donors who have an identifiable exposure risk to a TIA.
- Laboratory screening remains the key step in identifying donations from infected individuals.
- The implementation of a formal quality system with effective quarantine and disposal of unsuitable donations and products is critical for both ensuring high-quality laboratory screening and minimising the risk of releasing donations containing TIAs.
- The increasing development and use of effective and safe microbial inactivation procedures, and their application to a wider range of components, is

Practical Transfusion Medicine, 3rd edition. Edited by Michael F. Murphy and Derwood H. Pamphilon. © 2009 Blackwell Publishing. ISBN: 978-1-4051-8196-9.

an additional and developing strategy in reducing further any remaining risk of TIA in certain products.

• In many countries, the screening of donated blood for a minimum set of TIAs is mandatory.

• The identification of those infectious agents for which blood needs to be screened is based on prevalence and incidence data for the particular donor population, surveillance data for other potentially transmissible agents, the pathogenic potential of the agent, and any political, social or ethical considerations that may be relevant. Thus, in most countries blood is not screened for all potential TIAs identified. The selection of those infectious agents for which blood is screened is a compromise between evidenced clinical risk to recipients and available resources.

Transmissibility of infectious agents

The reasons why specific agents are transmissible and their specific characteristics need to be considered for a full understanding of TIAs. There are four main properties that generally need to be met for an agent to be transmitted by transfusion:

• it gives rise to asymptomatic infection;
• it is present in the bloodstream;
• it is transmitted parenterally; and
• it is able to survive during storage of the blood.

However, these are not absolute, and examples exist of agents that do not meet all of these criteria, yet are transmissible by transfusion

Asymptomatic infection

The agent must be capable of giving rise to asymptomatic infection in the infected individual, such that an actively infected and thus potentially infectious individual may present as a blood donor. Any potential donor who has any recognisable clinical symptoms which could be due to an infection should be deferred. However, this does assume that the donor selection and questioning procedures are adequate, and that the donor would declare any symptoms appearing in the few weeks before donation. Thus, any infectious agent that always gives

rise to clinical symptoms, i.e. a symptomatic infection, is very unlikely to be transmitted by transfusion because an infected donor should always be identified and deferred prior to donation.

Presence in the bloodstream

An infectious agent must be present in the blood of the donor at the time of donation, in an infectious or potentially infectious form, to be transmitted by blood transfusion. TIAs are carried in the blood in a number of different ways, depending on the particular agent and the stage of infection: free in the plasma, within the leucocytes (either as infectious virions or in a latent form) or within red cells.

Free in the plasma

Several viruses, bacteria and protozoa may be carried free in the plasma, as a means of directly infecting other tissues or as part of the life cycle of the organism when it is released from infected tissues into the blood.

Carried in leucocytes

Free virions or latent forms integrated into cellular nucleic acid can be carried in leucocytes. In some cases the same agent may be found in both forms, but at different stages of infection. Latent agents persist even in the presence of specific neutralising antibody. Although some types of leucocytes will actively engulf individual infectious agents in their role as scavengers, agents that can be found in leucocytes generally specifically infect these cells as part of their life cycle. Because leucocytes are nucleated and have a normal cellular cytoplasmic organisation, once latently infected the infection may persist for the life of the cell, and ultimately the life of the individual. However, reactivation can subsequently occur and may result in acute-phase infection.

Carried in erythrocytes

Some protozoan infections include a phase in which the agent is present and actively dividing in red cells. During this phase the agent usually matures into the next stage of its life cycle before being released from red cells, either while they are still circulating or in the liver or spleen.

Parenteral transmission

In general, only those infectious agents transmitted parenterally are considered to be TIAs and are of most concern in relation to the safety of donor blood. However, there are exceptions to this; for example hepatitis A virus (HAV) has been reported to be transmitted by transfusion. Although HAV is an enterovirus transmitted by the faeco-oral route and is not normally considered to be transmissible by transfusion, cases of transmission through large-pool plasma products as well as single-donor products have been reported.

Survival during storage

Blood and blood products may be stored in a number of different physical states (e.g. whole blood, plasma, high-concentration protein solution and lyophilised material) and at a number of different temperatures (-40 to $25°C$). Any agent present in donated blood must be able to survive at least some of these storage conditions and the conditions during processing in order to infect recipients of the products. Viruses are best suited to this, and certain viruses, if present in the original donation, may be found in virtually all products prepared. This is especially true of non-enveloped viruses such as HAV and parvovirus B19. Bacteria also persist but often they may also multiply during storage, and as they die leave endotoxins in the products, which can then rapidly cause severe illness in recipients. *Treponema pallidum*, the causative agent of syphilis, is one of the more unstable organisms and will usually survive for no longer than 72 hours at $4°C$.

Types of infectious agents transmitted

Viruses, bacteria and protozoa have been demonstrated to be transmitted by transfusion. Fungi have not been reported to have been transmitted, and there is still no totally objective and substantiated evidence that prions are actually transmitted although the circumstantial evidence is extensive. However, it is difficult to produce a definitive list of transmissible agents as increasing numbers of cases of transmission of unusual infectious agents are be-

ing reported in addition to the more common 'established' TIAs.

An important factor in the increasing exposure to a larger range of potentially transmissible agents is international travel. As travel increases, individuals are being exposed to an ever-increasing range of infectious agents that are not endemic, including many potential TIAs, which they would not encounter in their country of origin or residence. Migration of individuals from endemic areas with a high prevalence of infection is also a potential risk to blood safety in non-endemic areas, or even areas of lower endemicity. Thus, blood transfusion services, especially in countries whose donor populations travel extensively, face an expanding range of infectious agents, both newly emerging and re-emerging, that need to be considered to ensure a safe blood supply. Unfortunately, in vitro screening for many of these is either not practical or not appropriate, and donor selection processes are thus the key in the identification and deferral of 'at-risk' donors. Table 13.1 provides an up-to-date list of viral, bacterial and protozoan infectious agents reported to have been transmitted by transfusion or which are considered to be potentially transmissible.

Viruses

Hepatitis viruses

The hepatitis viruses are a diverse group of viruses, including hepadnaviruses, flaviviruses and picornaviruses, all of which have been transmitted by transfusion. Although hepatitis B (HBV) and hepatitis C (HCV) are transmitted parenterally and are typical candidate transfusion-transmissible viruses, hepatitis A (HAV) and hepatitis E (HEV) may also (rarely) be transmitted parenterally when sufficiently high titres of virus are present.

Hepatitis B virus

HBV is a DNA virus and a member of the hepadnavirus family. The infectious particle, the Dane particle, comprises the DNA genome encapsulated in core protein, which is then covered by an envelope of surface proteins. The hepadnaviruses are

Table 13.1 Infectious agents reported to have been transmitted by blood transfusion.

Viruses
Hepatitis viruses
  Hepatitis A virus
  Hepatitis B virus
  Hepatitis C virus
  Hepatitis D virus (requires co-infection with hepatitis B virus)

Retroviruses
  Human immunodeficiency virus 1 and 2 (plus other subtypes)
  Human T-cell lymphotropic virus I and II

Herpes viruses
  Human cytomegalovirus
  Epstein–Barr virus
  Human herpesvirus 8

Parvoviruses
  Parvovirus B19

Miscellaneous viruses
  GBV-C: previously referred to as hepatitis G virus
  TTV
  West Nile virus

Bacteria*
Endogenous
  Treponema pallidum (syphilis)
  Borrelia burgdorferi (Lyme disease)
  Brucella melitensis (brucellosis)
  Yersinia enterocolitica/Salmonella spp.

Exogenous
  Environmental species: *Staphylococcus* spp./*Pseudomonas*/*Serratia* spp.
  Rickettsiae: *Rickettsia rickettsii* (Rocky Mountain spotted fever), *Coxiella burnetii* (Q fever)

Protozoa
  Plasmodium spp. (malaria)
  Trypanosoma cruzi (Chagas' disease)
  Toxoplasma gondii (toxoplasmosis)
  Babesia microti/divergens (babesiosis)
  Leishmania spp. (leishmaniasis)

* For a detailed review of bacterial species and frequency in relation to blood transfusion, see Chapter 16.

characterised by the production of a vast excess of surface proteins, hepatitis B surface antigen (HBsAg) in the case of HBV, and these are released into the blood along with the infectious Dane particles.

The virus is transmitted parenterally and infection may follow one of the two courses: acute infection with the subsequent clearance of the virus and development of immunity (Figure 13.1) or chronic infection with persistence of virus replication for extended periods even during the lifetime of the individual (Figure 13.2). Chronic infection may resolve spontaneously and the individual may then develop immunity. Alternatively, a stable chronic infection may reactivate, resulting in a further acute episode.

Although HBV infection can lead to a severe disease, i.e. cirrhosis, hepatocellular carcinoma and liver failure, asymptomatic infections are very common, with most individuals resolving infection and

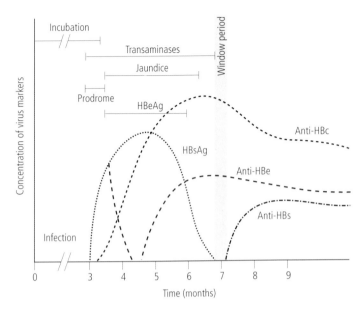

Figure 13.1 Markers of HBV infection during acute infection. Typical course of an acute infection with HBV. HBeAg, hepatitis Be antigen; HBsAg, hepatitis B surface antigen; anti-HBc, antibody to hepatitis B core antigen; anti-HBe, antibody to HBe; anti-HBs, antibody to HBsAg.

developing immunity without, or with only mild, symptoms.

Detection of HBV infection in donated blood is achieved by screening for HBsAg, the first serological marker to appear in the blood, and which persists throughout an active infection. The presence of HBsAg is prolonged (often for life) in chronic infection. Apart from anti-HBc (antibody to hepatitis B core antigen) the other markers of HBV infection are of value in confirming infection and determining the type and stage of infection, but have no role in the screening of blood donations for HBV.

Anti-HBc screening

For many years the subject of anti-HBc screening of donations, in addition to HBsAg, has been

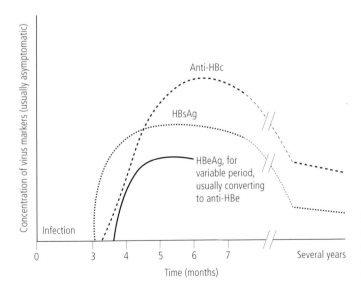

Figure 13.2 Markers of HBV infection during carrier state. Typical course of a chronic infection with HBV, leading to a carrier state (see Figure 13.1 for explanation of abbreviations).

considered. Before specific anti-HCV screening became possible, anti-HBc screening was considered as a possible surrogate marker for the causative agent of post-transfusion non-A, non-B hepatitis then seen in large numbers, but it was demonstrated subsequently that in most populations this strategy had little specific value.

It is argued that anti-HBc screening may have value in identifying the small number of donors who are either resolving an acute infection or clearing a chronic infection (see Figures 13.1 and 13.2). These donors are HBsAg negative on screening, but some may still have a low-level viraemia and potentially be infectious ('tail-end carriers'). Anti-HBc may be the only detectable circulating marker of infection in such individuals, and thus such donors may only be identifiable by anti-HBc screening. However, anti-HBc screening in this context is of value only if such situations can be shown to exist, and this is determined primarily by the incidence of HBV infection in the donor population. In addition, anti-HBc screening may be of value in the detection of HBV-infected donors who have mutant HBsAg (see section HBV Mutants). In cases of HBsAg mutations it is only the HBsAg protein that may be sufficiently altered in structure to render it undetectable by some HBsAg assays; the expression of the other markers of HBV infection expected in such individuals is unaltered.

The above situations could explain cases of post-transfusion HBV reported as resulting from the transfusion of donations screened as HBsAg negative where it is often not easy to demonstrate that the patient had no other risks of infection. However, a major issue with anti-HBc screening is the identification of those donors who are truly 'anti-HBc only' or who are naturally immune following infection earlier in life. It is generally agreed that individuals who are anti-HBc reactive with low-level anti-HBs (usually <100 mIU/mL, although there is little scientific evidence for the setting of this level) cannot be considered to be sufficiently immune to be used as donors. Currently a number of countries do screen all blood donations for anti-HBc but the value of this is debatable. However, anti-HBc screening is now a common practice, mandatory in

some countries, in the screening of tissue and stem cell donations.

HBV DNA screening

The screening of blood donations for HBV DNA has been considered to reduce even further the risk of transmission of HBV by reducing further the window period in early infection. However, early in infection the levels of HBV DNA are significantly lower than the other major TIAs and the sensitivity of the assays is only very marginally, if at all, greater than the current HBsAg assays. In situations where pools of samples are screened for viral nucleic acids, there would be no benefit from HBV DNA screening. In situations where individual donations are screened, the benefit would be marginal and certainly not cost-effective in terms of significant disease prevented. As mentioned above there is no value in HBV DNA screening with the current commercially available screening assays in the case of resolving acute infections, and anti-HBc would be a more reliable and cost-effective marker.

HBV mutants

There are currently two main groups of HBV mutants identified: the core group of mutants and the surface antigen mutants. The core mutants have normal HBsAg expression and are not currently considered to present any threat to the blood supply. However, the HBsAg group of mutants is of concern as HBsAg expression is altered such that some assays may fail to detect some examples. The extent of the problem is difficult to assess, and although mutants are being identified and variable reactivity with assays reported, their frequency is very low. A proportion of those that have been identified was a result of specific searches for such mutants and not as a result of transmissions from donations screened as HBsAg negative. There is no evidence currently available of a significant problem of post-transfusion HBV infection associated with HBsAg mutants.

Hepatitis delta virus

Hepatitis delta virus (HDV) is a small RNA virus, currently not firmly classified, that requires co-infection with HBV and replicates only in the hepatocytes. Although transmissible by transfusion, viral replication has an absolute requirement for co-infection with HBV and screening for HBsAg will also prevent transmission of HDV.

Hepatitis C virus

HCV is an enveloped RNA virus that has been classified as a separate genus within the flavivirus family. Although infections with HCV have been recognised for many years, the virus has only been identified and characterised within the last 20 years. It is transmitted parenterally and although there was initially some debate about the risk of transmission through sexual contact, the routes of infection are essentially the same as for HBV. Following infection there is an incubation period of about 3 weeks to 3 months prior to the appearance of HCV RNA and HCV antigen, and a further 0.5–4 weeks before the development of anti-HCV.

Infection with HCV can follow one of the two courses: acute infection followed by resolution of infection or chronic persistent infection. In about 40% of the cases, the infection is acute and resolves usually within a year. Whether true immunity follows the resolution of acute infection is not yet clear. Although HCV RNA is no longer detectable, the anti-HCV remaining may not protect the individual from subsequent re-infection. Although much is now known about the virus, the agent itself has still not been isolated and studied as an intact virion; HCV RNA and HCV antigen can be detected in the serum of infected individuals, but so far complete HCV virions have not been recovered.

Current knowledge about HCV and diagnostic assays that are now available derive primarily from isolation of the complete viral genome from human plasma and its in vitro expression and subsequent characterisation of the proteins expressed. The viral genome has been found to have certain areas with marked variation in the nucleic acid sequence, which has been shown to give rise to a number of distinct virus genotypes. Currently, six have been well characterised, and at least two more are being investigated. These genotypes tend to be geographically associated, and importantly do show some differences in the course and severity of in-

fection and in the response to interferon therapy, for example subtype 2 appears to be more resistant to current interferon therapy. Whether these variations are further reflected in the immune response to the virus, possibly a contributory factor to the classification of some HCV 'indeterminates', is not yet known.

The humoral immune response to HCV appears to be relatively weak compared with HBV and HIV; antibodies are not present at high titres and their reactivity against the currently identified individual epitopes is very variable. Our knowledge and understanding of the serology of HCV is based primarily on the reactivity of infected individuals against the specific and defined antigens used in current screening tests. This has limited the development of our understanding, because only a limited number of HCV-specific antigens are currently available for use in diagnostic tests.

Although the introduction of anti-HCV screening reduced dramatically the number of cases of post-transfusion HCV, occasional cases still occur. A feature of HCV infections is the window period during which HCV RNA is present prior to an immune response. Although donations collected from recently infected individuals may transmit HCV to recipients, the incidence of such HCV RNA-positive, antibody-negative donations is very low. Nonetheless, because of this the use of HCV RNA screening, currently using either individual donation testing or pools of samples (usually from 16 to 96), is increasing, since in countries with well-defined and resourced health care systems, blood transfusion services are under political and commercial pressure to improve further the safety of the blood supply. In many populations the cost of this appears to outweigh any benefit.

HCV antigen testing

Almost concurrent with the detection of HCV RNA is that of HCV core antigen (HCVcAg). The antigen is a normal constituent of the virion and conventional serological tests now exist to detect HCVcAg, both when complexed with specific antibody and when circulating in the plasma in the un-complexed form. In addition, in a similar way to HIV, high-quality HCV Ag-Ab combination assays are available for blood screening. Although not always correlating totally with viral RNA, HCVcAg can be detected, as expected, just as early during infection. In a number of studies using seroconversion panels where the early members were HCV RNA and antibody negative, HCVcAg was detected either at the same time as or within just a few days of viral RNA. This, of course, is not surprising as the antigen is an integral part of the virion. Any residual sensitivity difference between HCV RNA and HCVcAg detection is most likely to be due to the inherent sensitivity of the assay system rather than absence of antigen, i.e. failure to detect the low level of antigen present.

Thus, the detection of HCVcAg is a real alternative to the detection of HCV RNA in closing the antibody window period in HCV infection and increasing blood safety. Unfortunately, for many developed countries the appearance of the HCV combination Ag/Ab assays came too late, as the infrastructure for HCV RNA screening had already been developed and in most cases testing had started. Importantly, however, from a scientific and technical perspective, the detection of HCVcAg, either alone or in combination with Ab, is not only a totally acceptable alternative to nucleic acid detection but also technically easier to implement and sustain, and significantly cheaper. However, the litigious and regulatory nature of blood safety now generally outweighs any scientific values or judgement, and in countries where HCV RNA screening has already been introduced, it is very unlikely that it would be replaced by HCV Ag/Ab screening. Nonetheless, it is hoped that countries considering introducing HCV RNA screening would evaluate the potential of HCV Ag/Ab screening as an equivalent, but more cost-effective and technically simpler and therefore easier to control, methodology.

Hepatitis A virus

HAV is a picornavirus that has been classified as a separate genus, *Hepatovirus*. The virus is a non-enveloped RNA virus that is very stable and may persist in virally inactivated fractionated plasma products, especially those subjected only to solvent–detergent treatment.

The virus is normally only spread by the faeco-oral route, but some cases of transmission by blood products have been reported, e.g. by SD factor VIII preparations and occasionally by blood components. Natural transmission of HAV is dependent on poor sanitation and standards of hygiene; it has a very high prevalence (>90%) in most developing countries, but a falling prevalence in developed countries. Although the virus is normally excreted in highest titres in the faeces, in some individuals a high-titre viraemia may be present. While asymptomatic, such individuals may be the source of transmissions of HAV, and with the falling numbers of previously exposed (i.e. immune) individuals, neutralisation of any free virus in large-pool products may be incomplete.

The clinical symptoms of HAV resemble those of HBV, although the onset is usually more abrupt and the pre-icteric stage is less prolonged. Most infections occur in children and the severity of disease increases with age. About 0.1% of infections lead to death due to fulminant hepatitis. However, chronic infection does not develop, and most infected individuals recover completely with no long-term sequelae. Most infections last for about 1 month, although rarely some infections may relapse and last for as long as 6 months. After 2–3 weeks, IgM antibodies against HAV start to appear, followed by IgG anti-HAV. By about 6 months, the IgM antibodies disappear but the IgG titre stabilises, providing life-long immunity to HAV.

Hepatitis E virus

Hepatitis E was not recognised as a specific disease until 1980, when the viral agent was identified as the major cause of enterically transmitted non-A, non-B hepatitis. It is caused by a non-enveloped RNA virus which has characteristics similar to HAV and, although there are no specific data available, may also persist in virally inactivated fractionated plasma products, especially those subjected only to solvent–detergent treatment.

The virus is normally spread through the faeco-oral route, usually through sewage-contaminated water in areas of poor sanitation. However, sporadic cases do occur globally and it is considered that there is a global distribution of low pathogenicity strains. Additionally, transmission by transfusion has been reported in the UK. Although the virus is normally excreted in highest titres in the faeces, in some individuals a high-titre viraemia may be present. While asymptomatic, such individuals may be the source of transmissions of HEV; however, secondary transmission is rarer than with HAV.

An important additional consideration is the possibility of zoonotic spread. In non-endemic countries cases of HEV in individuals with no travel history have been reported, including fatal fulminant hepatitis. Several non-human primates are susceptible to infection and in the UK cases of HEV in non-travellers have been linked to infections in pigs.

The clinical symptoms of HEV resemble those of HAV and other types of acute viral hepatitis. It primarily affects young adults and is rare in children; infection is more severe in pregnancy, especially the third trimester. The incubation period following exposure ranges from 3 to 8 weeks, but then onset is abrupt; all patients are jaundiced and there are no extrahepatic features. Usually the disease clears within 1–4 weeks. HEV accounts for acute liver failure in endemic countries, and has been associated with fulminant hepatitis. Chronic infection does not develop. Virus excretion in stools persists for up to 2 weeks; HEV-specific IgM and IgG de-

velop and IgG persists, appearing to confer some short-term protection against re-infection.

Retroviruses

Human immunodeficiency virus

HIV is a retrovirus that primarily infects lymphocytes. The virus is transmitted parenterally mainly through sexual contact, mother-to-infant transmission and less commonly by blood or intravenous drug use. Unfortunately HIV has been transmitted through the transfusion of blood or products to thousands of people across the world.

The virus infects lymphocytes and integrates into the host cell DNA using the cellular machinery to replicate. Most HIV-infected individuals recover from this initial infection within 2–3 weeks, seroconvert and then remain asymptomatic often for extended but variable periods. However, during this period, individuals actually appear to undergo a persistent chronic infection, which causes a gradual decline in CD4 T-cell numbers. When these numbers fall below a certain level, the individual becomes susceptible to a number of infections and the symptoms marking the start of AIDS appear.

Following HIV infection, seroconversion occurs usually 1–3 months later (Figure 13.3). Prior to seroconversion, viral RNA can be detected in the

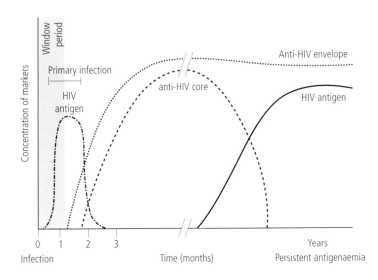

Figure 13.3 Serological markers of HIV infection. Note that the concentrations of HIV antigen are not on the same scale as for anti-HIV. Concentrations of the latter are much greater than those of the antigen.

bloodstream and proviral DNA can be detected in lymphocytes. In addition, 1–2 weeks before seroconversion, HIV p24 antigen can be detected. This is a viral core antigen and is one of the most abundant proteins produced by infected cells. As the antibody levels rise, the level of p24 antigen declines as it is bound by increasing levels of circulating antibody. Although not detectable by direct methods, HIV antigen production usually continues until AIDS develops.

A number of types and subtypes of HIV have been identified, and these may exhibit significant serological differences. The major division is into HIV-1 and HIV-2, and while there is significant serological cross-reactivity, there are also major differences and most anti-HIV tests used for blood screening incorporate antigens from both virus types. In addition, there are subtypes that also show some serological differences, although these are not so clear-cut. The identification of HIV-1 subtype O demonstrated the need for surveillance of these emerging types and subtypes because of its variable reactivity with the then current anti-HIV-1 and -2 assays. Today, all anti-HIV assays from the major international diagnostic manufacturers specifically detect subtype O, and no recent cases of failure to detect subtype O samples have been reported.

A significant proportion of blood donations in developed countries are now screened for HIV infection using combined HIV antigen–antibody combination assays, specific for HIV-1 and HIV-2. These assays are commonly referred to as enhanced antibody assays as generally they retain the sensitivity of the antibody-only assay, but the antigen component is slightly less sensitive than an antigen-only assay. They represent an effective compromise between having separate antibody and antigen assays, and running just one assay. There is significantly higher overall sensitivity at detecting HIV-infected donors than using only an antibody assay. However, in some countries, those with a high incidence of HIV in the population, the use of separate anti-HIV-1 and -2 and HIV p24 antigen assays is more appropriate as the probability of early infections is greater, the presence of HIV p24 antigen prior to the development of the humoral response,

and thus a higher sensitivity and broader screen is essential.

Additionally, in some countries HIV NAT is now routine, on both pools and individual donations. The value of HIV NAT is not yet clear in most countries where the incidence of HIV in blood donors is low and where blood is collected from low-risk donors. Although cases of HIV RNA-positive, antibody-negative donations are identified, the cost-effectiveness of HIV NAT is far from clear.

Human T-cell lymphotropic viruses (types I and II)

Human T-cell lymphotropic virus (HTLV)-I was the first human retrovirus identified. It is an oncogenic virus causing adult T-cell leukaemia and lymphoma (ATLL) and tropical spastic paraparesis, also known as HTLV-I-associated myelopathy. A second virus, HTLV-II, has also been identified in specific groups of individuals, for example intravenous drug users, although no significant disease process has yet been associated with this virus. Most infections with HTLV-I are asymptomatic. However, there is a small risk that disease may develop any time up to 40 years after infection. ATLL can present as an acute leukaemia of CD4 lymphocytes and death usually occurs within a year of the onset of symptoms. Tropical spastic paraparesis is a progressive disease involving the degeneration of neurones in the spinal cord, leading to gradual paralysis of the lower limbs. More recently, HTLV infection has also been associated with certain inflammatory diseases.

It is thought that HTLV is cell associated, infecting CD4 lymphocytes, and is transmitted in these cells parenterally via blood or semen, or from mother to infant via breast milk. Transmission by breast milk is a major route of infection in some areas where HTLV-I is endemic. Studies on the transmission of HTLV-I indicate that the virus is not normally transmitted in utero, but is transmitted in early life through breast milk equally to both male and female children. However, later in life sexual transmission is almost exclusively from males to females. Blood transfusion is another potentially significant route of infection. Early studies demonstrated the efficiency of transmission by blood transfusion, and that cell-free products, such as plasma, do not transmit infection. Fresh components from infected individuals are those most likely to transmit the virus.

Following infection with HTLV, there is an incubation period of 30–90 days before seroconversion. Prior to seroconversion viral RNA can be detected in lymphocytes. At the time of seroconversion, antibodies to HTLV appear and the detection of antibodies is used as the main diagnostic test for HTLV infection. After seroconversion the antibodies generally persist for life, even if clinical disease subsequently develops only much later. The serological responses to HTLV-I and HTLV-II are very similar, but like HIV-1 and HIV-2 there are sufficient differences to enable tests to be developed to specifically detect anti-HTLV-I and anti-HTLV-II, and thus discriminate between infections.

The potential significance of blood transfusion as a route of transmission has meant that in a number of endemic countries screening of donations for anti-HTLV-I and anti-HTLV-II has been carried out for some time. In some non-endemic developed countries with mixed populations screening has also been introduced, in some instances restricted to previously untested donors. In other countries debate continues over the need for, and value of, screening donations. A cost-effective approach to screening has been implemented in England, where a sensitive anti-HTLV enzyme immunoassay (EIA) is used to screen the pooled samples (pools of 48) that are prepared for NAT.

Herpes viruses

The human herpesviruses are a family of large DNA viruses that almost always give rise to latent infections following acute infection (Table 13.2). Their pathogenic and clinical significance vary from mild and insignificant to severe disease, often depending on the immune status of the individual. Transmission by blood transfusion of herpesviruses has been demonstrated clearly for human cytomegalovirus (HCMV) and Epstein–Barr virus (EBV). Transmission of the most recently identified herpesvirus, human herpesvirus 8 (HHV-8), is uncertain and currently under investigation. While transmission of

the other viruses in the family is less likely, it cannot be ruled out.

Human cytomegalovirus

HCMV is the herpesvirus of most significance in blood transfusion, and was previously transmitted widely, with serious consequences for some patients. The virus is widely distributed in populations, with increasing prevalence and lower age of infection in poorer socioeconomic conditions. Prevalence figures range from 20% (though falling) in industrialised countries to 90% or more in rural areas of economically restricted countries.

Although a serious infection in immunocompromised individuals, HCMV causes a largely asymptomatic infection in immunocompetent individuals, rarely with any significant long-term sequelae. The incubation period generally lasts from 1 week to 1 month, after which the infection normally lasts up to a month, but most often with no or only very mild and limited symptoms. Antibodies appear following resolution of infection and the development of the latent state of infection. Not only a significant proportion of donors but also a significant proportion of patients will have been exposed to the virus. However, patients who have not been previously exposed will normally only be at risk if they are immunosuppressed in any way.

The main reason for the significance of HCMV in transfusion medicine is because leucocytes (including lymphocytes, monocytes and neutrophils) are one site of latency of the virus. Transfusion of blood containing leucocytes has been shown to lead to HCMV infection. Although antibody to the virus can be demonstrated in previously infected individuals, these antibodies do not necessarily prevent recrudescence or re-infection, and re-activation of the latent virus may occur. As with most of the herpesviruses, the key trigger to re-activation/re-infection appears to be immunosuppression, whether due to specific immunosuppressive treatment or 'natural' immunosuppression.

Although previously screening for both specific IgM and IgG antibodies to HCMV was considered essential, it is now accepted that screening

Table 13.2 Human herpesviruses.

Designation	Sub-family	Common name	Transmission	Major disease
HHV-1	α	Herpes simplex type I	Respiratory Person–person contact with active lesions	Oral and ocular lesions Encephalitis
HHV-2	α	Herpes simplex type II	Respiratory Person–person contact with active lesions	Genital lesions
HHV-3	α	Varicella-zoster	Respiratory route	Chickenpox Shingles
HHV-4	γ	Epstein–Barr	Respiratory Person–person salivary contact	Glandular fever Implicated in Burkitt's lymphoma and nasopharyngeal carcinoma
HHV-5	β	Cytomegalovirus	Respiratory Person–person salivary contact Parenteral	Congenital infection: neural tube defects Infectious mononucleosis-type disease
HHV-6	β	Human herpesvirus 6	Currently unclear, probably respiratory Person–person salivary contact	Roseola Exanthem subitum
HHV-7	β	Human herpesvirus 7	Currently unclear, probably respiratory Person–person salivary contact	Roseola (reactivation of HHV-6)
HHV-8	γ	Human herpesvirus 8 Kaposi's sarcoma-associated herpesvirus	Parenteral Sexual	Kaposi's sarcoma Body cavity B-cell lymphoma

blood for IgG antibodies is effective in identifying previously exposed and thus potentially infectious donors. However, screening is not generally applied to all donations because the percentage of patients requiring screened blood is relatively low.

Epstein–Barr virus

EBV is the cause of infectious mononucleosis and is associated with other diseases, in particular Burkitt's lymphoma and nasopharyngeal carcinoma. Like HCMV, its sites of latency include leucocytes, in this case B cells, but recrudescence appears to be a lot less common. The virus is globally widespread, with prevalence levels from 40% in industrialised countries to more than 90% in economically restricted countries.

Only occasional cases of post-transfusion EBV infection have been reported. Donor screening is not performed and is considered to be of limited value because of the high prevalence of the virus and because donors with active infection, i.e. those with infectious mononucleosis, are generally symptomatic.

Human herpesvirus 8

HHV-8 (or Kaposi's sarcoma-associated herpesvirus), first isolated in 1994, is the most recently identified herpesvirus. Our knowledge and understanding of this virus are incomplete, and its significance to transfusion is unclear. It causes Kaposi's sarcoma, body cavity-based lymphoma and some severe forms of lymph node enlargement. Although clearly a different virus to HIV, there is a high frequency of HHV-8-related diseases among homosexually infected HIV patients. Infection rates vary significantly, ranging from less than 5% in northern Europe, 10% in the US and increasing through southern Europe into Africa where over 50% of some populations are infected.

The virus appears to be transmitted by both sexual and non-sexual routes, being more commonly transmitted through homosexual practices than heterosexual, but also through oral contact and even from mother to child at birth in higher prevalence countries. Transmission by organ transplantation has been reported, although it is rare, but this does suggest caution when considering transmission by blood transfusion.

Parvoviruses
Parvovirus B19

The parvoviruses are one of the smallest DNA viruses that infect humans. They are very stable non-enveloped viruses that are resistant to many chemical and physical inactivation techniques. Parvovirus B19 (human *Erythrovirus*) is the only definite member of the genus *Erythrovirus* (the virus replicates in erythroid progenitor cells).

Clinically, parvovirus B19 infection gives rise to the following:
• A range of generally mild symptoms including rash, vomiting, aching joints and limbs, fatigue, general malaise and leucopenia, and in many individuals the infection passes largely unnoticed.
• Aplastic crisis in sickle cell and thalassaemia patients, cases of chronic haemolytic anaemia and other conditions with red cell membrane defects. It may also cause aplastic anaemia in immunocompromised individuals.

• Severe foetal anaemia, death or malformation in infants infected in utero (mainly in the second trimester).

B19 is fairly widespread among the general population, with regular community outbreaks across most countries. The prevalence of antibody to B19 in blood donors ranges from 50 to 98% from developed countries to developing countries. It is transmitted mainly via the release of virus particles from the upper respiratory tract, but may also be transmitted parenterally, by blood transfusion, at times of high viraemia. Viraemia usually appears within the first week of infection and persists generally for 1–2 weeks, although longer term viraemia is not uncommon. The humoral immune response normally begins after 1–2 weeks with the appearance of IgM, followed closely by IgG antibodies. Chronic infections do not occur.

The detection of antibody to B19 indicates immunity to the virus. IgM testing may identify recently infected, and thus potentially still infectious, individuals. IgG antibodies persist for many years, possibly for life, and identify previously infected rather than infectious individuals.

B19 has been demonstrated to be transmitted by transfusion, although the significance of any resulting disease is related to the immune status of the patient transfused. There is little clinical significance in immunocompetent individuals, with a greater but still relatively low clinical significance in immunocompromised individuals.

Because of its low clinical significance, B19 is another virus, like GBV-C (see Section on GBV-C and HGV), that is clearly transmissible by transfusion but with limited clinical relevance. The only area of major concern is that of large-pool fractionated products, where because of its natural resistance to inactivation the virus can be found in some products in high titres during outbreaks. There is a concern that this may be of clinical relevance to immunocompromised patients receiving significant amounts of such products. Some fractionators have introduced lowered sensitivity NAT procedures to reduce the viral load prior to inactivation without excluding excessive numbers of donors. Parvovirus B19 over the recent years has been used as a model for viral inactivation procedures, because of its high resistance to many inactivation methods.

Miscellaneous viruses

There are a number of viruses that can be considered in this group: transmissible but which cause little or no clinical disease, or very restricted in their distribution or period of highest potential exposure. These viruses to a degree pose a dilemma as their significance varies significantly in different countries or even regions within a country, and to effectively remove the risk of their transmission from the blood supply may require significant intervention and resources, in some cases far in excess of any potential clinical benefits. In addition, some, like West Nile virus (WNV), are not persistent but can be more frequent in epidemic periods in certain countries.

GBV-C and hepatitis G virus

GBV-C and hepatitis G virus (HGV) are now known to have been simultaneous independent isolates of the same virus. Additionally, although originally called hepatitis viruses, there is doubt as to whether they do have any role in liver disease and their classification as a hepatitis virus may have been premature. In this text, the term GBV-C is used to refer to both the GBV-C and HGV original isolates.

GBV-C is a recently identified flavivirus that has been shown to be present at a relatively high prevalence and incidence worldwide. The virus is transmitted parenterally and viral RNA has been found at a high prevalence in the expected high-risk groups, such as transfused individuals, transplant recipients, intravenous drug users, haemodialysis patients, infants born to infected mothers and sexual partners of infected individuals.

The course of infection varies from an acute self-limited infection, with development of antibody to the viral envelope, to long-term chronic infection, with viral RNA production persisting for a number of years in the absence of an antibody response. Following infection, there is a short incubation period followed by the appearance of GBV-C RNA together with a rise in serum alanine aminotransferase, although the levels do not reach the high levels seen in HBV and HCV infections. In acute infection, the RNA levels start to fall 4–6 months after infection, and levels of antibody (specifically anti-E2) start to rise to a maximal level which may be maintained for 5 years or more. In a proportion of individuals, currently 20–40%, there is no clearance of the viraemia, antibody is not detected and a chronic infection is established.

A high proportion of infected individuals in the high-risk groups have also been found to be co-infected with HCV, but this is a consequence of the particular shared routes of infection. The virus has many general similarities with HCV in areas such as structure, genome organisation, epidemiology and general routes of infection, but there are also some significant differences, notably the lack of a core gene. GBV-C has been clearly demonstrated to be transmitted by transfusion, although any clinical significance associated with these transmission events has yet to be established.

The high prevalence of the virus in at-risk groups has not been shown to be, on its own, a significant contributory factor to any morbidity in infected individuals, nor does it exacerbate co-infection with HAV, HBV or HCV. The laboratory detection of active or recent infection is based on detection of viral RNA. Unlike HCV infection, specific circulating antibody has not been detected during the period of viraemia; the appearance of antibody appears to mark the clearance of viral RNA. The humoral immune response to GBV-C has not yet been characterised fully, but most of the seropositive individuals appear to produce antibodies only to the structural E2 antigen; humoral immunity to the non-structural proteins has not been found. In individuals on antiviral therapy viral RNA has been found to decline without the subsequent appearance of antibody.

Although a lot of information about the virus has been collected in a relatively short time, there is still a great deal that is unknown, for example whether significant clinical disease is associated with it and, especially, the apparent current lack of disease association following transmission by blood transfusion.

TT virus

TT virus (TTV) is a DNA virus that was first isolated in 1997 from a patient with post-transfusion hepatitis of unknown aetiology. The virus is non-enveloped and although it has some similarities with both parvoviruses and circoviruses, it is considered to be a member of a new virus family.

The prevalence of infection varies from 3 to 4% in blood donors in the UK and the US to as high as 80% in rural areas in some developing countries. Although transmitted parenterally, there is evidence of non-parenteral transmission and the contribution of each of these to transmission through populations is not fully understood. Transmission by blood transfusion has been demonstrated, and TTV has been cited as the cause of non-A–G post-transfusion hepatitis. However, the pathogenicity of TTV and specifically its role in liver disease is unclear. Generally infection is asymptomatic and detection in this situation is only possible through the use of molecular techniques; serological tests have not yet been developed. Because transmission is not exclusively parenteral, the significance of TTV to blood transfusion is unclear.

SENV

This virus is a relatively new DNA virus, a potential causative agent for chronic liver disease, with an assumed association with post-transfusion hepatitis. There have been two sub-types identified (SENV-H and SENV-D), and it appears to be distantly related to TTV. There are some indications that it might be of significance in cases of non-A–E post-transfusion hepatitis, although some studies have failed to show any significant differences in SENV prevalences in transfused and non-transfused individuals. Parenteral transmission thus may not be the major route of transmission of SENV. There have been no cases reported in the UK.

West Nile virus

WNV is a flavivirus primarily transmitted by mosquitoes. Birds act as intermediate hosts, in which viral titres reach high levels. Mosquitoes feeding on the birds can then become infected, completing the cycle. Although they become infected by mosquitoes, humans and those other large mammals that are infected appear to effectively stop the cycle of the virus because viral titres never rise above the threshold needed for feeding mosquitoes to become infected. Historically, WNV has caused epidemics across much of the world and a fatality rate of 5–15% has been seen. Currently, attention has been focussed on the US, since its first appearance in 1999 (see Chapter 16).

There is a defined viraemia following infection and prior to the development of the humoral response. The viraemia generally lasts no more than 28 days, usually a lot less, and is followed by the rapid appearance of IgM followed by IgG. Infection is often asymptomatic and there is no chronic stage. Although identification of infectious donors/donations is by NAT, the relatively short period of infectivity followed by immunity enables alternative strategies to be considered, i.e. the deferral of potentially exposed donors to beyond the viraemic period. However, the problem is identifying specific risk exposure; at-risk individuals need to be able to be identified clearly by the donor selection criteria adopted. Although there are specific geographical and seasonal factors, such a system is not exact and because of the high numbers of infected individuals who are asymptomatic, they may present with no identifiable risk factors and thus may not be deferred from donating. In the US, where the major problem with WNV currently resides, cases of transfusion transmission from donors in the early window period and tested by pooled NAT have been reported. Because viral titres are generally low in humans, individual donor NAT may be required.

SARS-CoV

Severe acute respiratory syndrome (SARS) is a respiratory infection caused by the newly emergent SARS coronavirus (SARS-CoV). The disease has severe morbidity and mortality, but presents with non-specific signs and symptoms and there is no clear-cut diagnostic approach to prospectively identify cases prior to the appearance of symptoms. The virus has a viraemic phase, which is found prior to symptoms and which persists into the symptomatic phase. Viraemic individuals may transmit if blood is collected during the early phase of infection prior to symptoms appearing. Screening of individuals for SARS-CoV is possible using NAT but is not practical bearing in mind the current geographical restrictions/exposure risk of the virus. Deferral of donors who may have been potentially exposed to the virus is currently the most effective way of minimising the risk of transmission.

Bacteria

The presence of bacteria in donated blood and tissues is assuming greater importance in transfusion medicine, because although it is uncommon, post-transfusion bacterial sepsis has a high mortality rate (see also Chapter 14). Furthermore, the potential for contamination is increasing because of the increased manipulation of blood during the preparation of blood components. Numerous instances of infected red cell products have been reported, and the storage of platelet concentrates at 20–24°C for up to 5 days has provided an ideal environment for the growth of any contaminating bacteria present.

There are two broad routes of bacterial contamination:

• endogenous contamination due to bacteria present in the donor's blood at the time of donation (bacteraemic donor), and which may include organisms such as *T. pallidum* and *Yersinia enterocolitica*; and

• exogenous contamination due to bacteria that have entered the blood pack from the environment during collection, processing or other handling, storage or transport, and which may include such organisms as *Pseudomonas* and *Staphylococcus*.

In either case, bacterial growth within the blood pack gives rise to endotoxins that are generally the major cause of the post-transfusion sepsis seen after transfusion of a contaminated unit. In these cases growth is restricted and the bacteria themselves do not survive past a few multiplication cycles, but the toxins they produce can have clinical significance.

Endogenous bacteria

If a donor is bacteraemic at the time of donation, except for certain diseases such as syphilis, it is most likely to be due to a low-grade asymptomatic infection, often with only a short period of bacteraemia.

Treponema pallidum (syphilis)

The spirochaete *T. pallidum* is the causative agent of syphilis. Treponemes:

• have thin flexible helical walls and are extremely motile;

• cannot be cultivated on artificial media although they can be cultivated in cell culture or in animals; and

• can be seen easily under dark-field microscopy.

Syphilis can follow several stages, leading to primary, secondary and tertiary syphilis following the initial infection. The primary site of infection is usually marked by a lesion known as a chancre, which is full of treponemes. Although this may heal and disappear completely, the regional lymph nodes may still be infected and continuing treponemal division may give rise to secondary syphilis and, if still untreated, to tertiary syphilis.

Because treponemes are released into the bloodstream as part of their life cycle, there is the potential for transmission by transfusion. They are particularly fragile, but can be transmitted by transfusion if they are present in the donation, and many transmissions were reported in the early days of blood transfusion. However, storage at 4°C soon destroys the organisms because they are very heat sensitive. It is generally considered that any spirochaetes present in the pack would be destroyed within 72 hours of storage at 4°C.

As spirochaetes can be seen only for short periods during infection, identification of infected individuals relies on serology. Blood is therefore screened using either non-specific tests for indirect evidence or specific tests for direct evidence (antibody to *T. pallidum*) of current or previous infection with *T. pallidum*. In countries with a low incidence of syphilis the vast majority of cases identified in blood donors are due to 'old' infections that have been treated successfully and present no risk of transfusion transmission, although some cases of recent primary acute syphilis are occasionally identified. In such countries, the value of continuing syphilis screening is often questioned as cases of post-transfusion syphilis are rare and any that may occur can be successfully treated with no lasting sequelae. However, syphilis screening of donated blood, no matter what the incidence in the donor population, has been considered to have value as a 'lifestyle' indicator, because individuals exposed to syphilis may also have been exposed to other sexually transmitted diseases and therefore should not donate.

Non-specific screening tests include simple and rapid tests such as the Venereal Disease Reference Laboratory (VDRL) test and rapid plasma reagin test, which essentially detect current or recent infection, measuring the amount of anticardiolipin free in the blood and produced in the early course of infection in response to the organism. Although non-specific cardiolipin tests may give rise to a high number of false-positive reactions, they are useful because they do give an indication of current status; in treated acute infections anticardiolipin titres fall and the tests become negative.

Specific screening tests detect antibody to *T. pallidum* and include both haemagglutination and EIA formats. Other tests in use, such as the *T. pallidum* immobilisation test or the fluorescent treponemal antibody absorption test, are primarily confirmatory tests.

Borrelia burgdorferi (Lyme disease)

Like syphilis, Lyme disease is caused by a spirochaete, *Borrelia burgdorferi*. The organism is carried by a number of insect vectors, mainly by ticks of the *Ixodes* genus, but it has been increasingly found in other blood-feeding insects such as horseflies and mosquitoes. It is likely that human transmission is possible via these routes. The disease was first identified around Lyme, Connecticut, in the US, but is now the most common tick-transmitted infection in the US, and is also known to be endemic in many other parts of the world. The disease is generally seasonal and marked by unique skin lesions, rash, fever and lymphadenopathy. This may progress to meningoencephalitis or myocarditis, and then arthritis. A high percentage of infected individuals develop chronic joint disorders.

Although no case of post-transfusion Lyme disease has yet been reported, the potential for transmission remains as *B. burgdorferi* can retain viability in blood stored for up to 6 weeks. EIAs are available which detect specific antibody against the organism, but as cases of spirochaetaemia are generally symptomatic, careful donor selection should ensure that any potential risk of transmission is minimised.

Brucella melitensis (brucellosis)

Brucellosis (undulant fever) is caused by the bacterium *B. melitensis* and has the following characteristics:

- It is usually acquired from an infected animal source.
- It is not usually transmitted from person to person, but because there is a period of bacteraemia, transmission by blood transfusion may occur and has been reported in endemic regions.
- It normally enters through the mucous membranes of the throat, migrates to the regional lymph nodes, where it multiplies before being released into the blood, from where it enters and resides in the reticuloendothelial systems of different tissues.
- Infection is characterised by general malaise and an undulating fever.
- Chronic infection normally follows, which may last for many years with bouts of sometimes quite serious illness.
- While the organism is prevalent in many parts of the world, brucellosis has only rarely been reported after transfusion. This may reflect poor reporting of post-transfusion infections and the true incidence of transmission may be at a higher level. The active deferral of donors at risk of exposure to, or previously infected with, *Brucella* should minimise any risk of transmission.

Yersinia enterocolitica

Yersinia enterocolitica is a Gram-negative bacterium that may be present as an asymptomatic bacteraemia in infected donors at the time of donation. The extent and significance of such infections is difficult to assess, as effective mass screening procedures are currently not feasible and only sporadic monitoring is performed. *Y. enterocolitica* has been recognised as a potentially serious microbial agent that may be present in donated blood.

It was thought that the organism persisted free in the blood, and because it was psychrophilic (able to grow at low temperatures) it was able to multiply in the blood pack during storage, eventually reaching high enough numbers to cause post-transfusion sepsis in the recipient. However, it is possible that in an infected individual the bacteria are phagocytosed but survive intracellularly in the circulating leucocytes. During storage of the blood, the natural breakdown of the leucocytes releases the bacteria, which are then able to grow at 4°C. This results in the build-up of large numbers of bacteria and their toxins in the stored unit, with the potential for causing both post-transfusion sepsis and septic shock in the recipient.

The screening of donations for *Y. enterocolitica* is not currently feasible; the deferral of potentially infected donors relies upon the routine donor selection procedures.

Other endogenous bacteria

Cases of post-transfusion sepsis caused by a number of other endogenous bacterial species are occasionally reported. Donors may have a transient bacteraemia, possibly as a result of:
- a low-grade gastrointestinal infection;
- following dental procedures; and
- a minor wound.

Donor bacteraemia may subsequently result in post-transfusion sepsis due to organisms such as *Salmonella*, *Campylobacter*, *Streptococcus* and *Staphylococcus*.

Exogenous bacteria

A number of bacterial species, for example *Pseudomonas*, *Serratia* and *Staphylococcus*, may be introduced into the blood pack from the environment during or after donation, either at venepuncture or during subsequent processing, storage or transportation of the blood. These environmental organisms are generally more likely to cause problems in blood components stored at higher temperatures, such as platelet concentrates, because they are potentially able to multiply to large numbers, producing high levels of bacterial toxins.

There have been many cases of post-transfusion septicaemia involving single or multiple recipients infected by the same source, and involving a large range of bacterial species. However, while a large number of bacterial species have been implicated, in most cases the precise source of the contamination could not be determined. Platelet concentrates are a common source of post-transfusion septicaemia, although the ratio of cases of sepsis to death is higher than with cases of post-transfusion septicaemia following transfusion of red cell concentrates.

Some years ago an outbreak of post-transfusion septicaemia due to *Serratia marcescens* was reported. The outbreak affected transfusion centres in both Denmark and Sweden and was traced to blood bags contaminated on their outer surfaces during manufacturing or packaging. Six patients were affected, one of whom died, and 4000 units of blood and an unknown number of platelet concentrates had to be discarded. Studies on the growth of *S. marcescens* in artificially infected blood packs have since demonstrated that not only does the organism grow well at both 4 and 22°C, but that natural protection mechanisms such as phagocytosis and complement-mediated killing are not effective in destroying it.

Rickettsiae

The rickettsiae are smaller than most other bacteria. They are most closely related to Gram-negative bacteria, but are unique in that they grow only inside animal cells. All rickettsial diseases are transmitted between animals via a blood-feeding insect vector, with the exception of Q fever.

Transmission of rickettsial infections by blood transfusion has occurred, but cases are extremely rare and only transmission of Q fever and Rocky Mountain spotted fever has been reported. It occurs because infectious organisms are shed into the blood, and donations taken during this phase of rickettsaemia may transmit the infection. However, most infections at this stage are symptomatic and donor selection procedures should identify any potentially infectious donors. Some laboratory screening tests are available but are very specialised and not ideally suited for the screening of blood donations.

Protozoa

Protozoan infections have always been a major problem in developing countries. However, with increased global travel and population migration, protozoan infections are now becoming a concern to all countries, and this concern extends to the safety of the blood supply.

Plasmodium spp. (malaria)

Protozoa of the *Plasmodium* species cause malaria. There are four known *Plasmodium* species that are agents of human malaria: *P. falciparum*, *P. malariae*, *P. vivax* and *P. ovale*. Although there are some basic similarities in the life cycles of the organisms and the clinical features of infection, there are also significant differences. The incubation periods range from 12 days for *P. falciparum*, 15 days for *P. vivax* and *P. ovale*, and as long as 30 days for *P. malariae*. In general, complications from *P. falciparum* infection are more serious than from the other three species and are often fatal.

The agent is transmitted to humans through the bite of the *Anopheles* mosquito, the life cycle of *Plasmodium* being split between the two hosts, with the sexual replication phase in the female mosquito and the asexual replication phase in the human. The merozoite form of the parasite infects the red cells, where it replicates, subsequently causing the red cell to burst, releasing more organisms into the blood. Only *P. malariae* persists for extended periods in humans (up to 30 years), while after 1–2 years plasmodia of the other three types normally die, and the individual, if not re-infected, becomes free from malaria.

The transmissibility of malaria by blood transfusion has long been recognised because of the erythrocyte phase of the life cycle, and cases of post-transfusion *P. falciparum* are often fatal due to the complication of cerebral malaria.

Immunity to plasmodia builds up in adults living in endemic areas, but is usually lost quickly upon moving to a non-endemic area. However, the recent development of immunity can be used to identify infected individuals by screening for specific antiplasmodial antibody. This has the greatest value when applied to individuals from low-prevalence areas who have travelled to endemic areas, and when sufficient time, to mount an immune response, has elapsed between returning from an endemic area and the screening being performed. Individuals from some endemic areas, where the exposure rate is high, may be found to be semi-immune, a situation in which parasites may be found circulating at the same time as antibody. Such individuals are among the highest risk for transfusion transmission as the antibody levels may fluctuate to below detectable. However, such individuals may be identified by geography alone and deferred permanently. Although direct detection of parasites in blood is possible, this is primarily a diagnostic test. In most cases such tests are far too insensitive to detect any but the most parasitaemic individual, generally in a period of crisis and hence symptomatic, and thus in most countries are of no value in the screening of blood donations.

Trypanosoma cruzi (Chagas' disease)

The protozoan *T. cruzi* causes Chagas' disease. The disease is confined mainly to the American subcontinent, where it is endemic in Latin America and increasing its presence in the southern states of the US as migrant workers from Latin America move north.

The agent is transmitted to humans by reduviid bugs (triatomides), who carry the parasites in their gut and excrete them in their faeces as they feed; the open feeding site acts as the site of entry for the parasite. Similarly to *Plasmodium*, the organism has a life cycle split between two hosts, the gut of the reduviid and the tissues and organs of humans. The blood acts as the transport system disseminating the organism around the body and provides a new source of organism for any feeding reduviids. Although the liver and spleen are usually infected, the most characteristic infected organ is the heart, and congestive heart failure plays a significant part in the morbidity and mortality of the disease.

Although transmission by reduviids is generally the major route of infection, blood transfusion is considered to be the second most important route of transmission in endemic areas. Donor selection can be problematical due to the high proportion of asymptomatic infections (>20%), and in vitro screening of all blood donations is carried out in some parts of Latin America.

This spread of the disease by travelling migrant workers is starting to affect other countries. Data from the US include the report of a case of endemic Chagas' disease in an infant in one of its southern states who had no identifiable risk of infection except insect bites. The risk of infection in travellers from non-endemic regions also has to be considered, and donor selection procedures amended accordingly.

Once infected, an individual generally remains infected for life, although the morbidity and mortality associated with Chagas' disease vary significantly. Like malaria, immunity to *T. cruzi* does occur, and can be used to identify individuals previously exposed to the organism and therefore not suitable as blood donors.

Toxoplasma gondii (toxoplasmosis)

Toxoplasma gondii, the causative agent of toxoplasmosis, is globally one of the most widespread vertebrate protozoan parasites; in some countries up to 95% of adults may have been infected with the parasite.

Members of the cat family are the hosts of *T. gondii*, and mice are thought to act as intermediate hosts helping to maintain its life cycle. The organism has a sexual replication phase in intestinal cells of cats and an asexual phase in another mammal. During this phase the sporozoites infect and multiply in a wide variety of other cell types, including those of the reticuloendothelial system, leucocytes and eventually the central nervous system (CNS). The acute infection in healthy individuals is generally asymptomatic and not associated with any morbidity. However, in immunocompromised individuals infection is far more severe, with the possibility of CNS involvement, myocarditis and pneumonia. Congenital infection can give rise to serious complications involving the liver and the CNS, and even abortion or stillbirth.

Transmission by blood transfusion has occasionally been documented in immunosuppressed individuals, including some fatalities, due to the presence of the organism in leucocytes.

Following resolution of acute infection, circulating antibodies appear but the organism persists latently in the circulating leucocytes, and reactivation has been reported. Although in vitro screening for antibody to *T. gondii* is available, selective donor screening and leucocyte depletion of blood components may be more appropriate for the small group of recipients with a significant risk of disease.

Babesia microti/divergens (babesiosis)

The tick-borne protozoan parasite *Babesia* (*B. microti* in North America and *B. divergens* in Europe) is the causative agent of babesiosis. The organism is transmitted by tick bite, and currently it is thought that the same reservoirs of Lyme disease are also the source of *Babesia*, and that the disease is restricted to the US and northern Europe. Babesiosis is generally symptomatic, although symptoms range from a mild to severe malaria-like illness with the red cells acting as sites of replication of the organism.

Studies with *B. microti* have shown that the organism can survive in red cells for at least 1 month under normal blood bank storage conditions and, like *Plasmodium*, can be transmitted by transfusion of blood from an infected asymptomatic individual. Identified transmissions are uncommon but not rare, as the disease is not widespread and symptoms are generally present, but no deaths have been reported. Although no cases of transfusion-transmitted babesiosis have been reported in Europe, it is quite likely that a number of cases have occurred and not been identified following asymptomatic infection in the recipient.

Laboratory screening is currently not possible and donor selection procedures have to be relied on to minimise any risks of transmission.

Leishmania spp. (leishmaniasis)

Infection with protozoa of the *Leishmania* spp. gives rise to leishmaniasis, which causes infection of the reticuloendothelial system and which exists in three main forms: cutaneous, mucocutaneous and visceral (kala-azar). It is thought that the basic differences between the three types of infection result from the differing ability of the *Leishmania* species to invade the body. Although a number of species exist, morphologically they are almost identical, and differences are apparent only when molecular techniques are used to examine their DNA.

The organisms are transmitted through the bite of infected sandflies of the genus *Phlebotomus*, but each *Leishmania* species is restricted to a particular *Phlebotomus* species. The reservoirs for the organism vary among different regions but include rodents and other small wild mammals, although in urban areas dogs and even humans can serve as reservoirs. The life cycle is split between the two hosts, with the flagellated forms in the sandfly and non-flagellated forms in the vertebrate host. The organism invades the reticuloendothelial system, where it replicates and is released back into the blood.

Although potentially a threat to the blood supply in endemic areas, parasitaemia is generally transient and at a low level, and consequently there is a low risk of transmission. This is supported by the lack of reports of transmission by blood transfusion even in endemic areas.

Laboratory screening is currently not possible, and donor selection procedures have to be relied upon to minimise any risks of transmission.

Prions

Prions have been included here as they have, in the shape of variant Creutzfeldt–Jakob disease (vCJD), had a significant impact on transfusion practice, at least in the UK, despite the absence of any firm evidence of transfusion transmission in humans.

Variant Creutzfeldt–Jakob disease

vCJD was identified in 1996 and is the most recently identified human prion disease (see also Chapter 15). Prion diseases occur in a number of animal species and occur when the naturally occurring benign form of the prion protein (PrP) changes to an insoluble protease-resistant form (PrP^{Sc}). This leads to the formation of plaques in the brain. vCJD differs from classical CJD in that the age of onset is earlier and disease progression is slower, and higher levels of PrP^{Sc} are found in the brain. Higher levels of PrP^{Sc} than in CJD have been found in tonsillar tissue, although these glycoforms differ from those found in the brain.

The demonstration of lymphoid association in scrapie, together with the finding of PrP^{Sc} in tonsillar tissue, has led to a relationship being postulated between PrP^{Sc} and B-lymphocytes.

Whilst the transmissibility of vCJD by blood transfusion has not been proven unequivocally, the transmission of scrapie and BSE in sheep has been demonstrated, and four human recipients of blood from vCJD infected donors have subsequently developed prion infection. The presence of 'infectious' prion in the blood is strongly suspected, but has not been demonstrated conclusively in anything but artificially produced situations.

Surveillance data on classical CJD are available and no cases of transmission have been found, even in multiply transfused individuals. However, there are differences between the two diseases and insufficient time has passed for similar analyses to be performed for vCJD. Any potential risk of transmission of vCJD by transfusion will be exacerbated if large numbers of the population prove to be infected, and monitoring of the epidemic in the human population is therefore essential.

At this time there is no suitable in vitro test that can be applied to donated blood to detect infected individuals, and currently the approach taken in the UK is to try to remove any agent present by leucocyte depletion of all donated blood, removing the cells possibly harbouring the agent, and the discard of UK plasma. However, experimental data supporting the benefit of this approach have not yet been obtained. Continued surveillance of vCJD is essential to determine if this approach to blood transfusion has been successful and has prevented transmission by transfusion.

Residual risk of transmitted infection

An essential part of the practice of transfusion microbiology today is to understand the overall effectiveness of the microbiology screening programme in place. Whatever the nature of the screening performed, the aim is to ensure that the blood and blood products transfused are as microbiologically safe as possible. In general, any properly designed and implemented blood screening programme should be effective in ensuring the safety of the blood supply by identifying donations from infected individuals. However, all screening programmes have their limitations. What is important is to understand and effectively quantify those limitations. The limitations are effectively represented by the calculation of the risk of the screening programme failing to identify an 'infectious' donation.

Residual risk is defined as the probability of an infectious donation not being detected by the screening programme in use. This risk arises because of a number of different compounding factors: the screening strategy implemented, the sensitivity of the screening assays used, the overall reliability of the laboratory practice and the probability of collecting a donation from a donor in the 'window' period of infection. In any well-designed and quality focussed screening programme, screening 'failures' (failing to detect a donation from an infected donor) are very rare. The main reason today for any such failure is when a donor has been recently (usually unknowingly) infected and they then donate. At that time the donation may be infectious, but the particular screening target for that particular infectious agent is not yet present at a detectable level. The donation will thus be 'screen negative' although potentially infectious. This is known as the 'window period' of infection; the period during which a donor may be infectious, yet undetectable on screening. The aim of all blood screening strategies is to reduce the window period as much as possible. To achieve this the factors that give rise to the window period must be understood, and the probability of collecting a donation from a donor in the window period quantified.

The window period is not primarily related to assay sensitivity per se – a number of factors are involved. The window period is a function of the biology of the infectious agent and the immunocompetence of the donor. Following exposure and infection, there is a (variable) time period before

there are sufficient 'target marker' to be detected. Even then, there is a finite level at which any marker becomes detectable, although this may be greater than the level required to transmit infection. The probability of encountering a window period donation is a function of the length of the window period, the incidence of infection in the donor population and the sensitivity of the screening assay used.

The residual risk of infection can be determined using the basic data generated through the screening programme. The estimates of residual risk are calculated using the original formula of Schreiber (see Further Reading) and are based on knowledge of the incidence of each transmissible infection in the donor population, the window period for each infectious agent and the inter-donation interval. Although these data are generally estimates in themselves, they are largely based on measurables which can be obtained by transfusion services from within their own screening systems. In brief, the residual risk increases as the incidence of infection and window period increase and the inter-donation interval decreases. The residual risk consequently decreases as the incidence of infection and window period decrease and the inter-donation interval increases.

In general, the data help to establish the overall effectiveness of the screening programme. More specifically, however, they can be used in a number of ways to both provide a base line for the 'current screening strategy' and predict the impact of changes to screening programmes, for example introducing an additional assay or changing an assay. In addition, the data can be extrapolated to help calculate the potential risk of a 'new' or 'emerging' infectious agent by comparing data for a similar existing agent.

Published residual risk analyses are now available for a number of countries, although their accuracy is very dependent on the quality of the data used in the calculations. Not all transfusion services have the infrastructure and quality systems to ensure the accuracy needed to generate reliable figures. Nonetheless these data are now being published and help to understand the actual levels of microbiological safety achieved in different

Table 13.3 UK residual risk data 2003–2004*.

PRIVATE	HIV		HCV		HBV	
	Per 10^6	$1/X \times 10^6$	Per 10^6	$1/X \times 10^6$	Per 10^6	$1/X \times 10^6$
Donations from all donors	0.19	5.22	0.03	29.03	2.02	0.50
Donations from new donors	0.44	2.26	0.15	6.79	6.11	0.16
Donations from repeat donors	0.16	6.16	0.02	46.99	1.54	0.65

* Data also include any additional risk due to test sensitivity and testing errors.

countries. Table 13.3 provides residual risk data for the UK.

Summary

Our knowledge and understanding of the range of infectious agents that can infect donated blood is relatively broad but is still growing. However, the clinical significance of infection by a number of these agents is still unclear and thought has to be given to the responses of blood transfusion services to this ever-increasing burden. If an infectious agent is not shown to be associated with pathogenicity and transmission events do not lead to clinical disease, should blood be screened for the agent? This question is currently being posed in response to the identification of GBV-C and TTV. However, how to respond is unclear and there is the ever-present danger of public pressure in response to perceived rather than actual risks. Blood transfusion services do have to be alert and actively monitor changes, but reacting to such pressures without due thought must be avoided. The calculation of residual risk is an important tool in understanding risk issues associated with the transfusion of blood and blood products and can be used to help predict the potential value and likely outcomes of implementing additional screening.

Key points

1 Good donor selection is critical to donation safety.

2 Although a number of infectious agents are potentially transmissible by transfusion, the number of agents that present a significant and continuous threat is relatively small.

3 Although good-quality and well-designed screening programmes are effective, occasionally a donation may be collected from an infectious donor who at that time is undetected by routine screening (window period of infection).

4 Bacterial contamination of products may be a greater day-to-day threat than the presence of viruses or parasites originating in the donor.

5 Residual risk analysis can be used not only to demonstrate the effectiveness of screening, but also to predict the impact changing an assay or introducing screening for a new infectious agent.

Further reading

Alter HJ. G-pers creepers, where did you get those papers? A reassessment of the literature on the hepatitis G virus. *Transfusion* 1997;37:569–572.

Arguin PM, Singleton J, Rotz LD *et al.* Transfusion-Associated Tick-Borne Illness Task Force. An investigation into the possibility of transmission of tick-borne pathogens via blood transfusion. *Transfusion* 1999;39:828–833.

Barbara J. Transfusion transmitted diseases: prions. In: *The Compendium*. Philadelphia: AABB, 1998, pp. 308–312.

Barbara JAJ, Regan FAM & Contreras MC (eds). *Transfusion Microbiology*. Cambridge: Cambridge University Press, 2008.

Boxall E, Herborn A, Kochethu G *et al.* Transfusion-transmitted hepatitis E in a 'nonhyperendemic' country. *Transfus Med* 2006;16:79–83.

Hollinger FB & Kleinman S. Transfusion transmission of West Nile virus: a merging of historical and contemporary perspectives. *Transfusion* 2003;43:992–997.

Ijaz S, Arnold E, Banks M *et al.* Non-travel associated hepatitis E in England and Wales: demographic, clinical and molecular epidemiological characteristics. *J Infect Dis* 2005;192:1166–1172.

Murphy MF. New variant Creutzfeldt–Jakob disease: the risk of transmission by blood transfusion and the potential benefit of leucocyte-reduction of blood components. *Transfus Med Rev* 1999;13:75–83.

Schreiber GB, Busch MP, Kleinman SH & Korelitz JJ. The risk of transfusion-transmitted viral infections. The Retrovirus Epidemiology Donor Study. *N Engl J Med* 1996;334(26):1685–1690.

UK SHOT data. Available at www.shotuk.org/ SHOTRE-PORT2004.pdf.

Williamson LM, Lowe S, Love EM *et al.* Serious Hazards of Transfusion (SHOT) initiative: analysis of the first two annual reports. *Br Med J* 1999;319: 16–19.

CHAPTER 14
Bacterial contamination

Patricia E. Hewitt
NHS Blood and Transplant, London, UK

Incidence of bacterial contamination

Bacterial contamination of blood components is responsible for more immediate morbidity and mortality than is transfusion-transmitted viral infection. Since 1995, bacterial contamination has been responsible for 29 of 50 (58%) transfusion-transmitted infections reported to the Serious Hazards of Transfusion (SHOT) scheme in the UK. Bacterial infection caused seven of nine deaths due to transfusion-transmitted infections in that period. Platelets were implicated in 25 of 29 cases of bacterial infection and the platelets were 3 days old or more in 23 of 25 cases. *Staphylococcus epidermidis* was isolated in 9 of 25 platelet cases. The French Blood Agency haemovigilance surveillance system attributed 16 deaths to bacterially contaminated blood components between 1994 and 1998, and 15.9% of all transfusion-related fatalities in the US in the years 1986–1991 were accounted for by this problem.

Although serious clinical sequelae of bacterial contamination after red cell transfusion are relatively infrequent, there is a much higher incidence after platelet transfusion. This is mainly due to the storage of platelets at a temperature (22°C) that supports bacterial survival or growth. In contrast, red cells are stored at 4°C, a temperature which does not support the growth of the majority of bacteria. Nevertheless, contamination of red cells does occur and can (rarely) lead to serious consequences. The prevalence of serious episodes is probably in the order of 1 in 5000 for platelet units and 1 in 500,000 (or less) for red cell units. Rarely, bacterial transmissions from cryoprecipitate and fresh plasma units have been reported due to contamination of the water baths used to thaw frozen units. Recipients of platelet transfusions, particularly those who require a prolonged period of support after chemotherapy or bone marrow transplantation, are exposed to significant risk during this period.

- The incidence of contamination assessed by routine bacteriological surveillance of red cell and platelet preparations has been reported as 0.4% in studies from Canada and Germany.
- Pooled platelet preparations have higher contamination rates than single-donor (apheresis) platelets. In a retrospective study at the NHS Blood and Transplant, North London Centre, the contamination rate of time-expired (i.e., >5-day old) pooled platelets was 0.7% compared with 0.4% for apheresis platelets. The incidence of reactions in recipients of pooled platelets was 1 in 4200 platelet transfusions in a study from the US and 1 in 2100 platelet transfusions in a prospective study in Hong Kong. In the latter study, each recipient was regularly evaluated for possible signs of a transfusion reaction, and observed reactions were investigated with bacterial cultures.

Practical Transfusion Medicine, 3rd edition. Edited by Michael F. Murphy and Derwood H. Pamphilon. © 2009 Blackwell Publishing. ISBN: 978-1-4051-8196-9.

• The incidence of reported reactions in transfusion recipients is much less than predicted from the figures obtained from routine surveillance monitoring of contamination rates of blood components or from the prospective clinical follow-up study from Hong Kong. Reasons for this discrepancy are discussed below.

Possible explanations for apparent infrequency of clinical events

• Non-pathogenic bacteria.
• Insufficient numbers of bacteria to cause clinical sequelae.
• Patients pre-medicated with steroids/antipyretics, which mask the typical signs of a reaction.
• Patients already taking antibiotics effective against the contaminating bacteria.
• Patients are immunosuppressed and expected to have infections, and episodes are therefore under-investigated/reported.

Factors contributing to frequency of bacterial contamination of platelets

• Storage conditions of platelets: at 22°C for 5 days.
• Many platelet preparations are pooled; pooling increases risk by increasing donor exposure.

Types of bacterial contaminants

Red cells (Figure 14.1)
• *Yersinia enterocolitica* (accounts for approximately 50% of reports).
• *Pseudomonas fluorescens*.
• *Serratia liquefaciens*.
• Other Gram-negative rods.
A number of factors contribute to *Y. enterocolitica* contamination of red cells:
• the bacterium can grow well at 4°C;

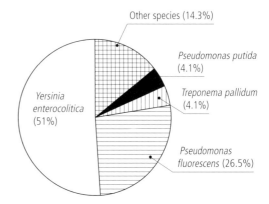

Figure 14.1   Bacterial species associated with sepsis from erythrocyte transfusions.

• donor leucocytes phagocytose living microorganisms in vivo and release them into the blood when the leucocytes disintegrate; and
• potent endotoxin is formed under the conditions of red cell storage.

Platelets (Figure 14.2)
• Coagulase-negative staphylococci.
• *Serratia marcescens*.
• Streptococci.
• *Bacillus cereus*.
• Gram-negative rods.
The contaminants reported as causing clinical reactions in platelet preparations differ from those

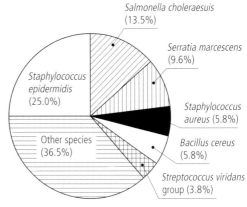

Figure 14.2   Bacterial species associated with sepsis from platelet infusions.

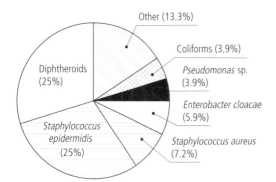

Figure 14.3   Bacteria isolated following monitoring of platelet products.

reported following routine bacteriological monitoring of platelets (Figure 14.3). This is largely accounted for by non-pathogenic bacteria detected during routine monitoring.

Sources of bacterial contamination

It is not always possible to identify the source of bacterial contamination, but cases should be carefully investigated, to cover the following areas:
• donor bacteraemia;
• skin contaminants on the donor's arm (the most common source);
• contamination of the pack or its contents at source (faulty manufacturing); and
• environmental contamination during collection, processing or storage (faulty heat seals, pin-hole defects, etc.).

Donor bacteraemia
• This is an uncommon source of bacterial contamination of blood components, since most bacteraemic individuals would not be fit enough to donate blood.
• Exceptions are usually due to 'episodic bacteraemia' in well individuals, for example transient bacteraemia following dental treatment or associated with a chronic low-grade infection such as osteomyelitis due to *Salmonella*.

• The other main source of bacteraemia in 'well' individuals is that associated with enteric infections, particularly *Y. enterocolitica* and, less commonly, *Campylobacter jejuni* and some *Salmonella*. These infections may give rise to mild non-specific symptoms of abdominal pain or diarrhoea, which would not necessarily be considered relevant in a healthy individual presenting as a blood donor. To exclude all donors with such symptoms in the period immediately preceding blood donation would result in the loss of significant numbers of blood donations that would present no risk at all.

Skin contamination of donor arm
• Inadequate skin cleaning, due to heavy bacterial contamination at the venepuncture site, the presence of bacterial spores not sensitive to the disinfectant used, or faulty technique.
• Scarring of the venepuncture site, more common in regular apheresis donors, preventing effective surface skin cleaning.
• Entry of a small core of skin from the venepuncture site into the phlebotomy needle and into the collection bag. The core may harbour bacteria that would not be affected by surface cleaning of the skin.

Contamination of pack and/or contents
• Case reports have previously cited contaminated anticoagulant fluid within the collection bag as the source of bacterial contamination.
• Other suggested routes of contamination have included grossly contaminated outer surface of packs/tubing, leading to contamination of the operator's hands, and contaminated vacuum tubes that were then used to collect samples from the primary pack after the collection was complete, leading to 'retrograde' contamination of the pack contents.

Environmental contamination
• Since sterile closed systems are used, blood contamination during storage and handling is thought to be very rare.
• Contamination of water baths used to thaw units of cryoprecipitate or fresh frozen plasma may

lead to entry of organisms into the pack, possibly through pin-hole defects or cracks in the plastic.

Clinical features of bacterial contamination

The symptoms of a reaction due to bacterial contamination usually appear immediately, during transfusion of the implicated unit (Table 14.1). Less often, symptoms are delayed until after the end of the transfusion. The most commonly reported symptoms and signs are:
- fever, temperature elevation usually greater than 2°C;
- chills, rigors;
- hypotension, collapse, shock;
- nausea, vomiting; and
- disseminated intravascular coagulation, intravascular haemolysis, and renal failure.

In anaesthetised patients, the clinical signs may be masked. Severe reactions are usually the result of endotoxins produced by contaminating bacteria during the storage period of the component.

Immediate management

- Stop the transfusion. *Note*: retain all packs for investigation.
- Give general supportive treatment, as required, which may include intravenous fluids, inotropic agents and diuretics to maintain urine output.
- Give broad-spectrum antibiotics until the results of blood cultures are known.
- Assess need for intensive care.
- Record carefully and accurately all actions taken.

Investigations

Patient
- Blood count, coagulation studies, urine output and blood cultures.

Blood pack
- Perform Gram stain for immediate evidence of bacterial contamination. This investigation is

Table 14.1 Transfusion reaction due to bacterial contamination: clinical example.

Clinical condition
48-year-old male; acute myeloid leukaemia
Admitted for isolation during neutropenic phase following fourth course of induction chemotherapy
Infected Hickman line site causing intermittent pyrexia
Pancytopenic: Hb 9.7 g/dL, WBC 0.3 × 10^9/L; platelet count 23 × 10^9/L

Management
Blood cultures and skin swabs taken; broad-spectrum antibiotics started
Uneventful transfusion of 2 units of red cells with an additional platelet transfusion
Continued intermittent pyrexia over following 24 h, Hickman site infection not controlled
Blood cultures repeated; started on second-line antibiotics
Continuing pancytopenia, but clinically stable
Further red cell and platelet transfusion prescribed
Collapsed during platelet transfusion with:
   copious diarrhoea
   tachycardia
   hypotension (blood pressure 70 mmHg systolic)
   epistaxis
   rigors; temperature 37°C
Treatment: transfusion discontinued, resuscitation with plasma expanders, blood and faeces obtained for culture
90 min later was alert, clinically recovered, blood pressure 120/80 mmHg, pulse rate 88 per min
Provisional diagnosis: severe platelet reaction or sepsis or haemolytic reaction. Platelet packs referred for culture
6 h after reaction developed haematuria; Hb 3.7 g/dL, platelet count 66 × 10^9 L. Sample taken for investigation of possible haemolytic transfusion reaction
18 h after reaction developed dyspnoea, oliguria, hypoxia
21 h after reaction developed petechial haemorrhage, peripheral oedema, thrombocytopenia, worsening hypoxia
Clinical diagnosis is septicaemia
Transferred to intensive care for respiratory and renal support; commenced on benzylpenicillin/metronidazole/ ciprofloxacin
Gram stain of remnants of platelet pack shows Gram-positive rods and Gram-negative organisms
Cultures of recipient's blood and contents of platelet pack yielded *Clostridium perfringens*. Further investigation revealed presence of toxin
Progressive multiorgan failure. Died 9 days after reaction
Cause of death: shock due to overwhelming septicaemia caused by infected platelet transfusion (toxin mediated)

relatively insensitive, but any contamination lead-ing to clinical symptoms will be significant and therefore readily detected.
• Culture pack contents, taking care not to con-taminate the pack during sampling.
• Inform the blood centre that supplied the pack as soon as bacterial contamination is suspected, as other components of the same blood donation may not yet have been transfused.
• Blood centres will generally require the pack to be returned for further investigation, including ex-amination for pack defects.

Source of contamination
• The blood centre will wish to investigate the pos-sible origin of any contamination by a systematic procedure addressing all the possible sources.
• The identity of the contaminating organism may indicate the likely source of the contamination and the priorities for investigation.

Measures to reduce the risk of bacterial contamination

Donor selection procedures
• Exclusion of donors at risk of bacteraemia, partic-ularly those who have had recent dental treatment (within 24 hours of donation).
• Questions to identify possible symptoms of *Yersinia* infection in donors are unlikely to be ef-fective, since the symptoms are non-specific.

Blood collection
• Avoidance of obviously scarred venepuncture sites.
• Attention to skin cleaning techniques, including evaluation of both the disinfectant solution and the technique of cleaning by monitoring of effective-ness through pre- and post-cleaning swabbing of the skin, training and regular retraining of staff.
• The use of collection devices that allow rejection of the first 20–30 mL of the donation or which di-verts this volume into a sampling device. There is evidence that this approach decreases the preva-lence of contamination.

Component storage times
• Bacterial proliferation in platelet preparations ex-hibits a lag phase of 24–48 hours. The incidence of significant levels of contamination increases steeply after 3 days of storage.
• In the mid-1980s, availability of improved plas-tics for the manufacture of platelet packs led to an extension of the shelf life of platelets in the US from 5 to 7 days. A dramatic increase in the number of severe reactions due to bacterial contamination led to a rapid return to the 5-day limit, which has not subsequently been changed (but see below).
• For red cells, where *Yersinia* is the major offend-ing organism, the current additive solutions and plastics used in packs allow a shelf life of 35 days. *Yersinia* exhibits a lag phase of 21 days, after which bacterial numbers and endotoxin production in-crease dramatically. Reduction of the shelf life of red cells to 21 days would be expected to signif-icantly reduce the problem, but would seriously jeopardise the availability of red cells for patients.

Component storage temperatures
The storage temperature of platelets is a significant factor in the risk of bacterial contamination suffi-cient to cause clinical symptoms. If the storage tem-perature could be reduced, then the risk of contam-ination would be reduced. Unfortunately, storage of platelets at lower temperatures significantly re-duces their haemostatic function and viability.

Pre-transfusion screening of components
There is evidence that the prevalence of significant contamination rises dramatically after 3 days of storage (for platelets) and 21 days (for red cells). It has been suggested that components stored for longer than these periods should be cultured before issue/transfusion. There are various meth-ods of detecting contamination, some of which (visual inspection, Gram staining) are relatively insensitive. There are automated techniques that might be appropriate for this situation, such as the BacT/Alert system (Organon Technika, Durham, NC). Other suggested strategies include ribosomal and polymerase chain reaction (PCR) assays. There are many unanswered questions, such as when

to sample, how to sample (without increasing the chance of contaminating the pack contents) and timing in relation to issue from the blood centre or prior to transfusion of the recipient. Conversely, sterility verification of platelet units could allow an extension of the current shelf life of platelets to 7 days, which would relieve the supply problems often encountered, and there would be a potential gain additional to patient safety. A variety of studies have shown that routine bacterial screening of platelets fails to detect all cases of bacterial contamination, probably related to low levels of contamination and/or the timing of sampling. Early sampling may lead to failure to detect low-level contamination and may not provide sufficient reassurance to extend the shelf life of the platelet product. Later sampling, while likely to be more efficient at detecting contamination, necessarily leads to delayed release of platelets for issue and use of 'older' platelets which may not be of optimum functionality. Nevertheless, bacterial screening of platelet components has been introduced into routine use in a number of blood services and further data about its usefulness in preventing serious adverse reactions, morbidity, and mortality in relation to platelet transfusions is being accumulated.

Leucocyte reduction

Phagocytosis appears to play an important role in the elimination of viable bacteria which might be present in a unit of blood. There is experimental evidence that leucocyte-reduction of cellular blood components reduces the level of bacterial contamination, and that such filtration should be carried out at least 8 hours after collection of the blood to allow sufficient time for phagocytosis to take place. There have been no prospective studies to determine the clinical efficacy of this strategy.

Photochemical decontamination of cellular blood components

Much development work is being carried out on the use of photodynamic methods for inactivation of bacteria. Such methods will also be effective against viruses and protozoa, and therefore present a real attraction in terms of blood component safety (see Chapter 21). Photodynamic methods include irradiation with ultraviolet B light, methylene blue, phthalocyanines, merocyanine 540 and a combination of psoralen and irradiation with ultraviolet A light. Data on the use of psoralen-treated platelets in animal models indicate that in vitro platelet function is maintained, as is in vivo platelet recovery and survival. Although other potential agents have been studied with similar results, clinical trials are clearly needed.

Summary

Unlike many other infectious risks of blood transfusion, bacterial contamination has continued to be a significant problem in recent years. Initiatives including leucocyte-reduction, diversion of the first 20–30 mL of the donation, bacterial screening of platelet preparations before issue and the investigation of potential methods for decontamination, are expected to have an impact in reducing serious reactions due to bacterial contamination. However, care must be taken not to ignore the primary problem, which is the source of contamination. Since the most common source is probably skin contamination of the donor arm, concentration on the basic procedure of skin cleaning prior to venepuncture and on evaluation of the effectiveness of such cleaning is a vital quality standard, which must not be ignored.

Key points

1 Always think about bacterial contamination in a case of immediate adverse reaction to blood transfusion.
2 Platelet transfusions carry the highest risk.
3 Prompt supportive and antibiotic treatment should be initiated in the event of such a reaction.
4 Remember that other blood component recipients may be at risk from the same blood donation.
5 Thorough investigation of the likely source most often points to skin contamination of the donor

arm but this may change as efforts are concentrated on reducing such contamination.

6 Pre-transfusion screening of platelet components is not guaranteed to detect all bacterial contamination.

7 The conditions necessary for the optimum detection of bacterial contamination have not yet been defined.

Further reading

Blajchman MA & Goldman M. Bacterial contamination of platelet concentrates: incidence, significance and prevention. *Semin Hematol* 2001;38(4 Suppl 11):20–26.

Blajchman MA, Goldman M & Baeza F. Improving the bacteriological safety of platelet transfusions. *Transfus Med Rev* 2004;18(1):11–24.

Hogman CF. Serious bacterial complications from blood components: how do they occur? [Editorial] *Transfus Med* 1998;8:1–3.

Jacobs MR, Palavecino E & Yomtovian R. Don't bug me: the problem of bacterial contamination of blood components – challenges and solutions. *Transfusion* 2001;41:1331–1334.

Sazama K. Bacteria in blood for transfusion: a review. *Arch Pathol Lab Med* 1994;118:350–365.

te Boekhorst PA, Beckers EA, Vos MC, Vermeij H & van Rhenen DJ. Clinical significance of bacteriological screening in platelet concentrates. *Transfusion* 2005;45:514–519.

CHAPTER 15

Variant Creutzfeldt–Jakob disease

Marc L. Turner

Edinburgh Blood Transfusion Centre, Royal Infirmary of Edinburgh, Edinburgh, Scotland

A variety of transmissible spongiform encephalopathies or prion diseases are described in animals and humans (Table 15.1). Scrapie, an endemic disease of sheep and goats, was first described over 250 years ago. Chronic wasting disease is spreading in deer and elk in the US. Bovine spongiform encephalopathy (BSE) was first described in cattle in the UK in 1986, though in retrospect the first cases probably appeared as early as 1982. It remains unclear whether BSE arose from scrapie in sheep or from a sporadic case of prion disease in cattle, but it is thought that it was transmitted through the food chain via rendered meat and bonemeal. In the UK over 180,000 clinical cases of BSE have been described, with around 300 cases in other European countries, and occasional cases elsewhere in the world, probably related to exported UK cattle or meat and bonemeal. The UK epidemic peaked in 1992 and has now subsided as a result of a ban on the use of ruminant protein in cattle feed. However, mathematical projections suggest that 1–2 million infected cattle could have entered the human food chain before showing evidence of disease. Unlike scrapie, BSE has proved itself capable of crossing species barriers by infecting a number of other animals including exotic and domestic cats (feline spongiform encephalopathy) and exotic ruminants in zoos (exotic ungulate encephalopathy).

In humans several forms of prion disease have been described. Sporadic or classical Creutzfeldt–Jakob disease (CJD) was first described in the early 1920s. It presents at a median age of 68 years as a rapidly progressive dementia with a duration of illness of around 6 months. The incidence of CJD is around 1 per million per annum throughout the world, with no clear link to the incidence of prion disease in other animals.

In the 1950s, a form of prion disease called kuru was described in the Foré people of the highlands of Papua New Guinea. This disease presented at a much younger age, with cerebellar ataxia as a prominent feature and a more prolonged clinical course. Kuru was transmitted from person to person probably through the cannibalistic funeral rites practised by the tribe at that time. It is informative to note that children died from kuru and that although cannibalistic feasts discontinued around 1959–1960, there are still occasional patients presenting with the clinical disease. This points to a very wide range of incubation periods, with an upper limit of 40–50 years or perhaps even beyond normal human lifespan.

In the 1980s a number of iatrogenic transmissions of CJD were described. These fell broadly into two groups. Direct central nervous systems (CNS) transmission due to contaminated neurosurgical instruments, EEG electrodes and dura mater grafts led to a rapidly progressive dementia reminiscent of sporadic CJD after a short incubation period of around 2 years and death within about 6 months of presentation. Peripheral transmission

Practical Transfusion Medicine, 3rd edition. Edited by Michael F. Murphy and Derwood H. Pamphilon. © 2009 Blackwell Publishing, ISBN: 978-1-4051-8196-9.

Table 15.1 Prion diseases.

Animals	Human
Scrapie	Sporadic Creutzfeldt–Jakob disease
Chronic wasting disease	Kuru
Transmissible mink encephalopathy	Iatrogenic Creutzfeldt–Jakob disease
Bovine spongiform encephalopathy	Variant Creutzfeldt–Jakob disease
Feline spongiform encephalopathy	Familial Creutzfeldt–Jakob disease
Exotic ungulate encephalopathy	Gerstmann–Sträussler–Scheinker disease
	Fatal familial insomnia

from cadaveric pituitary-derived growth- and follicle-stimulating hormone gave rise to a clinical picture reminiscent of kuru, with a prolonged incubation period of some 13–15 years.

Finally, a number of familial forms of CJD have been described including familial CJD, Gerstmann–Sträussler–Scheinker (GSS) disease and fatal familial insomnia (FFI), which arise due to polymorphisms in the gene for prion protein (PrP).

Prion diseases are therefore interesting from an aetiological perspective in that they can arise spontaneously, are transmissible and can also arise due to genetic polymorphism.

Variant CJD

The UK government instituted routine surveillance for CJD in 1989 in response to the BSE epidemic, with the aim of monitoring any change in the incidence or pattern of disease in the UK population. In 1995 the first cases of variant CJD were described. The clinical features differ from those of sporadic CJD. Patients are younger, with a median age at presentation of 28 years (range 12–74 years). They often present with behavioural change, such as depression and anxiety, or with dysaesthesia. Untreated, the disease progresses to cerebellar ataxia, involuntary movements, dementia and death over a period of 7–38 months. One hundred and sixty-six cases of variant CJD

have been described in the UK thus far, though the incidence of new cases appears to be falling. Elsewhere there have been 23 cases described in France, 4 in the Republic of Ireland, 3 in the USA, 2 in the Netherlands and Portugal, 4 in Spain and 1 each in Italy, Japan, Saudi Arabia and Canada. The American, Canadian, and two of the Irish patients spent a considerable time in the UK, whereas the others did not, and probably contracted the disease in their own countries. Though original estimates of the number of people who may eventually develop the disease gave very high upper limits, the recent downturn in the number of new cases in the UK has led to a revised prediction of just over 70 cases. However, a retrospective study of tonsil and appendix samples in the UK recorded 3 positive samples out of 12,600 tested, suggesting a prevalence of subclinical disease of around 1/4000 (95% confidence interval (CI), 1/1000 – 1/20,000). These individuals should be assumed to be at risk of passing infection to others via contaminated surgical instruments or blood transfusion.

A considerable amount of epidemiological, clinical, neuropathological and experimental data now supports the view that variant CJD is the same strain of disease as BSE, and that these are different from the prion strains which give rise to other forms of CJD in humans or scrapie and chronic wasting disease in animals.

Aetiology and pathophysiology

Prion diseases are associated with a change in the secondary structure of PrP. PrP is a widely expressed 30–35 kDa glycoprotein with two N-linked oligosaccharides. It is normally linked to the cell membrane by a glycosylphosphatidylinositol (GPI) anchor, though transmembrane anchorage has also been described. The normal secondary structure of PrP contains around 40% α-helices and 3% β-pleated sheets, with the membrane-distal part of the molecule largely unstructured. The development of prion disease is associated with a change in the secondary structure of the PrP glycoprotein, with an increase in the proportion of β-pleated sheets to some 40–50% of the molecule largely

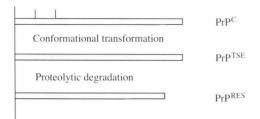

PrP^C

Conformational transformation

PrP^{TSE}

Proteolytic degradation

PrP^{RES}

Figure 15.1   The prion hypothesis. PrP^C(top) is a 30–35 kDa glycoprotein with two N-linked glycosylation sites, anchored by glycosylphosphatidylinositol to the cell membrane, with 40% α-helix and 3% β-pleated sheet. Prion diseases are associated with conformational change in the secondary structure, with an increase in the amount of β-pleated sheet to some 40–50% of the molecule (PrP^{TSE}) (middle). This changes the physico-chemical and biological properties of the molecule rendering it resistant to degradation by enzymes such as proteinase-K (PrP^{RES}) (bottom).

at the expense of the unstructured region (PrP^{TSE}) (Figure 15.1). This changes the physico-chemical characteristics of the molecule, giving it increased resistance to both physical and biological degradation. In vitro treatment with proteinase-K removes the membrane-distal part of the molecule, but is unable to digest the 30–32 kDa core (PrP^{Res}). PrP^{TSE} accumulates in vivo, leading to the deposition of amyloid plaques. The pathophysiology of the disease remains debated. Some authorities propose the presence of a small DNA molecule associated with PrP^{TSE} (termed a virion), but this has not yet been identified and the infectious agent does appear to be resistant to physical conditions that would normally degrade DNA. The prion hypothesis proposes that the abnormal isoform of the protein is itself the infectious agent, changing the structure of the normal form either through heterodimer formation or though a physico-chemical process of nuclear polymerisation.

Accumulation of amyloid plaques consisting of PrP^{TSE} leads to the classical neuropathological features of neuronal death, astrogliosis and spongiform degeneration of the CNS (plate 15.1 and 15.2). In sporadic, iatrogenic and familial forms of CJD, abnormal PrP accumulation appears to be confined to the CNS. In variant CJD, abnormal

PrP^{TSE} accumulation has been demonstrated in follicular dendritic cells (FDCs) in the tonsil, spleen, cervical, mediastinal, para-aortic and mesenteric lymph nodes and gut-associated lymphoid tissue of the appendix up to 2 years prior to the onset of clinical disease (plate 15.3). This observation is consistent with what we know about the pathophysiology of transmission of prion diseases by peripheral routes in experimental animals.

Experimental peripheral transmission of scrapie strains in murine models leads to the presence of infectivity and/or PrP^{TSE} in the spleen and lymph node from a very early stage of infection, well before detection of infectivity of PrP^{TSE} in the CNS. Interestingly, immunosuppression and splenectomy have long been known to decrease the efficiency of peripheral transmission, whereas irradiation and thymectomy do not. A series of experiments has demonstrated that mice with severe combined immunodeficiency are resistant to peripheral but not central prion challenge and that sensitivity is regained after allogeneic bone marrow transplantation. Similarly, PrP-negative mice with a PrP-positive CNS implant can be infected only by peripheral transmission following PrP-positive allogeneic bone marrow transplant, whereas PrP-positive mice develop resistance to peripherally transmitted disease following PrP-negative bone marrow transplant. Detailed knockout experiments have demonstrated that Rag 1, Rag 2 and μMT knockout mice are resistant to peripheral challenge whereas CD4, CD8, β-microglobulin and perforin knockout models display normal sensitivity. These data led to the suggestion that B-lymphocytes were essential to peripheral transmission whereas T-lymphocytes were not. However, B-lymphocytes are also essential for FDC survival and more recent studies have demonstrated that PrP-positive FDCs are essential to peripheral transmission whereas PrP-positive B-lymphocytes are not. Indeed, peripheral transmission can be inhibited even by temporary FDC inactivation by lymphotoxin β-receptor blockade and also by depletion of complement receptors. These data convincingly support the seminal role of FDCs in the early stages of peripheral transmission.

Assessing peripheral blood infectivity in animal models

It has been demonstrated that PrP is present in the peripheral blood of normal individuals at a concentration of 100–300 ng/mL, with the majority found in platelets and plasma. It has not, as yet, been proved possible to demonstrate accumulation of PrP^{TSE} in the peripheral blood of humans, though one study has demonstrated such accumulation in the peripheral blood of scrapie-infected sheep. Most of the information on peripheral blood infectivity comes from animal experiments where it has proved possible to demonstrate infectivity in the peripheral blood of sheep and rodents with experimental scrapie and BSE, and in rodents with experimental GSS, during both the clinical and incubation phases of disease. However, no infectivity has been demonstrated in natural scrapie in sheep and goats, natural transmissible mink encephalopathy or natural or experimental BSE in cattle. The reason for these differences is not clear. Levels of peripheral blood infectivity have been investigated in the Fukuoka-1 strain of GSS in experimental mice and have been found to be in the order of 100 infectious units/mL during the clinical phase of disease and 5–10 infectious units/mL during the incubation period. A fourfold to fivefold higher level of infectivity was demonstrated in the buffy coat (containing the leucocytes and platelets) compared with plasma. Plasma itself showed a 10-fold higher concentration of infectivity compared with any of the Cohn fractions in an experimental fractionation system. The distribution of infectivity in blood was similar during the incubation phase of disease. Similar findings have been described in the 263K scrapie hamster model, where little infectivity is associated with (purified) red cells or platelets, around 40% is associated with leucocytes and the remainder is in the plasma. Indeed, more recent data from the same group suggests that washing the leucocytes removes most of the associated infectivity.

In a different model, sheep experimentally infected with BSE or scrapie by oral ingestion have been bled during the incubation and clinical phases of disease and whole-blood donations administered intravenously to secondary recipients. Up to 50% of the secondary recipients in both cohorts have subsequently developed the relevant prion disease, amounting to proof of principle that certain forms of prion disease can be transmitted by blood transfusion.

Clinical transmission of CJD from the peripheral blood of patients

In humans, of 37 reported attempts to transmit sporadic CJD from peripheral blood of patients with clinical disease by intracerebral inoculation into rodents, there have been five positive reports. Interestingly, transmission of CJD from human peripheral blood to primates by intracerebral inoculation has not proved possible and this has thrown some doubt on the validity of the rodent data. Thus far, there have been no successful transmissions of variant CJD from human peripheral blood to rodents or primates.

There have been three anecdotal case reports of patients who have developed sporadic CJD some time after receiving blood components or plasma products. In none of these, however, has it been shown that the donors themselves developed CJD. In comparison a large number of epidemiological case-control, lookback and surveillance studies over the past 25 years have shown little evidence of increased risk of sporadic CJD in blood or plasma product recipients, even where a donor is known to have subsequently developed sporadic CJD.

There are now a number of patients identified with variant CJD who, in the past, were blood donors. Recipients of blood components and plasma products from these donors have been traced, and thus far three of their recipients have developed clinical variant CJD and one has shown evidence of abnormal prion accumulation in the spleen and a cervical lymph node, suggesting that this is actually quite an efficient route of transmission.

Strategies for risk containment

Blood services have felt it prudent to implement precautionary policies to contain the risk of

Table 15.2 UK criteria for excluding blood and tissue donors who have, or may have had contact with, sporadic, iatrogenic, or familial CJD.

Obligatory

Permanently exclude donors with CJD or other prion-associated disorder

Permanently exclude anyone identified at high risk of developing a prion-associated disorder

    Recipients of dura mater, corneal or scleral grafts

    Recipients of human pituitary-derived extracts such as growth hormone and gonadotrophins

    Individuals at familial risk of prion-associated diseases. This includes individuals who have had two or more blood relatives develop a prion-associated disease and individuals who have been informed that they are at risk following genetic counselling

Exceptions

Individuals who have had two or more blood relatives develop a prion-associated disease but who, following genetic counselling, have been informed that they are not at risk. This requires confirmation by the consultant with responsibility for donors.

---

transmission of variant CJD. However, such policies require careful evaluation, both in terms of likely efficacy in reducing the risk of secondary transmission by blood transfusion and in terms of the potential increase in other risks including that of blood shortages. Consideration also needs to be given to the cross-impact of different policies and the opportunity costs incurred.

Donor selection

The UK blood services use a number of criteria to exclude blood and tissue donors who may be at increased risk of sporadic, iatrogenic, or familial CJD (Table 15.2). There are no epidemiological risk factors described thus far that would discriminate a high-risk group for development of variant CJD within the UK. For example, there is no evidence that veterinary surgeons, cattle farmers, abattoir workers or others with high risk of exposure to infected bovine materials are at higher risk of developing variant CJD than the general population. In comparison, some individuals who have been vegetarians for prolonged periods have de-

veloped variant CJD. A number of countries have taken the precautionary step of excluding blood donors who have spent more than a defined period in the UK between the beginning of 1980 and the end of 1996. The defined period varies depending on the frequency and pattern with which indigenous donors visit the UK and the likely prevalence of subclinical variant CJD in the general population. These are factors which impact upon the efficacy of UK donor exclusion in terms of risk reduction and on the likely negative impact on the blood donor base.

Subsequent to the evidence of transmission of variant CJD by blood transfusion, the UK blood services moved in April 2004 to defer blood donors who have themselves received blood transfusions in order to reduce the risk that tertiary and higher-order transmissions would lead to a self-sustaining outbreak. This led to the loss of approximately 5–10% of the donor base.

Importation of blood components

An alternative approach would be to source blood components from countries with low incidence of BSE and variant CJD. It is impractical to source all red blood cell concentrates for the UK (some 2.5 million components per annum) from overseas volunteer non-remunerated donors. The short shelf life of platelet concentrates also mitigates against this approach. Consideration needs to be given to the risk of other infectious agents in the proposed alternative donor population and long-term security of supply. It is possible to source plasma from overseas since surplus clinical plasma is generated by red cell collection programmes and the product can be virus inactivated and cryopreserved for transportation with a 2-year shelf life.

In the UK it has been decided to import methylene blue-inactivated plasma for neonates and children up to 16 years of age. Neonates in particular receive a proportionately high number of blood components due to prematurity and surgery for congenital disorders. They are likely to have a low primary exposure to BSE through the food chain and they have the longest prospective lifespan during which to develop clinical variant CJD should they become infected. More recently solvent-detergent fresh frozen plasma has been imported for patients exposed to large volumes of plasma (such as patients undergoing plasma exchange for thrombotic thrombocytopenic purpura).

Development of peripheral blood assays for donor screening

There is no conventional immune response to prion infection and no DNA has been detected in association with transmission of these diseases. Hence, conventional serological and molecular approaches to the development of peripheral blood assays, utilised to such good effect in screening for microbiological disease, are not applicable to prion diseases.

A number of non-specific markers of CNS damage are known to be elevated in the peripheral blood of patients with CJD, including 14-3-3 and S100, but given that patients with CNS damage are excluded by donor selection criteria, it seems unlikely that these would have much to offer in the context of screening normal healthy blood donors.

Surrogate markers could allow exclusion of individuals at risk of development of variant CJD. Reduced transcription of erythroid differentiation-associated factors (EDAF) has been described in the bone marrow and peripheral blood of scrapie-infected sheep and rodents and of BSE-infected cattle. However, these finding do not appear to have been borne out in humans.

The gold standard would be, of course, infectivity bioassays. However, not only is it impractical to use such an approach for primary screening, but also, as noted above, infectivity is not detectable in the peripheral blood of patients with variant CJD despite the fact that it is clearly transmissible. This paradox is probably a reflection of the species barrier between rodents and man, but implies that total reliance will need to be placed on any in vitro assay since there may be no other way of establishing whether the test-positive individual is 'truly' infected or will develop clinical disease in the future.

Detection of PrP^{TSE} in the peripheral blood is the only practical way forward, although there are a number of fundamental problems. First is the analytical sensitivity likely to be required. If one assumes infectivity in human blood to be in the order of 1–10 infectious units/mL during the incubation period of disease (an extrapolation from the rodent models) and that the ratio of infectivity to PrP^{TSE} is similar to that seen in animal models, then the concentration of PrP^{TSE} in infected peripheral blood will be in the order of 0.01–0.1 pg/mL (in the context of 100–300 ng/mL of PrP^{C}). Moreover, there are uncertainties around the physico-chemical form of PrP^{TSE} in blood and indeed the exact relationship between PrP^{TSE} and infectivity. Nevertheless a number of assays are under development based on a combination of proteinase-K digestion, the use of chaotropic agents, high-affinity ligands or monoclonal antibodies as capture or detection agents and/or in vitro amplification, which are beginning to approach the levels of sensitivity required. Some of these approaches use PrP^{TSE} concentration steps to further increase the analytical sensitivity of the assay.

A second problem is the validation of such assays given that normally this would involve samples from patients with the disease in question. Variant CJD assays will have to be validated using animal model systems and human blood spiked with homogenised prion-infected tissues, given the limited volumes of blood available from patients with variant CJD.

Moreover, the diagnostic sensitivity and specificity of an assay is dependent not only on its analytical features but also on the population under study. An assay that has a high level of specificity in the clinical context of a patient with suspected disease may have a very low level of specificity (i.e. have a high false-positive rate) in the context of healthy blood donors. This point is made in Figure 15.2, which illustrates the consequences of screening 1 million blood donors with an assay with 99% sensitivity and specificity. Assuming a prevalence of subclinical variant CJD of 1 in 10,000 (as an example), around 99 infected individuals would be detected (true positives), whilst 1 would be missed (false negative). The majority

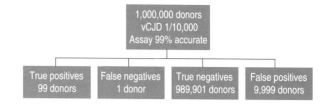

Figure 15.2   Likely impact of a putative variant CJD assay with 99% sensitivity and specificity.

- Negative predictive value: 99.99989%
- Positive predictive value: 0.98%

of donors would of course be true negatives, but a sizeable minority (just under 10,000) would be falsely positive. This brings into perspective the requirement for confirmatory assays, based on different analytical principles. Even with confirmatory assays it may still be very difficult to predict whether a test-positive individual will ever go on to develop clinical variant CJD (and/or whether they are infective to others).

Test-positive individuals would have to be informed and deferred. The psychological and social impact on the donor and the overall impact on donor recruitment and retention should not be underestimated.

Component processing

Universal leucocyte reduction was introduced in the UK in July 1998, predicated on the thesis that if variant CJD infectivity was present in the peripheral blood, it was likely to be mainly associated with the mononuclear leucocyte population. Mod-

ern leucocyte-depletion filters remove 3–4 $\log_{10}$ of leucocytes with no evidence of selective subset removal or cellular fragmentation. However, experimental studies in rodents suggest that only 40–70% of the infectivity in peripheral blood is removed by leucocyte reduction, with little impact on plasma-associated infectivity as expected. Under most scenarios, sufficient infectivity would therefore remain to allow transmission to a recipient. Several companies are now developing prion removal devices which may be able to remove additional 3 log infectivity from red cells concentrates and thereby impact on transmission risk (Table 15.3).

Plasma products

Plasma product recall is not indicated if a blood donor develops sporadic CJD, based on the accumulated clinical evidence of a low risk of transmission in lookback and surveillance studies. In December 1997 the UK Committee for the Safety of Medicines recommended product recall if a donor

Table 15.3 Likely impact of leucocyte reduction and prion reduction devices on variant CJD infectivity and transmissibility.

Log reduction in infectivity	Residual leucocytes	Residual plasma	Total residual infectivity	Risk of transmission
Leucodepletion alone	0.2	130	130.2	Certain
1 log	0.2	13	13.2	Certain
2 log	0.2	1.3	13.2	Certain
3 log	0.2	0.13	0.33	1/3
4 log	0.2	0.013	0.213	1/5

became infected with variant CJD in view of the uncertainties surrounding transmissibility of the disease. In Autumn 1999 the use of UK plasma for fractionation was discontinued altogether because of the recognition that a significant number of cases of variant CJD among donors would lead to multiple recalls and critical product shortages irrespective of the transmissibility of the disease. Other European plasma fractionation centres continue to use their own plasma.

Most studies suggest a significant reduction in infectivity by the Cohn fractionation process. Studies with 263K and 301V spikes using Western blot, DELFIA and infectivity bioassays as readouts suggest that cold ethanol precipitation, depth filtration, ion-exchange chromatography and nanofiltration all give several $\log_{10}$ reductions in infectivity titre, though whether these steps are additive is unclear. Criticisms of these studies surround the use of homogenised brain as the spike because infectivity may not be in the same physico-chemical form as that seen in naturally infected blood. The studies of Brown *et al.* referred to earlier, using plasma from mice infected with the Fukuoka 1 strain of GSS, have shown an overall reduction of up to 3–4 $\log_{10}$, though the starting levels of infectivity are low and so estimates of the reduction in infectivity by serial plasma processing steps are likely to be conservative.

A number of patients with variant CJD have donated plasma for product manufacture. The implicated batches have been identified and, where possible, the recipients traced, notified and managed as 'at risk for public health purposes'. No such recipients have thus far developed variant CJD.

Optimal use of blood components

There remains a need to reduce blood use and outdating both to manage the risk of unnecessary exposure to variant CJD and to reduce pressure on the blood supply at a time when significant reduction in the number of blood donors due to the introduction of new donor selection or screening criteria is a real possibility. Key issues to be addressed include better evidence of the efficacy of current clinical transfusion practice, reduction in blood outdate and discard rates, and adoption of approaches for blood conservation.

Cell, tissue and organ transplantation

Though the level of infectivity associated with other cell and tissue products is unknown, in almost all cases the mass of tissue transplanted is sufficiently large that the concentration of infection required to effect transmission would be well below the sensitivity of current assays. A precautionary assumption should therefore be made that these tissues will also transmit infection should the donor be infected.

Key points

1 To date, there have been four cases of variant CJD prion transmission by red cell components.
2 The prevalence of subclinical disease may be significantly higher than that suggested by the incidence of clinical cases.
3 A number of precautionary measures have already been taken including donor deferrals, universal leucocyte reduction and sourcing of plasma for fractionation from outwith the UK.
4 Further precautionary measures are under consideration including prion reduction filters and prion assays.
5 Such measures require careful evaluation in terms of likely efficacy, associated risks and opportunity costs.

Further reading

Brown P. The pathogenesis of transmissible spongiform encephalopathy: routes to the brain and the erection of therapeutic barriers. *Cell Mol Life Sci* 2001;58:259–265.
Brown P, Cervenakova L & Diringer M. Blood infectivity and the prospects for a diagnostic screening test in Creutzfeldt–Jakob disease. *J Lab Clin Med* 2001;137:5–13.

Brown P, Cervenakova L, McShane LM *et al.* Further studies of blood infectivity in an experimental model of transmissible spongiform encephalopathy with an explanation of why blood components to not transmit Creutzfeldt–Jakob disease in humans. *Transfusion* 1999;39:1169–1178.

Brown P, Rohwer RG, Dunstan BC *et al.* The distribution of infectivity in blood components and plasma derivatives in experimental models of transmissible spongiform encephalopathy. *Transfusion* 1998;38:810–816.

Brown P, Will RG, Bradley R *et al.* Bovine spongiform encephalopathy and variant Creutzfeldt–Jakob disease: background, evolution and current concerns. *Emerg Infect Dis* 2001;7:6–16.

Collee JG & Bradley R. BSE: a decade on. Part 1. *Lancet* 1997;349:636–641.

Collee JG & Bradley R. BSE: a decade on. Part 2. *Lancet* 1997;349:715–721.

Collinge J. Variant Creutzfeldt–Jakob disease. *Lancet* 1999;354:317–323.

Foster PR. Prions and blood products. *Ann Med* 2000;32:501–513.

Gregori L, McCombie N, Palmer D *et al.* Effectiveness of leucoreduction for removal of infectivity of transmissible spongiform encephalopathies from blood. *Lancet* 2004;364:529–531.

Hunter N, Foster J, Chong A *et al.* Transmission of prion diseases by blood transfusion. *J Gen Virol* 2002;83:2897–2905.

Llewelyn CA, Hewitt PE, Knight RS *et al.* Possible transmission of variant Creutzfeldt–Jakob disease by blood transfusion. *Lancet* 2004;363:417–421.

Macgregor I. Prion protein and developments in its detection. *Transfusion* 2001;11:3–14.

Peden AH, Head MW, Ritchie DL *et al.* Preclinical vCJD after blood transfusion in a PRNP codon 129 heterozygous patient. *Lancet* 2004;364:527–529.

Turner ML (ed.). *Creutzfeldt–Jakob Disease: Managing the Risk of Transmission by Blood, Plasma and Tissues.* Bethesda, MY: AABB Press, 2006.

CHAPTER 16

Emerging infections and transfusion safety

Roger Y. Dodd

American Red Cross, Jerome H. Holland Laboratory for the Biomedical Sciences, Rockville, Maryland, USA

The Institute of Medicine in the US has defined emerging infections as those whose incidence in humans has increased within the past two decades or threatens to increase in the near future. Emergence may be due to the spread of a new agent, the recognition of an infection that has been present in the population but has gone undetected, or the realisation that an established disease has an infectious origin. Emergence may also be used to describe the reappearance (or re-emergence) of a known infection after a decline in incidence. A proportion of such emerging infections have properties that permit their transmissibility by blood transfusion; perhaps the most notable example has been HIV/AIDS, although there are others, such as West Nile virus (WNV), babesia and malaria. This chapter will explain the basis for emergence of infectious agents and discuss their recognition and management in the context of the safety of the blood supply.

Emerging infections

There is no single reason to account for the emergence of infections, although it is possible to establish relatively broad groupings:

Practical Transfusion Medicine, 3rd edition. Edited by Michael F. Murphy and Derwood H. Pamphilon. © 2009 Blackwell Publishing, ISBN: 978-1-4051-8196-9.

- Failure of existing control mechanisms, including the appearance of drug-resistant strains, vaccine escape mutants or cessation of vector control accounts for a large group of agents.
- Environmental change can have profound effects, whether through global warming, changes in land utilisation or irrigation practice, urbanisation or even agricultural practices.
- Population movements and rapid transportation can introduce infectious agents into new environments where they may spread rapidly and without constraint, as has been the case for WNV in the US.
- Human behaviours can contribute in a number of ways; new agents have been introduced into human populations by contact with, or even preparation and consumption of, wildlife; many infections have been spread widely though extensive sexual networks, and armed conflicts have led to extensive disease spread.

Of course, many of these factors may also work in combination. Key points are that new or unexpected diseases can appear in any location at any time and that an appropriate understanding of the epidemiology of such diseases can assist in the development of appropriate interventions.

In order to be transmissible by transfusion, an agent must have certain key properties:

- Most importantly, there must be a phase when the agent is present in the blood in the absence of any significant symptoms. Until recently, it was generally thought that such infectivity would reflect a long-term carrier state for the agent in question, as exemplified by HIV, HBV or HCV, although there had been a few cases of transmission of hepatitis A virus, which provokes an acute infection with a relatively short period of asymptomatic viraemia. However, the finding of transfusion transmission of WNV showed that, in epidemic outbreaks, acute infections could be readily transmitted by transfusion.

• A secondary requirement is that the agent must be able to survive component preparation and storage.

• Finally, the agent should have a clinically apparent outcome in at least a proportion of cases of infection, or it will lack clear relevance to blood safety and its transmission will not generally be recognised. There are some examples of transfusion transmissible agents that do not seem to cause any significant outcomes, such as GB virus type C/hepatitis G virus (GBV-C/HGV) and torque tenovirus (TTV).

Table 16.1 lists a number of emerging infections that are known, or suspected, to be transfusion transmissible and also notes the factors thought to be responsible for their emergence.

Approaches to the management of transfusion-transmissible emerging infections

As far as it is possible, emerging infections that do, or may, impact on blood safety should be managed in a systematic fashion. In general, this will be the responsibility of agencies that are charged with the maintenance of public health, or the management of the blood supply or its regulation. However, there are a number of areas in which individual professionals can contribute. One of these is the first step, which is the recognition of a transfusion-transmitted infection and its subsequent investigation. It is, in fact, unlikely that the first occurrence of an emerging infection will be seen in a transfused recipient, so it is therefore important that there be a system of assessing the threat and risk of emerging infections for their potential impact on blood safety. This implies a process for evaluating each emerging

infection for its transmissibility by this route and for estimating the severity and potential extent of the threat. The risk assessment should help to define the need for and urgency of development and implementation of interventions to reduce the risk of transmission of the agent. Such interventions, if implemented, should be evaluated for efficacy and modified as appropriate.

Assessing the risk and threat of transfusion transmissibility

It is important to have a general awareness of the status of new and emerging infections, with particular reference to your own country or area. Such awareness may involve familiarity with a number of sources of information, ranging from news media, through alerts from local, national and global public health agencies, to specialised resources such as ProMED Mail (an Internet listserver and website that tracks and comments on disease outbreaks). Other tools are anticipated to become available; for example, the American Association of Blood Banks (AABB) is developing and will maintain a listing of potentially transfusion transmissible infectious agents that will be placed on a website: the listing will also contain much of the information discussed below, along with a ranking of threat level. Other agencies (for example, the Centers for Disease Control and prevention and the World Health Organization) provide general, current information about emerging infectious agents on their websites.

Table 16.2 outlines questions that serve to define the risk of transfusion transmission of each agent and the potential extent and severity of that risk. The primary question is whether or not the disease agent can, in fact, be transmitted by blood. As pointed out above, this is dependent on the presence of an asymptomatic phase during which the disease agent is present in the bloodstream. In some cases, of course, there may already be documentation of transfusion transmission of the agent in question, or there may be suggestive evidence, such as transmission by organ transplantation. However, in the latter case, such evidence may not be definitive, as rabies has been

Table 16.1 Selected emerging infections potentially or actually transmissible by blood transfusion.

Agent	Basis for emergence	Notes
Prions		
vCJD	Agricultural practice: feeding meat and bonemeal to cattle	Of most concern in UK; apparently coming under control
Viruses		
Chikungunya	Global climate change, dispersion of mosquito vector, travel	Rapid emergence in a number of areas, including Italy. Surveillance indicated
Dengue	Global climate change, dispersion of mosquito vector, travel	Similar properties to WNV; surveillance indicated
HBV variants	Selection pressure resulting from vaccination	Mutants may escape detection by standard test methods
HHV-8	Transmission between men who have sex with men and perhaps by intravenous drug use	Transmission by transfusion and transplantation known
HIV	Interactions with wildlife, sexual networks, travel	Classic example of an emerging infection
HIV variants	Viral mutation, travel	May escape detection by standard tests
Influenza	Pandemic anticipated as a result of antigenic change	Possible threat to blood safety, major impact on availability
SARS	Explosive global epidemic, wildlife origin, spread by travel	No demonstrated transfusion transmission, epidemic over
Simian foamy virus	Exposure to monkeys, concern about species jumping and mutation	Regulatory concern over blood safety, intervention in Canada
WNV	Introduction into the US (probably via jet transport), rapid spread across continent	Recognition of transfusion transmission in 2002 led to rapid implementation of NAT for donors
Bacteria		
Anaplasma phagocytophilum	Tick-borne agent expanding its geographic range	One potential transfusion transmission reported
Borrelia burgdorferi	Tick-borne agent expanding its geographic range and human exposure	No transfusion transmission reported
Parasites		
Babesia spp.	Tick-borne agent expanding its geographic range and human exposure	More than 60 transfusion transmission cases reported
Leishmania spp.	Increased exposure to military and others in Iraq, Afghanistan	Unexpected visceral forms potentially transmissible
Plasmodium spp.	Classic re-emergence, in part due to climate change, travel	Re-emergence threatens value of travel deferral
Trypanosoma cruzi	Imported into non-endemic areas by population movement	Transfusion transmissible, preventable by donor testing

transmitted by organ transplantation, but is almost certainly not transmissible by blood. The answer to this question is not always readily obtainable, but may often be inferred by considering what is known about the natural transmission route of the infection, or from the properties of closely related organisms. The duration of the blood phase of the infection will have a direct impact on the risk of transmission, reflecting the chance that an individual will give blood during the infectious phase.

Table 16.2 Key questions to assess risk of transfusion transmissibility of an infectious agent.

1. Have transfusion-transmitted cases been observed?
2. Does the agent have an asymptomatic, blood-borne phase?
3. Does the agent survive component preparation and storage?
4. Are blood recipients susceptible to infection with the agent?
5. Does the agent cause disease, particularly in blood recipients?
6. What is the severity, mortality and treatability of the disease?
7. Are there recipient conditions, such as immunosuppression, that favour more severe disease?
8. Is there a meaningful frequency of infectivity in the potential donor population?
9. Is this frequency declining, stable, or increasing?
10. Are there reasons to anticipate any changes in the frequency of donor infectivity?
11. What is the level of concern about the agent and its disease among professionals, public health experts, regulators, politicians, media and general population?
12. Are there rational and accessible interventions to eliminate or reduce transmission by transfusion?

The actual risk of transmission is a function of the frequency of the infection in the donor population and the length of the period of blood-borne infectivity. The period of infectivity may not, however, be identical to the period during which the infectious agent can be detected in the blood. For example, in the case of WNV, periods of viraemia in excess of 100 days have been measured occasionally, but the actual infectious period may be limited to the week or two prior to the appearance of antibodies. Another difficulty is that the frequency of disease and the frequency of infection may differ greatly, as is again the case with WNV. Nevertheless, it is abundantly clear that individuals who do not develop symptoms may be infectious via their blood donations. Consequently, it may be important to estimate the size of the infected (and infectious) population by laboratory testing rather than through disease reporting. Indeed, organised studies of prevalence rates of infection among donor populations have been used in many circumstances in order to assess the level of risk and to predict the impact of a testing intervention. Examples of this approach include studies on HTLV, trypanosomes (*T. cruzi*), babesia, and more recently, dengue virus, where assessments of the frequency of viraemia are proving valuable. Another important factor is the dynamics of the outbreak. Is the frequency of infection stable, or increasing, and if increasing, is change linear or logarithmic and what is the rate

of increase? Obviously, rapid increase, as seen in the case of WNV, would imply a need for a more rapid response than would a slow, linear increase, as in the case of *T. cruzi*.

The severity of disease that may result from a transfusion-transmitted infection is also an important guide to the extent and speed of implementation of any intervention. There are both objective and subjective aspects to such an assessment. Clearly, the severity of the disease and its associated mortality can be defined, but it may also be important to judge the public concern around the disease, which may be disproportionate to its actual public health impact. Another factor that is often presented as important is the extent to which a transfusion-transmitted infection might result in further or secondary infections. In actual fact, transmission of an infection by transfusion will almost certainly not lead to any magnification of an epidemic, but nevertheless, it is something that should be considered.

A word of caution is in order with respect to efforts to use modern laboratory methods to identify previously unrecognised infectious agents. There is increasing enthusiasm for this approach, but it is important to recognise that without any established relationship to a disease state, the results of such searches can be misleading. At this time, for example, it does not appear that either TTV or GBV-C/HGV have any relationship to any disease state and do not seem to offer risk to blood recipients, despite clear evidence of their transmissibility. It is unclear how many other such orphan viruses are awaiting discovery.

Recognition of transfusion transmission of emerging infections

There is no simple formula for recognising that a transfusion-transmitted infection has occurred, particularly in the case of a rare or unusual disease agent. Nevertheless, many such events have been recognised by astute clinicians. Knowledge of the potential for transmission of an emerging infection can be valuable and very likely contributed to the relatively early recognition of transfusion transmission of WNV. Unusual post-transfusion events with a suspected infectious origin should be brought to the attention of experts in infectious diseases or public health agencies for assistance in identification and follow-up. Appropriate investigation of illness occurring a few days or more after transfusion can reveal infections through identification of serologic or molecular evidence of infectious agents in post-transfusion samples. However, such detection is by no means definitive. It is helpful if a pre-transfusion patient sample is also available, as this will reveal whether the condition predated the transfusion. Also, recall and further testing of implicated donors will reveal whether one or more of them was the likely source of the infection. Ideally, if the responsible organism can be isolated from both donor and recipient, molecular analyses such as nucleic acid sequencing can demonstrate (or exclude) the identity of the agent from the two sources. There are significant problems in recognising that infections with a very long incubation period may have been transmitted by transfusion: this was illustrated by HIV/AIDS, which did not result in well-defined illness until many years after exposure. This prevented early recognition of transfusion-transmitted AIDS and further concealed the actual magnitude of the infectious donor population and of the population of infected blood recipients. This implies that, for

emerging infections that appear to have lengthy incubation periods, it would be wise to assess transfusion transmissibility by serologic or molecular evaluation of appropriate donor–recipient sample repositories, or to engage in some form of active surveillance such as that used to identify the transmission of variant Creutzfeldt–Jacob disease (vCJD) by transfusion in England. Haemovigilance programmes may contribute to the identification of post-transfusion infections, although they are generally designed to identify well-described outcomes.

Interventions

In the event that an emerging infection is found to be transfusion transmissible and public and professional concern implies a need to protect the safety of the blood supply, there are a number of interventions that could be considered.

A possible, but rather unsatisfactory approach is to focus on the recipient by diagnosing and treating cases that occur. This, of course, works only for treatable infections. It is de facto part of the approach to manage transfusion babesiosis in the US at this time.

Most interventions are focused on the donor or the donation. In the absence of a test, it may be possible to devise a question that would identify some proportion of donors at risk of transmitting the infection. Such measures are usually neither sensitive nor specific, but may have value, particularly where the disease is localised so that a travel history is sufficient to identify those at risk.

The development and implementation of a test for infectivity in donor blood is usually a more sensitive and specific approach than questioning and for some infections may be the only valid solution. In the past, serologic tests were relied upon, but now, nucleic acid testing is also available and may be a better solution, as was the case for WNV. Indeed, a test for WNV RNA was developed and implemented in less than a year in the US. However, this is not always the optimal solution. For example, some parasitic diseases in particular result in long-term, antibody-positive infection with very low levels of infectious agent in the bloodstream, resulting in only intermittent NAT-positive findings. This is particularly true of Chagas disease, and as most individuals were infected early in life, antibody tests are preferable for identifying potentially infectious donors.

An emerging technology that offers some promise is that of pathogen reduction, that is a treatment that inactivates infectious agents in blood while retaining the biological activities of the blood itself. Methods are currently available for plasma and for platelet concentrates and are in use in some countries. It should be noted that available methods may have differing efficacies for different infectious agents and that they may not be fully successful in eliminating very high levels of infectivity for some agents, although this has not been established in practice. A real disadvantage is that no method is currently available for red cells. A pathogen reduction method was implemented for platelets in the island of La Reunion during a large outbreak of chikungunya virus infection.

The precautionary principle is often cited when decisions about interventions to reduce the risk of transfusion-transmitted infections are discussed. In general, it is suggested that, in the absence of any specific information about the efficacy of an intervention, it is appropriate to implement it, as long as it does no harm. This position may be arguable, particularly as commentary on the precautionary principle suggests that it should not be invoked without some evaluation to assure that the measure is not extreme and does not exceed other measures taken in known circumstances. In fact, significant measures were taken to reduce the potential risk of transmission of vCJD even before it was known that it was transmissible by transfusion. It can be argued that subsequent events justified the precautions taken, but this may not always be the case.

Key points

1 Some emerging infections may threaten the safety of the blood supply.
2 Those responsible for maintaining the safety of the blood supply should be familiar with emerging infections.
3 Physicians responsible for the care of transfused patients should be alert for signs of unexpected infections.
4 The nature and extent of the safety threat offered by emerging infections may be assessed by examination of a fairly simple sequence of questions.
5 If interventions are needed, consideration should be given to the use of donor questions and/or laboratory tests.

Further reading

Alter HJ, Stramer SL & Dodd RY. Emerging infectious diseases that threaten the blood supply. *Semin Hematol* 2007;44:32–41.

Biggerstaff BJ & Petersen LR. Estimated risk of transmission of the West Nile virus through blood transfusion in the US, 2002. *Transfusion* 2003;43:1007–1017.

Dodd RY & Leiby DA. Emerging infectious threats to the blood supply. *Annu Rev Med* 2004;55:191–207.

Hewitt PE, Llewelyn CA, Mckenzie J & Will RG. Creutzfeldt-Jakob disease and blood transfusion: results of the UK Transfusion Medicine Epidemiology Review study. *Vox Sang* 2006;91:221–230.

Mackenzie JS, Gubler DJ & Petersen LR. Emerging flaviviruses: the spread and resurgence of Japanese encephalitis, West Nile and dengue viruses. *Nat Med (Suppl)* 2004;10(12):S98–S108.

Stramer SL, Fang CT, Foster GA, Wagner AG, Brodsky JP & Dodd RY. West Nile virus among blood donors in the United States, 2003 and 2004. *N Engl J Med* 2005;353:451–459.

Weiss RA & McMichael AJ. Social and environmental risk factors in the emergence of infectious disease. *Nat Med (Suppl)* 2004;10(12):S70–S76.

PART 3
Practice in blood centres and hospitals

CHAPTER 17

Regulatory aspects of blood transfusion

Joan Jones[1] *& Adrian Copplestone*[2]
[1]Welsh Blood Service, Cardiff, Wales
[2]Derriford Hospital, Plymouth, UK

Introduction

The first human transfusions were performed in 1667 by Richard Lower in London and by Jean-Baptiste Denis in Paris. Denis was charged following the death of a patient and this started the process of the regulation of transfusion. In recent years, an increasing number of laws, regulations and guidelines related to blood transfusion have been issued. Those working in transfusion services in blood centres and in hospitals have struggled to demonstrate their compliance with them. Because of the complexities of national legislation, this chapter concentrates on the regulatory position in the UK, but the same principles apply in most other countries (Table 17.1).

When considering the level of regulation, it is useful to distinguish the obligatory requirements from advisory guidance. However, when complications or mishaps of transfusion occur, regulatory authorities, the courts and the general public expect that all regulations and guidelines should have been followed.

Practical Transfusion Medicine, 3rd edition. Edited by Michael F. Murphy and Derwood H. Pamphilon. © 2009 Blackwell Publishing, ISBN: 978-1-4051-8196-9.

Legislation

Blood safety and quality regulations (2005)

The Blood Safety and Quality Regulations SI 50/2005 (BSQR) in the UK were introduced to implement a number of European Community Directives on Blood. The Directives which apply to blood are shown in Figure 17.1 and the inter-relation of the European Directives and their transposition into UK law in Figure 17.2. The BSQR were transposed into UK law in February 2005, to be implemented by November 2005. The regulations require institutions involved in the collection, testing, processing, storage and distribution of blood components (blood centres and hospitals that collect or manipulate the component) to be licenced. Autologous blood collections involving intra-operative and post-operative cell salvage are excluded from the regulations. Hospital blood transfusion laboratories are required to:

• maintain a quality management system (see below).

• ensure donor to recipient traceability; the records relating to these must be retained for 30 years; and

• comply with mandatory reporting requirements for serious adverse events (SAE) and serious adverse reactions (SAR) related to transfusion to the competent authority.

The competent authority for the UK (which oversees compliance with the regulations) is the Medicine and Healthcare products Regulatory

Table 17.1 Inspection requirements.

	UK	USA*	Canada†	Australia‡
Blood centres	Regulated/licenced by MHRA	Regulated/licenced by Food and Drug Admistration (FDA)	Regulated/licenced by Health Canada	Regulated by therapeutic goods administration (TGA) using Council of Europe Guide
Hospital transfusion laboratories	Licenced by the MHRA if components manipulated	Regulated/licenced by FDA if components manipulated	Regulated/licenced by Health Canada if product manufactured or transformed (to be implemented soon)	Accredited by NATA
	Regulated under BSQR by MHRA	Accredited by Arm of Federal Government or AABB or College of American Pathologists (COP)	Accreditation mandatory in some provinces	Some laboratories also licensed by TGA for manufacturing
	Accredited – CPA			
Patient bedside safety	Guidance BCSH and NPSA	The Joint Commission, AABB and/or CAP	Guidance Canadian Blood Standards	Hospital accreditation by various organisations, e.g. ACHS, using EQuIP standards. National professional guidelines widely used, e.g. ANZSBT-RCNA, but these are not currently standards
Transfer of blood between organisations	Regulated BSQR	Across State Line – licensed by FDA	Guidance Canadian Blood Standards	From blood centre to hospital: TGA as part of blood centre licence. At/between hospitals: covered by NATA/hospital accreditation
Haemovigilance	Mandatory – SABRE; Voluntary – SHOT	Fatalities – FDA; Incidents – some States	Voluntary Public Health Agency of Canada	National voluntary program in development. Individual state-based systems for incidents, serious reactions and fatalities – some mandatory, others voluntary

(Continued)

Table 17.1 *(Continued)*

	UK	USA*	Canada[†]	Australia[‡]
Traceability of blood components	Mandatory 30 years	At least 10 years	For blood centres: mandatory lifetime. For hospitals: varies by province in Quebec lifetime for hospitals	Mandatory, at least 20 years or indefinite
QMS	Mandatory for blood centres and hospitals – BSQR	Mandatory for blood centres; mandatory for hospitals if AABB accredited	Mandatory for blood centres; mandatory for hospitals if AABB accredited	Mandatory for licenced blood centres and accredited hospital/other laboratories

* Information supplied by James P. AuBuchon, MD.
[†] Information supplied by Pierre Robillard MD.
[‡] Information supplied by B Quested.
Abbreviations not given here are stated in the text: NATA, National Association of Testing Authorities; ACHS, Australian Council of Healthcare Standards; ANZSBT, Australian & New Zealand Society of Blood Transfusion; RCNA, Royal College of Nursing Australia.

Agency (MHRA). There is a requirement for annual re-certification by hospital blood transfusion laboratories and two-yearly inspections of blood establishments. They are responsible for all aspects of the collection and testing of human blood or blood components, whatever their intended purpose, and their processing, storage, and distribution, when intended for transfusion. They may undertake 'for cause' inspection visits of hospital blood transfusion laboratories and blood establishments and have the power to instigate a 'cease and desist' order if serious deficits are found or to prosecute the responsible person under criminal law. 'For cause' inspections are ad hoc inspections that are triggered as a result of, for example, safety and quality issues, suspected violations of legislation, and referrals by other member states. Such inspections may on occasions be carried out unannounced.

The MHRA also regulates the licensing of medical devices including much of the equipment used in

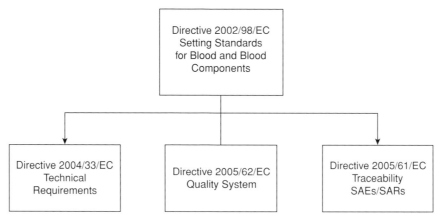

Figure 17.1 EU Directives which apply to Transfusion Laboratories.

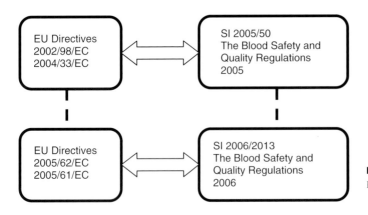

Figure 17.2 The inter-relationship between European Directives and the UK Law.

laboratories. All adverse incidents involving medical devices must be reported to MHRA as soon as possible, even if user error (rather than a device problem) is suspected.

Health service regulations

There are a large number of laws relating to the employment and safety that affect blood transfusion laboratories. In most hospitals, these are incorporated into corporate polices which need to be followed. In the UK, the majority of transfusion practice takes place in the National Health Service (NHS), but independent providers have similar requirements which fall into the following categories:
- Personnel
  - Equal opportunities
  - Mandatory professional registration, e.g. Health Professions Council
- Health and Safety
  - Health and Safety at Work Act
  - Employers Liability Act
  - Reporting of Injuries, Diseases and Dangerous Occurrences Regulations
  - Control of Substances Hazardous to Health Regulations
- Information Technology
  - Data Protection Act

Guidance that must be followed

Health Service Circulars (HSCs)

HSCs are formal communications, primarily to NHS chief executives, which usually contain a requirement for significant or urgent specific action. In England, to date there have been three HSCs which have impacted on the transfusion process, both within the blood transfusion laboratory and in clinical areas where blood is used. The most recent of these is HSC 2007/001 – *Better Blood Transfusion – Safe and Appropriate Use of Blood*.

The *Better Blood Transfusion* initiatives are in place to support the delivery of:
- safe transfusion practice;
- appropriate transfusion practice;
- ensuring that *Better Blood Transfusion* is an integral part of NHS care; and
- appropriate use of alternatives to transfusion.

The third HSC also calls for the avoidance of unnecessary blood transfusion in obstetric practice and the need to minimise the risk of haemolytic disease of the foetus and newborn. It also seeks to increase patient and public involvement in blood transfusion.

Wales, Scotland and Northern Ireland Health Departments have issued similar letters or set up similar programmes.

Other requirements

A recent development is the increase in requirements from other health service bodies.

National Patient Safety Agency (NPSA)

The NPSA is a Special Health Authority created to coordinate the learning from adverse incidents occurring in the NHS. As well as making sure that incidents are reported, the NPSA aims to promote an open and fair culture in hospitals and across the health service, encouraging doctors and other staff to report incidents and 'near misses' when things go wrong but do not cause clinical harm. *Safer Practice Notices* (SPNs) and alerts are published by the NPSA where risks are identified, and work is undertaken on producing solutions which can be adopted across the NHS.

In 2007, the NPSA published a *Safety Practice Notice (SPN 14): Right Patient, Right Blood*. This requires hospitals to undertake risk assessments on their current transfusion processes and review the feasibility of using:

• bar codes or other electronic identification and tracking systems for patients, samples and blood products (an electronic clinical transfusion management system);

• photo identification cards for patients who undergo regular blood transfusions; and

• a labelling system of matching samples and blood for transfusion to the patient concerned.

Organisations were to implement an action plan for competency-based training and assessment in relation to the following areas of practice:

• pre-transfusion sampling;

• collection of blood components from storage; and

• administration of blood components.

Laboratory accreditation

Within the UK there are two laboratory accreditation bodies, operating in complementary fields, the United Kingdom Accreditation Service (UKAS) and Clinical Pathology Accreditation (UK) Ltd (CPA). *The UK Accreditation Service (UKAS) is the accreditation body recognised by government to assess, against internationally agreed standards, organisations that provide certification, testing, inspection and calibration services.* UKAS and CPA have formed a partnership enabling the two organisations to cooperate on the development of accreditation policy, and this facilitates the exchange of best practice. Where appropriate, the activities of the two organisations will be aligned, thereby benefiting dually accredited organisations.

Table 17.2 CPA standards.

Standard	Area
A	Organisation and quality management systems
B	Personnel
C	Premises and environment
D	Equipment, information systems and materials
E	The pre-examination phase
F	Examination process
G	The post-examination phase
H	Evaluation and quality process

The partnership is aimed at strengthening the authority and reputation of accreditation both in the UK and internationally by bringing together these two organisations with established reputations in their respective fields. It is also a means of reducing the risk of fragmenting accreditation and avoiding proliferation of accreditation standards for laboratories.

CPA accreditation focuses on requirements for quality and competence as detailed in ISO 15189-2007 and laboratories are inspected on a two-yearly cycle under the standards outlined in Table 17.2.

Governance

Clinical governance

This is a framework through which NHS organisations are accountable for continuously improving the quality of their services and safeguarding high standards of care in which clinical care will flourish. This will also involve mechanisms for:

• reporting and investigating incidents or 'near miss' incidents;

• investigating and managing complaints;

• clinical audit;

• appraisal, induction and training of staff; and

• controlling policies and procedures used within the hospital or organisation.

When clinical incidents occur, they should be reported and investigated in a timely fashion. In SAE, e.g. the death of a patient or major ABO incompatible transfusion, the incidents should be reported immediately to the medical director. Transfusion incidents must be reported to MHRA via their on-line reporting system called SABRE (Serious Adverse Blood Reactions and Events) and to the Serious Hazards of Transfusion (SHOT) scheme. This is especially important when transfusion-related infections are suspected. Blood services should also be rapidly informed as other blood products from the donor can be quarantined, preventing harm to other patients.

Financial governance

Within an organisation there are usually strict rules controlling the purchase of equipment and reagents. For large procurement contracts, tenders will have to be sought following advertisement in the *Official Journal of the European Communities* (OJEC).

Insurance schemes, e.g. for risk management/clinical negligence

The NHS Litigation Authority (NHSLA) is a Special Health Authority, which was established in 1995 to administer the Clinical Negligence Scheme for Trusts (CNST) and provide a means for NHS organisations to fund the cost of clinical negligence claims.

The standards and assessment process are designed to: *provide a structured framework to focus effective risk management activities to deliver quality improvements in organisational governance, patient care and the safety of patients, staff, contractors, volunteers and visitors*
• *encourage and support organisations in taking a proactive approach to improvement*;
• *contribute to embedding risk management into the organisation's culture*;
• *assist in the management of adverse incidents and claims*.
Health care organisations often have rules applied to help reduce risks. In blood transfusion, this is often focussed on the training undertaken within an organisation.

External inspections of standards

In England, external inspection is undertaken by the Healthcare Commission (HCC), but most health services will have a similar body. The HCC exists to promote improvements in the quality of health care and public health in England and is a separate inspection body for both the NHS and independent health care. Other bodies with a right to inspection include the Health and Safety Commission, the Audit Commission and MHRA. 'Inspection' can be defined as a formal or official examination against established standards and 'accreditation' as the act of granting credit or recognition often against agreed standards.

Guidelines which should be followed

The British Committee for Standards in Haematology (BCSH) Blood Transfusion Task Force has, for many years, produced guidelines for good practice in transfusion medicine. They include:
• guidelines for the administration of blood and blood components and the management of transfused patients;
• guidelines for the clinical use of red cell transfusion;
• guidelines for the use of platelet transfusions; and
• guidelines for the use of fresh frozen plasma and cryoprecipitate.
The BCSH ensures that guidelines relating to transfusion are regularly reviewed and where required new guidelines are commissioned. Further guidelines will be published in the future and will be available on the BCSH website, www.bcshguidelines.org.

Other guidance can be found at:
• Handbook of Transfusion Medicine. Fourth Edition, 2007. www.transfusionguidelines.org.uk.
• Scottish Intercollegiate Guidelines Network. *Perioperative Blood Transfusion for Elective Surgery – A National Clinical Guideline*. Number 54. 2001. www.sign.ac.uk.
• The Association of Anaesthetists of Great Britain and Ireland. *Blood Transfusion and the Anaesthetist. Red Cell Transfusion.* 2001. www.aagbi.org/publications/guidelines.htm.
• The Association of Anaesthetists of Great Britain and Ireland. *Blood Transfusion and the Anaesthetist. Blood Component Therapy.* 2005. www.aagbi.org/publications/guidelines.htm.

The Joint National Institute of Biological Standards and Control and United Kingdom Blood Transfusion Services guidelines website (www.transfusionguidelines.org.uk) hosts the websites for the National Blood Transfusion Committee (NBTC) and the Regional Transfusion Committees (RTCs) as well as for Better Blood Transfusion Toolkit. Also hosted on this website is the outputs from the UK NHS Operational Impact Group, which provides specific information to hospital transfusion laboratories relating to:

- clarification of specific aspects of the BSQR;
- feedback from inspections; and
- support to laboratories in helping them achieve compliance to the regulations.

The problem with writing guidelines in transfusion medicine is that despite very large numbers of transfusions daily, the evidence base is relatively low (Chapter 47), leading to different groups producing conflicting guidance. In modern guideline production, the evidence for specific recommendations is graded (Table 17.3).

In the blood transfusion literature, there are relatively few randomised controlled trials (RCTs) and clinicians adhere firmly to their beliefs that a change in practice is inappropriate, when some RCTs have shown just the opposite (Chapter 48). The Systematic Review Initiative is a clinical research group established by the National Blood Service in 2002 to develop the evidence base for the practice of transfusion medicine, and the issue of how to get the most of the evidence base for transfusion medicine is discussed in Chapter 47.

How to cope with all the rules?

Standard operating procedures

Although there seems at first to be a bewildering array of rules to follow, most of them are fairly straightforward. Many of the laboratory standards overlap and the key is to make sure that all are carefully considered and addressed.

The way a laboratory or ward operates is by means of standard operating procedures (SOPs) which need to be available and easily readable by staff. Training is needed for all new members of staff and compliance audits will check whether they are being followed. When problems occur, it is important to look at the structure of the processes as well as the incident itself.

Quality management system

The quality management system (QMS) required for the BSQR is based on the principles of good manufacturing practice (GMP), and laboratories should refer to the Rules and Guidance for Pharmaceutical Manufacturers and Distributors published by the Pharmaceutical Press (referred to in the UK as the 'Orange Guide'). The main areas of GMP are identified in Figure 17.3. The BSQR indicates that a QMS should address:

- Personnel
  - Appropriately qualified personnel
  - Sufficient numbers
  - Training of SOPs
  - Regular competency assessments
  - GMP awareness training
- Premises and equipment
  - Designed and constructed to suit the intended operations
  - Facilitates workflow
  - Defined 'cold storage' facilities
  - Equipment validated to confirm it is 'fit for use'
  - Programme of planned preventative maintenance
- Documentation
  - Controlled document system
  - Written procedures and policies regularly reviewed
- Procedures
  - Procedures carried out according to documented instructions
  - SOPs covering all procedures within the laboratory
- Quality control (QC)
  - Documented internal QC
  - External review, e.g. NEQAS with all aspects of laboratory practice controlled and documented
- Control manufacture and analysis
  - Specific written contracts with suppliers

Table 17.3 Classification of evidence levels. (The system used to grade the evidence and guidance recommendations is that published by the US Department of Health and Human Services Agency for Healthcare Policy and Research (AHPCR).)

Level	Description
Ia	Evidence obtained from meta-analysis of RCTs.
Ib	Evidence obtained from at least one RCT.
IIa	Evidence obtained from at least one well-designed controlled study without randomisation.
IIb	Evidence obtained from at least one other type of well-designed quasi-experimental study*.
III	Evidence obtained from well-designed non-experimental descriptive studies, such as comparative studies, correlation studies and case studies.
IV	Evidence obtained from expert committee reports or opinions and/or clinical experiences of respected authorities.

Classification of grades of recommendation

Recommendation grade	Evidence
A	Requires at least one RCT as part of a body of literature of overall good quality and consistency addressing specific recommendation. *(Evidence levels 1a, 1b)*
B	Requires the availability of well-conducted clinical studies but no RCTs on the topic of recommendation. *(Evidence levels IIa, IIb, III)*
C	Requires evidence obtained from expert committee reports or opinions and/or clinical experiences of respected authorities. Indicates an absence of directly applicable clinical studies of good quality. *(Evidence level IV)*

* Refers to a situation in which implementation of an intervention is outwith the control of the investigators, but an opportunity exists to evaluate its effect.

○ Supply of blood components to other facilities will be covered by a service level agreement
• Complaints and product recall
  ○ Effective recall procedure
  ○ Evidence of undertaking this shall be available
• Self-inspection
  ○ Ongoing process of 'self-inspection' to verify compliance with GMP
  ○ Formal record of non-compliances
  ○ Evidence of corrective actions
In addition to these, the BSQR has two annexes related to QMS which cover:
• Computer systems
• Validation and qualification

Traceability

BSQR requires hospital transfusion laboratories to 'maintain, for not less than 30 years, the data

needed to ensure full traceability of blood and blood components, from the point of receipt of the blood or blood component by the hospital blood bank'.

Haemovigilance

BSQR requires that there are procedures in place for quality assurance within the transfusion laboratory for the reporting of SAE and SAR.

Who will be inspected?

Hospital blood transfusion laboratories are required to complete an annual form, developed by the MHRA, in which the laboratory indicates their compliance with the regulations. The form is reviewed by the Inspectorate division of the MHRA,

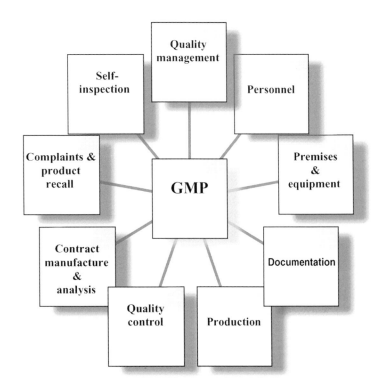

Figure 17.3 Good manufacturing practice (GMP).

and those laboratories where there is deemed non-compliance are inspected, and some others for the QC of the inspection process.

Practical points in relation to regulatory inspections

Preparing for inspections
- Ensure all paperwork is in place and the laboratory is clean and tidy.
- Review the answers you provided on the compliance form.
- Where processes, systems, etc., have progressed since the completion of the compliance form, ensure this information is made available for the inspectors.
- Where you know you are not compliant, have a prepared action plan.
- Be realistic when identifying the time required to plan and deliver the actions.

The inspection itself
- Ensure there is a room the inspectors can use with hot and cold drinks available, a table and chairs and where there is some peace and quiet to review paperwork.
- There will be an opening meeting where the inspectors will introduce themselves.
- The inspection is all about obtaining information, witnessing tasks being performed and reviewing documented procedures.
- The inspector will also want to review the systems and processes in place for:
  - Traceability
  - Storage and distribution
  - Review of SAE/SAR reporting
  - Crossmatching/automation
- This list is not exhaustive and the inspectors may wish to look at any system/laboratory process.
- There will be a closing meeting by the inspector where they will present their findings and notification of the next steps.

○ Presentation of findings
○ Opportunity for establishment to provide further information
○ Acceptance of findings
○ Notification of next steps

Learning from problems

Recognising and learning from errors is an important aspect of a quality system. A programme of 'self-inspections' of critical areas (GMP audits) will allow the laboratory to identify quality failings and undertake a programme to rectify all non-compliances. It is important to understand:
• Why the error occurred?
• Was this a 'system' error or a human error?
• How could these be prevented in the future?
• What is the risk to patient safety?
• What corrective actions and preventive actions can be introduced?

Key points

1 Quality is the responsibility of all staff working in the transfusion laboratory.
2 There are a large number of regulations which cover the management of transfusion practice within a hospital (or in a community setting).
3 A systematic approach is required to ensure that current policies and practices are up to the standard required and they are regularly reviewed.
4 Laboratory and clinical practice needs to be audited to ensure compliance.
5 Incidents need to be fully investigated to ensure that the underlying cause is determined and corrective actions are taken.

Further reading

Council of Europe Directive 2002/98/EC, Directives (2004/33/EC, 2005/61/EC & 2005/62/EC). Available at http://ec.europa.eu/health/ph_threats/human_substance/legal_blood_en.htm. Accessed 16 December 2008.

Department of Health. HSC 2007/001: *Better Blood Transfusion – Safe and Appropriate Use of Blood.* Available at http://www.dh.gov.uk/en/Publicationsandstatistics/Lettersandcirculars/Healthservicecirculars/DH_080613. Accessed 16 December 2008.

Diamond LK. A history of blood transfusion. In: Wintrobe MM. (ed.), *Blood Pure and Eloquent.* New York: McGraw-Hill Book Company, 1980, pp. 663–665.

Hebert PC, Wells G, Blajchman MA et al. A multicenter, randomized, controlled clinical trial of transfusion requirements in critical care. Transfusion requirements in critical care investigators, Canadian critical care trials group. *N Engl J Med* 1999;340:409-417.

National Patient Safety Agency Safer Practice Notice (14) Right Patient, Right Blood. Available at http://www.npsa.nhs.uk/patientsafety. Accessed 16 December 2008.

The Blood Safety & Quality Regulations 2005 No. 50 as amended (the principal Regulations, amending Regulations (SI 2005/1098, SI 2005/2898, SI 2006/2013 & SI 2007/604). Available at http://www.opsi.gov.uk/stat.htm. Accessed 16 December 2008.

Rules and Guidance for Pharmaceutical Manufacturers and Distributors Edited 2007. Compiled by the Inspection and Standards Division, Medicines and Healthcare products Regulatory Agency (MHRA), London, UK. ISBN:978 0 85369 719 0.

The Systematic Review Initiative. Available at http://www.transfusionguidelines.org.uk. Accessed 16 December 2008.

CHAPTER 18
The role of haemovigilance in transfusion safety

James P. AuBuchon
University of Washington; Puget Sound Blood Center, Seattle, Washington, USA

Introduction

The quality improvement movement in health care has engendered many adages in the last decade while increasing our ability to improve the delivery of services and patient outcomes. One of these is especially pertinent to haemovigilance: If you can't measure it, you can't improve it. This concept sums up the rationale behind the creation of a haemovigilance system in most developed nations over the last decade and the excitement associated with the data they are generating. By defining the frequency of the problems encountered in the transfusion system and our failures to achieve the desired goal of safe and efficacious transfusion *every time*, we can begin to identify where our attention and resources should be directed in order to allow transfusion medicine to participate fully in modern medicine's attempt to provide care through robust systems that yield dependable outcomes.

Although different entities have applied slightly different definitions to haemovigilance, that of the European Haemovigilance Network (EHN) is one of the most encompassing:

Haemovigilance is a set of surveillance procedures covering the entire transfusion chain (from the donation of blood and its components to the follow-up of recipients of transfusions), intended to collect and assess information on unexpected or undesirable effects resulting from the therapeutic use of labile blood products, and to prevent the occurrence or recurrence of such incidents.

Recognition that transfusion hazards can accrue from any of the multiple steps along the complex pathway from donor selection to recipient transfusion requires that a haemovigilance system maintain a broad, all-encompassing scope in order to define these risks. Also important is the inclusion of the expectation that steps will be taken to reduce these risks, since merely collecting data will not prompt improvements in the transfusion system. In essence, then, haemovigilance systems provide the engine through which transfusion systems can improve their services and outcomes.

Origin and impetus

Haemovigilance systems arose out of a confluence of events that questioned the safety of the health care system to deliver treatment without causing unnecessary harm and the ability of the blood supply system to deliver units of minimal

Practical Transfusion Medicine, 3rd edition. Edited by Michael F. Murphy and Derwood H. Pamphilon. © 2009 Blackwell Publishing, ISBN: 978-1-4051-8196-9.

risk. Increasing recognition that the reliability of medical care systems is suboptimal has led to broad efforts to reduce the substantial risks associated with delivery of all aspects of health care. These efforts alone might have stirred blood bankers into action, but the earlier public debates, commissions of inquiry, and prosecutions (and convictions) stemming from how the nascent HIV risk of the 1980s had been handled provided additional impetus for the field to assess the safety of its services through ongoing risk assessment measures. As the infectious disease risks of HIV and HCV that had been captivating our attention through the 1980s and 1990s were documented to have been greatly diminished through concerted multifaceted interventions, the field of transfusion medicine felt increasingly able to re-direct its attention to problems that had been known to exist for many years but that had never been definitively and effectively addressed.

The legal framework and the organisational structure of these systems vary from country to country. The first system, that in France, was established as a mandatory system in which the reporting of all untoward outcomes from transfusions was required. The second system implemented arose through the efforts of transfusion medicine professionals in the United Kingdom and was organised through the Royal College of Pathologists as a voluntary reporting system focussed on Serious Hazards of Transfusion (SHOT). Subsequently, systems have been created and implemented in most developed nations as a hybrid of these approaches. Some of these reside within and derive reporting mandates from a national ministry of health while others are primarily organised through professional societies or the country's blood collection system with sharing of data to all concerned parties. The European Community currently requires implementation of a haemovigilance system in each member state with reporting to a central office. Although each country's system has characteristics unique for its own health care and transfusion systems, they bear multiple similarities and have yielded similar results, as will be discussed in the next section.

Table 18.1 Important features of a haemovigilance system.

Confidentiality of submitted data
Broad participation, supported by education
Non-punitive evaluation of data
Reporting of *rates* of occurrences
Sufficient detail to make effective recommendations for improved practices
Focus on improved safety and outcomes
Simple and efficient operations
Sustainable organisation

Key elements and residual questions

The structure and content of haemovigilance systems varies by country, but the successful show several similarities in important facets of their philosophy and function (Table 18.1).

Detection and reporting of adverse events

Common to all haemovigilance systems is development and/or application of a system to capture events of interest directly from the side of the transfusion recipient or the hospital transfusion service. Many of the countries that first implemented haemovigilance systems had most of their transfusion expertise headquartered in blood centres and few transfusion medicine specialists located in hospitals. They generally did not have a history of capturing transfusion reaction events in real time for investigation, accumulation and (local) analysis. To provide information for the new haemovigilance network, France identified a 'rapporteur' or 'haemovigilance officer' in each hospital (usually a physician, such as a haematologist or anaesthesiologist), the UK trained a cadre of nurses as 'specialised practitioners of transfusion', and Québec established a network of 'transfusion safety officers' (TSOs, usually nurses) in the larger hospitals that also oversaw reporting of events from nearby smaller facilities. In countries with a more established transfusion medicine professional presence at the hospital level, these new assignments or positions would not be required. For example, the haemovigilance reporting system in the US is being based on the pre-existing transfusion reaction reporting system extant in hospitals of all sizes that reports to the hospital's transfusion service and to the facility's transfusion committee.

For any reporting system to be reliable, those charged with capturing the event must be cognisant of the commonly recognised signs and symptoms of transfusion reactions as well as remaining alert to events that 'just don't seem right' during or after a transfusion. Simply dismissing an unusual sign or an unexpected symptom as causally unrelated to the transfusion will deprive not only the patient of steps that might prevent a recurrence in a future transfusion but the transfusion system of the knowledge of an event that might disclose a significant new phenomenon. Ensuring that those likely to be the first to identify problems with a transfusion will report the occurrence is a critical first step in creating and maintaining a useful and credible haemovigilance system. Tying haemovigilance reporting to a bedside system that captures standardised and complete data from every transfusion undoubtedly improves the penetration of the system and the believability of the data it generates, as well.

Despite the diligence of such efforts, however, haemovigilance systems will always be challenged to tally untoward outcomes that occur long after a transfusion because of the loss of an obvious temporal relationship (Table 18.2). For example, identifying transfusion transmission of an infectious disease would require recognition of the lack of other means of transmission to the recipient and relative rarity of the disease entity in order for the transfusion connection to be recognised, and then the physician caring for the patient would need to contact the transfusion service in order for an investigation and possibly a report to the haemovigilance system to be generated. Haemovigilance-like investigations led to the detection of transmission of West Nile virus (WNV) through transfusion relatively early in the US outbreak of this disease, but making the connection between poor patient outcome and transfusion exposure of an organ donor would have been much more difficult had the incubation period been longer. Additional utility of a haemovigilance system is seen, however, through real-time assessment of regional risk through donor testing and revision of donor testing protocols in response to this information, as is being done in the US.

Scope of reporting

The scope of haemovigilance systems, however, is varied (Table 18.3). The SHOT system clearly specifies its interest only in the *serious* hazards and precludes reporting febrile and urticarial reactions, for example. This restriction provides natural focus on the hazards that have the largest potential impact on a particular recipient but at some risk of missing events of lesser morbidity that may affect a larger number of patients or that may be harbingers of more serious sequelae later after transfusion. The more common approach of seeking to capture all transfusion reactions, on the other hand, risks 'system fatigue' from overwhelmed personnel or

Table 18.2 Limitations of haemovigilance systems.

Incomplete reporting
Detection of transfusion relationship of late events, including infections
Limited details
Variation in terminology and definitions
Influence of health care system's or institution's 'culture' regarding compliance, process improvement and reporting

Table 18.3 Variations among haemovigilance systems.

Scope	Serious events or all events?
	Events causing harm or also 'near-miss' events?
Breadth	Labile transfusible components
	Plasma derivative products
	Tissues and/or organs for transplantation (biovigilance)
Analysis	System level
	Institutional level
	Comparison with all hospitals in the system
	Comparison with (anonymous) peer institution subset

reporting and analysis tools through which events of major clinical significance are obscured from view by the more numerous but less-informative reports of 'minor' events.

The extension of haemovigilance systems to incidents that are not directly associated with a reaction or an untoward outcome for a recipient is an important means of detecting problems in the transfusion *system* and preventing these from harming patients. Whether called an incident, a deviation or an error, these failures to adhere to standard procedures may represent human frailty or limitations, inadequate training, unique features of a patient's situation or a combination of factors that aligned with weak points in the transfusion process. The most notable among these has been patient and sample identification errors in pre-transfusion testing. Inclusion of 'near-miss' events where the error is detected and remedied and/or where it does not cause harm to the recipient quickly causes such occurrences to become the most commonly reported events in a haemovigilance system. Although these occurrences may individually appear to be of minor importance, they represent a critical view into the workings of a transfusion system and allow preventive actions to be taken to bolster system safeguards.

Analysis of incident reports

The ability of an individual hospital or some other relevant unit of the health care system to assess the outcomes of its transfusions is important in addition to the national review of problems in the transfusion system. At the smallest division in which policies are common and practice is (presumed to be) universal, an analysis of reports of transfusion reactions and transfusion practice should be undertaken in order to understand how this microsystem compares to the larger whole. In most situations, this analysis would be at the hospital level since enforcement of uniformity of practice outside of one's immediate reach is often difficult. Identification of where one's system is not being applied faithfully is critical knowledge that can be used to strengthen the system and remove ambiguity or opportunities for imprecise or incorrect actions to occur (or at least to go unnoticed). The individual hospital

that participates in a national haemovigilance system that captures these kinds of data can benefit by comparing their experience to that of others working in the same type of system. Understanding where in the transfusion chain differences in practice are occurring may identify those steps in the process that are truly critical to be performed with a high degree of fidelity and in identifying transfusion practices associated with superior outcomes.

Whether dealing with clinical events, such as transfusion reactions, or near-miss incidents, a standardised lexicon must be adopted. Clear and precise definitions must be utilised, and terms resistant to misinterpretation must be employed to decrease the chance of a misapplication of a classification scheme that would degrade the value of the system's data. The importance of this standardisation for comparison between systems was recognised early on by the EHN, and a working party of the International Society of Blood Transfusion (ISBT) has been developing definitions of transfusion reactions that could be used to achieve commonality and facilitate meaningful comparisons of data between countries. Some systems have taken the additional step of interposing a review of the details of a reported event to ensure that it meets the definitions used in that system. While this rigor adds robustness to the reports of the system, larger systems or those with relatively fewer resources need to depend on participants' accurate application of the definitions embedded in the classification scheme.

There are several features of haemovigilance systems and hospital 'cultures' that are presumed to be associated with higher rates of reporting compliance. The degree to which an institution focusses on outcome improvement and adherence to policies is probably an important determinant of the acceptance of a reporting system such as represented by a haemovigilance system. Related to this may be the extent to which an 'open learning culture' is supported in the institution. Similarly, the more that 'incidents' are recognised as failures of the (imperfect) system rather than of those working within it, the more likely that staff will feel comfortable reporting the occurrences. When these reports lead to improvements in the process (and particularly when those affected by the incident have been able to participate in the improvement of the transfusion system), the satisfaction that is generated also empowers further reporting toward the end of improving operations and outcomes.

How to encourage active participation in haemovigilance?

This leads naturally to a discussion of whether reporting to a haemovigilance system should be 'voluntary' or 'mandatory'. In all likelihood, a mixture of incentives is most salutary. Error reporting will suffer in a system where reporting may be 'required' but more frequently leads to punishment of those caught in a cumbersome, error-prone system than to change in that system. The lack of non-punitive reporting would clearly limit the ability of the haemovigilance system to effect improvements. A non-punitive approach to reporting – for the individual reporting the case as well as for those involved in it and the institution itself – is essential to compliance. On the other hand, voluntary reporting, even when coupled with confidentiality safeguards, is unlikely to attract respondents unless the importance of their actions is well understood and they see the fruits of their efforts through system reports and process changes. All systems have noted continual rise in the number of reports submitted over their first few years, as more staff 'on the front lines' become aware of the system, its importance and the logistics of reporting; those systems with more extensive educational infrastructure appear to have the most rapid attainment of extensive penetration. Endorsement of participation by a professional association or the ministry of health may boost participation, particularly if the system is easy for participants to use and has already established its credibility. In a legal system where the involved person or institution is subject to liability damages from an 'error', assurance of confidentiality for the details of the report and freedom from compelled disclosure are absolutely essential for enabling reporting. Even if no harm befell a patient from an incident, an institution would understandably require assurance that its 'dirty laundry' could not be used against it by a plaintiff's attorney alleging a pattern of inappropriate practices.

Data management

Simplicity of reporting is also the key to high participation rates. Most haemovigilance systems began with paper reports but are converting or have converted to electronic submission systems. This approach not only facilitates data management by the coordinating office but also simplifies the reporting mechanism for the participant; an intelligent, web-based data capture system could display only those items that were pertinent to the case's report as it unfolded rather than frightening a respondent with multiple pages of data elements, many of which would not be pertinent in any one particular case. Such a system could also check for completeness and prevent logging of an incomplete case or check for internal congruity in a case and prevent clearly erroneous entry errors. The extent to which a system wishes to go to ensure that its definitions are being followed may be dependent on assumptions made about the support available for data entry. For example, does the system require entry of pre- and post-transfusion temperatures and check to see if the definition of a febrile transfusion reaction has been met, or does the system expect that the respondent is applying the definition correctly? The former approach would provide better assurance of data integrity but would require more time for data entry.

Optimally, the national haemovigilance system would be interfaced to a facility's internal error management software (such as MERS-TM) and be able to accept the report of the necessary elements of a case automatically. Most haemovigilance systems have not reached that level of sophistication, but centrally coordinated health care systems may be able to integrate laboratory information, error management and haemovigilance systems to accomplish this. Since the capabilities of many transfusion services to analyse and report their experience with incidents and events are limited in their laboratory information system, the ability of the national haemovigilance system to construct the tables and graphs illustrating the experience of the reporter's institution and overlay the system's experience (in aggregate form or from institutions with similar characteristics) may reward (and thus encourage) participation.

The extent of data collection ultimately affects the richness of the system's data. The more detail of an incident or a reaction that is captured by a system, the greater the impact on policy development the system may offer. Capturing detail about where an incident occurred may help identify 'high-risk clinical areas', and identifying the steps in the transfusion process that were vulnerable to error will similarly help direct attention to the part of the transfusion process where improvements will have the greatest impact. Performance of a root-cause analysis is beyond the purview of a national haemovigilance system, but capturing the results of such an analysis and estimating the probability of a recurrence and its impact can also help focus attention on 'big payoff' targets.

A critical category of data elements in a haemovigilance system is the 'denominator data'. Although tallying the number of units of each component type transfused or the number of pre-transfusion specimens tested does not inform us about transfusion safety, this information is essential in turning reported occurrences into rates. Only through a comparison of the rates of events can we compare meaningfully across institutions and countries of different sizes and different transfusion activity levels. As different countries – or, indeed, different regions within one country – account for outdated and discarded units differently, depending solely on reports from blood centres for component volumes may lead to inaccuracy in calculation of transfusion rates.

Breadth of the system

An analogous consideration is the breadth of the system: What products should be included in the system's tracking? The EHN's definition of haemovigilance focusses on labile components, but there remains much to be learned about the use of and reactions to plasma derivative products, and in some jurisidictions, these are handled through the same transfusion service system. In such a case, as in Canada, valuable information can be gleaned

through extending the system to these additional components. Should haemovigilance systems be further expanded to incorporate tissues and organs to become *bio*vigilance systems? The principles of haemovigilance – including product traceability, learning from one's practice and a commitment to continual improvement – are applicable to transplantation as well as to transfusion, and transfusion services handle these products in some countries, as well. Efforts to create systems applicable to tissues have already begun in earnest in the US, again spurred by safety concerns, and marrow transplant organisations have for many years been tracking the outcomes of their efforts in order to find keys to improving patient outcomes. The extent to which these efforts will be interdigitated with haemovigilance systems rather than standing alone as complimentary systems will be determined by the extent to which the participating institutions and physicians contribute directly to both fields and whether their systems are mutually supportive. At the least, transfusion medicine specialists should be aware of these parallel efforts in related fields so that, whenever possible, their systems can be made compatible and congruent, even if not communicating directly.

However, inclusion of donor operations should be regarded as an integral to a haemovigilance system. Not only are there important donor and patient safety elements to be gleaned from taking a holistic view of the transfusion process, but a system that spans the same vein-to-vein reach of the transfusion process will be better positioned to 'connect the dots' and unravel dilemmas and inform policy changes. Already enlightening have been data on the frequency of post-donation reaction rates with different blood volumes collected and delineation of the rate of post-donation death among donors assumed to be healthy. As with the recipient-focussed end of the system, standardised terminology and definitions are needed to ensure comparability of recorded observations.

Learning from experience

Haemovigilance systems are sufficiently mature in multiple countries that the medical literature is providing an increasing number of reports of their observations. By their nature, these are observational, but they still provide interesting insights into the problems faced by different transfusion systems and the risks borne by their donors and recipients. It is beyond the scope of this chapter to attempt to replicate all the available data, but the reader is referred to several recent, thorough reports to understand the scope of information available (see Further Reading).

Several important, common themes are evident from reviewing these data, and some of these observations have led to recommendations that have improved transfusion safety, the intention of haemovigilance systems in the first place.

1 Transfusion of the incorrect unit or component is the most frequent system problem encountered. The problem may manifest as the patient not receiving precisely the component (sub)type that was ordered or may manifest as a fatal haemolytic transfusion reaction. Clearly, inadequate and/or inaccurate identification of the patient or sample/unit at the time of pretransfusion sampling and at transfusion are frequent problems that defy simple solutions but that merit more attention and more capable technology. As shown in the Canadian experience, almost half of all high-severity incidents were related to pre-transfusion sample collection, and a third of all high-severity events where harm occurred were associated with transfusion of the incorrect unit.

2 The greatest mortality risk in most systems currently appears to be transfusion-related acute lung injury (TRALI), although assessment of the frequency of this complication is complicated due to subtle differences in the definitions applied and understanding that significant 'under-recognition' is undoubtedly occurring. This highlights again a potentially important role for TSOs in clinician education for the benefit of the transfusion recipient as well as for improved reporting and understanding of the reaction.

3 Data from haemovigilance systems have been helpful not only in defining the frequency of bacterial contamination of platelets but also in investigating the frequency of certain types of contamination after identification of a cluster of incidents and

in documenting the effects of implementing interventions to address the problem.

Several applications of haemovigilance data from the SHOT system have been particularly noteworthy in improving the safety of that transfusion system and show the power of haemovigilance systems when their data are applied thoughtfully through evidence-based recommendations (see Further Reading). Reports of mistransfusion due to identification problems continued unabated until the recognition that delineation of the problem alone would not effect an improvement. Subsequent implementation of augmented approaches to patient, sample and unit identification was associated with, for the first time, a decline in the number of reported deaths due to mistransfusions. Similar results of interventions have been reported from other systems, such as in France, where ABO-incompatible transfusions were reduced by three-quarters.

Similarly, recognition of the magnitude of the problem posed by TRALI and the high frequency of association of TRALI cases with the plasma of female donors prompted the UK's National Blood Service to reduce the proportion of plasma for transfusion coming from female donors with a subsequent marked reduction in the number of deaths attributable to TRALI.

Haemovigilance data have also led to some unexpected, intriguing observations. Thirteen fatal cases of graft-versus-host disease (GVHD) were reported in a 10-year time span through SHOT, all of them prior to the implementation of universal leucoreduction and all but two of them in patients who did not meet usual indications for use of irradiated components. Also, universal leucoreduction was associated with a marked reduction in the number of post-transfusion purpura (PTP) cases reported and an apparent shift of these from predominantly red cell recipients to include more platelet recipients (57% from 3%). This information may be useful in exploring the pathophysiology of these reactions and provide information that may be relevant to blood supply systems not currently employing this approach to component production. Without a haemovigilance system operating 'in the background' to amass this experience, these findings might have been missed due to the relative infrequency of GVHD and PTP.

Haemovigilance systems could also be applied to address important yet unanswered questions through the large number of events that they track. For example, the utility of routine pre-medication with antipyretics and antihistamines remains an open question, and a haemovigilance system could seek to generate a database of sufficient size to address this issue. Similarly, the large experience of one or multiple nations might be able to determine whether the incidence of TRALI is affected by all the plasma in a platelet unit originating from a single donor versus multiple but smaller exposures. There is also considerable interest in applying the power of a haemovigilance system's large purview for 'Phase IV' or 'post-marketing surveillance' studies to help assess the safety of new interventions, such as pathogen inactivation. This could be accomplished through ensuring that appropriate questions were included on the post-transfusion report form completed by transfusionists or through targeted studies utilising special reporting tools.

Although the stated intention of haemovigilance systems is to improve the safety of transfusion, such systems are also excellently positioned to improve the practice of haemotherapy through the assessment of patient outcomes. There remains wide variation in the application of indications for transfusions, and the lack of adoption of published guidelines is sometimes blamed on lack of evidence of their clinical applicability. The data necessary to address these questions are not readily available to most transfusion services at present, but further expansion and integration of laboratory information systems with electronic medical records and linkage with recipient registries may allow future versions of haemovigilance systems wider access to data that could address these and other important transfusion-related questions.

Key points

1 'If you can't measure it, you can't improve it', but measurement alone will not improve systems.

Concerted action to improve transfusion systems and reduce transfusion risks is necessary.
2 Haemovigilance systems are most effective when they are based on data reported by clinical practitioners trained to be observant for transfusion-related problems and reported consistently using standardised nomenclature and definitions.
3 Including 'near-miss' incidents in haemovigilance reporting provides insights into weak points of the transfusion process and the opportunity to improve the system by reducing the potential for human error to cause harm.
4 The most common problem reported across multiple haemovigilance systems is the transfusion of an 'incorrect blood component', and the most dangerous problems encountered frequently relate to sample and patient identification errors.
5 Recognition of serious problems followed by action directed at their cause can improve transfusion safety, as has been seen in steps taken to reduce the frequency of TRALI and ABO-related acute haemolytic events.
6 Haemovigilance systems may be extended to provide important information about haemotherapy decisions and follow-up of new transfusion approaches.

Further reading

AuBuchon JP & Whitaker BI. America finds hemovigilance! *Transfusion* 2007;47:1937–1942.

Callum JL, Kaplan HS, Merkley LL *et al.* Reporting of near-miss events for transfusion medicine: improving transfusion safety. *Transfusion* 2001;41:1204–1211.

Callum JL, Merkley LL, Coovadia AS, Lima AP & Kaplan HS. Experience with the medical event reporting system for transfusion medicine (MERS-TM) at three hospitals. *Transfus Apher Sci* 2004;31:133–143.

Engelfriet CP & Reesink HW. Haemovigilance. *Vox Sang* 2006;90:207–241.

Faber JC. The European blood directive: a new era of blood regulation has begun. *Transfus Med* 2004;14:257–273.

Faber J-C. Work of the European haemovigilance network (EHN). *Transfus Clin Biol* 2004;11:2–10.

Stainsby D, Jones H, Asher D *et al.* (on behalf of the SHOT Steering Group). Serious hazards of transfusion:

a decade of hemovigilance in the UK. *Transfus Med Rev* 2006;20:273–282.

Rebibo D, Hauser L, Slimani A, Hervé P & Andreu G. The French haemovigilance system: organization and results for 2003. *Transfus Apher Sci* 2004;31:145–153.

Robillard P, Chan P & Kleinman S. Hemovigilance for improvement of blood safety. *Transfus Apher Sci* 2004;31:95–98.

Williamson LM. Transfusion hazard reporting: powerful data, but do we know how best to use it? *Transfusion* 2002;42:1249–1252.

Williamson LM, Stainsby D, Jones H *et al.* (on behalf of the Serious Hazards of Transfusion Steering Group). The impact of universal leukodepletion of the blood supply in hemovigilance reports of posttransfusion purpura and transfusion-associated graft-versus-host disease. *Transfusion* 2007;47:1455–1467.

CHAPTER 19

Donors and blood collection

William Murphy[1,2] *& Ellen McSweeney*[1]
[1] Irish Blood Transfusion Service, National Blood Centre, Dublin, Ireland
[2] School of Medicine and Medical Science, University College, Dublin, Ireland

Collecting blood from people for transfusion to others is not optional – it is an essential part of health care. A developed health care system needs to provide approximately 30–40 therapeutic units of red cells and up to five therapeutic doses of platelets annually per thousand of the population it serves. There is no satisfactory alternative therapy in most cases, and no prospect of any such alternative emerging soon.

Blood donors: paid, directed, payback and altruistic

People can be motivated to donate blood in three different ways: (1) as a direct response to the needs of an individual they care about, (2) for an economically valued reward, or (3) as an altruistic act. All three methods are in wide use today. All have their drawbacks. However, it has by now become clear that societies that succeed in establishing a mature programme of altruistic donations generally gain a more secure and stable supply of safer blood for transfusion than those that do not. There is compelling evidence that the incidence and prevalence of infectious diseases are higher among donors who donate for personal economic gain. There is also

Practical Transfusion Medicine, 3rd edition. Edited by Michael F. Murphy and Derwood H. Pamphilon. © 2009 Blackwell Publishing, ISBN: 978-1-4051-8196-9.

some evidence that individuals who are directly approached by a relative or friend to donate for a particular patient are more likely to withhold critical information about their personal infectious risk history that may compromise the safety of the recipient of the donation.

Motivation, recruitment and retention of altruistic donors are not easy or cheap. In most developed nations 5% or less of the population donates per year. While donors will queue for hours in times of clear perception of need, such as in a major disaster, most of the time blood services need to work hard to maintain supply. Establishing a mature altruism-based blood donation and collection programme requires a high degree of social cohesion and an immense effort in education and communication. Maintaining a programme once it is established may also need considerable effort and expense. Many successful national or regional programmes based on altruism were set up around the middle of the twentieth century, at a time of national need in conflict or post-conflict. The appeal of sharing health and well-being was relatively easily conflated with national military or civil requirements at that time. Countries that did not establish altruism-based blood services to begin with have tended to find it much more difficult to establish one afterwards, and often remain dependent on non-altruistic donations. Huge efforts are currently being made to redress this throughout the developing world, often directed towards younger adults (Chapter 24).

Paying blood donors will provide a supply of blood, but it requires enough people in the population for whom the payment on offer provides sufficient motivation. Students or other economically marginalised individuals will often provide blood or plasma for payment, but the strategy will limit overall supply where there are not enough economic marginals in the community to respond. In more developed economies the balance of high demand for blood for transfusion with limited numbers of people who will be motivated by the rewards on offer often makes paying for donations an inadequate strategy. In addition, paying for blood also undermines the alternative, more successful motivation of altruism in these economies.

Apart from the problems of supply, paid donors are, in general, a less safe source than volunteer donors. Data comparing disease markers between paid and non-paid donors reflect this. In an analysis of 28 published data sets, it was found that while the incidence of disease markers had diminished over the years between 1977 and 1996 for paid and unpaid donors alike, unpaid donors were on average 5–10 times safer than paid donors and that this difference had not changed over time. The logic is compelling: people who genuinely feel well, and have no great incentive to donate other than genuine regard for their fellow humans, will tend not to withhold risk information, or at least not return regularly even if they do. People who need money or items of small economic value at the level they may be offered by blood services will have more pressing needs and are more likely to withhold relevant risk information. In addition, increased at-risk exposure from drug addiction or sex working occurs more frequently at the lower economic margins of a westernised society.

A system of directed and payback donations, where donors are recruited among the relatives and friends of the patient requiring blood transfusions, also provides some supply. Such an approach will generally be insufficient to support a well-developed health care system, and is prone in places to covert paying to donors, including professional donors.

Risks to the blood donor

Blood donation is generally very safe. Most people can readily tolerate venesections of approximately 10% of their blood volumes without apparent harm or significant physiological compromise. However, it is not a trivial undertaking and requires considerable care to minimise the risk to the donor. This is particularly the case since there is no proven health benefit to the donor except in the treatment, inadvertent or otherwise, of haemochromatosis. The risks associated with blood donation are listed in Table 19.1.

It is unlikely that the risks to blood donors can ever be reduced to zero. Coupled with the societal necessity for blood donations, this places a significant ethical burden on blood services to use their best endeavours to reduce the risks. This includes particular attention to detail, careful collation and analysis of data on the incidence and nature of adverse events or reactions, and proper management of the information derived, for example by sharing and comparing data among blood services to identify and promote best practices. The uneven risk-to-benefit ratio for blood donors also places an ethical responsibility on health care givers, the users of blood donations, to avoid wastage and unnecessary use of blood transfusions.

Donor selection and exclusion

Prospective blood donors are subjected to a process, often specified in national legislation, intended to minimise the risks to the donor and to the eventual recipient of the donated blood. This involves a donor history to identify clinical conditions in the donor that may suggest increased risk to the donor of a serious adverse event/reaction if the donation goes ahead, or any recognisable risk in the donor for transmitting infectious agents to the recipient. Infectious risks from donors are listed in Table 19.2, along with available donor exclusion strategies to address these risks.

In some services the donor undergoes some form of physical examination, but this is often cursory

Table 19.1 Adverse events or reactions in blood donors.

Type of event or reaction	Incidence
Vasovagal events or reactions Dizziness, nausea, simple fainting, severe faint with prolonged loss of consciousness and convulsions; associated trauma from falls or vehicle accidents.	*1.3 per 100 attendees for all vasovagal events or reactions
Needle injury To the vein, causing pain and bruising, which may be extensive, thrombophlebitis, thrombosis	*1 in 1500 attendees for all grades of bruising and haematoma
To the artery, causing extensive bruising, fistula, aneurysm, distal ischaemia, compartment syndrome	*1 in 28,000 attendees for all arterial punctures
To the nerve, causing pain, and motor and sensory loss, which can be prolonged	*1 in 9700 attendees for all nerve injuries
To a tendon, causing acute and intense pain.	
Serious cardiovascular events or reactions Angina, myocardial infarction, cerebrovascular accident.	Very rare; may or may not be causally related to the donation; always associated with underlying pre-existing disease
Iron deficiency with or without anaemia Even in the absence of anaemia, tissue iron deficiency may be associated with mild disturbance of cerebral function such as impaired concentration, and with sleep disturbance/restless legs	Unknown incidence; requires systematic study by blood services
Allergic reactions/anaphylaxis Reactions may be to the skin preparation materials or adhesives, or to latex in the attendants' gloves.	Rare
In apheresis donors in addition to the above Citrate toxicity from the anticoagulant	
	Mild reactions are common; severe reactions are rare, and usually but not invariably happen if apheresis is continued in the presence of worsening mild reactions
Thrombocytopenia and protein deficiency from excessive platelet or plasma donations respectively	Rare and easily prevented
Allergic reactions to ethylene oxide used in the sterilisation of the harness	Rare
Haemolysis/air embolus due to errors in the procedure or problems with the manufacturing of the harness	Very rare
For granulocyte donors: allergic reactions to hetastarch if used as a sedimentation agent, or adverse drug reactions to steroids or growth factors used to raise the donor's leucocyte count	Mild reactions including bone pain are common with the use of growth factors and steroids in donors. Many blood services do not provide granulocytes by apheresis. Pooled buffy coats provide an alternative that is logistically simpler, safer for the donor, and may be equally efficacious

Where marked with an asterisk, the figure is from Crusz T. *Blood Matters* 2007;22. See Further Reading.

Table 19.2 Infections risks from blood donors.

Categories of risks	Examples of infections	Donor exclusions that may reduce risk
Failure of a test to detect an infectious agent where it should have done so: while this risk is very low, it is not zero, and provides a reason to continue strict exclusion practices in the presence of increasingly sensitive testing methods	HIV 1 & 2, Hepatitis C, Hepatitis B	Excluding at-risk donors identified by questions about risk activities in the past: e.g. drug use or high-risk sexual activity at any time in the past
Window-period infections: a donor is infectious with an agent for which the donation is routinely tested, but the infection was acquired so recently that the donor does not yet have detectable infectivity in the blood	HIV 1 and 2, Hepatitis C, Hepatitis B	Excluding at-risk donors identified by questions about risk activities in the recent past: e.g. recent at-risk sexual activity, recent tattoos or piercings or recent invasive procedures
Infections for which donors are not routinely tested	Malaria, West Nile virus, Chagas' disease, visceral leishmaniasis, vCJD, dengue	Excluding donors, where possible, on the basis of travel or previous residence. This is very difficult in areas of high prevalence and endemicity, and requires additional testing where possible
	Any recently acquired infection that the donor has not yet cleared and that may have a viraemic or bacteraemic phase	Excluding donors on the basis of a recent history of any febrile illness; excluding donors who have recently had a live virus vaccination
Known diseases in the donor's past that may have an unknown transmissible element	Cancer, autoimmune diseases	Excluding donors with a previous history of cancer, with the exception of some localised and cured forms Excluding donors with a history of multi-system autoimmune disease
Risks from unrecognised yet-to-emerge infectious agents	In the recent past HIV and HCV were extensively spread by blood transfusions before the true nature of the diseases became apparent. A similar fate could have arisen with vCJD.	Excluding donors with a history of conditions strongly associated in the past with the early and extensive spread of emerging diseases with long incubation periods. Such donors include sex-workers and intravenous drug users More contentiously, excluding men who have previously had sex with men at any time in their past. Excluding donors who have previously received blood transfusions. Excluding xenotransplant recipients.
Risk from transmissible spongiform encephalopathies	All prion diseases are considered to have the possibility of an infectious blood phase	Excluding donors who have a strong family history of spongiform encephalopathy Excluding donors who have been treated with human-derived pituitary hormones or dura mater Outside the UK and Europe, exclusion on the basis of residence in higher risk countries during the BSE epidemic In some European countries previous recipients of blood transfusions are excluded to try to limit the risk of transfusion-acquired vCJD

and abbreviated and, among altruistic donors at least, is of doubtful value in someone who has provided satisfactory answers to a detailed history.

Donors generally undergo a measurement of their haemoglobin level at some point, either prior to the donation or, in some countries, on a sample taken at the same time as the donation. This measurement of haemoglobin serves two purposes – it provides some protection to the donor against having a pre-existing anaemia made worse by donating, and it helps ensure that the final therapeutic product will have a minimum red cell content. It might also help prevent acute adverse reactions or events in the donor, but there is no evidence that this is the case. The cut-off levels for the allowable haemoglobin level in the donor vary between blood services and regulatory authorities and are empirically derived. Often, as in the European Union (EU) rules (Directive 2004/33/EC, see Further Reading) a different level is used for males and females, with the allowable minimum haemoglobin level set 1 gm/dL higher for males than for females. Haemoglobin levels vary in the same individual between capillary and venous blood, with the seasons and with the time of day, and with posture and activity. In addition, measuring haemoglobin levels may not provide adequate protection against pre-anaemic iron deficiency.

Iron deficiency in blood donors

Blood donation results in significant iron loss of approximately 200–250 mg per donation; iron deficiency in the absence of anaemia may be common among donors, particularly mothers or menstruating females, and can cause symptoms such as poor concentration and sleep disturbances. This aspect of the practice of blood donation has received insufficient attention to date in many countries, with a reliance on haemoglobin levels to determine iron status. Iron deficiency also arises in donors of plasma or platelets by apheresis due to the red cell losses from the frequent blood samples, and from the inevitable small residual amounts of blood in the collection harness. A study of 1535 male and 1487 female Australian blood donors showed that 5.3% of males and 18.9% of females who met the EU criteria for haemoglobin levels were iron deficient as de-fined by a serum ferritin level of less than 12 µg/L. The prevalence of iron deficiency among the general female population in Australia is 5–7% and is negligible among the general male population (Farrugia, 2006).

Iron deficiency among donors may be prevented or treated by adequate intake of oral iron. However, optimum regimens for iron prophylaxis or therapy among blood donors have not been generally defined, and practice varies considerably. Options include regular measurement of blood or plasma indices of iron deficiency, routine provision of iron supplements, particularly to female donors, and dietary advice. Fears about the risk of serious iron toxicity in children who accidentally take a donor's iron tablets are probably well founded: iron should be dispensed with adequate warnings, packaging and advice when it is supplied. In addition, iron should not be given routinely to donors unless haemochromatosis has been excluded.

Increasing awareness of the necessity to prevent, detect and treat iron deficiency in advance of anaemia in regular donors is likely to result in modifications to practice in the future. Additional large-scale studies and technical developments are required to optimise the approach to screening donors to prevent morbidity from anaemia and iron deficiency, while allowing useful donations to proceed from perfectly well donors with physiologically lower levels of circulating red cells.

Where a blood service is subject to mandatory, legally binding regulations, donor exclusions may be specified by law. In the EU the specifications are generally interpreted as a minimum requirement by the member states or the national blood services; in the US and other jurisdictions, in contrast, the specifications are generally regarded as a maximum requirement by the blood service operators, who rarely add to them on their own initiative. The EU requirements for permanent and temporary exclusion of donors are listed in Table 19.3; the blood services in many countries routinely exceed these requirements, sometimes on the basis of local epidemiological risks, and sometimes on the basis of national or regional perceptions of best practice. Exclusions on the basis of sexual risk, travel, haemochromatosis or previous transfusions vary

Table 19.3 Deferral criteria for donors of whole blood and blood components (European Commission, 2004).

1. Permanent deferral criteria for donors of allogeneic donations

Cardiovascular Disease

Prospective donors with active or past serious cardiovascular disease, except congenital abnormalities with complete cure

Central nervous system disease

A history of serious CNS disease

Abnormal bleeding tendency

Prospective donors who give a history of a coagulopathy

Repeated episodes of syncope, or a history of convulsions

Other than childhood convulsions or where at least 3 years have elapsed since the date the donor last took anticonvulsant medication without any recurrence of convulsions

Gastrointestinal, genitourinary, haematological, immunological, metabolic, renal, or respiratory system diseases

Prospective donors with serious active, chronic, or relapsing disease

Diabetes If being treated with insulin

Infectious diseases

Hepatitis B, except for HBsAg-negative persons who are demonstrated to be immune

Hepatitis C

HIV-1/2

HTLV I/II

Babesiosis (*)

Kala-azar (visceral leishmaniasis) (*)

Trypanosomiasis cruzi (Chagas' disease) (*)

Malignant diseases except *in situ* cancer with complete recovery

Transmissible spongiform encephalopathies (TSEs), (e.g. Creutzfeldt Jakob Disease, variant Creutzfeldt Jakob Disease)

Persons who have a family history which places them at risk of developing a TSE, or persons who have received a corneal or dura mater graft, or who have been treated in the past with medicines made from human pituitary glands. For variant Creutzfeldt Jacob disease, further precautionary measures may be recommended.

Intravenous (IV) or intramuscular (IM) drug use

Any history of non-prescribed IV or IM drug use, including bodybuilding steroids or hormones

Xenotransplant recipients

Sexual behaviour

Persons whose sexual behaviour puts them at high risk of acquiring severe infectious diseases that can be transmitted by blood

2. Temporary deferral criteria for donors of allogeneic donations

2.1. *Infections:* Duration of deferral period

After an infectious illness: prospective donors shall be deferred for at least 2 weeks following the date of full clinical recovery. However, the following deferral periods shall apply for the infections listed in the table:

Brucellosis (*): 2 years following the date of full recovery

Osteomyelitis: 2 years after confirmed cured

Q fever (*): 2 years following the date of confirmed cured

Syphilis (*): 1 year following the date of confirmed cured

Toxoplasmosis (*): 6 months following the date of clinical recovery

Tuberculosis: 2 years following the date of confirmed cured

Rheumatic fever: 2 years following the date of cessation of symptoms, unless evidence of chronic heart disease

Fever > °C: 2 weeks following the date of cessation of symptoms

Flu-like illness: 2 weeks after cessation of symptoms

Malaria (*):

– individuals who have lived in a malarial area within the first 5 years of life:

3 years following return from last visit to any endemic area, provided person remains symptom free; may be reduced to 4 months if an immunologic or molecular genomic test is negative at each donation;

(Continued)

Table 19.3 *(Continued.)*

- individuals with a history of malaria: 3 years following cessation of treatment *and* absence of symptoms. Accept thereafter only if an immunologic or molecular genomic test is negative;

- asymptomatic visitors to endemic areas: 6 months after leaving the endemic area unless an immunologic or molecular genomic test is negative;

- individuals with a history of undiagnosed febrile illness during or within 6 months of a visit to an endemic area: 3 years following resolution of symptoms; may be reduced to 4 months if an immunologic or molecular test is negative.

West Nile Virus (WNV) (*): 28 days after leaving an area with ongoing transmission of WNV to humans.
2.2. *Exposure to risk of acquiring a transfusion-transmissible infection*

- Endoscopic examination using flexible instruments,

- mucosal splash with blood or needlestick injury,

- transfusion of blood components,

- tissue or cell transplant of human origin,

- major surgery,

- tattoo or body piercing,

- acupuncture unless performed by a qualified practitioner and with sterile single-use needles,

- persons at risk due to close household contact with persons with hepatitis B:

  Defer for 6 months, or for 4 months provided a NAT test for hepatitis C is negative.

- Persons whose behaviour or activity places them at risk of acquiring infectious diseases that may be transmitted by blood.

  Defer after cessation of risk behaviour for a period determined by the disease in question, and by the availability of appropriate tests.

2.3. *Vaccination*
Attenuated viruses or bacteria: 4 weeks.
Inactivated/killed viruses, bacteria or rickettsiae: No deferral if well.
Toxoids: No deferral if well.
Hepatitis A or hepatitis B vaccines: No deferral if well and if no exposure.
Rabies: No deferral if well and if no exposure. If vaccination is given following exposure defer for 1 year.
Tick-borne encephalitis vaccines: No deferral if well and if no exposure
2.4. *Other temporary deferrals*
Pregnancy: 6 months after delivery or termination, except in exceptional circumstances and at the discretion of a physician.
Minor surgery: 1 week
Dental treatment:
Minor treatment by dentist or dental hygienist (NB: Tooth extraction, root-filling and similar treatment is considered as minor surgery): defer until next day.
Medication: Based on the nature of the prescribed medicine, its mode of action and the disease being treated.

(Continued)

Table 19.3 (*Continued.*)

---

3. Deferral for particular epidemiological situations

Particular epidemiological situations (e.g. disease outbreaks):

Deferral consistent with the epidemiological situation. (These deferrals should be notified by the competent authority to the European Commission with a view to Community action.)

4. Deferral criteria for donors of autologous donations

Serious cardiac disease: Depending on the clinical setting of the blood collection.

Persons with or with a history of

    – hepatitis B, except for HBsAg-negative persons who are demonstrated to be immune

    – hepatitis C

    – HIV-1/2

    – HTLV I/II

Member States may, however, establish specific provisions for autologous donations by such persons.

Active bacterial infection.

The tests and deferral periods indicated by an asterisk (*) are not required when the donation is used exclusively for plasma for fractionation.

from country to country in the EU, while remaining within the legal specification defined in the EU Directives.

The blood collection/donation process

Assessing the donor, collecting and storing the information obtained, collecting the unit of blood and the accompanying blood samples, and storing and transporting the collected blood are all critical manufacturing steps in the preparation of the final therapeutic product. The entire process needs to be controlled within a functioning quality system, while maintaining the humanity of the process, and especially the dignity of the donor. The venue must be clean, warm, but not excessively so, uncluttered, bright and without excessive noise. Staff should not be distracted or distressed by extraneous events. There must be appropriate space available for confidential discussions between donors and staff. The flow of the donor from reception through registration, interview, haemoglobin check if done, and venesection should be orderly and unidirectional. Allocation of numbers and labels for the units collected must be rigorously controlled; mix up in labels between units or between samples is a potentially fatal error. Materials used in the collection clinic – bags, antiseptic wipes, mixer-weighers, haemoglobinometers etc. – must all be controlled.

Several blood services do not take a blood collection from a donor on their first attendance. Instead, they take a sample for blood group, blood count and virus screen. This practice almost guarantees that a unit of blood will not be mislabelled with the wrong ABO group provided an automated check against historical donor records is in place; it also provides some protection against window period donations from people who are donating for the purposes of getting an HIV or hepatitis test. It is however very costly – a significant proportion of blood in most services come from first time and once-only donors.

Preparation of the venepuncture site must also be rigorously controlled to reduce the risk of bacterial contamination; this is discussed in Chapter 14. This process and indeed all collection activities should be subject to regular audit.

Donors may be recruited or retained to donate for apheresis as well as, or instead of, whole blood.

Apheresis may be for red cells, usually as a double dose from larger donors, platelets or plasma, or combinations of these. Donor acceptance or rejection criteria are broadly the same, though plasma donors may be exempted for some infectious risks (Table 19.3). Platelet and plasma donation intervals are shorter. Since patients receiving apheresis platelets, and to a lesser extent apheresis red cells, receive fewer donor exposures, there is a clear benefit to using these components as much as possible. For selected products, such as HPA-1a negative platelets, apheresis is the only viable approach. Apheresis is generally a more expensive method of providing components than whole blood collection and processing, but the economics vary from place to place. In addition, apheresis donation can be a very effective way of maximising the return to a blood service from many of its committed donors.

Much of the plasma used in the manufacture of blood products comes from apheresis donors, many of whom are paid, and who donate every few weeks. Populations of paid plasma donors have a higher prevalence and incidence of infectious disease markers than non-remunerated donors, but since the early 1990s blood product manufacture has had a very good safety record from the point of view of transmission of infectious diseases. This has been achieved by increased donor screening and exclusion procedures, advances in testing, including the introduction of nucleic acid testing for viruses, and effective methods of pathogen removal or inactivation, such as pasteurisation, solvent detergent treatment and nanofiltration. As things stand at present, supply of manufactured blood products worldwide could probably not be maintained without paid plasma donation, though several countries have in the past, and several still do, supplied their national needs for blood products from non-remunerated donors.

Obligations to donors

Although donors are well and are not seeking care, they are subjected to a health care intervention from the moment they begin to complete the history questionnaire. The blood service enters a contract with them and develops an ethical obligation to them from the very start of the first attendance. The service's main duty of care is to the recipient of the donation, and it cannot compromise that, but it has obligations to the donor that must also be discharged. Donation is not a right, but rights accrue to the donor once the process is embarked upon.

The donor has a right
- to confidentiality and autonomy;
- to informed consent;
- to protection from harm – this includes not being made to feel unhealthy when they are merely outside of donation specifications;
- to receive the results of tests when these are of significance to their health;
- they are entitled to receive direction and counselling around the results of such tests;
- they must be protected as much as possible from adverse events or reactions by the use of adequate facilities, adequately trained staff, provision of clear and accurate information, and 24-hour access to advice after donation.

In turn, donors are required
- to be truthful in their answers to the screening questions – in some countries this obligation is explicitly stated to have the force of the law behind it; and
- to inform the blood service if any change arises in their health after they have donated.

In some services, donors are also provided with a form or a phone number they can use if they have knowingly withheld important information during the screening process that they have been too embarrassed to give at interview. This process, termed confidential unit exclusion, is still in use in some countries. It may provide some protection against donations in the window period, but it may also encourage donors to withhold information at the point where it should be given; this in turn would compromise blood safety.

Donors also have some rights in relation to the use of their donation – the consent that they give must include the possibility that the donation may not be used for the therapeutic use that they assume, but that it might expire unused, or be used for control purposes. Where a unit of blood is collected specifically for control, test or calibration purposes, the donor is entitled to be asked to give explicit consent for that. In addition, the health care providers should take account of the unique nature of the medicine that they are using, and ensure ethical and appropriate use.

Key points

1 The incidence and prevalence of infectious diseases are higher among donors who donate for personal economic gain.
2 Iron deficiency in the absence of anaemia may be common among donors and may cause symptoms such as poor concentration and sleep disturbances.
3 Assessing the donor, collecting and storing the information obtained, collecting the unit of blood and the accompanying blood samples, and storing and transporting the collected blood are all critical manufacturing steps in the preparation of the final therapeutic product.
4 The donor has a right to confidentiality and autonomy, informed consent, and protection from harm.
5 Clinicians should take account of the unique nature of blood components as a medicine, so as to avoid wastage and ensure appropriate use.

Further reading

Council of Europe: Final report – Collection, testing and use of blood and blood products in Europe in 2003. Strasbourg, Council of Europe Publishing. Available at http://www.edqm.eu/medias/fichiers/2003_Report_on_the_collection_testing_and_use_of_blood_and_blood_products_in_Europe.pdf.

Crusz TAM. Adverse events of blood donation. *Blood Matters* 2007;22. NHS Blood and Transplant. Available at www.blood.co.uk/pdfdocs/blood_matters_22.pdf. Accessed December 2008.

European Commission. Commission Directive 2004/33/EC of 22 March 2004 implementing Directive 2002/98/EC of the European Parliament and of the Council as regards certain technical requirements for blood and blood components. *Official Journal of the European Union* 2004;L91:25–39.

Farrugia A. Iron and blood donation – an under-recognised safety issue. *Dev Biol (Basel)* 2006;127:137–146.

ISBT Working Party on Haemovigilance. Standard for Collecting and Presentation of Data on Complications Related to Blood Donation. 2007. Available at www.isbt-web.org/documentation. Accessed December 2008.

Sebok MA, Notari EP, Chambers LA, Benjamin RJ & Eder AE. Seasonal temperature variation and the rate of donor deferral for low haematocrit in the American Red Cross. *Transfusion* 2007;47:890–894.

Van der Poel CL. Remuneration of blood donors: new proof of the pudding? *Vox Sang* 2008;94(3):169–170.

Van der Poel CL, Seifried E & Schaasberg WP. Paying for blood donations: still a risk? *Vox Sang* 2002;83(4):285–293.

CHAPTER 20

Blood donation testing and the safety of the blood supply

David Wenham[1], Lisa Byrne[2] & Simon J. Stanworth[3]

[1]NHS Blood and Transplant, Colindale, London, UK
[2]NHSBT/HPA Infection Surveillance Scheme, NBS, Colindale, London, UK
[3]NHS Blood and Transplant, John Radcliffe Hospital, Oxford, UK

Introduction

This chapter describes the aims and methods of laboratory testing of blood donations. It focuses not only on the range of tests currently employed but also on operational aspects crucial for the safe and efficient application of this process to the thousands of samples received in a blood centre laboratory each day. Testing is dealt with under three headings:

- red cell serological testing;
- microbiological testing; and
- operational and quality control issues.

Red cell serological testing

In the UK and most countries it is mandatory to test every blood donation for:

- ABO blood group;
- RhD blood group; and
- presence of irregular red cell antibodies.

In practice, most UK blood services also perform full Rh and Kell typing on all donations.

The results from these grouping tests are necessary as baseline information for safe transfusion practice in order to reduce the risk of premature destruction of the transfused donor red cells in a recipient's circulation due to immunological incompatibility towards the major red cell antigens.

Samples

Tests are carried out on anticoagulated venous blood samples collected at the time of donation. The samples are identified by a unique bar-coded identification system, which in most countries is an International Society for Blood Transfusion (ISBT) 128 number consistent with the aims of international conformity in blood group labelling and which ensures that each donation has a unique number.

The UK Blood Transfusion Service Guidelines ('Red Book') provide specifications and guidance on the testing reagents required for blood grouping, as described in the following sections.

ABO grouping

Donor red cells are tested with monoclonal anti-A and anti-B antibodies, which are capable of detecting all subgroups of these red cell glycoproteins. A reverse grouping is also performed by testing the donor plasma with A_1, A_2, B, and A_1B reagent red cells.

Most blood services make use of automated systems for serology testing where batched samples

Practical Transfusion Medicine, 3rd edition. Edited by Michael F. Murphy and Derwood H. Pamphilon. © 2009 Blackwell Publishing, ISBN: 978-1-4051-8196-9.

are divided into separate microtitre plate wells. The test results are read photometrically and the pattern of results obtained from testing donor red cells and donor plasma analysed by microprocessors to establish the ABO blood group result for a particular donation. In the case of repeat donors, such a system also allows the results for ABO groupings to be compared with those generated previously.

In the case of first-time donors, the ABO and RhD groups are tested twice and validated only when the two sets of results are in agreement.

RhD grouping

RhD grouping is performed by testing donor red cells with two different monoclonal anti-D reagents. These two reagents are selected with the requirement for high sensitivity in order to optimise the detection of weak or partial D-bearing red cells. This would include all the weaker Rh variants, including category D^{VI}. It is felt to be essential that blood services correctly identify all such red cells as RhD positive in view of the highly immunogenic capability of the Rh system.

Detection of irregular blood group antibodies

Donor samples are tested to exclude the presence of red cell antibodies that could cause reduced red cell survival or haemolysis when transfused into recipients whose red cells are positive for the relevant antigen(s). This is a screening and not an antibody identification step and involves the testing of donor plasma with a group O R_1R_2 K-positive red cells which are also positive for the majority of other red cell antigens thought to be clinically significant.

It is essential that all Rh and Kell antibodies above a threshold level of detection should be identified. The control system for UK blood services is set at a level of 0.5 IU anti-D, which is a higher threshold than that defined for hospital blood bank practice (0.1 IU). However, blood services are largely concerned with the detection of high levels of antibodies; weak antibodies will be considerably diluted during processing or transfusion. In contrast, hospital blood bank practice initially requires stringent detection of any antibodies in a potential recipient, irrespective of the level.

Blood for neonatal transfusion is tested for irregular antibodies to a higher level of sensitivity over standard testing, in order to further minimise the very small risk of transfusion reactions due to passive transfer of antibodies in this specific group of patients.

Most automated blood-grouping processes are based on the detection of antibodies on enzyme-treated red cells at 30°C. These techniques are known to be less sensitive for antibodies such as anti-Fy, anti-N, anti-M and anti-S. Clearly, antibodies directed against blood group antigens not present on the screening cells will not be detected, but these may not be clinically significant and are a lower priority in donation testing for the reasons mentioned above. However, the screening cells chosen do ensure that Rh and Kell antibodies are detected, as these antibodies have very occasionally been found to cause passive transfusion reactions.

High-titre anti-A and anti-B

Standard practice in hospitals is to transfuse group-specific red cells to all recipients. Group O red cells may also be transfused to certain groups of patients, such as neonates and patients requiring urgent transfusion, before their blood group is known. However, it is recognised that some group O donors may have high titres of anti-A and anti-B in their plasma that could cause lysis of A and/or B cells, particularly where large volumes of plasma are transfused, e.g. fresh frozen plasma (FFP) and platelet transfusions, or after exchange transfusion of red cells. In practice, because most red cell packs are stored in optimal additive solutions for preservation, the amount of plasma after dilution ultimately transfused is very small.

Plasma containing high-titre haemolysins can be screened in the blood service laboratory by observing the reactions between donor plasma and a diluted sample of reagent A1B red cells, and the products labelled accordingly. Recent refinements to testing for high-titre haemolysins include methods to assess only the more clinically relevant IgG (rather than a combination of IgG and IgM) fraction. There is no standard method of testing for high-titre haemolysins and the acceptable cut-off titre varies greatly with the technique used, thereby requiring local assessment of the procedures used. In practice, an automated system lends itself to universal testing of all donations for high-titre anti-A and anti-B, not just from group O donations. Very occasionally, high-titre anti-A may be found in group B donations (and vice versa).

Supplementary testing

Not infrequently, anomalies appear in some of the above test results and will preclude accurate grouping of a donation. For example, it has been estimated that 1 in 10,000 blood donors have a positive direct antiglobulin test (DAT) at the time of donation, which could interfere with the above assays. Weakly positive DAT may not be detected in the routine grouping test, which is based on a control channel for donor red cells mixed with inert serum. These donations may cause problems in hospital blood banks, since they would appear incompatible after cross-matching by indirect antiglobulin test (IAT). Subsequent donations from these donors will be 'flagged' and monitored as the positive DAT may be transient.

In many cases where samples give anomalous automated blood-grouping results, the blood service laboratory has to resort to manual techniques to correctly identify the blood group or antibodies. In general, only antibodies reacting in the IAT are considered to be clinically significant. It is standard practice to establish whether the corresponding blood group antigen is absent from the donor's red cells. In the case of identified anti-D or anti-c, quantitation of the antibody is performed because in those cases where levels are found to be not significantly raised, the red cells may still be released for transfusion, since during component preparation the antibody-containing plasma may be replaced with optimal additive medium.

Phenotyped red blood cells

Many blood centres also undertake a more comprehensive red cell antigen phenotyping service in order to identify donors whose red cells could be used for transfusion to recipients whose plasma is known to contain clinically significant blood group antibodies or to patients at high risk of forming multiple alloantibodies, e.g. sickle cell disease. This may involve screening up to 10–15% of samples from all donations received at the laboratory in a day, and should ensure that most requests for antigen-negative blood from hospitals can be met. In particular, testing for S, s, $Fy^{a/b}$, $Jk^{a/b}$, Kp^a and Lu^a in these red cells is often performed, as well as an additional sickle test to identify the presence of HbS (see below). Where donations are tested and found negative for the antigens listed above, this information is printed on the blood group label to aid hospitals with selection of blood for patients with antibodies.

In selected donations further specific red cell phenotyping may be arranged. Individuals tested for HbS on the basis of their ethnic origin could be screened for the U antigen, which is far more likely to be absent in Afro-Caribbeans than in Caucasians. This facilitates the provision of U-negative blood required for transfusion to those individuals who have developed anti-U, which is a clinically relevant antibody.

As mentioned, testing is performed to identify donations positive for HbS, in order to ensure that this blood is not transfused either to adults with sickle cell disease or to neonates during exchange transfusions. The need for a sickle cell screening test in a blood service will depend on the prevalence within the donor population. An additional consideration is the need to provide counselling support to inform donors found to be carriers of HbS. Of recent interest, it has been found that sickle-trait (HbAS) blood significantly interferes with the function of the filters currently used for leucocyte depletion (Chapter 21). Such 'failed' donations would be discarded, but the pattern of red cell antigens in these individuals could be unique and very useful as a transfusion resource.

Microbiological testing of blood donations and donor counselling

A wide range of infectious agents has been documented as transmissible by blood transfusion and these are described in Chapter 13. Donor selection criteria and the use of established guidelines to defer individuals at risk of infection by these agents are the important first steps aimed at reducing the risk of collecting blood donations with the potential to transmit infection. This is particularly important with respect to the collection of blood from donors in the 'window period' of an infection who may be asymptomatic and infectious, but without the viral load, with regard to hepatitis B surface antigen (HBsAg), or level of antibodies, with regard to hepatitis C virus (HCV) or human immunodeficiency virus (HIV) or human T-cell leukaemia/lymphoma virus (HTLV), to be detected by serological screening tests.

The laboratory screening tests form the core of the process to identify infected blood components prior to transfusion. From the perspective of the transfusion recipient, sensitivity is the most important criteria for a laboratory screening test, i.e. it will accurately identify most, if not all, infected donations. Maximal sensitivity in a test has to be balanced against specificity. However, many of the newer techniques and kits currently used in blood centres show remarkably high levels of both specificity and sensitivity. Indeed, risks of viral transmission by blood products remain extremely low (see Chapter 13). All positive screening tests require further confirmatory or reference testing to establish whether the result represents a genuine positive case.

It must be appreciated that in contrast to blood grouping, in which every sample produces a grouping result, most reports generated in microbiological screening are negative, and this has implications for quality control. On the other hand, blood centres screen large numbers of samples, which means that even though the screen tests exhibit high sensitivity and specificity, there will be significant numbers of samples from donors being identified as reactive on initial screening but where subsequent reference tests are found to be negative (i.e. false positives).

Screening results found to be initially and then repeatedly reactive on further testing (carried out because some initial reactive screen results may reflect assay or instrument-related problems) will be followed up by reference laboratory testing. The number of these repeat-reactive samples far exceeds the numbers of confirmed positives (see later section about results from screen tests). However, donors need to be aware that their blood has been found to be repeatedly reactive in one of the microbiological screen tests, although the likelihood is that the reactive result represents false positivity. This can be a complicated issue to explain and should be undertaken only when it has been confirmed that the reactive result represents false positivity. Blood centres must also develop strategies for dealing with donors found to be confirmed positive (sometimes unexpectedly) and for initiating the counselling and involvement of specialist treatment centres as required.

Principles of the screen test methodology

Most viral serology tests are based on immunoassay principles, using enzyme or chemiluminescent techniques of detection. Donor plasma is mixed first with captured antigen of the virus and then with antigen/antihuman globulin specific for the presence of antibody to the infectious agent. Detection may involve a conjugate linked to an enzyme, usually peroxidase, which can be detected photometrically after addition of substrate which produces colour, or by chemiluminescence, in which the optical measuring device detects photons emitted by the chemiluminescent reaction. Other changes to the methodology include improved ways of presenting the captured antigen and the use of antibodies to detect both an IgG and IgM immune seroconversion response to the virus. These changes aim to enhance the detection of the earliest possible immune responses to infection. Additional strategies aimed at reducing the window period of detection entail the development of even more sensitive techniques for detection of specific antibodies and the development of screen assays to look for the viral antigen itself or the nucleic acid. In the US, HIV antigen (p24) testing is now a standard part of blood donor testing and in many countries a 'combination' assay that can detect both HIV antibody and antigen has been introduced. Many countries including the UK have now

Table 20.1 Screening tests in transfusion microbiology.

	Test	Microorganisms
Generally mandatory (where affordable)	HBsAg*	HBV
	Anti-HIV-1, -2 and -0* (in some countries, only HIV-1 poses a threat)	HIV-1, HIV-2 and HIV-0
	Anti-syphilis*	*Treponema pallidum*
	Anti-HTLV*	HTLV-I (and cross-reactivity for HTLV-II)
Mandatory in some countries	Anti-HCV*	HCV
	Anti-HBc	Surrogate tests for non-A, non-B hepatitis. Anti-HBc will detect some
	Alanine aminotransferase	HBsAg-negative, HBV-infected donors
	HIV antigen (p24)	HIV
	NAT testing	HCV; other agents to follow
Discretionary	Anti-CMV	CMV
	Anti-malaria	*Plasmodium* species
	Anti-Chagas' disease	*Trypanosoma cruzi*
	Specific antibodies (hepatitis B, varicella-zoster)	High-titre immunoglobulins

* Mandatory screening tests for all blood donations in the UK.
CMV, cytomegalovirus; HBsAg, hepatitis B surface antigen; HBV, hepatitis B virus; HCV, hepatitis C virus; HIV, human immunodeficiency virus; HTLV, human T-cell leukaemia/lymphoma virus; NAT, nucleic acid amplification technology.

developed programmes to use nucleic acid amplification technology (NAT testing) on pooled samples of donor plasma to detect viral-associated DNA or RNA (see p 206).

Screening tests

Table 20.1 lists the screening tests used in transfusion microbiology. These tests have been divided into those mandatory in the UK, those mandatory in other countries and those used on selected groups of donors, as discussed later. Screening tests for specific antibodies, such as anti-hepatitis B and anti-varicella-zoster, are performed by some blood services in order to identify donors whose plasma may be collected for issue as high-titre specific immunoglobulin. The final decision to implement a particular screening test in a country will depend on a number of factors, including the prevalence of the infectious disease in the donor population. For example, following extensive discussion, testing for HTLV was introduced as an additional centralised test in the UK, although the prevalence of this in-

fection is considered low in comparison with other countries.

Testing for hepatitis B does not involve detection of antibody but direct detection of HBsAg. Some of the issues concerning the limitations of testing for HBsAg alone are discussed in Chapter 21.

Laboratory screening for infection by *Treponema pallidum* (syphilis) remains mandatory in many countries including the UK. Actual risks of transmission are low for many reasons, and treponemes survive for only short periods at the low temperatures used for red cell storage. Nevertheless, the incidence of syphilis is rising in different areas of the world and it can be argued that syphilis screening of donated blood is of value as a lifestyle indicator, since individuals exposed to syphilis may also have been exposed to other sexually transmitted diseases.

Immunological responses to cytomegalovirus (CMV) infection are detected by the presence of CMV antibodies in donor blood. As CMV is a latent infection, the presence of antibody indicates not only a previous but also a current and

Table 20.2 Donation testing data (UK and Ireland), January 2006 to December 2006.

Assay	No. of donations tested	Initially reactive		Repeatedly reactive		Confirmed positive		Rate per 100,000 donations
		No	%	No	%	No	%	
HBsAg	2,650,068	3496	0.13	1352	0.05	82	0.0031	3.09
Anti-HCV	2,649,459	2481	0.09	1712	0.06	86	0.0032	3.25
Anti-HIV	2,641,633	5279	0.20	1934	0.07	28	0.0011	1.06
Treponemal antibodies	2,652,999	3566	0.13	1730	0.07	96	0.0036	3.62

Adapted from *NBS/HPA Infection Surveillance Scheme Data*.

potentially infectious state. Screening is undertaken on both random donations and selected previously negative donations. Being a cell-associated virus, it is to be expected that leucocyte depletion should significantly reduce the risk of CMV transmission by blood components. However, as for all procedures and tests, there is a 'failure' rate (albeit very low) and it remains a controversial issue whether leucocyte-depleted blood components provide equal or lesser risk of CMV transmission compared with antibody testing.

As a consequence of the measures taken to minimise the potential risk of transfusion-transmitted variant Creutzfeldt–Jakob disease (vCJD) (see Chapter 15), plasma for younger-aged recipients in UK is imported from the US for use as products such as FFP (and cryoprecipitate). Such plasma will be subjected to the same microbiological screening tests as for other blood products derived from UK-sourced plasma and will be virally inactivated using a methylene blue technique.

Results from screen tests in the UK

Tables 20.2 and 20.3 show the results obtained by screening and confirmatory testing on donations in the UK and Ireland. In the case of screening tests (Table 20.2), the results were taken over a period of 1 year in 2006. By comparison, the data on confirmed cases were derived over a period of just over 10 years (Table 20.3). The tables highlight two points:

• First, confirmed cases are a small percentage of the numbers of initial reactive results.

• Second, the frequency of confirmed cases shows a wide variation between new and repeat donors, with a greater frequency of confirmed positives amongst donations from new donors. In 2006, approximately 10% of donations were from new donors, whereas they accounted for 83% of donations with detected markers of infection; the frequency of detection was approximately 40-fold higher in donations from new donors compared with donations from repeat donors. This forms the

Table 20.3 Confirmed positive rates (1 in X donations), from 1 October 1995 to 31 December 2006.

	Scotland		UK (except Scotland) plus Ireland	
	New donors	Repeat donors	New donors	Repeat donors
HBsAg	5,236	75,678	3,394	180,558
HCV	1,458	24,991	2,202	69,445
HIV	23,946	168,657	20,956	209,951
Syphilis	10,155	46,270	5,874	65,262
HTLV1	186,017	314,479	9,915	90,849

* HTLV data from 1 August 2002 to 31 December 2006
Adapted from *NBS/HPA Infection Surveillance Scheme Data*.

basis for preferentially processing donations from repeat as opposed to new donors for use in selected at-risk groups of recipients such as infants and neonates in order to further minimise the risk of transmitted infection.

However, the data from these tables also indicate the importance of having systems in place to continuously monitor infections in donors. For example, although there has been no overall trend in the frequency of HIV markers over the period of surveillance, an increase in the frequency of confirmed HIV infection among repeat donors has been observed since 2002. In 2006, 52% of HIV-infected donors were newly tested for HIV; there was a 14-fold difference in the frequency of HIV in donations from new donors compared with repeat donors, the lowest observed difference of all markers monitored by the surveillance scheme.

Between 1996 and 2006, the frequency of all markers of infection among donations from new and repeat donors declined, mostly attributed to a fall overall in HBV and HCV detection. This decline was more gradual from 2002 onwards, reflecting the higher frequency of markers of HBV and trepenomes among donations from new and repeat donors (mostly attributed to a rise in infections in male donors). Despite evidence of improved microbial safety of blood, infections in donors remain a concern for patient safety, and therefore it is important to carefully monitor infections in donors in order to inform donor selection and transfusion practices and allow for measures of the microbial safety of blood to be made.

Nucleic acid amplification technology

The application of polymerase chain reaction (PCR) or transcrition-mediated amplification methodology has the theoretical potential of identifying viral agents in the blood at the earliest possible stages of infection, since the sensitivity for detection is significantly higher than that obtained even by antigen assays. The window period of infection is longest for HCV (75 days compared with 21 days for HIV), and this has been one factor in driving the recent introduction of NAT testing for HCV in the UK. All plasma products, including FFP, must now be derived from pools of plasma found negative for HCV RNA before issue for clinical use. NAT testing for HIV remains under consideration in the UK but is undertaken by other European blood services.

A number of operational, technical and economic factors have raised concerns about the actual effectiveness of NAT testing, despite the potential benefits. Some of these issues include the following:

• staff training, in view of the general complexity of this form of testing;
• the need for scrupulous methods to avoid cross-contamination;
• appreciation of the time constraints inherent in obtaining NAT results and which crucially may be after the issue of blood components (currently often only 1 day); and
• cost analyses, which take into consideration the implications of patenting of the PCR methodology and the operational requirements for traceability of reactive results to the single donation level.

These issues are linked to the approach taken by most blood centres undertaking NAT testing, which is now based on testing pooled samples of approximately 50 donations. Such a system must allow traceability, but could also affect the potential sensitivity of the assay for a number of reasons including dilution and the presence of inhibitors within some donor serum samples. Risk estimates had previously suggested that around 1 in 250,000 donations will be derived from HCV-seroconverting donors in the window period. However, recent results obtained after the introduction of NAT testing in the UK indicate that the proportion of samples that are NAT positive but antibody negative may be considerably lower, of the order of 1 in 1 million. This reduction in apparent risk following the introduction of a new test is a not uncommon feature of microbiological testing, since the parameters used to develop a level of risk in the first instance tend to be based on less accurate initial input data. In many respects, if we aim towards a system of zero risk, screen testing for microbiological agents should be based around both NAT testing and antibody testing. However, the details of the benefits and the cost-effectiveness of such an approach is beyond the scope of this chapter (but see Further Reading).

A final consideration affecting the whole role of NAT testing for transfusion microbiology concerns the increasing application of validated specific viral inactivation steps within component processing. Effective inactivation would have the advantage of destroying transmissible viral agents for which there is currently no suitable test or those which are presently uncharacterised. In contrast, piecemeal addition of NAT testing for new agents would clearly require prior identification and characterisation of the virus.

Quality framework and operational issues

Ultimately, the microbiological and blood group safety of the blood supply depends on the input and interaction of a number of quality and operational factors.

The quality system needs to meet the requirements of a 'Competent Authority' under EU blood safety directives. Inspections are carried out by the Medicines and Healthcare products Regulatory Authority (MHRA) in the UK and appropriate authorities in other countries. Testing must be performed only by staff trained in approved standard operating procedures (SOPs). Document control systems must be in place to ensure only current procedures are used and any changes documented and approved. Any errors that occur in laboratory procedures must be logged using a quality incident report (QIR) system which requires corrective and preventative action to be taken.

Fully automated sample and test processing is now a standard practice in the UK blood centres for both microbiology and blood grouping. Systems in use may vary from modular to fully integrated, but all have specific sample identification and a system for tracking the sample throughout the testing procedure in order to provide a complete audit trail and documented evidence of testing to statutory requirements.

Operational advantages of automation include:
- better reproducibility;
- lower staff costs; and
- the ability to cope with high volume.

Test result interpretation and decision-making must be performed electronically by a data management system that can transfer individual results to a main computer. This integrated computer system will provide facilities that cover the whole blood donation process, providing essential controls and operational information to ensure safe working practices. Test results can be compared with previous laboratory findings and medical history to ensure that any hazardous material cannot be issued to hospitals.

Automated equipment must be validated before use and serviced and maintained to manufacturers' recommendations. Logs of servicing and regular calibration checks must be kept to provide evidence of satisfactory operational performance.

Several critical steps are involved in the performance of microbiological assays and blood-grouping tests. These need to be monitored, verified and logged by the testing processors. Microbiology test kit suppliers are now required to provide assays that have sample addition monitors and coloured reagents; these can be measured photometrically on the test processor and provide evidence in an event log that the critical steps have been performed and that the tests are valid. Appropriate quality control samples are essential. There are nationally agreed standards for all mandatory microbiology assays, and these must be performed with each batch of tests as 'go–no-go' controls, providing documented evidence of satisfactory test-run sensitivity. These standards are supplied by the National Institute of Biological Standards and Controls (NIBSC), are low-level positive controls and are used to monitor and validate day-to-day performance. They are also used to assess new batches of test kits prior to use within the laboratory, although acceptance testing of kits has now also been streamlined and centralised in the UK. Records of test results must be maintained in a readily accessible archive, usually in both paper and electronic format. In the UK, a fully traceable archive of all samples tested must be maintained for a minimum of 3 years.

The levels of process control now employed by the blood centre donation testing laboratories give a very high level of confidence that the test result for a donation is both valid and correct and that any potentially hazardous material will be discarded. Ultimately, the critical measure of the quality of microbiological screening must be the rate of post-transfusion infection. It is therefore very important that good links are maintained with hospitals so that possible post-transfusion infections are reported and fully investigated.

Key points

1 In the UK and most other countries, it is mandatory to test every blood donation for ABO blood group, RhD blood group and presence of irregular red cell antibodies.

2 Plasma containing high-titre haemolysins may also be screened in the blood service laboratory (e.g. by observing the reactions between donor plasma and a diluted sample of reagent A_1B red cells).

3 Donor selection criteria and the use of established guidelines to defer individuals at risk of infection by these agents are the important first steps aimed at reducing the risk of collecting blood donations with the potential to transmit infection.

4 A wide range of infectious agents have been documented as transmissible by blood transfusion, and laboratory screening tests form the core of the process to identify infected blood components prior to transfusion.

5 Many of the newer techniques and kits currently used in blood centres to identify infected blood components show remarkably high levels of both specificity and sensitivity. For known agents, risks of viral transmission by blood products remain extremely low.

Further reading

Barbara J, Ramskill S, Perry K, Parry J & Nightingale M. The National Blood Service (England) approach to evaluation of kits for detecting infectious agents. *Transfus Med Rev* 2007;21(2):147–158.

Campell-Lee SA. The future of red cell alloimmunization. *Transfusion* 2007;47:1959–1960.

Dow B. Microbiology confirmatory tests for blood donors. *Blood Rev* 1999;13:91–104.

Drew WL & Roback JD. Prevention of transfusion-transmitted cytomegalovirus: reactivation of the debate? *Transfusion* 2007;47:1955–1958.

Guidelines for the UK Blood Transfusion Services, 6th edn. London: HMSO, 2002.

Infection Surveillance Annual Report 2006. London. The National Blood Service and Health Protection Agency (Centre for Infections), November 2007. Available at http://www.hpa.org.uk/infections/topics_az/BIBD/publications.htm.

Katz LM, Cumming PD & Wallace EL. Computer-based blood donor screening: a status report. *Transfus Med Rev* 2007;21(1):13–25.

Kiely P & Wood E. Can we improve the management of blood donors with nonspecific reactivity in viral screening and confirmatory assays? *Transfus Med Rev* 2005;19(1):58–65.

O'Brien SF, Ram SS, Vamvakas EC & Goldman M. The Canadian blood donor health assessment questionnaire: lessons from history, application of cognitive science principles, and recommendations for change. *Transfus Med Rev* 2007;21(3):205–222.

Van den Burg PJ, Vrielink H & Reesink HW. Donor selection: the exclusion of high risk donors? *Vox Sang* 1998;74(Suppl 2):499–502.

Webert KE, Cserti CM, Hannon J et al. Proceedings of a consensus conference: pathogen inactivation – making decisions about new technologies. *Transfus Med Rev* 2008;1:1.

Zou S, Fang CT & Schonberger LB. Transfusion transmission of human prion diseases. *Transfus Med Rev* 2008;1:58.

CHAPTER 21

Production and storage of blood components

Rebecca Cardigan[1] *& Lorna M. Williamson*[2]

[1]NHS Blood and Transplant, Cambridge, UK
[2]University of Cambridge; NHS Blood and Transplant, Cambridge, UK

Whole blood and its processing to components

Guidelines from the UK, Council of Europe and AABB define a blood donation as 450 mL $\pm$ 10% of blood collected into citrate anticoagulant also containing phosphate and dextrose. There are no absolute indications for transfusion of whole blood, and the vast majority of blood units collected in the UK are processed to components – red cell and platelet concentrates, and plasma. Such plasma is suitable for either fractionation to plasma derivatives, or freezing as whole fresh frozen plasma (FFP).

Component production from whole blood consists of centrifugation to separate out plasma and cells of different density, followed by manual or automated transfer of components from the primary collection pack to transfer packs. Collection and transfer packs are manufactured as a single closed unit to maintain sterility.

Whole-blood donations from which platelets are to be harvested must be held and processed at 20–24°C, but, for other donations, pre-processing storage and centrifugation can be at either 20 or 4°C. Some countries hold all blood overnight at 20°C prior to component production. This yields components of high quality but is not yet permitted in the US because of concerns regarding bacterial proliferation.

There remains a small but finite risk of transmission of viruses via single-unit or small pool blood components. Unlike fractionated plasma products, blood components are not yet routinely subjected to a virus inactivation step. Techniques for doing so are now available for FFP and platelets and are under development for red cells. These are discussed in the appropriate sections below.

Collection of components by apheresis

Apheresis involves separation of the blood into components during collection on specially designed equipment, the harvesting of specific blood elements, and return of the rest of the blood to the donor. Because there is less loss of iron, plasma and platelet apheresis donors can donate monthly, and plateletpheresis permits collection of 1–3 adult doses/procedure, depending on the platelet count of the donor. Apheresis has been regarded as a more risky procedure than whole-blood donation, and tended to be undertaken only in donor clinics with trained nursing and medical staff available. However, apheresis equipment has developed into small portable machines drawing only a low extracorporeal volume so that they can be used safely on mobile sessions. Such equipment can

Practical Transfusion Medicine, 3rd edition. Edited by Michael F. Murphy and Derwood H. Pamphilon. © 2009 Blackwell Publishing, ISBN: 978-1-4051-8196-9.

be programmed flexibly to collect red cells and platelets/or plasma, with double-dose red cells being another option. An advantage of red cell collection by apheresis is that the haematocrit and haemoglobin content is much more consistent and predictable than in those produced from whole-blood donations. In addition, double-dose red cells could reduce the number of donors to whom recipients are exposed, which may be particularly relevant for transfusion-dependent and paediatric patients. Thus, the distinction between whole-blood donation and apheresis is becoming less, and it is likely that 'near donor processing' will expand in future years.

Quality monitoring

Specifications for the key parameters of each component type are generally set out in a national guideline such as the *Guidelines for the Blood Transfusion Services in the United Kingdom*. For other variables, there is freedom to set local specifications, which should be defined in a compendium by the manufacturing blood service.

In the UK, 1% of components produced are subjected to quality monitoring, although for those which are produced only occasionally, a set number each month must be tested. For key parameters, 75% of units tested must fall within the specification limits, although a different approach is applied to monitoring of leucocyte removal.

Leucocyte depletion of blood components

Many developed countries (although notably not the US) have implemented universal leucocyte depletion of components. In the UK and Ireland, the risk that variant Creutzfeldt–Jakob disease (vCJD) might be transmissible by blood, and in particular by leucocytes, was the major factor in this decision in 1998 (Chapter 15). In other countries, additional benefits, such as a reduction in immune-related complications and removal of cell-associated viruses, were considered equally important. Adverse immunological effects attributed to leucocytes include HLA alloimmuni-

sation, transfusion-associated graft-versus-host disease and immunosuppression, which in turn may lead to increased postoperative sepsis and tumour recurrence. However, universal leucocyte depletion may remove some of the beneficial effects of transfusion-induced immunomodulation, such as improved survival of transplanted kidneys, and suppression of Crohn's disease. These are discussed in detail in Chapter 10.

Production of leucocyte-depleted blood components

Leucodepletion (LD) is completed prior to component storage while the cells are still intact, usually within 48 hours of donation. For whole-blood donations this is achieved by filtration, whereas an LD step by centrifugation/elutriation is integral to some apheresis technologies. Mechanisms of leucocyte removal are thought to include platelet activation, causing secondary adhesion of granulocytes and monocytes, direct adhesion, and physical trapping of the more rigid lymphoid cells in the fibre of the filter. Most whole-blood LD filters remove >2 logs of platelets in addition to >4 logs leucocytes; therefore, only FFP and red cells can be produced from leucocyte-depleted whole blood (Figure 21.1). Leucocyte-depleted whole blood is then subjected to a single 'hard' centrifugation step (see Figure 21.1a), followed by expression of the plasma to yield red cells and plasma which are both leucocyte-depleted. Additive solution may be added to the red cells at this stage. To produce platelet concentrates, each component (red cells, plasma or platelets) must be filtered after their separation from whole blood (Figure 21.1). In this process, termed 'bottom-and-top' (BAT) processing (see Figure 21.1b), a 'hard' centrifugation step is followed by expression of the plasma from the top of the pack and removal of the red cells through the bottom of the primary pack into a transfer pack containing an additive solution. The buffy coat remains in the primary pack and this may be used as a start material for platelet production (see below). The same processing options apply for non-leucocyte-depleted components, except that the filters are omitted. The red cells and plasma can then be passed separately through leucocyte-depleting

(a) Whole-blood filtration

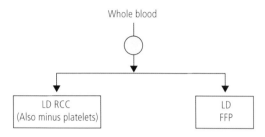

(b) Component filtration

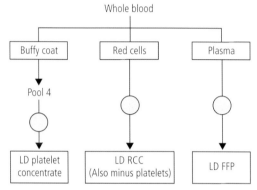

Figure 21.1 (a) Production of red cell concentrates (RCC) and plasma from blood donations, (b) Production of red cell concentrates, platelet concentrates and plasma from blood donations.

filters. LD results in a 10–15% loss of volume of whole-blood or processed component, but has minimal adverse effects on the quality of blood components.

Quality monitoring of leucocyte-depleted components

The specification for LD blood components reflect the current capability of LD systems, the fact that only a fraction of components are tested for residual leucocytes, and that the limit of sensitivity of current counting methods is around $0.3 \times 10^6/U$. Residual leucocytes can be counted by flow cytometry; microscopic methods using large-volume counting chambers (Nageotte) are not suitable for large-scale use. Studies using either flow cytometry or quantitation of mRNA encoding markers of leucocyte subsets suggest that all leucocyte depletion methods remove $3–4_{10}$ logs of all granulo-

cytes, monocytes and both B and T lymphocytes. In filtered red cells, most residual leucocytes appear to be granulocytes. Specifications set by the UK, and Council of Europe and AABB appear different, but are in fact broadly similar (Table 21.1). Quality monitoring of leucocyte depletion systems once implemented involves testing 1–5% of each component type produced, and plotting the results on a statistical process-monitoring chart. Systems with either poor overall capability or outliers giving a bimodal result distribution require 100% of components to be counted and are therefore best avoided. Guidelines for implementing quality monitoring of leucocyte depletion are published by the Biomedical Excellence for Safer Transfusion (BEST) Collaborative (see Further Reading).

Despite advances in technology, LD systems occasionally fail. The risk that an LD system will result in blood components being issued that fail to meet the required specification for residual leucocytes is dependent on a number of factors: the capability of the LD system, potential manufacturing defects in the LD filter or pack system, the proportion of components that are tested for residual leucocytes and donor-related causes. Although most donor-related causes of filter failure are poorly understood, it is known that donors with sickle cell trait are more likely to either block LD filters or fail to leucocyte deplete, and 100% of these donations are therefore usually assessed for residual leucocytes.

Removal of cell-associated viruses and prions by leucocyte depletion

Viruses associated with different leucocyte subtypes include cytomegalovirus (CMV, mainly in monocytes) and other DNA herpes viruses such as Epstein–Barr virus and human herpes virus 8 (in B cells) and T-cell viruses, such as human T-cell leukaemia virus I and II. Most studies of pre-storage leucocyte depletion have demonstrated its efficacy in preventing transfusion-transmitted CMV, but a recent study has suggested that if enough patients are studied, a small increase in risk might emerge. Bedside filtration appears to be unreliable in this regard. The Council of Europe, the AABB and the British Committee for Standards in Haematology all consider that components leucocyte depleted

Table 21.1 Specifications for leucocyte-depleted blood components.

	UK	Council of Europe/ European Directive	AABB
Level of residual leucocytes	$<5 \times 10^6$/U	$<1 \times 10^6$/U	$<5 \times 10^6$/U for red cells and apheresis platelets $<8.3 \times 10^5$/U for PRP platelets
% of components in which this must be attained	99	90	95
Statistical confidence that this is attained	95%	Not stated	Not stated

at source are equivalent in safety to those tested as CMV seronegative. However, this view has not been endorsed by either the FDA or the UK guidelines for the transfusion services. A Consensus Conference in Canada concluded that it would be premature to discontinue CMV testing, which continues to be performed by most transfusion services. Information on removal of other viruses by leucocyte depletion is limited, although one study of HTLV-I removal showed incomplete clearance of virus from some asymptomatic carriers by leucocyte depletion. Studies in a rodent red cell transfusion model of vCJD suggest that leucocyte depletion only reduces infectivity by 42%.

Red cell components (for specifications, see Table 21.2)

For the vast majority of red cell units, an additive solution containing adenine is added following separation to achieve a haematocrit of 50–70% and maintain red cell quality during storage. Red cells used for intrauterine transfusions (IUT), and exchange or large volume transfusion to neonates, are normally stored or reconstituted in 100% plasma due to concerns over potential toxic effects of some of the constituents of additive solutions. The most important changes which occur during storage are loss of intracellular potassium and a reduction in red cell recovery following transfusion. Red cell concentrates in additive solution have a 35–42-day shelf life (depending on the storage solution), at a controlled temperature of 2–6°C. Red cells which are stored only in plasma

have a 28-day shelf life. To minimise the possibility of bacterial proliferation and maintain viability, red cells should be removed from refrigeration as little as possible. For patients with severe febrile or anaphylactic reactions to red cells or those with immunoglobulin A (IgA) deficiency, red cells are washed and re-suspended in saline. The objective of washing is to remove as much plasma as possible, as such reactions can be due to antibodies to plasma proteins. At least one closed system for cell washing is now available, which allows red cells to be stored after washing, albeit with a shortened shelf life. Red cells from donors with rare phenotypes or from occasional patients with multiple red cell alloantibodies, for whom provision of compatible donor blood is extremely difficult, can be stored frozen for 30 years. Prior to transfusion, frozen red cells are thawed and washed to remove the cryoprotectant used to store them.

Pathogen inactivation in red cells

Red cells present a particular challenge for pathogen inactivation. Photochemical methods suitable for platelets and plasma cannot be applied to red cells because of the high degree of light absorption by haemoglobin. A number of compounds which do not depend on light activation are in development or in clinical trial, but none is yet available for routine use.

Prion reduction in red cells

Since leucocyte depletion alone is unlikely to render units free of PrP^{sc}, there is considerable

Table 21.2 Specification and typical values for volume and haemoglobin content for LD red cell components

| | Specification | | | | | | Typical values* | | |
| | Volume (mL) | | | Hb content (g/unit) | | | | | |
	UK	EU	AABB	UK	EU	AABB	Vol (mL)	Hb (g/unit)	Plasma vol (mL)
Red cells in additive solution, LD all methods	>75%; 220–340 mL	NS	NS	>75%; >40 g	>40 g	NS	284 ± 25	56 ± 7	17
Red cells in additive solution, LD, apheresis	>75%; 220–340 mL	NS	>95%; >128 mL red cells	>75%; >40 g	>40 g	>95%; >42.5	273 ± 17	53 ± 4	22
Red cells in plasma, LD for exchange	NS			>75%; >40 g	NS		321 ± 27	60 ± 6	116
Red cells in additive solution, LD buffy coat removed	As above						250 ± 19	49 ± 6	6
Red cells in additive solution, LD	As above						304 ± 17	58 ± 5	28

*Based on UK quality monitoring data.

interest in alternative methods to reduce the risk of transmission of vCJD by transfusion. Filters that remove prion protein from red cell concentrates are well advanced in their development, with the P-Capt filter system developed by PRDT in collaboration with Macopharma now licenced in Europe. A filter for red cells developed by Pall is currently being redesigned following breakthrough transmissions in some of their animal studies. As yet, there are no prion removal filters for whole blood, platelets or plasma. The filtration systems for red cells require prior leucocyte depletion, so are associated with a further 10–15% loss of haemoglobin. Prion removal and leucocyte depletion may be combined into one filter in the future, with several companies working on such an approach. On the basis of current working assumptions on levels of infectivity and prevalence of infection in the UK population, it is predicted that at least 3 log removal of infectivity (in addition to LD) would be needed to provide clinical benefit in terms of preventing transmission of vCJD. The P-Capt prion removal filter removes 3–4 logs of infectivity from red cells spiked with scrapie-infected hamster brain and >1.2 log (to below the limit of detection) of infectivity from the blood of hamsters infected with scrapie. The P-Capt filter has been shown to have negligible effect on the in vitro quality of red cells, the expression of common red cell antigens or recovery of red cells following transfusion to healthy volunteers. A clinical study is now underway in surgical patients, with a further planned in transfusion-dependent recipients, designed to detect increased rates of adverse events or red cell alloimmunisation with prion-filtered red cells. The UK transfusion services have also commissioned an independent assessment of the efficacy of prion reduction, since data to date has been generated solely by the manufacturers. Prion removal technologies would therefore appear to offer great promise in reducing the risk of vCJD by transfusion. However, decision-making regarding their implementation will require careful consideration of the costs and benefits involved, and what role they will play if and when it becomes possible to test donors for vCJD.

Platelet concentrates

Platelet production and storage

Platelets may be produced either from whole-blood donations or by apheresis, in which platelets with or without plasma are collected, and the red cells returned to the donor. Specifications for platelet yield and residual leucocyte count are similar for the two methods (see Table 21.3). Apart from exposing the patient to fewer donors, and the possibility of HLA/HPA matching with the patient, apheresis platelets are not intrinsically of higher quality. Platelet production from whole blood may be carried out either from pooled buffy coats generated by bottom and top processing or from platelet-rich plasma (PRP) as an intermediate step (Figure 21.2). Buffy coat-derived platelets have long been favoured in Europe, and are now standard in the UK, while the PRP method is standard in North America. Leucocyte depletion by filtration may be routinely incorporated into either process. An adult therapeutic dose of platelets (2.5–3.0 × 10E11) can be manufactured from buffy coats, or by the PRP method, from four to six whole-blood donations. In contrast, with the appropriate selection of donors according to platelet count and haematocrit, one, two or even three adult doses can be harvested from a single apheresis donor during one collection procedure. In the US, platelet apheresis donors were for a time-administered RhTpo to boost platelet yields. This is no longer permitted as safe practice (Chapter 43), and has never been practiced in the UK.

Platelets are stored with agitation in incubators set at 20–24°C for up to 5 days. Platelet concentrates should never be placed in the refrigerator as this impairs platelet function. Some countries routinely store platelets for 7 days, provided these are screened for bacterial contamination (Chapter 14). With pre-storage leucocyte depletion and the improved gas exchange offered by modern storage packs, platelets stored for 7 days in plasma maintain their in vitro function well, and several countries are performing additional clinical studies to assess the functionality of platelets stored beyond 5 days. During storage, platelets undergo a fall in pH

Table 21.3 Specification and typical values for volume and platelet content for LD platelet components.

Platelet processing method	Number of donors per dose	Specification						Typical values*	
		Volume (mL)†			Platelet content (× 10⁹ per unit)				
		UK	EU	AABB	UK	EU	AABB	Volume (mL)	Platelet content
PRP	5–10	—	>40 mL per 60 × 10⁹ platelets	Not specified	—	>60	>55‡		
Apheresis	1–2	Locally defined	>40 mL per 60 × 10⁹ platelets	Not specified	>240§	>200	>300‡	198 ± 15	288 ± 38
Buffy coat-derived pooled	4–8	Locally defined	>40 mL per 60 × 10⁹ platelets	Not specified	>240§	>60 per single-unit equivalent	—	297 ± 38	330 ± 52

* Based on UK quality monitoring data.
† The volume is also partly dictated by a requirement to keep the pH of platelet components within specified limits during storage.
‡ >90% of components must meet this criterion.
§ >75% of components must meet this criterion.

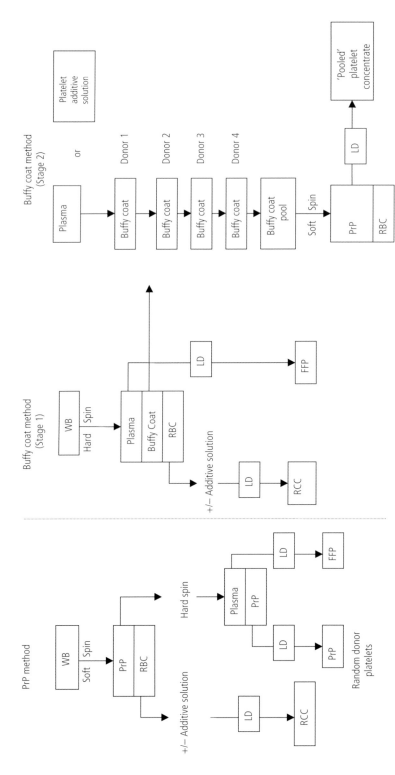

Figure 21.2 Production of platelet components from whole blood.

due to accumulation of lactate, express increased surface expression of activation markers such as P-selectin (CD62P), and change shape from discoid to round. Many different laboratory assays have been advocated to monitor development of this so-called 'platelet storage lesion' but few have been demonstrated to correlate with in vivo survival. pH remains the only quantitative change which must be monitored routinely and must be above 6.4 at outdate. Visual inspection to look for the 'swirling' effect of discoid platelets has been recommended, but this is highly subjective and changes only when the platelets have been grossly damaged.

For patients with severe anaphylactic-type reactions, which are usually due to plasma proteins, it is possible to prepare platelets to be virtually plasma free using one of a number of new platelet additive solutions. This product is sometimes referred to as 'washed platelets', although washing is unnecessary and may lead to platelet activation. These solutions differ from red cell additive solutions, in containing some or all of potassium, acetate, citrate, phosphate, gluconate and chloride. Platelets in 100% additive solution have only a 24-hour shelf life, but a number of countries have begun to produce platelets in a mixture of 30% plasma and 70% platelet additive solution. This strategy makes more plasma available for fractionation and allows a normal 5-day shelf life. Data to day 7 and beyond are limited. These solutions have great potential, but require careful validation, which may need to include volunteer and patient studies.

Pathogen reduction in platelets

A group of compounds called psoralens have been developed for their virus and bacterial killing properties, and a system for pathogen inactivation of platelet concentrates using a second-generation psoralen called amotosalen (S-59), has been licenced in Europe. Psoralens form adducts with DNA and RNA; when activated by exposure to ultraviolet light A (UV-A), binding becomes irreversible and nucleic acid replication is blocked. Amotosalen/UV-A treatment results in a high degree of killing of the major transfusion-transmitted viruses HIV, HCV and HBV, including intra-cellular

pathogens such as CMV and HTLV. There is, however, no effect on prions, which lack nucleic acid. Additional properties of S-59 photoinactivation include killing of Gram-positive and Gram-negative bacteria, inactivation of the antigen-presenting cells important in HLA alloimmunisation, and inhibition of the donor T-cell proliferation which characterises transfusion-associated graft-versus-host disease (TA-GVHD). Thus, there could potentially be multiple benefits from this approach, and in clinical trials of S59 photoinactivated platelets, it was considered unnecessary to perform gamma irradiation for prevention of TA-GVHD. Randomised clinical trials, performed on >500 patients, have shown that S59-treated platelets, whether prepared by apheresis or from pooled buffy coats, are effective in preventing haemorrhage in thrombocytopenic patients with haematological malignancies. However, platelet increments and inter-transfusion intervals were less favourable than in control patients, raising the possibility that increased numbers of platelet units might be required to support such patients. This question can be answered only by further large-scale clinical studies. Other systems for pathogen reduction in platelets are also in development. One particularly interesting approach is to use riboflavin (vitamin B_2) with light activation, as there is no need for a post-treatment removal step, but data from clinical studies using this system are not yet available.

Fresh frozen plasma

Definition and specification

FFP is the plasma from a single donation, usually 250–300 mL, which has been frozen soon after collection (usually within 8 hours) without pooling to a core temperature of less than -30°C. To minimise virus risk, FFP is not manufactured from first-time donors in the UK. FFP can also be derived from apheresis collections, in 300 or 600 mL volumes. It is used primarily as a source of multiple coagulation factors in situations such as massive transfusion, disseminated intravascular coagulation and liver disease (Chapter 29). The permitted shelf life depends on storage temperature, e.g., less than

Table 21.4 Specifications and typical values for residual cellular and coagulation factor content of frozen plasma components

Specification	Residual cellular content ($\times 10^9$/L)[*]			Coagulation factor content		
	UK[†]	EU	AABB	UK[†]	EU	AABB
FFP	Platelets <30	Platelets <50 Red cells <6	None	FVIII > 0.70 IU/mL	FVIII > 0.70 IU/mL	None
Cryoprecipitate	None	Platelets <50 Red cells <6	None	Fibrinogen >140 mg/unit FVIII > 70 IU/unit	Fibrinogen > 140 mg/unit FVIII > 70 IU/unit	Fibrinogen > 150 mg/unit FVIII > 80 IU/unit
Cryoprecipitate-depleted plasma	None	Platelets<50 Red cells<6	None	None	None	None
Typical values[‡] FFP	Residual cellular content Platelets <3 × 10^9/L Red cells 0.63 ± 0.50 × 10^9/L		Coagulation factor content FVIII 1.19 ± 0.40 IU/mL		Total volume (mL) 272 ± 17	
Cryoprecipitate	—		FVIII 182 ± 71 IU/unit; Fibrinogen 471 ± 199 mg/unit		40 ± 5	
Cryoprecipitate-depleted plasma	—		–		305 ± 31	

[*] Specifications for residual WBC are as per Table 20.1.
[†] >75% of components must meet these criteria.
[‡] Based on UK quality-monitoring data.

−30°C for 24 months. In Europe, FFP must be monitored for levels of factor VIII (Table 21.4). Although most FFP is prescribed for patients with normal or elevated factor VIII levels, it is selected for quality-monitoring purposes, as it is labile and hence sensitive to exposure to adverse conditions. FFP is thawed (in a protective overwrap to prevent bacterial contamination) in a water bath; purpose-designed microwave ovens are also available. Once thawed FFP can be stored at 4°C for at least 24 hours.

Virus inactivation

Two virus-inactivated FFP preparations are now available in the UK – methylene blue (MB) treated and solvent–detergent (SD) treated, with other systems in development. Both methods offer good virus protection, but are associated with loss of clotting factors. Another system for treatment of single units of plasma, based on the use of Amotosalen, has now been licenced in Europe. This offers an alternative to MB FFP for single-donor virus-inactivated FFP and cryoprecipitate and is currently under consideration in the UK. The key features of MB FFP and SD FFP and Amotosalen FFP compared with untreated FFP are shown in Table 21.5.

MB is a phenothiazine dye which, when exposed to white light, generates reactive oxygen species which damage nucleic acids, preventing viral replication. Treatment is applied to single unpooled units of plasma and requires prior removal of white blood cells (WBC) by filtration or freeze–thawing. The MB is contained in or added to the integral pack system, mixed with the plasma, and then placed on a light box for activation. The MB is removed using an adsorption filter prior to transfusion to the patient, leaving residual MB concentrations of <0.3 μM. At these concentrations,

Table 21.5 A comparison of Standard FFP with Methylene Blue treated FFP, Amotosalen treated FFP and Solvent Detergent treated FFP

	Standard FFP	Methylene blue FFP	Amotosalen FFP	Solvent detergent FFP
Source	UK donors, all previously virus tested. Single-unit format	US volunteers donors, all male. Single-unit format	Not yet available in UK. Single-unit format	Non-UK donors; pools of up to 380 L (600–1500 ABO identical donations)
Donation testing:				
Serology	HIV, HBV, HCV, HTLV	HIV, HBV, HCV, HTLV	HIV, HBV, HCV, HTLV	HIV, HBV, HCV, HTLV
Genomic	HCV	HCV, HIV	HCV, HIV (depending on source)	HAV, HCV, B19, HIV, HBV
Virus risk				
HIV 1 + 2	1:10 million	No proven cases reported to date for HIV, HBV, HCV (1 possible HCV transmission)	No data	No reported transmissions to date of HIV, HBV, HCV in SDFFP- or SD-treated plasma products
Hepatitis C	1:50 million			
Hepatitis B	1:1.2 million	No greater than for standard FFP. None reported to date		None reported
Hepatitis A	Rare event			Batch withdrawals due to possible B19 content. Seroconversion in patients no greater than with untreated FFP
Parvovirus B19	Rare event			
Volume	180–300 mL + 50 mL paediatric size	235–305 mL + 50 mL paediatric size	As for FFP	200 mL; no paediatric size
Coagulation factor content	Variable between units. 75% units >0.7 IU/mL VIII	Variable between units. 75% units fVIII >0.5 IU/mL; all other factors >0.5 IU/mL; no reduction ATIII, protein C, protein S. No coagulation factor/complement activation	Variable between units. 20–25% loss of FVIII, no reduction ATIII, protein C, protein S. No coagulation factor activation	Constant within batch. All factors >0.5 IU/mL.
Cryoprecipitate/ cryosupernatant	Available	Cryoprecipitate available 2008	Both possible	Not available

(Continued)

Table 21.5 (*Continued*)

	Standard FFP	Methylene blue FFP	Amotosalen FFP	Solvent detergent FFP
Residual additives	None	<0.3 μM MB. No toxicity seen or predicted at this level, even in premature neonates	<0.6 μM, no toxicity predicted	<2 μg/mL TNBP*; <5 μg/mL Triton-X 100. Residual levels not toxic
Allergic reactions	May be reduced by leucocyte depletion	Reactions attributable to cells would be expected to be reduced		Probably less frequent than FFP
Mild	1%	No data		
Severe	0.1%	No data		
Adverse reactions due to antibody:		As for standard FFP	As for standard FFP	Pooling reduces all of these risks
Red cell	Tested for high-titre anti-A,B	Not tested for high-titre anti-A,B		High-titre anti-A, B not a problem since donations pooled
TRALI	<1 case/year since preferential male FFP introduced	None reported to date		Rare
Thrombocytopenia	Very rare			None proven
Cellular content	Leucocyte depleted; RhD matching not recommended	Leucocyte depleted; RhD matching not recommended	Leucocyte depleted; RhD matching not recommended	No intact cells or fragments; no need to RhD match
Product licence Indications	Not required	Medical device; CE marked As for FFP	Medical device; CE marked As for FFP	Licenced, batched product As for FFP
Usage to date	300,000 units/year in the UK	>1,000,000 units in Europe	180,000 units in Europe	3,000,000 units in Europe

no toxicity has been demonstrated or is predicted. Glucose 6 phosphate dehydrogenase deficiency is not a contraindication to use of this product.

There is approximately 30% loss of activity of factors VIII and XI, and of particular note is the effect of MB on fibrinogen, with up to 30% loss of activity. It is, however, unclear as yet whether these changes require increased volumes of the product to be prescribed.

SD treatment can be applied only to pools of several hundred ABO-identical units; as the treatment destroys the lipid envelope of red cells, no RhD matching is required. Exposure to SD destroys the lipid envelope of the human immunodeficiency virus (HIV) and hepatitis B and C viruses, and no such transmissions have been reported. Non-lipid-coated viruses such as parvovirus B19 and hepatitis A are not specifically inactivated, but their titre may be reduced in downstream processing. In addition, plasma pools with high genomic titres of these viruses are rejected, and pools contain specified levels of viral antibodies, which may be at least partially protective. No increase in clinical cases of hepatitis A virus or B19 in SD FFP recipients is evident. Concerns have been expressed in the US that SDFFP might be associated with increased thrombotic risk in certain clinical situations, attributed to loss of proteins C and S during SD treatment. However, these complications have not been prominent in recipients of SDFFP manufactured by the European method, which results in greater preservation of these proteins. A variant of SDFFP in which ABO groups are mixed is in development. By neutralisation of A and B substances by anti-A and anti-B, it is intended to produce a 'universal FFP' which could be given to patients of any ABO group.

vCJD and FFP

In animal studies, plasma was found to contain infective prion. Therefore, a precautionary measure for the UK was announced in 2002 whereby FFP for children born on or after 1 January 1996 would receive FFP imported from the US, where the incidence of BSE is negligible, with no human cases of vCJD. This was implemented in 2004, with plasma coming from volunteer donors extensively tested

for transfusion-transmitted viruses, including West Nile virus. Plasma is pathogen inactivated by the MB process on arrival in the UK. In 2005, the use of imported MB FFP was extended to patients under the age of 16.

Cryoprecipitate and cryosupernatant

Cryoprecipitate is manufactured by slowly thawing single units of FFP overnight at $4°C$. This precipitates out the so-called cryoproteins, namely factor VIII, fibrinogen, fibronectin and factor XIII. By removing most of the supernatant plasma ('cryosupernatant'), a component providing a high concentration of these clotting factors is obtained (Table 21.4). Although originally developed for factor VIII deficiency (haemophilia A), most cryoprecipitate is now prescribed to treat congenital or acquired hypofibrinogenaemia, usually in the context of liver disease, disseminated intravascular coagulation or massive transfusion. An adult dose of 10–12 packs is generally indicated once the fibrinogen level falls to $\ll 0.5 - 1.0$ g/L. Pools of 5 units of cryoprecipitate are now available in the UK. An alternative product would be a virus-inactivated fibrinogen concentrate, but none are yet licenced in the UK. Cryosupernatant has been used successfully as a replacement fluid in plasma exchange procedures for thrombotic thrombocytopenic purpura (TTP). It was thought to have theoretical advantages over FFP, possibly because it lacks the highest molecular weight multimers of von Willebrand factor, although recent studies suggest that FFP is equally effective. It is now rarely used in the UK since the UK Departments of Health now recommend that patients with TTP are treated using SD FFP.

Virus inactivation of cryoprecipitate and cryosupernatant

Production of cryoprecipitate from SD FFP has been performed experimentally. Such cryoprecipitate contains insufficient von Willebrand factor to treat patients with von Willebrand's disease. Fibrinogen levels are reduced but acceptable. Manufacture of cryoprecipitate from MB plasma is under assessment, but is challenging because of the fibrinogen loss in the start plasma, potentially altered recovery in the cryoprecipitation process, and the inhibitory effect of MB on fibrin polymerisation. However, laboratory studies using newer assays of coagulation suggest that this product results in the formation of a robust clot.

Granulocytes for transfusion

The use of transfused granulocytes is now uncommon. They are sometimes used for severely neutropenic patients (granulocyte count $<0.5 \times 10^9$/L) with focal bacterial or fungal infection refractory to antimicrobial therapy, but there are difficulties in obtaining sufficient functional cells from donors and administering them frequently enough to the patient. Production options have been to use 10 or 12 buffy coats from random donors, or to harvest apheresis granulocytes from family members using a red cell sedimenting agent such as hydroxyethyl starch. Animal studies suggest that $>1 \times 10^{10}$ granulocytes once or twice daily are required to treat an adult, but apheresis usually produces no more than 0.5×10^{10}/dose. Therefore, unstimulated apheresis granulocytes are directed towards children, in whom an adequate dose can be achieved, with adult patients receiving buffy coat-derived granulocytes. A pooled granulocyte component made from 10 buffy coats has been developed in the UK and is currently being assessed in clinical studies. The main advantage of the pooled component over standard buffy coats is a reduction in red cell contamination and volume, and that it is issued as a single unit.

There has been renewed interest in the use of granulocytes by studies of granulocyte colony-stimulating factor (G-CSF)-mobilised granulocytes collected by apheresis. Administration to the donor of a single subcutaneous injection of 10 µg/kg G-CSF plus oral dexamethasone 8 mg 12–24 hours prior to apheresis raises the peripheral leucocyte count to $>25 \times 10^9$/L. This, coupled with Pentaspan sedimentation, allows collection of a therapeutic dose of granulocytes of $5–20 \times 10^8$ granulocytes/kg body weight of the recipient. This can result in a measurable rise in the peripheral granulocyte count in the patient and recovery of migrated cells from saliva. Clinical trials of such granulocytes are ongoing. At present, use of G-CSF for granulocyte collection is permitted in volunteer donors unrelated to the patient in the US but not in the UK.

All granulocyte preparations should be released for issue as soon as possible after collection, which may mean that certain time-consuming screening assays such as HCV genome testing cannot be done prior to release. They must be gamma irradiated to prevent TA-GVHD, and should be administered to the patient without delay. If a short period of storage is unavoidable, this should be at 22°C without agitation. Because of red cell contamination, a red cell cross-match should be performed.

Components for intrauterine transfusion and for neonates and infants

General requirements (see Table 21.6)

In the UK, such components are not manufactured from 'first-time' donors, or haemoglobin sickle heterozygous donors and cellular components are manufactured only from CMV antibody-negative donors. FFP has not been shown to transmit CMV so provision of CMV antibody-negative FFP is not critical. For components other than those in additive solution, they must be free of clinically significant red cell antibodies, including high-titre anti-A and anti-B. Gamma-irradiation is required for intrauterine and exchange transfusions. 'Top-up' red cells transfusions need be irradiated only if there has been a previous intrauterine transfusion (IUT) or if the component is prepared from a family member. Family donations are not encouraged except in rare cases of foetomaternal alloimmunisation where the infant's requirements cannot be met from donor blood. Although components are leucocyte depleted at source, they should still be administered through a 170–200-µm filter to remove any microaggregates formed during storage.

Intrauterine transfusions

Red cells are given in utero to treat severe fetal anaemia due to haemolytic disease of the

Table 21.6 UK specifications for red cells for intrauterine transfusion (IUT), exchange/large volume transfusions and 'top-up' transfusions for neonates.

	IUT	Exchange transfusion	Top-up transfusion
Previous virology-negative donation in previous 2 years	Yes	Yes	Yes
Free of high-titre anti-A, anti-B	Yes	Yes	No
Use of additive solution permitted	No	No	Yes
Leucocyte depleted	Yes	Yes	Yes
Gamma-irradiation	Yes	Yes	No
Haemoglobin S negative	Yes	Yes	Yes
CMV seronegative	Yes	Yes	Yes
Shelf life	24 h post-irradiation and <5 days total	24 h post-irradiation and <5 days total	35 days

newborn (HDN) or parvovirus B19 infection. Red cells for IUT are prepared from blood <5 days old to a haematocrit of >0.7–0.9, and gamma irradiated. They should be administered within 24 hours of irradiation, and always by the end of day 5.

In cases of foetomaternal alloimmunisation to platelets, weekly transfusions of selected platelets (usually HPA-1a and HPA-5b negative) are given in utero to minimise the risk of bleeding associated with fetal blood sampling (Chapter 5). Apheresis of genotyped donors is used to produce a platelet 'hyperconcentrate' of >120 × 10^9 platelets in 60 mL of plasma.

Exchange/large volume transfusion of neonates

This is undertaken to treat hyperbilirubinaemia due to either haemolytic disease or prematurity (Chapter 26). Either whole blood or partially packed red cells with a haematocrit of 0.6 may be used. Red cells in additive solution are not recommended by some paediatricians, because of concerns regarding the adverse effects of mannitol, but some countries use this component for exchange transfusion without apparent problems. The same concerns have been expressed over the choice of component for other large volume transfusions in neonates, such as for cardiac surgery or extracorporeal membrane oxygenation. However, some cardiac centres have switched to red cells in SAGM without apparent problems.

Top-up transfusions for neonates

Premature neonates are among the most heavily transfused patients in any hospital. Most red cell transfusions are given to replace repeated samples taken for laboratory testing. As each infant may require multiple small transfusions, adult packs are split into four to eight 'paedipacks' of 30–60 mL, which are allocated to one infant for the duration of transfusion dependence. Such a strategy reduces donor exposure considerably. For these small volume transfusions, red cells in additive solution may be used, up to the normal 35-day shelf life. Gamma-irradiation of these is not required in the UK, unless there has been a previous IUT or the blood comes from a family member. Studies of RhEpo in premature infants have not convincingly shown a reduction in transfusion requirements.

Platelet concentrates and FFP

These are most simply prepared from apheresis donations. Multiple aliquots can be allocated to the same infant if required. An alternative strategy for platelets is to prepare a platelet concentrate from a single buffy coat, or from a unit of whole blood using the PRP method. These components are generally used for sick babies with multiple coagulation defects. Platelets from a panel of HPA-1a and 5b-negative donors are available 'off the shelf' for rapid availability for suspected cases of neonatal alloimmune thrombocytopenia (Chapter 5).

Key points

1 There are no recognised indications for the trans-fusion of whole blood, and therefore blood is sep-arated into its components for transfusion (red cells, plasma and platelets).
2 Blood components can be produced from whole-blood donations or collected directly from the donor by apheresis technology.
3 In the UK, all blood components are leucocyte depleted.
4 Systems are now available in Europe to inacti-vate pathogens in plasma or platelet components prior to storage.
5 Filters have been developed that are designed to remove prion protein from red cells to reduce the risk of transmission of vCJD.

Further reading

British Committee for Standards in Haematology. Guide-lines on the clinical use of leucocyte-depleted blood components. *Transfus Med* 1998;8:59–71.

British Committee for Standards in Haematology. Guide-lines for the use of platelet transfusions *Br J Haematol* 2003;122:10–23.

British Committee for Standards in Haematology. Trans-fusion guidelines for neonates and older children. *Br J Haematol* 2004;124:433–453.

British Committee for Standards in Haematology. Guide-lines for the use of fresh-frozen plasma, cryoprecipi-tate and cryosupernatant. *Br J Haematol* 2005;126:11–28.

Council of Europe. *Guide to the Preparation, Use and Qual-ity Assurance of Blood Components*, 13th edn. Strasbourg: Council of Europe Publishing, 2007.

Dumont LJ, Dzik WH, Rebulla P, Brandwein H, and the members of the BEST Working Party of the ISBT. Practical guidelines for process validation and process control of white cell-reduced blood components: re-port of the Biomedical Excellence for Safer Transfu-sion (BEST) Working Party of the International Society of Blood Transfusion (ISBT). *Transfusion* 1996;36:11–20.

Klein HG, Anderson D, Bernardi MJ et al. Pathogen in-activation: making decisions about new technologies – preliminary report of a consensus conference. *Vox Sang* 2007;93:179–182.

McClelland DBL. (ed). *Handbook of Transfusion Medicine*, 3rd edn. London: The Stationery Office, 2001.

Pamphilon DH. Viral inactivation of fresh frozen plasma. *Br J Haematol* 2000;109:680–693.

Pamphilon DH, Rider J, Barbara JAJ & Williamson LM. Prevention of transfusion-transmitted cytomegalovirus infection. *Transfus Med* 1999;9:115–123.

United Kingdom Blood Transfusion Services/National In-stitute for Biological Standards and Control. *Guide-lines for the Blood Transfusion Services in the United Kingdom*, 7th edn. London: The Stationery Office, 2005.

CHAPTER 22

Medicolegal aspects of transfusion practice

Patricia E. Hewitt
NHS Blood and Transplant, London, UK

Ethical principles

The International Society of Blood Transfusion (ISBT) some years ago instituted a code of ethics setting out the guiding principles for blood donation and transfusion. Following revision, this code of ethics has been adopted by the World Health Organization (WHO). It has also been used to support ethical standards in the drafting of the European Blood Directive. It is recommended that all blood transfusion provision is in accordance with the principles included in this code. The main provisions are listed below.

- There should be no coercion to donate blood.
- Both donors and recipients must be adequately informed.
- Confidentiality must be maintained.
- Adequate standards should be enforced.
- Clinical need must be the determinant of transfusion therapy.

Quality guidelines

Uniformity and process control can be achieved by compliance with detailed quality guidelines. The *Guidelines for the Blood Transfusion Services in the*

Practical Transfusion Medicine, 3rd edition. Edited by Michael F. Murphy and Derwood H. Pamphilon. © 2009 Blackwell Publishing, ISBN: 978-1-4051-8196-9.

United Kingdom and the *American Association of Blood Banks Technical Manual* are two examples of such documents. Although such guidelines do not possess legal status, they set out the requirements to be met for good manufacturing practice. Deliberate non-compliance would be regarded very seriously. Unavoidable non-compliance should be carefully documented and should include a clear explanation of the reasons for non-compliance.

Regulatory framework in the UK

The regulatory framework in the UK is briefly described. Similar arrangements will be in place in all developed countries.

Medicines Act 1968

The Medicines Act provides the framework for the regulation and control of all dealings with medicinal products. Prior to the Blood Safety and Quality Regulations (2005), both cellular and fractionated blood products were included within the terms of the Act. Fractionated products (e.g. albumin, coagulation factor concentrates and intravenous immunoglobulin preparations) are individually licenced. The provision of labile blood components (red cells, platelets, fresh frozen plasma) was enabled by means of an organisational licence awarded to individual blood centres by the Medicines and Healthcare Products Regulatory

Agency (MHRA) following appropriate inspection and demonstration of compliance with the standards of good manufacturing practice. Such inspections of 'blood establishments' are now covered under the Blood Safety and Quality Regulations.

Consumer Protection Act 1987

The Consumer Protection Act creates a strict liability action against manufacturers and suppliers when physical injury or property damage is caused by a defective product.

The Consumer Protection Act 1987 was enacted as a result of a European Community Directive in 1985 and clearly includes within its terms the provision of all blood and blood products. Its premise is the principle of product liability, that is that there is no need to prove that a negligent action has taken place, but merely that the end product is defective and has caused harm. In Section 3 (1) of the Act, a 'defect' is defined as follows: 'There is a defect in the product...if the safety of the product is not such as persons generally are entitled to expect...' Blood providers can be held liable under the terms of the Act as producers, suppliers or keepers. The liability therefore extends from the blood centre producing the product to the hospital blood transfusion laboratory which stores and issues products. There are possible defences within the terms of the Act, such as the 'state-of-the-art defence'. In essence this means that if a product is found to be defective based on current knowledge, that information cannot be used to prove that the same product was defective sometime previously when the current knowledge was not available (Table 22.1). This defence was not held to apply in the case of the hepatitis C litigation in England, since the defect (the transmission of hepatitis C) was apparent at the time of the claimants' transfusions (1988–91), although the means of detecting the defect (the availability of a hepatitis C test) was not necessarily available during the whole period.

NHS Act 1999

This Act modernised the NHS in England, Wales and Scotland. Raising standards in the quality of NHS care are at its heart. A statutory duty of quality is placed on all NHS providers, monitored by

Table 22.1 Relevant UK statutes.

Act	Terms
Medicines Act 1968	Regulates medicinal products
Consumer Protection Act 1987	Encompasses all aspects of provision of blood and blood products from donation to hospital blood bank
NHS Act 1999	Concentrates on clinical use of blood

Blood Safety and Quality Regulations 2005 regulates collection, testing, processing and storage of blood, traceability, reporting of adverse events and quality systems.

means of the Healthcare Commission. Additionally, the National Institute of Clinical Excellence (NICE) ensures that minimum standards of health care are developed throughout the UK. The spur to set up these statutory provisions had been inequality in care. All aspects of health care, including blood transfusion, will no doubt in time be scrutinised; the emphasis is likely to be on clinical aspects of transfusion therapy.

European Blood Safety Directives (2002/98)

The European Blood Safety Directive (2002/98) sets standards relating to blood collection, testing, processing and storage. A 'daughter' Directive (2004/33) lays out technical requirements in support of these standards. Together, the two directives were transposed into UK law as the Blood Safety and Quality Regulations 2005, which came into force on 8 February 2005. Two further 'daughter' Directives (2005/61 and 2005/62), which cover aspects of traceability, reporting of adverse reactions and events, and specifications for quality systems, came into force by separate amending legislation in 2006.

These new regulations impose safety and quality requirements on human blood collection, testing, processing and storage. The requirements apply to all 'blood establishments', which include the blood transfusion services in England, Scotland, Wales, and Northern Ireland. In addition, the collection and processing of blood components within hospital premises confers the status of 'blood establishment' upon the hospital, bringing such activities and premises under the control of the regulations. The regulations replace some of those (in relation to inspection, licencing and accreditation) previously covered under the Medicines Act. They lay down a requirement for inspection not less than every 2 years by the regulatory authority (MHRA). Failure to comply with the licencing regulations can lead to the imposition of a fine or closure of an organisation, and, in the worst cases, a fine or imprisonment for the designated 'responsible person' of the blood establishment.

Many of the provisions of the regulations, such as traceability, reporting of adverse events and specifications for quality systems, also apply to hospital blood transfusion laboratories. The regulations have had wide-reaching implications for both blood services and hospital blood transfusion laboratories.

Duty of care

Putting aside the ethical principles, quality guidelines and regulatory frameworks described above, there remains the clear duty of care which must be at the heart of the provision of blood transfusion. This duty must be according to an accepted standard. At present, the standard is determined according to the Bolam principle: 'The test is the standard of the ordinary skilled man exercising and professing to have that special skill.' This defines the standard as that of a responsible body of doctors skilled in the same specialty. The standard of care can be supported by the application of professional guidelines, although currently the latter have no legal standing. The duty of care of blood services, according to the defined standard, is both to the blood donor and to the recipient patient.

Duty to the donor

The two general principles that underpin blood donation are that there should be every effort to ensure no harm to the health of the donor and no risk to the health of the recipient patient. The duty to the donor includes compliance with strict medical selection procedures. The donor should be informed about the screening tests performed on the donation and should provide a written consent to testing. Information should be provided on situations that could potentially pose risk to the donor, for example the administration of growth factors prior to stem cell donation or the use of general anaesthetic during bone marrow donation. In these instances, a donor would need to consent formally to the procedure. The blood services in the UK make leaflets available at all routine blood donation sessions, to inform prospective blood donors of relevant issues. Additionally, the blood service has a duty to maintain the confidentiality of a donor, particularly in the event of a recipient patient being harmed by blood obtained from a single donor. The duty of care to the donor also extends to the clinician prescribing the blood, to ensure appropriate use, particularly as that donation is provided on a voluntary basis with no expectation of monetary gain.

Duty to the recipient patient

In the UK the standard of care for patients receiving blood transfusion is addressed under the legislation referred to above. It is suggested that, as a minimum, this standard of care should include the provision of adequate information to the recipient patient and ensuring appropriate clinical use of individual blood components.

Consent to transfusion

Any patient being asked to consent to a medical treatment or investigation has the right to be informed of the aims, benefits and risks of the treatment, and to be given details of any alternatives. Without such information, consent is not valid. The standard NHS 'Patient agreement to investigation or treatment' form includes a section completed by the health professional who has the discussion with the patient. This section documents that an explanation has been given to the patient about the proposed investigation or treatment, including the possibility of extra procedures which may be found necessary, and blood transfusion is specifically mentioned at this point. The patient signs a general consent to the procedure/investigation described, embracing the possibility of additional procedures, but has the opportunity to list any procedures for which he or she withholds consent without further discussion.

The patient must have the capacity to consent. No doctor should force a competent adult to accept any treatment even if that adult's decision appears to be irrational. An adult could be incapacitated and therefore unable to give consent because of loss of consciousness or mental retardation. In general, no other person can give consent on behalf of an incapacitated adult. (In some countries, e.g. Scotland, the power of *parens patriae* applies, where another adult can take responsibility as a parent for an incapacitated individual.) Prior wishes may be taken into consideration where the adult has previously been competent and the treatment is regarded as non-controversial. Treatment may be given to an adult incapable of consenting if the treatment is urgent and in the patient's best interests. In an elective situation, however, it would be best to seek a ruling from a court of law. The General Medical Council has published a comprehensive guide to consent and this is recommended for more detailed reading (Table 22.2).

In the case of children, the Family Law Reform Act 1969 makes it lawful for a minor to consent to, or refuse, treatment when he or she reaches the age of 16 years. In the case of a child below 16 years of age, the parents usually give consent, although such children are able to give valid consent in their own right if they are capable of understanding clearly the nature of the proposed treatment. Here, a difficulty could be where parents have specific religious beliefs that prevent them from consenting to blood transfusion for their child. In this instance, a doctor can decide to provide a treatment, including blood transfusion, in the child's

best interests. The treatment must be carried out in order to save life or to ensure improvement of or to prevent deterioration in the physical or mental health of the child. This would form the basis of a doctor's individual decision during an emergency situation, but in the case of a planned blood transfusion it would be appropriate to seek a ruling from a court of law. In these circumstances it is recommended that the doctor's medical defence body is consulted for advice on how to proceed.

For consent to be informed and valid, it must be based on adequate information. Attempts have been made to define what constitutes adequate information, and it is legally acceptable that the explanation need not include all the potential adverse consequences if the risk of them occurring is small or immaterial. Minor insignificant reactions to transfusion occur relatively commonly, whereas the risk of complications with serious or fatal long-term consequences, e.g. transmission of HIV, is extremely low. However, there is heightened public awareness of such low risk, and it is therefore appropriate for these events to be included in a preliminary explanation. Again, the standard that applies in the UK is that of a responsible body of skilled doctors, the Bolam principle. In the US, however, a different rule applies, the standard being judged according to that which a prudent patient would think relevant to receive, a situation which is likely to develop within the UK in the next few years.

There must be no coercion in obtaining consent. A competent adult is able to accept or refuse treatment even if that decision could lead to harm or indeed death. If an individual doctor decides to treat an adult without consent, then that doctor should be prepared to explain and justify the decision.

Jehovah's Witnesses

Jehovah's Witnesses, because of their religious beliefs, will never accept normal blood transfusion therapy, although in appropriate circumstances could find cell salvage in continuous circulation acceptable. Many Jehovah's Witnesses carry an Advance Medical Directive which states the

Table 22.2 Informed consent must include these elements.

Capacity to understand
Should be based on adequate information
Should be obtained without coercion

---

individual's views and requirements to be followed in the event that the individual is unconscious or otherwise unable to express his or her views. Where the situation is one relating to a competent adult, as long as it is clear that there is no coercion, the decision to refuse treatment must be respected, even if it would lead to harm or indeed death of the patient. In an emergency situation, if the patient is unconscious and therefore incapacitated, then prior previously held beliefs must be taken into account and blood transfusion should not be prescribed if those beliefs made it clear that it was unacceptable. In the situation of a child, where the parents' religious beliefs could prevent the child from being given a necessary blood transfusion, it would be advisable to seek a proper legal ruling, which would usually mean the child becoming a ward of court and therefore decisions on the treatment being taken by the court.

Patient recourse

Despite compliance with standards and appropriate care, things do, and will, go wrong. In some countries, for example New Zealand and the Scandinavian countries (Sweden, Norway, Finland and Denmark), compensation for medical accidents is provided under a 'no-fault' system. However, in most countries there is a need to prove liability. In these circumstances, liability will rest either with the individual doctor or with the health employer if vicarious liability applies (this is the current position in the UK for all NHS work). There have been examples of no-fault compensation awarded in the UK in specific circumstances, for example the Vaccine Damage Payment Scheme, which provides payment of a fixed lump sum where serious mental or physical damage has been caused by the administration of specified vaccines. A vCJD compensation scheme, administered by the vCJD Trust, was set up to provide payments for people infected with vCJD through exposure to bovine products, or otherwise through exposure to BSE or vCJD within the UK. This scheme therefore covers individuals believed to have been infected through UK blood transfusions. Specifically in relation to

blood transfusion, there are schemes (the MacFarlane Trust and the Eileen Trust) for recipients infected with HIV through the use of plasma products and through blood transfusion both before and after the introduction of mandatory screening of the blood supply in the UK. These were ex gratia payments to those affected, with the government emphasising that they should not be regarded as an admission of liability or as compensation, but as a response to a particular and tragic situation. Requests for similar treatment for individuals infected with other agents, such as hepatitis B and C, were, at first, refused. However, a scheme known as the Skipton Fund was subsequently set up for recipients who had been infected with hepatitis C through treatment with NHS blood products, although only those transfused prior to the introduction of testing of blood donations in September 1991 qualify for such payments. Similar treatment does not apply to recipients infected with other agents through blood transfusion, although such cases are small in number. It becomes difficult to explain the different treatments of patients who have suffered apparently similar unfortunate and unexpected adverse effects through treatment with blood transfusion.

A patient who has suffered harm can bring an action either in medical negligence or under product liability. If brought in negligence, there would be a need to prove a breach in the duty of care, and that the breach directly caused harm to the patient. If brought under product liability, negligence need not be present; a defective product must have directly caused the harm (Table 22.3).

An example of an action that could be brought under medical negligence would be that of the transfusion of a unit of red cells to the wrong recipient patient because of failure to check patient identification. Here, there would be a clear breach of the duty of care, that is in checking the patient identification against the red cell unit, and it would also be simple to demonstrate that harm, in the form of a haemolytic transfusion reaction, had occurred as a direct result of the breach. The recipient patient would be able to seek damages for the injury and compensation for any consequent financial loss. A further example would be where a blood

Table 22.3 Comparison of medical negligence versus product liability.

Medical negligence	Product liability
Duty of care	Defective product
Breach of the duty	Harm caused directly by the defect
Harm caused directly by the breach	

transfusion recipient acquired an infection from the blood transfusion, and where the blood transfusion only became necessary because of negligent treatment of the underlying medical condition.

Cases of product liability in relation to blood transfusion in Europe are few. The most notable case was that of a number of recipients (114) in England and Wales who brought a claim under the Consumer Protection Act in 2000–2001. In his judgement, Burton found that the Blood Service was liable for the damage because the product (i.e. the blood) did not provide the safety that the consumer (patient) was 'generally entitled to expect'. The claimants were awarded damages on a provisional basis according to the damage (extent of hepatitis C disease) present at the time of the action. Provisional damages allow for the claimants to return with a future claim should their medical condition deteriorate. This case has attracted much attention within Europe and will surely be used as a precedent in future claims. Other case law within Europe is scarce, although some European countries (e.g. France and the Scandinavian countries) provide for no-fault compensation in relation to infection acquired through medical treatment. The judgement in the hepatitis C litigation was not appealed. Similar claims in relation to transfusion-transmitted infection have been settled in the absence of any successful challenge to the ruling.

Key points

1 All those involved in the provision of blood and blood components must be aware of the relevant regulatory framework(s).

2 Those prescribing blood transfusion must be aware of consent issues.

3 Valid consent is based on having relevant information.

4 A competent adult can choose to refuse blood transfusion, despite the likely consequences, and that choice must be respected.

5 No-fault compensation/payment schemes apply for some transfusion complications in the UK, but not for all.

6 The Consumer Protection Act has opened the door for claims from blood transfusion recipients without the need to prove negligence.

Further reading

A and others v National Blood Authority [2002] 3 All ER 289.

American Association of Blood Banks. *Technical Manual*, 15th edn. Bethesda, MA: AABB, 2005.

Bolam v Friern Barnet Hospital Management Committee [1957] 2 All ER 118.

Braithwaite M & Beresford N. *Law for Doctors: Principles and Practicalities*. London: Royal Society of Medicine Press, 2002.

General Medical Council. *Seeking Patients' Consent: The Ethical Considerations*. London: GMC, 1999.

Gillick v West Norfolk and Wisbech Area Health Authority [1984] 3 All ER 402.

Goldberg R. Paying for bad blood. Strict product liability after the hepatitis C litigation. *Med Law Rev* 2002;10:165–200.

Grubb A & Pearl DA. *Blood Testing, Aids and DNA Profiling*. Bristol: Family Law (Jordan and Sons Ltd), 1990.

Guidelines for the Blood Transfusion Services in the United Kingdom, 7th edn. Norwich: The Stationery Office, 2005.

NHS Conferation. The coming year in Parliament for health. Briefing 1998; Issue 24.

The Consumer Protection Act 1987. In *Halsbury's Statute of England*. London: HMSO. F v West Berkshire Health Authority [1989] 2 All ER 545.

UK Blood Safety and Quality Regulations (BSQR). Available at www.opsi.gov.uk/si/si2005/20050050.htm. accessed is January 2009.

Warden J. HIV infected haemophiliacs: 90 million more. *Br Med J* 1989;299:1358.

Williams FG. Consent for transfusion. *Br Med J* 1997;315:380–381.

CHAPTER 23

Blood transfusion in hospitals

Sue Knowles[1] & Geoff Poole[2]
[1] Epsom and St Helier University Hospitals NHS Trust, Surrey, UK
[2] Welsh Blood Service, Bridgend, Wales

Transfusion medicine in a hospital setting is focussed on ensuring that a patient receives the correct blood component support which is clinically indicated, in a safe, timely and cost-efficient manner and that transfusion reactions are recognised and managed effectively. Specialists in all branches of medicine and surgery are involved in prescribing blood components and the transfusion process itself involves multiple steps and the cooperative action of several groups of staff.

In a modern health care setting, patients still die from lack of transfusion support. Massive haemorrhage continues to be the second most common direct cause of maternal death in the UK, resulting in 14 deaths between 2003 and 2005, and a fatality rate between 1 in 600 and 1 in 800 cases of obstetric bleeding. Some instances are due to the patient's refusal to accept blood component support or a failure to recognise the clinical signs of internal bleeding. However, others can be attributed to either a lack of knowledge of the local massive transfusion protocol or a failure of communication between the obstetric and haematology teams in implementing the protocol.

Patients are frequently overtransfused. Transfusion-associated circulatory overload (TACO) has been an overlooked complication of blood transfusion which can be difficult to distinguish from transfusion-associated acute lung injury (TRALI). In critically ill patients in an intensive care unit setting, it can occur following 1 in 350 units of blood components transfused. In the 2006 Serious Hazards of Transfusion (SHOT) report, there were two deaths and three cases of morbidity due to TACO as a direct result of errors made in the transfusion process.

Mistransfusion, i.e. giving the patient the incorrect unit of blood, resulting in an ABO-incompatible transfusion, is another frequent cause of mortality and morbidity resulting from blood transfusion. Mistransfusion is the result of human error that can occur at any step in the transfusion process, and is often due to failures to comply with clerical or technical procedures or the use of systems that are either poorly constructed or not understood. Multiple errors can be made in the transfusion process, some of which can be detected during an effective bedside check at the time of administering blood. It has been observed that as many as 1 in 19,000 red cells are given erroneously and 1 in 33,000 will involve ABO-incompatible units. Estimates of mortality due to mistransfusion range from 1 in 600,000 units to 1 in 1.8 million.

While there has been enormous progress made and resources given to reduce the risks of transfusion-transmitted infections, there is little evidence from serial annual haemovigilance reports that the safety of blood transfusion in a hospital setting is improving. Although there are numerous guidelines and directives available, and an

Practical Transfusion Medicine, 3rd edition. Edited by Michael F. Murphy and Derwood H. Pamphilon. © 2009 Blackwell Publishing, ISBN: 978-1-4051-8196-9.

Table 23.1 Errors in the transfusion process and some potential outcomes.

Problem	Outcome
Unnecessary prescriptions	Transfusion-associated circulatory overload
	Patient subjected to other unnecessary risks
	Wastage of blood components
Failure to prescribe specialist components	Risk of, for example transfusion-associated graft-versus-host disease
Failure to keep blood in a controlled environment	Wastage of blood components
Incorrect interval between sampling for pre-transfusion testing and transfusion	Potential for acute and delayed haemolytic transfusion reactions
Sample for pre-transfusion testing taken from incorrect patient. Transposition of samples or other errors in the laboratory. Incorrect unit of blood collected for and/or administered to the patient	Mistransfusion and potential for an ABO- or RhD-incompatible transfusion
Insensitive techniques in pre-transfusion testing	Potential for acute and delayed haemolytic transfusion reactions
Poor laboratory stock control	Wastage of units
	Inappropriate use of group O and national shortages of that group
Delays in provision of blood components in an emergency	Patient morbidity due to hypoxia or coagulopathy

understanding of measures which can be taken to improve transfusion safety, in practice an effective transfusion quality framework is required to minimise the risks of transfusion in a hospital setting and to ensure that the supply of donated blood is managed effectively (Table 23.1). This in turn requires committed leadership and adequate resources.

Key features of hospital transfusion governance

In the UK, the Blood Safety and Quality Regulations (BSQR) (SI 2005 50) require that blood establishments and hospital blood banks maintain quality systems based on good practice, and this is interpreted by the Notified Body (regulator), the Medicines and Healthcare products Regulatory Agency (MHRA), as meaning good manufacturing practice (GMP). The BSQR require that:
• laboratory staff are appropriately qualified and trained;
• validated processes are used;
• documentation on operational procedures, guidelines, manuals and reporting forms is maintained;

• full traceability of blood and blood components is maintained for 30 years;
• the regulator is informed of all serious adverse events and reactions via the Serious Adverse Blood Reactions and Events (SABRE) reporting tool; and
• specific requirements for the storage, transport and distribution of blood are met.

However, this regulation does not extend to practice in clinical areas, and other measures are needed to ensure that all processes, systems and policies that influence the quality and governance of transfusion practice are optimised and working as expected (Figure 23.1). Recommendations for practice are derived from the literature, including lessons learnt from haemovigilance and external quality assessment (EQA) schemes. These are translated into professional guidelines, or action plans and standards required by government agencies, who in turn assess compliance. Professional bodies promote best practice through training, education and communication, and all groups of staff should have regular appraisals, which where appropriate should include the satisfactory completion of recognised continuous professional development.

In England, the Healthcare Commission is responsible for promoting improvements in the

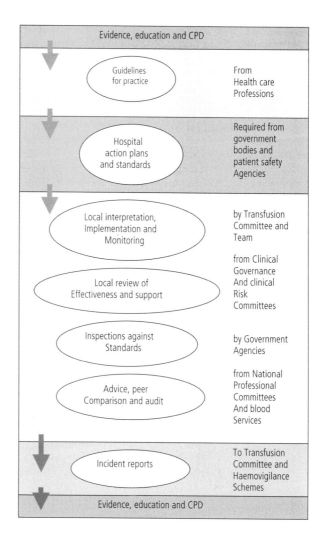

Figure 23.1 Schematic showing key elements of a transfusion governance framework.

quality of health care. Many of the core standards for governance and risk assessment are applicable to blood transfusion, including those requiring hospitals:

• to identify and learn from all patient safety incidents and other reportable incidents and make improvements in practice;

• to ensure that patient safety notices, alerts and other communications concerning patient safety, which require action, are acted upon within required timescales;

• to require that professionally qualified staff continuously update skills and techniques relevant to their clinical work; and

• to require that professionally qualified staff participate in regular clinical audits and reviews of clinical services.

Specifically, the National Patient Safety Agency in England in 2006 issued a safety notice requiring competency-based training and assessment for all staff involved in blood transfusion, a bedside identity check for administering blood that matches the blood pack with the patient wristband (excluding compatibility form or case notes) and a formal risk assessment of the alternative means of confirming patient identity

The National Health Service Litigation Authority also inspects acute English hospitals against risk management standards, which include blood transfusion. Hospitals are expected to have a transfusion policy and to provide evidence of implementation and of processes to monitor its effectiveness.

Hospital transfusion committee

The Hospital transfusion committee (HTC) is the focal point for overseeing transfusion practice. In the US, an HTC has been a requirement since 1972 for hospital accreditation by the Joint Commission on Accreditation of Healthcare Organizations. English NHS health circulars on *Better Blood Transfusion* first appeared in December 1998, with subsequent updates in 2002 and 2007, and these describe the functions and organisation of HTCs. To be effective, the HTC requires a dedicated hospital transfusion team (HTT) consisting of a lead consultant for transfusion, transfusion practitioner(s) and blood bank manager, and adequate resources, including IT and clerical support to facilitate data retrieval and audit. The HTT will have responsibility for implementing the objectives of the HTC. Given the importance of the HTC with respect to clinical governance, it has to be incorporated into the hospital frameworks for clinical governance, performance and risk management. The HTC has the remit to promote best practice, review clinical transfusion practice, monitor the performance of the hospital transfusion service, participate in regional or National initiatives and communicate with local patient representative groups as appropriate. The following list illustrates some of the specific functions of the HTC:

• To ensure that local policies and procedures are in place, based on national guidelines and regulations, and updated as required. These should include the following:

　a the administration of blood and blood components and the monitoring of the transfused patient, including the collection of samples for compatibility testing and the management of acute adverse reactions;

　b a maximum surgical blood ordering schedule (MSBOS);

　c the appropriate and safe use of blood components and blood products;

　d indications for specialist blood components (gamma-irradiated, CMV seronegative and phenotyped);

　e management of massive transfusion;

　f the application of blood conservation measures including the use of cell salvage and pharmacological agents;

　g the management of Jehovah's Witness and other patients refusing blood support.

• To agree to a strategy for the education and training and competency assessment of all staff involved in blood transfusion and to monitor compliance.

• To agree an annual local audit plan, to review the results of these and national audits and to provide feedback to relevant staff.

• To organise continuing education in transfusion medicine for all members of the hospital staff involved in prescribing or administering blood.

• To ensure that investigations and, as appropriate, root cause and trend analyses are conducted of 'near misses' and adverse events or reactions, which in turn will focus the need for further education or amendments to existing procedures.

• To ensure that transfusion incidents; adverse events and reactions are reported to the relevant national haemovigilance schemes.

• To review performance regularly, e.g. incidents, proportion of staff competency-assessed, wastage rates, inappropriate blood component usage and utilisation of blood components by directorate, user or surgical procedure.

• To review the operational effectiveness of the service, e.g. response times for emergency requests, elective work undertaken on call, crossmatch to transfusion ratios for individual surgical procedures and users.

• To develop and formalise contingency and emergency planning.

• To review quality assurance measures including performance in external quality assessment schemes and the outcome of accreditation inspections and other external audits.

• To review the adequacy and timely provision of blood and blood components from the blood establishment.

• To review the adequacy of diagnostic reference services and consultant advisory services.

• To ensure that patients undergoing transfusion are provided with access to information in relation to the risks and benefits of transfusion, and to blood avoidance strategies.

• To ensure that an audit trail of documentation exists to trace the ultimate fate of all blood components received.

Composition

A chairperson should be appointed by the hospital chief executive and should have a good understanding and experience of transfusion medicine practice. Ideally, the chairperson should not be the consultant responsible for the hospital transfusion laboratory, who could be perceived to have a vested interest.

The following membership is suggested:

• representatives of major speciality users of blood in all directorates;

• lead consultant haematologist for blood transfusion;

• hospital blood bank manager;

• specialist practitioner(s) of transfusion;

• senior nursing officer;

• representative from clinical risk management;

• representative of junior medical staff;

• representative of hospital management;

• local blood centre consultant (ex officio); and

• other representatives may be co-opted as required, e.g. from medical records, portering staff, clinical audit, training or pharmacy.

Administration of blood and blood components and the management of the transfused patient

This process involves several steps:

• counselling the patient of the need for a blood transfusion, when alternative approaches (salvaged blood, iron and/or RhEpo) are insufficient or inappropriate for their circumstances;

• the prescription of blood and blood components;

• requests for blood and blood components;

• sampling for pre-transfusion compatibility testing;

• collection and delivery of blood and blood components from transfusion issue refrigerator to clinical care area;

• administration of blood and blood components; and

• monitoring of transfused patients.

Errors occurring at blood sampling, collection and administration can lead to patient misidentification and an ABO-incompatible transfusion (Chapter 7). Successive haemovigilance reports confirm that the majority of these errors occur in clinical areas. Prescription errors, however, lead either to a failure to provide specialist components or to an inappropriate blood transfusion and the potential for TACO. The latter has occurred when transfusions have been given on the basis of spuriously low haemoglobins either taken from drip arms or measured by gas analysers, or when there has been an error in prescribing the volume of blood component to be transfused or the rate of transfusion. A failure to monitor the transfused patient, particularly in the first 15 minutes of receiving each unit, can lead to a life-threatening reaction being overlooked and delays in resuscitation.

The hospital should have written procedures to cover all these steps, to which the relevant staff are trained and assessed. The responsibilities, actions, documents and potential errors are provided in Tables 23.2–23.7. The prescription chart, the donation numbers of components transfused and the nursing observations related to the transfusion should be kept in the patient's medical case notes as a permanent record. Since the BSQR require a complete audit trail of blood to the patient's bedside, many hospitals complete this by returning a signed and dated compatibility form or compatibility label to the transfusion laboratory.

Technologies to reduce patient misidentification errors in administering blood

Additional manual systems of patient identification

Sets of red labels with the same unique number can be allocated to a transfusion episode. A label can be incorporated into an additional patient wristband

Table 23.2 Prescription of blood and blood components.

Responsibility	Action	Document	Potential errors
Medical officer	Ensure patient is aware of the need for a blood transfusion and has read and understood information related to the risks and benefits of transfusion	Patient information leaflet Hospital consent form	Failure to take account of patients' religious beliefs or other views
	Prescribe component, any specialist requirements, quantity, and duration of transfusion		Prescription chart. Unnecessary prescription, in the failure to follow hospital guidelines or as a result of an error in baseline blood count or coagulation screen. Lack of awareness of or failure to prescribe specialist components
	Document rationale for transfusion	Patient case notes	

Related hospital procedures and documents
Guidelines for the use of blood and blood components, including specialist components
Practice guidelines/procedures for individual diseases/treatments

at the time of phlebotomy, affixed to the request form, sample tube and into the current medical notes, and the unique number can also be printed onto the compatibility labels and compatibility report form. At the time of administration, the additional unique number provides a supplementary means of cross-checking.

Bar-coded patient administration systems

The use of hand-held computers and portable bar code label and wristband printers provide the means for improving patient identity and patient safety. For example, at the stage of sample collection, the phlebotomist's and patient's identity can be scanned and a bar-coded label generated at the bedside to attach to the tube. In the laboratory, the allocated unit is labelled to incorporate the patient's unique identification bar code and the unit number. At the time of administration, the member of staff is prompted by the hand-held computer to scan their own identification bar code, the

bar-coded patient wristband, the compatibility label and the unit number. The computer confirms whether the unit is correct for the patient and also provides prompts to check for special requirements, pre-transfusion observations and the expiry date of the pack.

Influencing clinical practice

There are several potential factors that influence transfusion medicine practice and decision-making:
- physician knowledge;
- physician perception based on clinical experience;
- peer pressure and feedback;
- effectiveness of the hospital governance framework;
- educational prompts at the time of the decision;
- financial pressures or incentives; and

Table 23.3 Requests for blood and blood components.

Responsibility	Action	Documentation	Potential errors
Doctor or registered nurse	State full patient identification, location, diagnosis, details of type and quantity of component and time required. State previous obstetric and transfusion history when requesting red cells	Written/electronic request form or laboratory telephone log in an emergency	Incomplete or incorrect patient information leading to failure to recognise historical laboratory record, recording requirement for specialist components or phenotyped units
			Failure to request specialist components
			Failure to comply with hospital MSBOS
Hospital blood transfusion laboratory staff	Review historical record and whether a further sample for pre-transfusion testing required	Previous laboratory record	Patient identification error in transcribing telephone request
			Failure to locate/heed information contained in historical record
			Failure to request a new sample in a recently transfused patient and potential for overlooking newly developed red cell antibodies

Related hospital procedures and documents
Timing of pre-transfusion sampling with respect to previous transfusion
Maximum surgical blood ordering schedules (MSBOS)

• public and political perceptions and the fear of litigation.

Improving transfusion medicine practice within a hospital community requires a planned consistent approach which is endorsed and implemented through clinical governance.

Guidelines, algorithms and protocols

Guidelines are defined as systematically developed statements to assist practitioner and patient decisions about appropriate health care for specific clinical circumstances. Controlled data are unavailable to assess the impact of professional guidelines, but most would agree that nationally derived documents rarely lead to change unless there is a local implementation and dissemination strategy, which requires time and resources.

Developing a local strategy to implement the guidelines is a useful opportunity to gain ownership, in that it can provide educational opportunities in examining the evidence basis, and identify dissension and other local barriers to its implementation, e.g. staff resources, laboratory turnaround times.

Local groups should adopt the recommendations of pre-existing guidelines but customise them for local use. This may involve separating a guideline into several sections or incorporating some of its recommendations into other local protocols for specific conditions, e.g. a fresh frozen plasma guideline incorporated into the protocol for the management of disseminated intravascular coagulation, massive haemorrhage and obstetric haemorrhage.

Table 23.4 Sampling for pre-transfusion compatibility testing.

Responsibility	Action	Documentation	Potential errors
Medical, nursing or phlebotomy staff, authorised and trained	Direct questioning of patient to provide surname, first name and date of birth when judged capable. Check that details given match those on patient wristband and on request form		Patient misidentification as a result of failing to positively identify patient or as a result of wristband missing or with incomplete information
	Take blood sample and immediately label at bedside with the required patient information	Sample labelled and signed	Patient misidentification as a result of: • Pre-labelled sample tube with another patient's ID • Labelled away from the bedside with another patient's ID • Addressograph label affixed from incorrect patient
Hospital blood transfusion laboratory staff	To determine that sample labelling meets requirements for pre-transfusion testing. If unacceptable, to inform requester of the need for another sample	If unacceptable, to document reasons and log accepted	Potential to issue inappropriate unit if inadequately labelled samples Failure to provide blood in a timely manner if clinicians unaware of the need for another sample

Related hospital procedures and documents
Hospital sample labelling policy
Hospital policy for allocation and maintenance of unique patient identifiers and for resiting wristbands in theatre or intensive care

Table 23.5 Collection and delivery of blood and blood components from transfusion issue refrigerator to clinical care area.

Responsibility	Action	Documentation	Potential errors
Staff authorised and trained	Take documentation bearing patient identification to the issue refrigerator Check that unit removed and accompanying blood transfusion compatibility form bear the identical patient identification details	Prescription chart or a completed collection slip	Incorrect unit collected if no documentation bearing patient ID Incorrect unit removed
	Record time and sign that correct unit has been collected		Lack of audit trail from failure to sign out unit from issue refrigerator

Related hospital procedures and documents
Hospital blood collection policy

Table 23.6 Administration of blood and blood components.

Responsibility	Action	Documentation	Potential errors
Doctor or registered nurse	At the bedside, direct questioning of patient to provide surname, first name and date of birth when judged capable. Check that this identity is identical with documents	Prescription chart	Unit transfused to wrong patient if unit checked away from bedside or no verification of patient identity
		Compatibility form (if used) Compatibility label Patient's wristband	
	Check that blood group is compatible	Compatibility form (if used)	Incorrect ABO/D group transfused if failure to detect laboratory grouping or labelling error
		Compatibility label Base label on blood pack	
	Check that special requirements are fulfilled	Prescription chart	Inappropriate component transfused if failure to note laboratory issuing error
		Blood pack	
	Check that unit of blood has of not passed its expiry date, and it is intact with no evidence visual discolouration		Failure to note transfusion of time-expired component
			Failure to note unit potentially contaminated with bacteria
	Document date and time of commencement of unit and sign	Compatibility form and/or prescription chart	
	Retain donation number in patient record	Label/sticker on prescription chart or in main body of case record	Failure to complete audit trail

Related hospital procedures and documents
Hospital blood administration policy

Experience in other medical fields has also demonstrated that embedding the recommendations of a guideline into documents in use at the time of the clinical consultation/decision can significantly improve compliance. Examples of this approach could include:
• listing the indications for specialist blood components on the blood transfusion request forms or electronic request screens;
• listing the nursing actions to be taken in the event of a transfusion reaction on a specific transfusion observation chart; and

• detailing the checks to be made on the compatibility form prior to administering blood.

Intraoperative algorithms for the use of platelet concentrates and fresh frozen plasma to correct microvascular bleeding during and after cardiac bypass surgery have also proved to be successful in reducing inappropriate use of these components, when combined with near-patient testing and the rapid availability of results to feed into the decision tree.

The local documents should be incorporated into the transfusion policy and disseminated alongside

Table 23.7 Monitoring of transfused patients.

Responsibility	Action	Documentation	Potential errors
Staff authorised and trained	Measure temperature, pulse and blood pressure before the start of each unit	Observation chart, recording date and time	In absence baseline observations, cannot detect any change giving a warning of a transfusion reaction
	Explain to the patient possible adverse effects to be reported and keep patient under close visual observation in first 15–20 min of each unit		Patient not aware of symptoms to be reported that can provide first warning of a transfusion reaction
	Measure temperature and pulse 15 min after start of each unit	Observation chart, recording time	In absence early observation, potential to miss a serious transfusion reaction
	Measure temperature, pulse and blood pressure at the end of each unit	Observation chart, recording time	In absence of timed final observation, cannot know whether any subsequent changes in patient's condition are temporarily related to an ongoing transfusion

Related hospital procedures and documents
Hospital policy on monitoring transfused patients
Management of transfusion reactions

training events for all involved staff. A list of relevant guidelines is included at the end of this chapter.

Audit

The audit cycle consists of defining the area to be studied and comparing observed practice with a standard (Figure 23.2). Analysis of the findings should lead to recommendations for improved practice, which may include a revision of the content and clarity of the standard.

The audit process has been criticised since it has been said to consume considerable resources and result, at best, in only a transient change in clinical behaviour. However, audits frequently fail because the cycle is not completed, i.e. when the results and educational messages are not disseminated and discussed by those whose practice could be improved, when no analysis is undertaken of the corrective actions which should be introduced to improve practice, and no resources are provided to implement the actions identified.

Audits can also be made more effective when they are conducted repeatedly or on an ongoing basis.

Audits can be conducted retrospectively or prospectively. If adopting a prospective approach in monitoring the appropriateness of the requests for blood components, this can be considered to be intrusive and potentially delay the delivery of patient care, but does prevent unnecessary transfusion. Immediate retrospective audit of component utilisation does not prevent unnecessary transfusion but, if conducted in a timely and individual fashion, can provide effective educational feedback and a sustained change to a physician's prescribing habit. Ongoing computerised prospective or retrospective auditing, using agreed algorithms, is the only realistic way of monitoring and providing individual clinician feedback on the inappropriate use of blood components.

Regular audit cycles have been shown to improve compliance with the bedside procedures for administering blood. Regular audits of an MSBOS

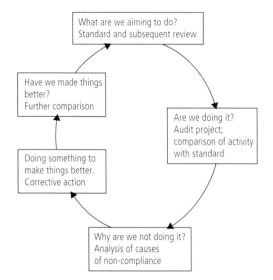

Figure 23.2 The audit cycle.

are essential if the schedule is to be kept in line with changing practice.

Audits that involve several health care organisations are particularly effective since peer pressure is applied in comparing practice. Participating hospitals' results can be made anonymous for all other participants. The National Blood Service in England has organised audits of compliance with the *Better Blood Transfusion* Health Service Circulars, the blood administration process, the use of blood components and overnight red cell transfusions. In future, the Healthcare Commission will be notified of hospital participation.

Surveys

Many activities which fall under an 'audit' banner are not comparing practice with a standard but are monitoring or surveying practice. These activities, many of which can be quantified, often lead to the development of quality indicators or performance indicators. Trend analysis, or comparison of one organisation with another or one blood user with another, is a powerful means of exerting peer pressure and influencing practice (benchmarking).

Performance indicators or benchmarking can be applied, for example, to:

• percentage of patient wristband errors;

• percentage of mislabelled samples;

• hospital blood wastage;

• percentage of group O usage;

• number of units crossmatched to number of units transfused (C:T) ratio;

• red cells used per surgical procedure (for each surgical team);

• percentage of primary arthroplasties requiring allogeneic transfusion;

• percentage of patients receiving platelets after coronary artery bypass grafting; and

• percentage of patients with refractory anaemia having received a trial of treatment with RhEpo.

National schemes

A number of national schemes in the UK set out to monitor or assure transfusion practice. Such schemes can be used to influence policy and educate users within hospitals. They are generally made anonymous to encourage full participation. National schemes include the following (but note that the devolved NHS administrations in Northern Ireland, Scotland and Wales may have additional or alternative schemes):

• The SHOT haemovigilance scheme was launched in November 1996. It is a voluntary system for collecting data on serious adverse events and near misses in the transfusion of blood and blood components. It produces an annual report of its findings and recommendations.

• EQA schemes, for example the National External Quality Assessment scheme in blood transfusion laboratory practice, provide 'clinical' material to laboratories on a regular basis. Laboratory results are returned to the scheme organisers for analysis and collated reports are disseminated to users.

• The Blood Stocks Management Scheme collates and publishes through its website details of blood stock inventory and wastage and allows participants to compare their practice with that of comparably sized hospitals.

Public and political perceptions and fear of litigation

The knowledge that human immunodeficiency virus (HIV) could be transmitted by blood transfusion in 1982 led to a decline in the use of allogeneic red cells in the US, from 12.2 million units in 1986 to 11.4 million units in 1997. This decline is even more significant if the growth and ageing of the population in the US during this period are taken into account. Over the same period, autologous donations increased by a factor of more than 30. Individual physicians were sued in the US if their patient contracted HIV through the blood supply and their transfusion was not clinically indicated.

Concern about variant Creutzfeldt–Jakob disease (vCJD) being transmissible through blood led in 1998 to the Department of Health in the UK requiring that all hospitals should have HTCs, implement good transfusion practice and that they should have explored the feasibility of cell salvage. Universal leucocyte depletion of blood, when introduced in the UK in 1999 as a preventive measure for vCJD, led to a significant increase in the price of red cells, and encouraged a more judicious approach to transfusion and the use of transfusion alternatives. As a consequence, total red cell usage in the UK reached a plateau between 2000 and 2001 and has subsequently fallen by up to about 5% per year, despite the increase in surgical procedures performed over this period.

Local investigation and feedback following 'near misses' and serious adverse events

The UK SHOT scheme defines a 'near miss' as any error which, if undetected, could result in the determination of a wrong blood group, or the issue, collection or administration of an incorrect, inappropriate or unsuitable component but which was recognised before transfusion took place. 'Serious adverse events' must also be reported to the MHRA in the UK – these are any untoward occurrences associated with the collection, testing, processing, storage and distribution of blood or blood components that might lead to death or life-threatening, disabling or incapacitating conditions for patients or which results in, or prolongs, hospitalisation or morbidity. Systematic root cause analysis of these incidents provides the opportunity to understand the weaknesses in systems and processes. Corrective action can then be taken to minimise the occurrence of a critical incident. Identified weaknesses include staff misconceptions or ignorance, defective or risky protocols or processes.

Sample errors, most importantly those where the tube is labelled with the intended patient's details but is subsequently found to contain blood from another patient, are the most common detectable errors in the SHOT 'near miss' scheme. These inevitably arise as a result of a failure to systematically and positively identify the patient at the bedside. Corrective action should involve counselling and educating the individual concerned who failed to comply with the correct procedure. However, any investigation will also uncover compounding latent factors contributing to the event, which need to be collectively understood and addressed, for example:
• the practice of not positively identifying patients, since health care workers perceive this as denoting an inadequate knowledge of the patients under their care;
• reduced junior doctors' hours and shift patterns of all those involved in direct patient management, leading to unfamiliarity with patients; and
• patient 'hot bedding' in the UK, which frequently leads to pre-operative patients having to be sampled for pre-transfusion testing before case notes are made available on the wards or wristbands are applied.

Sadly, exposure to avoidable patient morbidity or fatality is often the trigger for affecting the local medical and nursing community's perception of the risks of blood transfusion and for instigating a change in procedures.

Education and continuing professional development

Education of all individuals in the transfusion process has been difficult to achieve in the UK until it was made an integral part of a hospital-documented mandatory training programme and subject to external inspection. However, it requires a considerable dedicated resource and a flexible and pragmatic approach to accommodate shift patterns, staff shortages and agency staff. Observational competency assessment is more readily achieved with the help of 'champions' in every clinical area and knowledge-based assessments can be facilitated by web-based training programmes.

Education is an essential component of every strategy to gain clinician compliance with clinical procedures and guidelines and to modify practice as a result of audit, surveys or investigations into errors. Educational interventions have been found to be more successful when they are interactive, focussed on a specific objective and directed at groups of individuals with reflections on their own practice.

Continuing professional development schemes exist for the various professional groups involved in health care. The schemes vary but all are intended to encourage knowledge acquisition. In a typical scheme, such as the one introduced by the British Blood Transfusion Society in April 2001, members keep a portfolio in which accredited activity in educational, professional and vocational areas is recorded.

Maximum surgical blood ordering schedule

This is a table of elective surgical procedures that lists the number of units of blood routinely crossmatched for each. The number of units allocated takes into account the likelihood of the need for transfusion and the response time for receiving blood following an immediate spin crossmatch or electronic issue. An MSBOS reduces the workload of unnecessary crossmatching and issuing of blood, and can improve stock management and wastage.

The successful implementation of an MSBOS depends on all parties agreeing to the tariff, the education of junior staff, the confidence of senior staff that there is a robust system for accessing blood promptly when there is unexpected blood loss and the ability to override the tariff when there are reasons to indicate that greater blood loss will occur. A tariff is constructed by:
- analysing each surgical procedure in terms of the C:T ratio;
- managing procedures with a C:T ratio greater than 2, i.e. a low probability of transfusion, with

Table 23.8 Maximum surgical blood order schedule (general surgery).

Operation	Units crossmatched or group and screen (G & S)
Adrenalectomy	3
Colectomy	2
Cholecystectomy	G & S
Gastrostomy, ileostomy, colostomy	G & S
Gastrectomy (partial)	G & S
Liver biopsy	G & S
Mastectomy	G & S
Oesophagectomy	4
Pancreatectomy	4
Parathyroidectomy	G & S
Partial hepatectomy	6
Splenectomy	2
Thyroidectomy	G & S
Vagotomy	G & S
Bile duct stricture repair	3

a group and screen, and issuing blood only when there is a need for transfusion; and
- allocating an agreed number of units for procedures with a C:T ratio of less than 2.

In recipients with red cell alloantibodies, consideration should be given to the time taken to acquire and crossmatch antigen-negative units. An overall C:T ratio of 1.5 for elective surgery is achievable when the laboratory is centrally issuing blood. However, lower ratios would be possible with remote electronic issue in theatre suites. An example of an MSBOS is provided in Table 23.8.

Pre-transfusion compatibility testing

This testing comprises:
- determination of the ABO and D group of the recipient;
- a screen for red cell alloantibodies reactive at 37°C in the plasma of the recipient;
- a check for previous records or duplicate records, and comparison of current with historical findings (these elements comprise a group and screen);

- identification of the specificity of any alloantibody detected in the antibody screen;
- selection of blood of an appropriate blood group or extended phenotype;
- a serological or electronic crossmatch; and
- labelling of the blood with the recipient's identifying information.

Detection of red cell antigen–antibody reactions

The phenotyping ('blood grouping') of red cells and the detection of red cell alloantibodies depend on interpretations of serological interactions between red cell antigens and antibodies. Various serological methods and test systems are available to demonstrate these interactions, and these must be optimised in order to obtain the appropriate sensitivity and specificity for their intended clinical use. Failure to follow the instructions provided by reagent manufacturers can lead to incorrect conclusions.

Test methods have been developed to allow the detection of antibodies of different isotypes. Antibodies that have specificities for red cell antigens are usually IgG or IgM. IgM antibodies are pentameric molecules that can cross-link between antigens on adjacent cells, thus causing direct agglutination of red cells. Conversely, IgG antibodies are monomeric, and although they are divalent, the distance between the Fab regions on a single IgG molecule is in general insufficient to allow direct agglutination to take place, as there are stronger intercellular repulsive forces between red cells at these distances. Methods such as the indirect antiglobulin test (IAT) (which uses a secondary antibody; see Figure 23.3) or the enzyme method (which uses proteolytic enzymes such as papain to cleave negatively charged, hydrophilic residues from the red cell membrane) must therefore be used to detect most IgG red cell antibodies.

Test systems for the detection of serological reactions can be classified into three broad categories.

Liquid-phase systems

Liquid-phase systems rely on the visualisation of haemagglutination reactions in individual glass/plastic tubes or 96-well microplates. The pres-

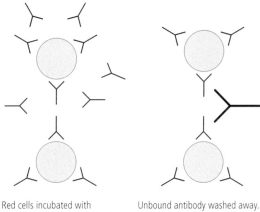

Red cells incubated with serum containing IgG antibody

Unbound antibody washed away. Anti-human globulin added to precipitate cells

Figure 23.3 Indirect antiglobulin test.

ence or absence of agglutinated red cells distinguishes positive and negative reactions, allowing the grading of reaction avidity according to the strength of haemagglutination. These liquid-phase systems are more commonly used for blood grouping than for antibody screening, as IgM blood-grouping reagents can be used in simple, rapid and direct agglutination methods. IAT methods using red cells suspended in a low-ionic-strength solution remain the gold standard for the detection of clinically significant red cell alloantibodies, although these methods require meticulous attention to procedure, in particular during the washing phase to remove unbound IgG.

Column-agglutination systems

The introduction of column-agglutination systems during the last decade has resulted in a very significant change to routine laboratory practice in the UK. One of these systems, first described by Lapierre in 1990, uses a plastic card containing six channels, each of which contains a mixture of Sephadex and Sephacryl gels. This gel mixture is formulated to allow the passage of unagglutinated cells but not of agglutinated red cells. Positive reactions are therefore distinguished by agglutinates at or near the top of the gel column and negative reactions appear as buttons of red cells at the bottom (Figure 23.4). A similar column-agglutination

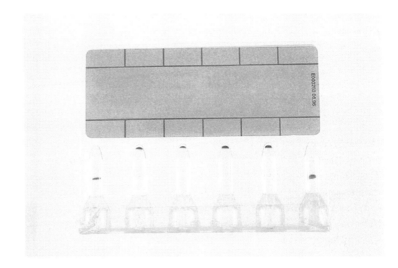

Figure 23.4 Column-agglutination technology. Positive results are seen in the first and last columns.

method involving a glass microbead density barrier in place of a gel is also available.

Reagent (IgM) antibody can be incorporated into the gel or bead columns, allowing phenotyping to be undertaken simply by the addition of test cells to the top of the column. Similarly, the IAT can be performed in columns containing antiglobulin reagent to which plasma and reagent red cells are added. Because plasma proteins are less dense than the gel, a washing phase is not needed. This property and the relative stability of the reaction end point give column agglutination methods a degree of simplicity and reliability not achieved by other methods.

Solid-phase systems

These systems are based on 96-well microplates and provide another alternative to the tube or column IAT. Although differing in detail, all these methods achieve a positive reaction end point that is characterised by a monolayer of red cells across the surface of the microplate well. A discrete button of red cells at the bottom of the well indicates a negative reaction (Figure 23.5). Solid-phase systems suffer from the disadvantage that they require carefully standardised centrifugation and washing steps; however, unlike the situation with liquid-phase test systems, fully automated equipment allows these steps to be performed safely and consistently without operator intervention.

Reduction of error in pre-transfusion compatibility testing

An analysis of cases in the UK during 1996–2006 where blood components had been mistransfused showed that laboratory errors were implicated in up to 34% of incidents. Many of these laboratory errors were due to the transposition of samples or to simple human error in the setting up or interpretation of tests. Provided that the correct laboratory identifier (as a bar code) is placed on the patient's sample, these errors can be avoided by using a fully automated system that is interfaced to the blood transfusion laboratory computer. The basic features of a fully automated ('walk away') system should include:

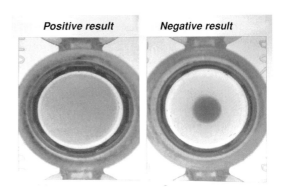

Figure 23.5 Solid-phase technology.

- trays or carousels to stack samples;
- automated liquid handling and other robotic operations;
- devices to ensure that positive sample identification is maintained;
- clot sensor and liquid level alarms;
- an optical device to record reaction patterns; and
- a comprehensive system management software that interprets reaction patterns and flags discrepant results.

Automated systems can utilise solid-phase microplate or column-agglutination technology.

Where full automation is not available or cannot be used for the whole process (as is currently the case with antibody identification), steps must be taken to minimise the occurrence of error or minimise its impact. A high standard of training and participation in internal and external quality assessment schemes, and strict adherence to validated documented procedures are among the measures that reduce the occurrence of human error. The most critically important procedure in the blood transfusion laboratory, the determination of the ABO group, should be performed by two people (except in urgent situations) if there is no record of a grouping result from a previous sample. Similarly, the determination of a D group should be performed in duplicate, in the absence of full automation.

ABO and D grouping
- The patient's red cells should be tested against monoclonal anti-A and anti-B grouping reagents.
- The patient's serum/plasma should be tested against A_1 and B reagent red cells, except in neonates.
- The expected reaction patterns in ABO grouping are illustrated in Table 23.9.

- The patient's red cells should be tested with an IgM monoclonal anti-D reagent, which does not detect the 'partial D' group, DVI.
- ABO and D groups must be repeated when a discrepancy (anomaly) is found. Repeats should be performed using a fresh suspension of washed cells. An autocontrol should be included.

Antibody screening
- The IAT performed at 37°C is the best method available for the detection of red cell antibodies of clinical importance. It is simple (especially when using a column-agglutination system), has an appropriate level of sensitivity and has a high degree of specificity.
- The patient's serum/plasma should be tested against two or more 'screening cells' using the IAT.
- The reagent red cells used for screening should between them express antigens reactive with all clinically significant antibodies; ideally the phenotypes R_1R_1 or $R_1{}^wR_1$ and R_2R_2 should be represented in the screening cell set. It is recommended that the following phenotypes should also be represented: Jk(a+b−), Jk(a−b+), S+s−, S−s+, Fy(a+b−), Fy(a−b+).
- Antibody screening is the most reliable and sensitive method of detecting a clinically significant antibody, since stronger reactions may be obtained with cells having homozygous expression of the antigen and the red cells are preserved in a medium to minimise loss of antigens during the storage period.
- Antibody screening performed in advance of the requirement for transfusion also provides the laboratory with time to identify the specificity of the antibody and, when clinically significant, to select antigen-negative units for crossmatching.

Group	Anti-A	Anti-B	A_1 cells	B cells	O cells
A	+++	−	−	+++	−
B	−	+++	+++	−	−
O	−	−	+++	+++	−
AB	+++	+++	−	−	−

Table 23.9 ABO grouping patterns.

Antibody identification

- When an antibody has been detected in the screening test, the specificity should be determined by testing the patient's serum/plasma against a panel of reagent red cells of known phenotypes.
- In addition to the IAT, other methods (e.g. using enzyme-treated red cells) may be helpful, particularly when a mixture of antibodies is present.
- The specificity of the antibody can be determined when the serum/plasma is reactive with at least two examples of red cells bearing the antigen, and non-reactive with at least two examples of red cells lacking the antigen.
- When one antibody specificity has been determined, it is essential that additional clinically significant antibodies are not overlooked. Multiple antibodies can be confirmed only by choosing red cells that are antigen negative for the recognised specificity but positive for other antigens to which clinically significant antibodies may arise.

Autoantibodies

These may be suspected when the patient's serum/plasma reacts with all cells used in the reverse ABO group or with all cells in the antibody identification panel including the patient's own red cells. Not all autoantibodies give rise to haemolysis.

Serological investigations should focus on obtaining the correct ABO and RhD group of the patient and on excluding the presence of underlying alloantibodies.

Cold-type autoimmune haemolytic anaemia

- The red cells should be washed at 37°C for performing the direct antiglobulin test (DAT), which will usually be strongly positive due to coating with C3d.
- Underlying alloantibodies can be excluded by using cells and serum separately warmed to 37°C.

Warm-type autoimmune haemolytic anaemia

- The red cells will usually have a positive DAT due to coating with IgG with or without complement. Rarely, the red cells may be coated with IgA or IgM and IgG.
- Underlying alloantibodies may be detected following the removal of autoantibodies from the pa-

tient's serum. This may be achieved either by absorbing the serum with the patient's own red cells (e.g. using a combination of papain and dithiothreitol 'ZZAP' to elute the autoantibody and enzyme treat the red cells) or if the patient has been recently transfused, with red cells of similar phenotype (if already known) or with two or more examples of red cells of known phenotypes.

Selection of red cells for transfusion

- Red cells of the same ABO and D group as the patient should be selected, except in a life-threatening situation before the patient has been grouped. In this case, group O should be used; if the patient is a pre-menopausal female, group O, D-negative should be used. Group-specific units should be provided as soon as the patient's group is known.
- The selection of blood for patients with red cell alloantibodies is summarised in Table 23.10. However, in life-threatening situations, the immediate need for red cell transfusion may necessitate the use of incompatible units.
- Units for fetal or neonatal exchange transfusions should be selected to be compatible with the maternal serum/plasma.
- Pre-menopausal females should ideally receive K-negative red cells, and R_1R_1 units if they are c-negative.
- Patients with a lifelong dependency on red cell support should receive red cells matched for Rh antigens and K (see Chapter 27).
- Recipients of ABO- and D-incompatible allogeneic haemopoietic stem cell grafts will need to be transfused with red cells of the donor group in the case of a minor ABO mismatch, or group O in the case of a combined ABO mismatch. D-negative red cells should also be selected for D-positive recipients of a D-negative donation (see Chapter 27).

The laboratory also has the responsibility for ensuring that requests for irradiated or CMV seronegative units are fulfilled and that the patient's record is 'flagged' for this requirement.

Serological crossmatch

Crossmatching techniques have been simplified in recent years, and only the immediate spin

Table 23.10 Recommendations for the selection of blood for patients with red cell alloantibodies.

	Typical examples	Procedure
Antibodies that could be considered clinically significant	Anti-D, -C, -c, -E, -e Anti-K, -k Anti-Jk^a, -Jk^b Anti-S, -s, -U Anti-Fy^a, -Fy^b	Select ABO-compatible, antigen-negative blood for serological crossmatching
Antibodies directed against antigens with an incidence of <10%, and where the antibody is often not clinically significant	Anti-C^w Anti-Kp^a Anti-Lu^a Anti-Wr^a (anti-Di3)	Select ABO-compatible blood for serological crossmatching
Antibodies primarily reactive below 37°C, and never or only very rarely clinically significant	Anti-A$_1$ Anti-N Anti-P$_1$ Anti-Le^a, -Le^b, -Le^{a+b} Anti-HI (in A$_1$ and A$_1$B patients)	Select ABO-compatible blood for serological crossmatching, performed strictly at 37°C
Antibodies sometimes reactive at 37°C and clinically significant	Anti-M	If reactive at 37°C, select ABO-compatible, antigen-negative blood for serological crossmatching If unreactive at 37°C, select ABO-compatible blood for serological crossmatching, performed strictly at 37°C
Other antibodies active by IAT at 37°C Indirect antiglobulin test	Many specificities	Seek advice from blood centre

crossmatch and the IAT crossmatch remain in common use.

The IAT crossmatch can be abolished when antibody screening is performed with screening cells that share apparent homozygous expression of common antigens capable of stimulating clinically significant antibodies, and the patient's serum/plasma has never been found to contain clinically significant antibodies. An exception to this rule should be made for patients who have received an ABO-incompatible solid organ transplant and who may develop an IgG anti-A or anti-B produced by passenger lymphocytes. Several retrospective and prospective studies have shown that there is negligible risk in omitting the IAT crossmatch. Although up to 0.2% IAT crossmatches may reveal an unpredicted incompatibility, few of these transfusions result in haemolysis. Antibodies directed against low-frequency antigens may be missed, but the majority of these are naturally occurring and do not cause patient morbidity.

If the IAT crossmatch is omitted, there must be some check included to detect ABO incompatibility. The immediate spin crossmatch (i.e. agglutination in saline following a 2–5 minutes incubation) is a serological check that can be used. However, this technique is fallible when the patient has low levels of anti-A or anti-B and, unless ethylenediamine tetra-acetic acid (EDTA) saline is used, false-negative results may also arise as a result of steric hindering of agglutination by C1. False-positive crossmatches arising from rouleaux or cold agglutinins not detected in the antibody screen have the potential to delay the issuing of compatible units.

The limitations of the immediate spin crossmatch have heralded the acceptance of electronic issue as an alternative method of preventing the release of ABO-incompatible units of blood.

Electronic issue

Electronic issue should only be used for detecting ABO incompatibility between the donor unit and the patient sample that was submitted for pre-transfusion testing. There are several essential requirements for adopting this approach, which are common to the various professional standards.

• The computer contains logic to prevent the assignment and release of ABO-incompatible blood.

• No clinically significant antibodies are detected in the recipient's serum and there is no record of previous detection of such antibodies.

• There are concordant results of at least two determinations of the recipient's ABO and D groups on file, one of which is from a current sample.

• Critical elements of the system (application software, readers and interfaces) have been validated on-site and there are mechanisms to verify the correct entry of data prior to release of blood, such as the use of bar code identifiers to enter information when it cannot be automatically transferred. Fully automated blood grouping and antibody screening, although not a requirement in current UK guidelines, is strongly recommended.

Electronic issue has been routinely practised in Sweden for over 10 years, during which time one error has been noted due to an incorrectly labelled unit of blood, which was supplied by a small non-computerised blood centre.

Electronic issue has several potential advantages:

• reduced technical workload;

• rapid availability of blood;

• improved blood stock management and reduced wastage;

• less handling of biohazardous material;

• elimination of unwanted false-positive results in the immediate spin crossmatch; and

• ability to issue blood electronically at remote sites, using trained non-laboratory staff.

This last characteristic has allowed the development of networked electronic blood release systems. When the patient details are entered, the system checks that the criteria for electronic issue are fulfilled and lists the compatible units available in the remote site blood refrigerator. The bar codes of the unit selected are scanned into the computer and, if ABO and D compatible, a compatibility label is printed that is attached to the unit and rescanned. This step generates a second label, or compatibility form, which is signed by the clinical staff at the time of the transfusion.

Key points

1 The transfusion process is unique since it links one sector of the community (the donors) with another (the patient) in an altruistic, potentially life-saving activity and it also links many grades of staff across a health care organisation.

2 For many patients, there is still no substitute for human-derived blood components.

3 Prescribers of blood components have a moral obligation to the donors to ensure that the donations are used appropriately.

4 Prescribers of blood components also have a duty of care to their patients to ensure that the benefits of the transfusion outweigh the risks.

5 There are many different members of staff involved in the hospital transfusion process, which provides too many opportunities for human error to prevail.

6 Investment in a quality infrastructure, computerisation and automation is essential to prevent errors in this process.

Further reading

Audet AM, Greenfield S & Field M. Medical practice guidelines: current activities and future directions. *Ann Intern Med* 1990;113:709–714.

Department of Health. *Better Blood Transfusion*. HSC 2007/001. London: HMSO, 2007.

Dzik WH, Corwin H, Goodnough LT *et al.* Patient safety and blood transfusion: new solutions. *Transfus Med Rev* 2003;17:169–180.

Eisenstaedt RS. Modifying physicians' transfusion practice. *Transfus Med Rev* 1997;11:27–37.

McClelland DBL (ed.). *Handbook of Transfusion Medicine*, 4th edn. Norwich: TSO, 2007. Available at www.transfusionguidelines.org.

Heddle NM, O'Hoski P, Singer J, McBride JA, Ali MA & Kelton JG. A prospective study to determine the safety of omitting the antiglobulin crossmatch from pretransfusion testing. *Br J Haematol* 1992;81:579–584.

Jensen NJ & Crosson JT. An automated system for bedside verification of the match between patient identification and blood unit identification. *Transfusion* 1996;36:216–221.

Judd W.J. Requirements for the electronic crossmatch. *Vox Sang* 1998;74(Suppl 2):409–417.

Klein HG & Anstee D. *Mollison's Blood Transfusion in Clinical Medicine*, 11th edn. Oxford: Blackwell Publishing, 2005.

Research Unit of the Royal College of Physicians. *Audit Measures for Good Practice in Blood Transfusion Medicine*. London: RCP Publications, 1995.

Serious Hazards of Transfusion. *Annual Report 2006*. Manchester: SHOT Office, 2006. Available at www. shotuk.org.

Turner CL, Casbard AC & Murphy MF. Barcode technology: its role in increasing the safety of blood transfusion. *Transfusion* 2003;43:1200–1209.

Guidelines

British Committee for Standards in Haematology. The administration of blood and blood components and the management of transfused patients. *Transfus Med* 1999;9:227–238. Available at www. bcshguidelines.com.

British Committee for Standards in Haematology. Guidelines for compatibility procedures in blood transfusion laboratories. *Transfus Med* 2004;14:59–73. Available at www.bcshguidelines.com.

British Committee for Standards in Haematology. Guidelines for policies on alternatives to allogeneic blood transfusion. 1. Predeposit autologous blood donation and transfusion *Transfus Med* 2007;17:354–365. Available at www.bcshguidelines.com.

British Committee for Standards in Haematology. The specification and use of information technology systems in blood transfusion practice. *Transfus Med* 2007;17:1–21. Available at www.bcshguidelines.com.

CHAPTER 24

Blood transfusion in a global context

David Roberts[1], Jean-Pierre Allain[2], Alan D. Kitchen[3], Stephen Field[4] & Imelda Bates[5]

[1]University of Oxford; NHS Blood and Transplant and Department of Haematology, John Radcliffe Hospital, Oxford, UK
[2]NHS Blood and Transplant; Division of Transfusion Medicine, Department of Haematology, University of Cambridge, Cambridge, UK
[3]National Transfusion Microbiology Laboratory; NHS Blood and Transplant, Colindale, London, UK
[4]Welsh Blood Service, Pontyclun, Cardiff, Wales
[5]Liverpool School of Tropical Medicine, Liverpool, UK

Introduction

'17% of the world's population has access to 60% of the global blood supply'

Inequality in the provision of 'safe blood' round the world mirrors the unequal distribution of almost all other resources crucial for effective health services or indeed for health itself. Unfortunately, in many countries, providing safe blood is made more difficult by lack of donors and the high frequency of transfusion transmissible infections. At the same time, the problems posed by the poor supply of blood are compounded by the frequent need for urgent life-saving transfusions in childbirth, in children with malaria and the increased demand for HIV/AIDS patients.

The purpose of this chapter is not to guide those developing transfusion services in less affluent countries but to inform a wider audience of the problems faced in the development of effective transfusion services in these countries. A secondary aim is to stimulate some debate and analysis of the problems faced by transfusion services globally. Finally, a short chapter must be selective and our choice of topics and examples, and their solutions reflect our own experience in Southeast Asia and sub-Saharan Africa.

Blood safety

A safe and rapid supply of blood is an essential part of medical services. Unsafe blood supply is costly in both human and economic terms. Transfusion of infected blood not only causes direct morbidity and mortality in the recipients, but also has an economic and emotional impact on their families and communities and undermines confidence in modern health care. Those who become infected through blood transfusion are often infectious to others and contribute a significant secondary wave of iatrogenic infections. Investment in safe supplies of blood is cost-effective for every country, even those with few resources.

The World Health Organization (WHO) has identified four key objectives for blood services to ensure that blood is safe for transfusion:

• Establish a coordinated national blood transfusion service that can provide adequate and timely supplies of safe blood for all patients in need.
• Collect blood only from voluntary non-remunerated blood donors from low-risk populations and use stringent donor selection procedures.

Practical Transfusion Medicine, 3rd edition. Edited by Michael F. Murphy and Derwood H. Pamphilon. © 2009 Blackwell Publishing, ISBN: 978-1-4051-8196-9.

• Screen all blood for transfusion-transmissible infections and have standardised procedures in place for grouping and compatibility testing.
• Reduce unnecessary transfusions through the appropriate clinical use of blood, including the use of intravenous replacement fluids and other simple alternatives to transfusion, wherever possible.

The WHO also emphasises that effective quality assurance should be in place for all aspects of the transfusion process, from donor recruitment and selection, through infection screening, blood grouping and blood storage, to administration to patients and clinical monitoring for adverse events.

It is axiomatic that transfusion medicine is a distinct and multi-disciplinary sector of the health service and should be incorporated into national health plans. It is the responsibility of governments to develop policies and legislation that will facilitate the development of a national transfusion service and ensure that the blood transfusion process and its associated quality assurance programmes are of a high standard.

However, it must be realised that in some areas such as sub-Saharan Africa, transfusion is almost exclusively an emergency measure to treat patients with extreme, life-threatening anaemia. This situation has two important consequences:

• Blood is considered a therapeutic commodity with little more regard from the medical community and government than drugs delivered by the pharmacy.
• Whole blood is an appropriate choice, helping in reducing the cost of transfusion (sparing component preparation expenses).

The WHO has provided a recommended structure of national blood transfusion services. They suggest that at the national level the transfusion service should have a medical director, an advisory committee and clear national transfusion policies and strategies with the appropriate statutory instruments to ensure the national coordination and standardisation of blood testing, processing and distribution. Notwithstanding these recommendations, transfusion activities must be integrated with other services at local and national levels.

There has been some progress to realise WHO's recommendations for a national blood programme. In Africa, in 2002 the WHO estimated that among the 46 member states in the African continent, only 14 had a national blood policy and just six had a policy to specifically encourage and develop a system of voluntary non-remunerated donation. In the most recent survey, in 2007, 40/41 African states had a national blood policy, but only 56% (23/41) countries were able to implement their polices.

It is worthwhile reflecting on why the development of national transfusion services has not been achieved. A key reason is that it is logistically complex. Management skills to run such services are lacking. There has been an understandable emphasis on primary health care over the last 25 years, and this may have diffused interest in hospital-based, curative medicine. A second reason may be the high cost of blood transfusion in relation to disposable income and health care budgets. The average annual income in sub-Saharan Africa is in the range of $ 400–1000, and a unit of blood costs $ 10–20 in a hospital service and $ 60–100 in a centralised service. Blood is therefore an expensive commodity in relation to the annual per capita budget for health care in these countries and it remains to be seen if blood costing more than $ 50 per unit when produced in centralised, externally funded units is sustainable. Precise cost–benefit analyses for the use of blood have not been done. Nevertheless, blood transfusion for severe malarial anaemia and severe haemorrhage can be life saving, and it seems plausible that the cost of transfusion probably approaches the generally accepted cost–benefit range of $ 1 per year of life saved for health interventions in the poorest countries.

To prepare enough safe blood in a sustainable fashion, African countries need to develop their own ways to produce it. Uncritical adoption of external advice and models may lead to unsustainable and inappropriate solutions. What then are the models of transfusion services in Africa and what are the consequences for the timely supply of safe blood?

Organisation of transfusion services in sub-Saharan Africa

African countries have developed a variety of systems to try to achieve a sustainable safe blood

---

Box 24.1 Case studies – examples of blood transfusion systems in sub-Saharan Africa

Integrated National Blood Service – Ivory Coast

Côte d'Ivoire blood service was created in 1992 with substantial subsidies from the European Union. A National Blood Transfusion Centre is located in Abidjan, the capital, with three smaller provincial centres. In addition, blood depots are located in hospitals of five other main cities. For a population of 12 million, approximately 80,000 units of blood were collected in 2002, mostly from volunteer blood donors recruited amongst secondary school students (>60%), although 24% of them were first-time donors.

Any hospital in the country can access the blood supply free of charge to the hospital and the patients. The government allocates funding. Less than 20% of the blood is processed into blood components that are mostly used in the capital. Antibodies to HIV, HCV as well as HBsAg are tested by EIA in the capital. The recurrent cost per unit produced is estimated at $40.

Regional hospital - Ghana

In a 1200-bed hospital, the current demand for blood products is, in adults, whole blood for acute anaemia or massive haemorrhage and in children 200 ml plasma-depleted red cells for anaemia related to malaria, sickle cell disease or thalassaemia. Approximately 10,000 candidate donors are screened per year and 7000 blood units are available for clinical use. Patients' families are asked to pay $14 for a unit of blood and $7 if the blood is replaced. Volunteer blood is primarily collected in secondary schools (80% of total volunteer donations). Anti-HIV, HBsAg and anti-HCV are screened pre-donation with high-performance rapid tests so that blood bags (representing one third of the total consumable budget) are not wasted. Furthermore, deferred donors can be identified, informed and counselled, and contribute to a decreasing prevalence of viral markers in volunteer donors.

Rural community hospital – Zimbabwe

This 40-bed hospital is too isolated to conveniently order and receive blood from the regional hospital centre and has to rely on its own resources to produce the 100–200 blood units per year they need. They have procured the blood bags and the anti-HIV and HBsAg rapid tests from the regional blood centre. Because of the small demand, collecting and keeping a refrigerated blood stock is neither feasible nor economical. The staff have designed an alternative strategy called 'blood club'. The local population was informed about transfusion through village meetings and sketches presented by the local drama group, which illustrated situations involving the need for blood and blood donors. Volunteers who agreed to join the club were registered and tested for blood group and HBsAg. HBsAg negative volunteers (80%) are called upon if blood is needed in the hospital. When a patient needs blood, the blood group is determined and two blood group-matched volunteers are brought to the hospital and tested for anti-HIV. Blood is then collected from a HIV-negative donor. The patient's family are charged $9 for each unit of blood.

---

supply. These vary from large, modern, national blood centres to locally organised donor programmes for individual district health care facilities.

A minority of countries have invested significant resources in transfusion services, often with financial support and advisers from European governments, United States Agency for International Development (USAID) or non-governmental organisations (NGOs), including Red Cross, Red Crescent, Family Health International and the Safe Blood for Africa Foundation. In these countries, there has been a commitment to establishing centralised systems based on the example of wealthy nations (Box 24.1). These centres typically collect over 10,000 units a year, use automated equipment and produce some blood components. Blood

donor recruitment, screening and processing of donated blood, are carried out in specifically designed premises away from the hospitals where blood is transfused.

However, the majority of countries in sub-Saharan Africa do not operate a centralised transfusion service. Each hospital recruits blood donors and processes blood for transfusion. These hospitals often handle less than 1000 units a year and experience difficulties in standardisation, quality assurance and in maintaining supplies of high-quality reagents.

Recruiting voluntary donors from the community is complex and expensive and depends on regular education programmes, collection teams, vehicles and cold storage. It is proving very difficult to expand the number of volunteer donors. Indeed, over the last 15 years, there has been increasing difficultly in persuading donors to donate, as fear of knowing one's HIV test result has become more widespread. There are also cultural beliefs surrounding blood donation that inhibit donors coming forward. Some of these appear to be misinformation about donating blood (e.g. 'men will become impotent if they donate blood'; 'HIV can be caught from the blood bag needle'). It is worth noting that similar problems faced widespread acceptance of blood donation when Percy Oliver and Geoffrey Keynes began to establish the first blood banks of volunteer donors in London over 70 years ago.

There are, however, other cultural beliefs that are much more complex and related donors' to deep-seated and ethnographically diverse understanding of the value of blood to the individual and to society, e.g. blood is related to kinship or personal health. Understanding local beliefs surrounding blood and blood donation is likely to be important to develop effective services.

As volunteer donors are in short supply, family members are frequently used to provide blood for their relatives in hospital. In 2002, in Africa as a whole, WHO estimated that over 60% of blood originated from replacement/family donors. In sub-Saharan Africa the proportion of blood derived from replacement donors is certainly higher. These replacement donors should be family members, but relatives may not only be reluctant to donate for the reasons discussed above, but are also open to exploitation by 'professional donors' who charge relatives a fee to donate in their place. Finally, replacement donors have significantly higher seropositive rates than volunteer donors for HIV, hepatitis B and C and syphilis. Many viral infections such as HTLV-I and HTLV-II and human herpesvirus-8 occur during infancy and have similar prevalence in replacement and volunteer donors. There are therefore several reasons to reduce replacement donors in sub-Saharan Africa (and elsewhere), but many obstacles must to be overcome to achieve these goals. Local transfusion systems allow many patients to survive serious illness and are often maintained by dedicated staff

in difficult circumstances. However, even with the best input from local staff, these district services experience problems of supply and safety.

The supply of blood

Patients in poorer countries usually present late in the course of their disease, and the delays and lack of stored blood inherent in the replacement donor system mean that patients may die before a blood transfusion can be organised. By the time a donor has been found, screened and venesected, and the blood is transfused into the patient, several hours or even days can elapse. A survey of the blood supplied by a dedicated district service in East Africa showed that the average delay in sourcing blood for children with severe malaria anaemia was 6 hours. Anecdotal evidence suggests that in some areas and at some times in many areas blood may not be available at all. Finally, locally based services at regional or national centres have difficulty in separating blood, even into simple fractions such as red cells, platelets and plasma, to provide specific components if needed.

Testing and storage of donor blood

Local blood transfusion services encounter many problems, including lack of funding, insufficient training, poor management, frequent failure to supply reagents and consumables, and breakdown of the cold chain mostly related to frequent power cuts. Blood frequently has to be collected in small hospital-based units often with no dedicated staff and no specifically allocated budget. In the year 2000, the WHO review estimated that 25% of the blood in sub-Saharan Africa was not tested for anti-HIV and that blood transfusion was the origin of 5–10% of new HIV infections. Since then, a lot of investment had gone into providing HIV, HBsAg and to some extent HCV tests. The latest survey shows that >98% of blood is tested for HIV. The residual risk of HBV infection remains substantial because of donations containing undetected low level of

HBsAg or occult HBV DNA. Recent estimates of the residual risk of HIV transmission are 1:2600–6000, Hepatitis C 1: 400–1500 and Hepatitis B 1: 300–500, when using Enzyme Immunoassay (EIA) screening.

The cost of local blood supply

When a transfusion service is provided by individual hospitals, it places an enormous burden on laboratory resources. There has been almost no research into the cost of setting up and running transfusion services in resource-poor countries. One survey showed that in a typical district hospital in southern Africa, the overall cost of the transfusion service, including consumables, proportional amounts for capital equipment, staff time and overheads, was 36% of total laboratory costs. Each unit of whole blood cost the laboratory approximately $ 20 to collect and process.

The cost of a national service is even greater because of the additional costs of quality assurance, local education programmes, dedicated collection team(s), vehicles and cold storage. In addition, a national service has to solve the very real practical problems of maintaining regular distributions of sufficient quantities of blood to remote facilities. It is also frequently observed that the creation of a national service creates internal migration of technical staff from hospitals to national or regional centres. One solution to this would be to train staff specifically for the processing, testing and issue of blood and so release the time of valuable, skilled hospital staff.

Clinical use of blood

In contrast to Europe, most transfusions in sub-Saharan Africa are given for life-threatening emergencies, most often anaemia in children or pregnant women and haemorrhage following childbirth or trauma. Transfusions are administered to children predominantly for malaria-related anaemia and can undoubtedly reduce the mortality of children with severe anaemia. Many clinical guidelines, albeit based on consensus opinion rather than well-defined evidence, suggest transfusions are indicated if Hb < 4 or 5 g/dL with symptoms of decompensation. Even in areas of high HIV prevalence, young children generally have a relatively low risk of becoming naturally infected with HIV and potentially have a long life expectancy. Pregnant women are the second most common recipients of blood particularly for haemorrhagic emergencies. Significant quantities of blood are also used in trauma, surgery and general medicine. There are neither systematic reviews nor international guidelines covering the use of blood in these specific contexts, and few audits of blood use. The scope for improving clinical practice and reducing unnecessary transfusion through education and the use of guidelines is probably substantial

The problems surrounding the rapid supply of a safe supply of blood have led to the use of autologous blood transfusion. There are logistical and training problems to be overcome. However, small programmes have been established for autologous transfusion of elective surgery patients at district hospitals.

Putting the WHO objectives into practice: improving the supply, safety and use of blood in sub-Saharan Africa

Some countries have used external funds to establish an integrated national service, but few have been able to make the transition to a sustainable, national transfusion service in the absence of external funding. Moreover, in several countries, external funding for ten or more years has failed to develop a functioning national transfusion service, and these failures have led some funders withdrawing grants to national transfusion services. However, some recent success has been achieved in developing a transfusion service in several centres in Nigeria (see Box 24.2). The alternative is that, in many areas, transfusion services have to be optimised within the existing general hospital budget. Whatever sums are available the specific, often interconnected problems, surrounding the supply, safety, cost and use of blood must be addressed. There has to be a balance between providing an

---

Box 24.2 Towards development of a National Transfusion Service in Nigeria

Nigeria, the most populous country in Africa, had in 2004 a highly fragmented hospital-based transfusion system. There was little coordination from the central government and most of the blood came from replacement and paid donors. Testing for transmissible disease markers was inconsistent and poorly controlled. The current practice of family replacement donors in hospital-based blood service is the most economical option, but in the face of high child and maternal mortality rates the blood supply has proved to be insufficient. There was therefore the need to change practice.

Safe Blood for Africa Foundation with a grant from USAID established a demonstration blood service in capital Abuja. This service collected its blood from voluntary unremunerated donors in the local community. The blood was tested for HIV, Hepatitis B and C, labelled with ISBT 128 compliant labels and distributed to the local hospitals. A simple but effective quality management system was established with standard operating procedures written and followed. A validated transfusion computer system was installed which only allowed release of validated units of blood to hospitals. The objective of this project was to be the model for other centres throughout the country. The Federal Ministry of Health soon established regional centres in Kaduna, Owerri, Port Harcourt, Ibadan Maiduguri and Jos, and has a long-term plan to roll out further centres in future. The Minister of Health also established an expert committee which drafted a national blood policy and national guidelines for the standards for the practice of transfusion in Nigeria. Safe Blood for Africa Foundation provided technical assistance for the establishment of these centres and provided training to the staff in all elements of transfusion.

The major problem was to recruit blood donors. The youth were encouraged to donate with the establishment of a Club 25 programme. There was active promotion through the media and was highlighted by a televised donation by the President on the occasion of the official opening of the Abuja centre. A problem encountered was the high number of donors presenting with haemoglobin levels below the required standard of 12.5 g/dL. This is probably a reflection of the poor health status within the community.

---

ideal integrated national service and the more pragmatic solutions afforded by local services.

Improving the blood supply and the safety of the donor pool

Careful donor selection is crucial not only to improve the supply of blood but also to reduce transfusion-transmitted infection risk (see Box 24.3 and Table 24.1). The selection of volunteer donors from lower risk populations is considered the most effective approach and considerable effort has been devoted to promoting voluntary, repeat donations. However, in most parts of Africa, replacement donors are the main resource. They are typically young males in the high-risk bracket of HIV infection or other sexually transmitted viruses. As the availability of replacement donors is limited, the most effective way to improve the availability and safety of blood is to recruit volunteer donors. In practice these are secondary school students with median age ranging between 16 and 20 years. They are younger, have a greater proportion of females, and are 5–10 times less likely to be infected with HIV than replacement donors. Experience has shown that while recruiting volunteer donors in schools can be relatively inexpensive, making them into repeat donors is difficult and expensive.

Several strategies have been devised to encourage repeat voluntary donors and thus reduce the risk of virus carriage. In Zimbabwe, Pledge 25 Club, a program using education and incentives to attract school students to give blood 25 times, has been successful. Similar, less ambitious schemes, for example a 'Club 5', could also be effective. The WHO slogan of 'Safe blood starts with me' has also resulted in educational programmes around the world. These schemes can be complemented by strategies to recruit donors from faith-based organisations or collaborating with radio stations to organise and promote blood donations. The success of well-organised requests for blood donors has been proven in some campaigns but remains to be tested in many countries where national calls for donors have not been made in the absence of centralised blood transfusion services. [11]

The best use of fluid replacement regimes for severe haemorrhage requires further study. At

---

Box 24.3 Epidemiology of blood-borne infections in sub-Saharan Africa

HIV

The overall prevalence of HIV antibody in sub-Saharan Africa ranges between 0.5 and 16%. In donors, it tends to remain below 5% in West Africa, below 10% in East and Central Africa and above 10% in southern Africa.

Hepatitis B

Chronic hepatitis B prevalence, indicated by the presence of circulating HBsAg, ranges between 5 and 25% of the population including blood donors. This high prevalence is due to (vertical) transmission at birth or (horizontal) infection in infancy and the virtual absence of national vaccination programs. Infection after the age of 10 is uncommon. HBsAg is more prevalent in West Africa (10–25%) than in East or Central Africa (5–10%); the lowest prevalence is found in southern Africa (5% or less).

Hepatitis C

Antibody to HCV is not routinely screened for in many parts of Africa, but the prevalence of this infection ranges between 0.5 and 3% and reaches 10–15% in Egypt. The prevalence may be high locally, suggesting the importance of specific factors such as various types of injections, past diagnostic or vaccination campaigns contributing to spread the infection.

Other infections

Most countries in sub-Saharan Africa do not screen for *HTLV* since the prevalence is low (<2%).

Although the risk of acquiring syphilis from infected blood is low, most blood banks in sub-Saharan Africa do screen for *Treponema pallidum*. Fresh blood is potentially infectious for syphilis, but storage at 4°C can inactivate the bacterium.

Malaria can be transmitted by transfusion. In areas of low or no malaria transmission, screening for the parasite is important, as recipients are likely to have no immunity. In countries where malaria is highly endemic, the prevalence of *Plasmodium* in donor blood is often very high (16–40%) and excluding donors with low-grade parasitaemia is often impracticable and pre-emptive treatment of patients receiving transfusion with anti-malarial drugs often an unfortunate necessity.

Residual risk of transfusion transmission of blood-borne viruses

Improving the size and reliability of the donor pool affects not only the supply but also the safety of blood. In particular, a previously screened donor pool would reduce the substantial residual risks of transfusion-transmitted infection due to the window period for HIV and HCV and occult chronic carriage for HBV (HBsAg negative/DNA positive).

The present residual risk of viral transmission by transfusion has been assessed for HIV. In studies conducted in Kenya, Zambia and the Democratic Republic of the Congo, the risk of HIV transmission by transfusion was estimated to be between 1 and 3%, related in part to prevalence, but also to test performance, storage conditions and staff training. The residual risk of HBV infection remains substantial because of donations containing undetected low level of HBsAg or occult HBV DNA. This risk remains high for children below the age of 10 but the problem is at least in part mitigated by the very high prevalence of adult recipients carrying HBV markers (60–90%). Precise estimates of the residual risk of HIV transmission in Ivory Coast in 2002–2004 were 1:2600–6000, HCV 1: 400–1500 and HBV 1: 300–500, when using EIA screening.

These figures represent the risk of the respective infection even when using the best EIAs. This residual risk emphasises the pressing need to improve the safety of the donor pool, to develop cheap and reliable nucleic acid testing and to optimise the use of blood.

---

the same time, other novel solutions are being sought to alleviate the shortage of blood. It may be feasible to use placental blood as an accessory source of blood to transfuse small children in malarious areas. The placenta containing this blood is normally discarded after delivery. However, the high haematocrit and easy availability may make it suitable for small-volume emergency transfusions if blood can be collected free of bacterial contamination. In the long term, artificial blood substitutes could provide a useful alternative to allogeneic blood transfusion during acute illnesses. However, they remain expensive and have only limited approval pending further

Table 24.1 Prevalence of transfusion-transmissible agents in sub-Saharan African blood donors.

Country	Year collected	Prevalence (%)					
		Anti-HIV	HBsAg	Anti-HCV	HTLV	Syphilis	Malaria
Benin	1998	0.5–3	12	1.4–2.3	0.3–5.4		33.5
Botswana	2000	10	5	1			
Cameroon	1994–1998	4.1–5.8	10–16	1.6			
Ghana	1998–2002	1.7–3.8	15	1.7–8.4	0.5	13.5	
Kenya	1995–1998	4.5–3.0	4.2–3.9	1.5–1.8			
Malawi	2000	10.7	8.1	6.8	2.5		
Nigeria	2004–2005	2.0	9.9	1.9		0.5	
RDC	1998	6.4	9.2	4.3			
Republic of South Africa*	2001	4.5	5	0.5			
Tanzania	1998	8.7	11	8–10.3	0	12.7	
Togo	1995–2000			3.3	1.8		
Uganda	2000	3.9–5.4					
Zambia	1991–1995	8–16	6.5				
Zimbabwe	1997	8.8	2.5–15.4		0.1		

* Donors of African origin.

randomised trials of their safety and efficacy (see Chapter 35).

Improving screening for blood-transmitted infections

Test sensitivity is critical in the face of high prevalence rates for HIV, HBV and HCV (Box 24.3 and Table 24.1). These high prevalence rates pose a very substantial danger and a major logistic and technical challenge to those trying to provide safe blood. Even with the best available testing procedures there remains a substantial residual risk of HIV transmission in the order of 1 in 3000 though the failure to detect seronegative early HIV infection in the pre-seroconversion window period (see above). In these situations, the prevalence rate may be reduced by 90% in repeat donors, reinforcing the value of a stable donor pool.

The techniques used for screening must be considered carefully to ensure effective screening of the particular donor population and the skills of the staff involved. Nucleic acid testing is highly effective and has been introduced in a few centres. However, widespread use of NAT remains neither affordable nor practical for most centres and countries. Cheaper and/or simplified methods to perform NAT testing would be useful.

New approaches adapted to local situations appear promising. In small blood banks, the expensive microtitre plate systems used post donation can be replaced by cheaper, more cost-effective, high-performance rapid tests performed pre- or post-donation. Pre-donation testing provides the advantages of reducing material waste and easy, on-site communication with deferred donors who, otherwise, could not be reached. There are fears that pre-donation testing may reduce the willingness of donors to come forward, although published data did not find evidence of this. At present, WHO does not recommend pre-donation testing. There is a diversity of opinion and some consider that WHO and aid agencies need to show flexibility and consider the benefits of multiple strategies adapted to local needs rather than recommending rigid models designed for totally different populations, staff and resources.

Some new technology is on the horizon. Rapid immunochemical and nucleic acid dipsticks are being developed for blood-borne pathogens and may cut the cost of pre- and post-donation testing to a tenth of present costs. Clearly, these and other inexpensive and effective testing technologies, as well as pathogen inactivation techniques, directed towards the needs of developing countries should become a major target of external support.

The WHO has established systematic evaluations of both EIA and rapid tests to guide developing countries in their choice of tests. These evaluations include test costs. Many rapid tests for anti-HIV and HBsAg and fewer for anti-HCV are available, but sensitivity and specificity, ease of use and cost vary greatly. Some of these tests are performed in one single step with results obtained in 10–20 minutes using whole blood, plasma or serum samples. The best assays have sensitivity similar to EIA for anti-HIV, detect 1 ng/mL of HBsAg and have >95% sensitivity for anti-HCV and >98% specificity.

Reducing the cost of transfusion services

The challenge for Africa is that safe blood should be available for health services and individuals even when resources are extremely limited. The majority of a blood unit cost originates from imported goods such as equipment, blood bags, grouping and screening assays. Staff costs are a relatively small proportion of the overall costs because salaries are low and because negligible resources are put into staff training, supervision and auditing mechanisms. According to published studies, a unit of blood from a hospital-based service may cost between $10 and 40, but even $10 is not affordable by most families in sub-Saharan Africa.

Because transfusion is such an expensive service, the costs often have to be subsidised by aid packages, external agencies or governments. Resources for transfusion services are often vulnerable to fickle, political and non-sustainable fluctuations. Developing systems that rely more on local resources means that in the long term they may be more dynamic, productive and sustainable. Certainly, much more research is needed comparing the cost-effectiveness of various strategies to supply safe blood to patients in poor countries.

Improving the clinical use of blood: guidelines for transfusion practice

The use of simple guidelines can reduce unnecessary transfusions and many institutions in sub-Saharan Africa and Asia have developed guidelines

to promote rational use of blood transfusions and blood products. The scope for improvement in clinical practice is great. For example, strict enforcement of a transfusion protocol in a Malawian hospital reduced the number of transfusions by 75% without any adverse effect on mortality.

The principles underlying most transfusion guidelines are similar and combine a clinical assessment of whether the patient is developing complications of inadequate oxygenation, with measurement of their haemoglobin (as a marker of intracellular oxygen concentration). In sub-Saharan countries, the recommended haemoglobin threshold for transfusions is often well below that which would be accepted in more wealthy countries. In the US, anaesthetists suggest that transfusions are almost always indicated when the haemoglobin concentration is less than 6 g/dL whereas in many African countries transfusions are recommended for children at haemoglobin concentrations less than 4 g/dL, provided there are no other clinical complications.

Ensuring that the transfusion guidelines are implemented is extremely difficult for poorer countries without formal monitoring and auditing systems. This is particularly problematic if the quality of haemoglobin measurements is not assured. Studies have shown that if clinicians do not have confidence in haemoglobin results, they will rely entirely on clinical judgement to guide transfusion practice and this can lead to significant numbers of inappropriate transfusions. In a typical district hospital in Africa the cost of providing a unit of blood is approximately 40 times the cost of a quality-assured haemoglobin test. Investment in improving the haemoglobin testing therefore has the potential for significant cost-saving downstream in the much more expensive transfusion process as well as reducing the risk of transfusion-related infections.

Conclusion: the future of blood transfusion in a global context

Fulfilling the first WHO objective of establishing 'a coordinated national blood transfusion service that can provide adequate and timely supplies of safe blood for all patients in need' has proved to be very difficult in many countries even given substantial external funding. Nevertheless, some countries have made progress and have recently established national transfusion services. On the other hand, progress has been made by developing local services and there has to be a balance between providing an ideal integrated national service and the more pragmatic solutions afforded by local services. There remains considerable scope to optimise fluid management regimens and to reduce unnecessary transfusions through the appropriate clinical use of blood and products.

Increased blood supply depends on the recruitment of voluntary non-remunerated donors. The examples and discussions in this chapter have centred on Africa, but the same considerations apply to many of the poorer countries in Asia and Latin America. Here, there are wide variations in resources available for health care not only between but also within countries.

In all countries, increased blood supply depends on the recruitment of volunteer donors and this should become priority for policy development and resource allocation. A reliable and expanded donor pool will not only provide a life-saving therapy but also improve safety. Resources must be made available by governments to ensure that the essential supplies are available, such as blood bags, grouping reagents and test kits, and laboratory and blood bank management systems also need to be improved to ensure effective testing and processing, and the maintenance of the cold chain. Hospitals and other health facilities could cooperate to directly purchase cheap, high-quality tests adapted to their needs.

There is currently a feeling of guarded optimism about the future of blood safety in developing countries. The recent increase in allocation of resources for the prevention of HIV across the world, including the investment by governments of wealthy countries and contributions from international and private agencies, have begun to recognise the importance of reducing HIV transmission through blood but run the risk of neglecting other basic laboratory services, e.g. blood-grouping and haemoglobin measurements. Parallel to the price reduction for anti-viral drugs, the cost of screening

tests supplied to developing countries has also decreased. The high cost of anti-HCV testing will soon be reduced when the patent expires. Also possible methods of pathogen inactivation applicable to whole blood are being developed that could, in one step, reduce or eliminate the risks of viral, bacterial and parasitic infections. More effective and efficient methods for testing blood are to be welcomed. The real challenge will be to integrate improvements in the supply and safety of blood in sustainable, coordinated national transfusion services.

Key points

1 In the last 5 years, nearly all African states had a national blood policy, but just over half have been able to implement their polices.
2 The main obstacles to implementation are a lack of trained staff, the high cost of blood in relation to the health care budgets and recruitment of donors.
3 In the absence of centralised services, facilities rely on blood collected by hospitals from family or replacement donors.
4 High rate of chronic viral infections in the populations implies that the residual risk of infection of HIV and Hepatitis B infection remains substantial with EIA testing.
5 Several initiatives are being trialled to improve the supply and/or safety of blood by encouraging repeat voluntary donors, reviewing donor testing strategies, developing systems that rely more on local resources, using umbilical cord blood and researching methods for low-cost NAT testing.
6 There are few guidelines covering the use of blood and few audits of blood use and the scope for improving clinical practice and reducing unnecessary transfusion is probably substantial.

Further reading

Allain JP, Candotti D, Soldan K *et al.* The risk of hepatitis B virus infection by transfusion in Kumasi, Ghana. *Blood* 2003;101:2419–2425.

Bates I, Manyasi G & Medina Lara A. Reducing replacement donors in sub-Saharan Africa: challenges and affordability. *Trans Med* 2007;87:434–442.

Bates I, Mundy C, Pendame R *et al.* Use of clinical judgement to guide administration of blood transfusions in Malawi. *Trans R Soc Trop Med Hyg* 2001;95:510–512.

English M, Ahmed M, Ngando C, Berkley J & Ross A. Blood transfusion for severe anaemia in children in a Kenyan hospital. *Lancet* 2002;359:494–495.

Fairhead J, Leach M & Small M. Where techno-science meets poverty: medical research and the economy of blood in The Gambia, West Africa. *Soc Sci Med* 2006;65:1109–1120.

Field S and Allain J-P. Transfusion in sub-Saharan Africa does a Western model fit. *J Clin Pathol* 2007;60:1073–1075.

Hassall O, Ngina L, Kongo W *et al.* The acceptability to women in Mombasa, Kenya, of the donation and transfusion of umbilical cord blood for severe anaemia in young children. *Vox Sang* 2007; 94(2):125–131 .

Lackritz E, Campbell C & Ruebush T. Effect of blood transfusion on survival among children in a Kenyan hospital. *Lancet* 1992;340:524–528.

Matee MIN, Magesa P & Lyamuya EF. Seroprevalence of HIV, hepatitis B and C viruses and syphilis infections among blood donors at the Muhimbili National Hospital in Dar es Salaam, Tanzania. *BMC Public Health* 2006;6:21.

Ouattara H, Siransy-Bogui L, Fretz C *et al.* Residual risk of HIV, HVB and HCV transmission by blood transfusion between 2002 and 2004 at the Abidjan National Transfusion Centre. *Trans Clin Biol* 2006;13:242–245.

Owusu-Ofori S, Temple J, Sarkodie F, Candotti D & Allain JP. Pre-donation testing of blood donors in resource-poor settings. *Transfusion* 2005;45:1542–1543.

World Health Organization. Blood Transfusion Safety and related web pages. Available at http://www. who.int/ bloodsafety/en/; http://www.afro.who.int/ bls/pdf/ blood_safety_report_07.pdf. Accessed at 12 January 2008.

PART 4
Clinical transfusion practice

CHAPTER 25

Good blood management: the effective and safe use of blood components

Brian McClelland[1] *& Tim Walsh*[2]

[1] Scottish National Blood Transfusion Service, Protein Fractionation Centre, Edinburgh, Scotland
[2] Department of Anaesthetics and Intensive care, Royal Infirmary, Edinburgh, Scotland

Introduction

This chapter focuses on clinical decisions about transfusion of blood components and emphasises the importance of restricting the use of blood components to situations in which there are good grounds for believing that transfusion is likely to offer a real benefit to the patient.

Although in a country like the UK, the risks associated with receiving a transfusion are very small in the context of all the risks of hospital care, there is a high level of concern to avoid the well-publicised risks of transfusion. It is important, therefore, that patients and the wider public understand that transfusion, like all medical interventions, can never be free of risks. It may be helpful when considering risks and benefits to think of a transfusion as a transplant of human tissue, and not as a drug.

Information and consent

Patients who are able to communicate must be informed about the benefits, risks and choices for their treatment. The pre-admission clinic for elective surgery is an ideal opportunity to include in-

Practical Transfusion Medicine, 3rd edition. Edited by Michael F. Murphy and Derwood H. Pamphilon. © 2009 Blackwell Publishing, ISBN: 978-1-4051-8196-9.

formation about transfusion as part of the information given to the patient about the whole process of care. Formal consent for transfusion is not required in the UK, but the prescriber has a professional duty to make sure the patient knows if transfusion is intended. The patient should be made aware of the reasons why transfusion may be prescribed, that there may be risks both of receiving blood and, in some circumstances, of not receiving it. Whatever method is used, the patient's clinical record should record that information about transfusion has been given and that the patient's questions have been answered.

Evidence for effectiveness

Effectiveness – the measure of how much a treatment can help the patient – is a balance of the benefits and the risks. Many of the conventional and widely taught indications for transfusing blood components are not supported by reliable evidence of clinical benefit. It is important to take a critical approach to prescribing blood components. Guidelines for practice must reflect the best available evidence for clinical effectiveness.

There are still few good randomised controlled clinical trials of some of the main uses of transfusion, and recent high-quality trials tend to challenge conventional beliefs in the effectiveness of transfusion therapy (Chapter 46). Systematic

Table 25.1 Clinical effectiveness of conventional transfusion practices: the evidence may challenge conventional wisdom.

Human albumin and artificial colloids for infusion in critically ill patients[*][†]
Meta-analysis of clinical trials show no evidence to suggest benefit from
   The use of albumin vs. use of crystalloid
   The use of artificial colloids vs. use of crystalloid
Controversy continues about the suggestion that the use of albumin may increase mortality
The SAFE study randomised 6997 patients requiring resuscitation, 3500 to receive saline and 3497 to receive 4% albumin[§]
Deaths: saline group 729, albumin group 726 (relative risk of death 0.99, 95% CI 0.91 –1.09; $P = 0.85$)
There were no significant differences between the groups in new single-organ or multiple-organ failures, days spent in
   ICU, days in hospital, days on ventilator or days of renal replacement therapy
Conclusions: In patients in the ICU, use of either 4% albumin or normal saline for fluid resuscitation results in similar
   outcomes at 28 days

Red cell transfusion[‡]
838 sick patients in ITU
Randomised to transfuse to maintain Hb at 7–9 g/dL or 10–12 g/dL
Mortality at 30 days
   7—9 g/dL: 19%
   10–12 g/dL: 23%

---

[*]Cochrane Injuries Group Albumin Reviewers. Human albumin administration in critically ill patients: systematic review of randomised controlled trials. *Br Med J* 1998;317:235–240.
[†]Schierhout G & Roberts I. Fluid resuscitation with colloid or crystalloid solutions in critically ill patients: a systematic review of randomised trials. *Br Med J* 1998;316:961–964.
[‡]Hébert Wells G, Blajchman MA *et al.* A multicentre, randomized controlled clinical trial of transfusion requirements in critical care. *N Engl J Med* 1999;340:409–417.
[§]Finfer S, Bellomo R, Boyce N, French J, Myburgh J & Norton R, SAFE Study Investigators. A comparison of albumin and saline for fluid resuscitation in the intensive care unit. *N Engl J Med* 2004;350:2247–2256.

review (usually with an analysis of the pooled results) of clinical trials or other studies is an important way of examining the basis of current practice (Chapter 47). An example is the uncertainty revealed by systematic reviews of studies on the effects of various intravenous replacement fluids on mortality in severely ill patients, summarised in Table 25.1. The value of a large well-designed trial in resolving such uncertainty is illustrated by the SAFE trial in almost 7000 patients, which showed equivalent outcomes with no excess mortality or morbidity in patients resuscitated with 4% albumin compared with those randomised to receive normal saline. Subsequent sub-group analyses have also challenged conventional wisdom by finding an association between albumin use and adverse outcomes in head trauma when compared to saline resuscitation.

The value of systematic review evidence as a guide to best practice depends on the quality of the original trials and also on whether they reflect current clinical practice. They may identify therapies that are effective, ineffective or harmful but, as in the case of a recent systematic review of studies on the effects of fresh plasma transfusion, may also show that the available trials are simply inadequate to identify the clinical situations in which a blood component or product is beneficial or harmful.

Risks of transfusion

Chapters in Part 2 of this book deal with the specific infective and immunological risks associated with transfusion. In addition, there are a number of recent reports of adverse effects of transfusion found based on analyses of large clinical databases of patients who have undergone cardiac surgery. Many of these use propensity matching of patients to try to match cohorts who have similar risk factors in all areas except exposure to transfusion, thereby creating a 'virtual' randomised trial from non-randomised data. Many of these studies report an increase in all-cause mortality that has been interpreted as being associated with transfusion. Although such studies are useful, they risk providing misleading results due to confounding among factors such as severity of surgical bleeding with the use of transfusion, or factors that have not been included in the analyses. However, the number of such studies with similar findings, combined with the suggestive evidence from one large randomised trial that there may be higher mortality in more liberally transfused patients, should raise concerns and stimulate further well-controlled prospective studies that could detect adverse effects of transfusion on major clinical outcomes.

Which patients receive transfusions?

Transfusion of whole blood originated with the management of major bleeding in obstetrics trauma or surgery. In countries such as the UK, platelet and red cell support has become an essential support for the management of many malignant conditions. However, the 'epidemiology' of blood use is changing, and an increasing proportion of red cell transfusions is being prescribed for older patients, often with multiple pathologies, including for example chronic liver disease. In contrast, in many parts of the world a large proportion of blood is used for urgent management of life-threatening anaemia in infants and children often associated with malaria and for symptomatic treatment of anaemia associated with human immunodeficiency virus (HIV) therapy. The following sections outline some general principles that apply to all patients who may need transfusion, and some that relate to the specific broad categories of patients.

Good blood management

The guiding principle is that allogeneic (donor) blood should be prescribed only when the clinician is satisfied that it is likely to offer the patient a worthwhile benefit, or that the risk of not transfusing is likely to be greater than the risk of transfusing. However, as with much wise clinical advice, it can be extremely difficult to put this into effect.

Decision-making is straightforward when a patient has major haemorrhage, bleeding associated with profound thrombocytopenia or severe, disabling anaemia associated with cancer chemotherapy. However, many transfusions are given in situations where it is extremely difficult to estimate the probability that the patient will benefit. The challenge in clinical practice is to make this judgement where there is real uncertainty. An example is the decision whether or not to transfuse an elderly patient with a moderately low haemoglobin (Hb) concentration in the postoperative period. Retrospective studies of patients operated on for hip fracture reveal great variability in the use of perioperative red cell transfusion. There is at present no substantial evidence to tell us whether such patients (or a subgroup) are likely to do better if they are 'transfused up' or if they are allowed to remain moderately anaemic. Two pilot randomised controlled trials in hip-fractures patients examined the effect of alternative transfusion protocols (transfuse at a 'trigger' level of 10 g/dL *versus* transfuse only for symptoms). The use of the 10 g/dL trigger resulted in more transfusion (Table 25.2). The FOCUS study in the US plans to enroll 2600 patients to test the clinical outcomes of these alternative transfusion regimes.

From a public health perspective, good blood management embraces wider issues such as anaemia prevention through programmes on nutrition, malaria, HIV infection, parasite infestation and so on.

Blood management in elective surgery

In elective surgery, the low blood requirements of some surgical teams probably reflects their attention to the many individual elements of management that may greatly influence the need to transfuse. Many studies continue to show that there are large differences in the use of blood components for a given surgical procedure in apparently similar patient populations managed in different

Table 25.2 Influence of changing the 'transfusion trigger' on blood use in hip fracture patients: data from two pilot clinical trials.

Results

Location	Scotland*		United States	
Number eligible	73		192	
Number consented	61		143	
Postoperative Hb < 10 g/dL, >8 g/dL	23		96	
Randomised	9	9	40	40
Arm of trial	Trigger	Symptom	Trigger	Symptom
Completed protocol	9	9	37	35
Transfused: n (%)	9 (100)	1 (11)	39 (98)	19 (45)

The trial design was: patients admitted for repair of hip fracture (mean age 85 years) were randomised to either: 'symptomatic' (transfuse if symptoms or if Hb below 8 g/dL and clinician wishes to transfuse) vs. 'trigger' (transfuse to maintain Hb just above 10 g/dL).
*Two patients randomised in this series are included among the 80 randomised patients in the US study.
Data from: Carson JL *et al.* A pilot randomized trial comparing symptomatic vs. hemoglobin-level-driven red blood cell transfusions following hip fracture. *Transfusion* 1998;38:522–529; and Palmer JB *et al.* Hip fracture and transfusion trial (HATT) (abstract). *Transfus Med* 1998;8:36.

hospitals (Figure 25.1). This can only partly be explained by obvious factors such as the patient's age, gender and preoperative Hb concentration or by reported surgical variables such as blood loss or duration of operation. The use of blood conservation technologies (Table 25.3) may reduce the need for allogeneic transfusion especially where surgical blood usage is high (Chapter 33). These methods reduce the use of allogeneic transfusion but may have other consequences. For example, pre-deposit autologous transfusion usually increases the total amount of red cell units transfused when both autologous and allogeneic units are counted. It is also important to note that reductions in red cell transfusion are much more evident in studies that record a high blood use in the control group. In other words, some surgical teams manage their patients using transfusion infrequently and without recourse to any of the above blood-sparing methods. Transfusion and the decision to transfuse cannot be considered in isolation. Attention to the many aspects of the patient's management that influence the need for blood replacement is at least as important as the use of specific blood-sparing methods and may prove to be safer and more cost-effective.

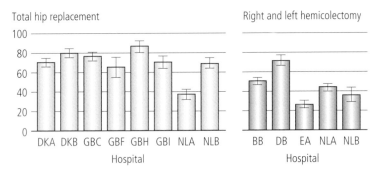

Figure 25.1 Proportion of operated patients perioperatively transfused with red cell units in each hospital, after adjustment for age, gender, preoperative haematocrit, and blood loss in THR (total hip replacement) and COLE (right and left hemicolectomy). Each hospital is identified by a country code followed by a letter, e.g. NL (Netherlands), hospital A (NLA). (Adapted from Sanguis Study Group. *Transfus Med* 1994;4:251–268.)

Table 25.3 In elective surgery the use of autologous blood and/or drugs reduces bleeding and RhEpo reduces the use of allogeneic transfusion.

Intervention	Type of surgery	No. of trials	No. of patients	Exposure to allogeneic (donor) blood. Odds ratio (95% confidence interval)
Autologous techniques				
PAD	Miscellaneous	6	933	0.17 (0.08–0.32)
ANH	Miscellaneous	16	615	0.31 (0.15–0.62)
ANH	Miscellaneous, methodologically sound	8	NR	0.64 (0.31–1.31)
Cell salvage				
Washed	Orthopaedic	7	429	0.39 (0.30–0.51)
Unwashed	Orthopaedic	9	733	0.35 (0.26–0.46)
Unwashed	Cardiac	12	899	0.85 (0.79–0.92)
Drugs				
Aprotinin	Cardiac	45	5808	0.31 (0.25–0.39)
Desmopressin	Cardiac	12	793	0.98 (0.64–1.50)
Tranexamic acid	Cardiac	12	882	0.50 (0.34–0.76)
Aminocaproic acid	Cardiac	3	118	0.20 (0.004–1.12)
RhEpo + PAD	Orthopaedic	11	825	0.42 (0.28–0.62)
RhEpo + PAD	Cardiac	5	224	0.25 (0.08–0.82)
RhEpo alone	Orthopaedic	3	684	0.36 (0.24–0.56)
RhEpo alone	Cardiac	2	245	0.25 (0.06–1.04)

ANH, acute normovolaemic haemodilution; NR, not recorded; PAD, preoperative autologous blood donation.

Adapted from Laupacis A & Fergusson D, for the International Study of Perioperative Transfusion (ISPOT) Investigators. Drugs to minimize perioperative blood loss in cardiac surgery: meta-analyses using perioperative blood transfusion as the outcome. *Anesth Analg* 1997;85(6):1258–1267.

Adapted from Huët C, Salmi LR, Fergusson D, Koopman-van Gemert AW, Rubens F & Laupacis A, for the International Study of Perioperative Transfusion (ISPOT) Investigators. A meta-analysis of the effectiveness of cell salvage to minimize perioperative allogeneic blood transfusion in cardiac and orthopedic surgery. *Anesth Analg* 1999;89(4):861–869.

Transfusion protocols or local practice guidelines

A systematic review of the effects of clinical transfusion protocols indicates that the use of a protocol that, for example specifies guideline Hb concentrations for transfusion and a plan for routine Hb or haemostasis checks at relevant stages can be a useful way to help reduce large and unexplainable variations in practice. Recorded Hb values and transfusion data provide objective data for clinical quality assurance.

Blood management targets and interventions: elective surgery and emergencies

• Optimise the haemoglobin concentration before planned surgery.

  ○ detect anaemia, identify cause and treat;
  ○ haematinics;
  ○ RhEpo with iron.
• Optimise iron stores before surgery, even if patient not anemic.
• Optimise haemostasis before planned surgery.
  ○ identify congenital coagulation disorders;
  ○ withdraw drugs that impair haemostasis (if safe to do so).
• Improve haemostasis during surgery.
  ○ anaesthetic techniques;
  ○ surgical techniques;
  ○ positioning;
  ○ antifibrinolytic drugs;
  ○ avoid hypothermia;
  ○ collect and re-infuse blood lost during surgery;
  ○ intraoperative blood salvage.

Autologous transfusion techniques are described in Chapter 34.

Erythropoietin (RhEpo, epoietin, human recombinant erythropoietin)

This is a peptide hormone, normally made in the kidney (Chapter 43). The therapeutic product is made by genetically engineered expression of the human erythropoetin gene. There are currently three products licenced in the UK, with some differences in the licenced indications. RhEpo is a potent stimulator of erythropoiesis although some recent evidence suggests that it may also have other physiological effects. Effective use in the surgical context may require parenteral iron administration.

RhEpo, like red cell transfusion, has its risks. If the Hb concentration is raised too rapidly, or too high, the risk of hypertension and thrombosis increase. These complications are a reminder that even infrequent adverse events due to alternatives to conventional transfusion must not be ignored.

Parenteral iron preparations are often used with RhEpo to deliver the iron required for rapid erythropoiesis.

Pharmacological agents used to reduce surgical bleeding

These are aprotinins which affect platelet function and fibrinolysis, tranexamic acid and ε-aminocaproic acid (EACA) (inhibitors of fibrinolysis), and desmopressin (1-deamino-8-D-arginine vasopressin or DDAVP) which acts centrally to increase plasma factor VIII levels. Recent (and controversial) observational studies have suggested that aprotinin may be associated with poor outcomes in cardiac surgery patients. A large randomised trial comparing the efficacy and safety of different antifibrinolytic treatments in high-risk cardiac surgery patients (the BART trial) was recently terminated because of excess mortality with aprotinin, despite clear evidence of a blood sparing effect. At the time of writing aprotinin cannot be recommended in this setting until further information is available from this important trial. These agents are described in detail in Chapter 36.

Recombinant factor VIIa

This product is effective for haemophilia patients with inhibitors. It can also be used to control massive surgical, traumatic or obstetric bleeding although it is not licenced for these indications and its effectiveness remains a matter of controversy (Chapter 36). Because there may be risks of thrombotic complications and the drug is currently extremely expensive, hospitals have special procedures for making it available, for example by consultation with a haematologist with an interest in haemostasis.

A 'total quality management' approach to minimise anaemia, bleeding and the need for transfusion

Individual surgical teams can manage their patients to minimise the need for transfusion without recourse to specific 'blood-sparing' technologies. This may reflect the use of protocols to guide transfusion decisions, and a commitment to attend to the many individual details of management that can reduce the need for blood replacement (Chapter 33).

A quality assurance system for management of anaemia and bleeding in surgery could be defined as an integrated approach that covers all aspects of management that influence the quality of care provided for the patient and ensures that they are consistently, correctly handled.

Indications for the use of blood components

Red cells and whole blood (Table 25.4)

Acute anaemia and bleeding: clinical assessment and the decision to transfuse

The generally accepted reason for transfusing red cells is to increase the circulating red cell mass as a means of improving oxygen supply to the tissues. On this basis, transfusion is indicated only if reduction in oxygen supply causes a clinically significant problem, and if it is likely that oxygen supply will be improved by a rapid increase in red cell mass. Current practice in surgery and critical care in developed countries, much influenced by one large trial on ICU patients (Table 25.1), is to adopt Hb

Table 25.4 Use of red cell components.

To increase circulating red cell mass with the intention to relieve clinical features caused by insufficient oxygen delivery in special situations such as in sickle cell disease and thalassaemia (see Chapter 10)		
Examples of clinical quality assurance indicators: red cell prescription indicator	Observed	
Patient records contain correct details of red cell transfusion	95% of records	
Hb value recorded before transfusion	90% of records	
Patient records contain a stated reason for transfusion	23%	
'Avoidable' red cell transfusion	% of red cell transfusions	
Percentage of red cell units given that result in a discharge of Hct above 33%	23% (lowest clinical unit)	
82% (highest clinical unit)		
Red cell transfusion during patient admission for specified procedure	Percentage transfused	Units of red cells per transfused patient
Colectomy	0–79 (41)	0.3 (1)
Transurethral resection of prostate	0–46 (17)	0–1 (0.5)
Coronary artery bypass graft	17–100 (83)	0–6 (3)
Repair of abdominal aortic aneurysm	64–100 (83)	0–6 (3)
Primary unilateral hip arthroplasty	29–100 (81)	0.5 (2)

Adapted from The Sanguis Study Group. Use of blood products for elective surgery in 43 European hospitals. *Transfus Med* 1994;4:251–268.

concentrations of 7–8 g/dL as the threshold below which transfusion is indicated.

Recent studies raise some questions about both the above rationale for red cell transfusion and the adoption of this threshold Hb concentration. When resting subjects are intentionally haemodiluted to very low Hb concentrations, evidence of myocardial ischaemia is rare and only appears at Hb concentrations of 5–6 g/dL. When stable ICU patients were transfused with 2 units of red cells at an Hb of 8–9 g/dL, there was no observable improvement in any of the ICU measures of systemic or regional oxygenation. These findings appear to suggest that even lower Hb thresholds could be appropriate for red cell transfusion, at least in some patient groups. On the other side of the debate, it is known that athletes' performance improves objectively when Hb concentrations are raised to the high normal range by autologous transfusion or RhEpo.

In some clinical situations, the Hb concentration may be a poor indicator of the need to restore red cell mass by transfusion. After major surgery, there may be a period when Hb concentration is lowered by the effects of haemodilution as well as blood loss and must be interpreted in the light of the patient's fluid status. In practice, the decision to transfuse is also influenced by known and estimated blood loss and by the clinical judgement of the risk of further bleeding.

Chronic anaemia

Patients with chronic renal failure have improved clinical outcomes if Hb concentrations are maintained in the region of 11 g/dL. Clinical experience, backed by at least one study, is that many chronically anaemic patients including those with malignant disease have an improved quality of life if Hb concentrations are kept nearer the normal range. It is not yet known whether such patients benefit equally when the Hb concentrations are maintained by RhEpo treatment or by red cell transfusion.

The available evidence does not allow us to conclude that the conservative transfusion guidelines currently recommended for surgical and critically ill patients are suitable for patients with chronic anaemia due to a serious underlying disorder. Current guidelines therefore advise that for surgical or critically ill patients with evidence of heart disease, transfusion at a Hb concentration around 10 g/dL is a reasonable compromise until better evidence is available.

Clinical factors relevant to the decision to transfuse (Table 25.5)

One way to aid clinical decision-making is to summarise the factors that are most important in making the decision into a simple checklist or algorithm that can be used (on paper or in the head) to help to focus the decision on whether or not to transfuse. Figure 25.2 is an illustration of this approach.

Single unit transfusion of red cells?

Dogmatic statements have often been made that there is no case for giving a single unit transfusion. This dogma should be ignored. For example, in the case of a 45-kg patient with hypoxic signs or symptoms attributed to a Hb concentration of 7 g/dL, a single unit of red cells may be quite sufficient to relieve symptoms (and raise the Hb concentration by 1–2 g/dL).

Whole blood versus red cell concentrate

(Table 25.6)

The doctrine of blood component therapy (together with the requirement for plasma for fractionation) has encouraged the almost universal use of red cell concentrates in most developed countries. Whole blood may be entirely appropriate for a patient with acute bleeding who requires both red cells and expansion of plasma volume. The clinical experience of military surgical teams is that the early administration of plasma with red cells (in approximately equal volumes) appears to be associated with better achievement of haemostasis. In cases when disseminated intravascular coagulation (DIC) contributes to the blood loss, it may be entirely logical to use whole blood (or leucocyte-depleted whole blood) since it contains at least a part of the total dose of fibrinogen and stable clotting factors that the patient requires and can reduce the need for plasma units from other donors. The suggestion that whole

Table 25.5 Factors in deciding whether a patient needs transfusion.

Blood loss
External bleeding
Internal bleeding – non-traumatic, e.g. peptic ulcer, varices, ectopic pregnancy, antepartum haemorrhage, ruptured uterus
Internal bleeding – traumatic, chest, spleen, pelvis, femur(s)
Red cell destruction, e.g. malaria, sepsis, HIV
Haemolysis, e.g.
Malaria
Sepsis
HIV

Cardiorespiratory state and tissue oxygenation
Pulse rate
Blood pressure
Respiratory rate
Capillary refill
Peripheral pulses
Temperature of extremities
Dyspnoea
Cardiac failure
Angina
Conscious level
Urine output

Haemoglobin estimate
Clinical
    Tongue
    Palms
    Eyes
    Nails
Laboratory: haemoglobin or haematocrit (PCV)

Patient's tolerance of blood loss and anaemia
Age
Other conditions, e.g. diabetes, pre-eclampsic toxanaemia, renal failure, cardiorespiratory disease, chronic lung disease, acute infection, treatment with β-blockers
Anticipated need for blood
Is surgery or anaesthesia anticipated?
Is bleeding continuing, stopped or likely to recur?
Is haemolysis continuing?

blood may be appropriate for some patients will be seen by some as highly controversial, although in many parts of the world it is widely used.

In the UK, because of concerns that plasma may contain infectivity for vCJD, every effort has been made to minimise the transfusion of plasma from

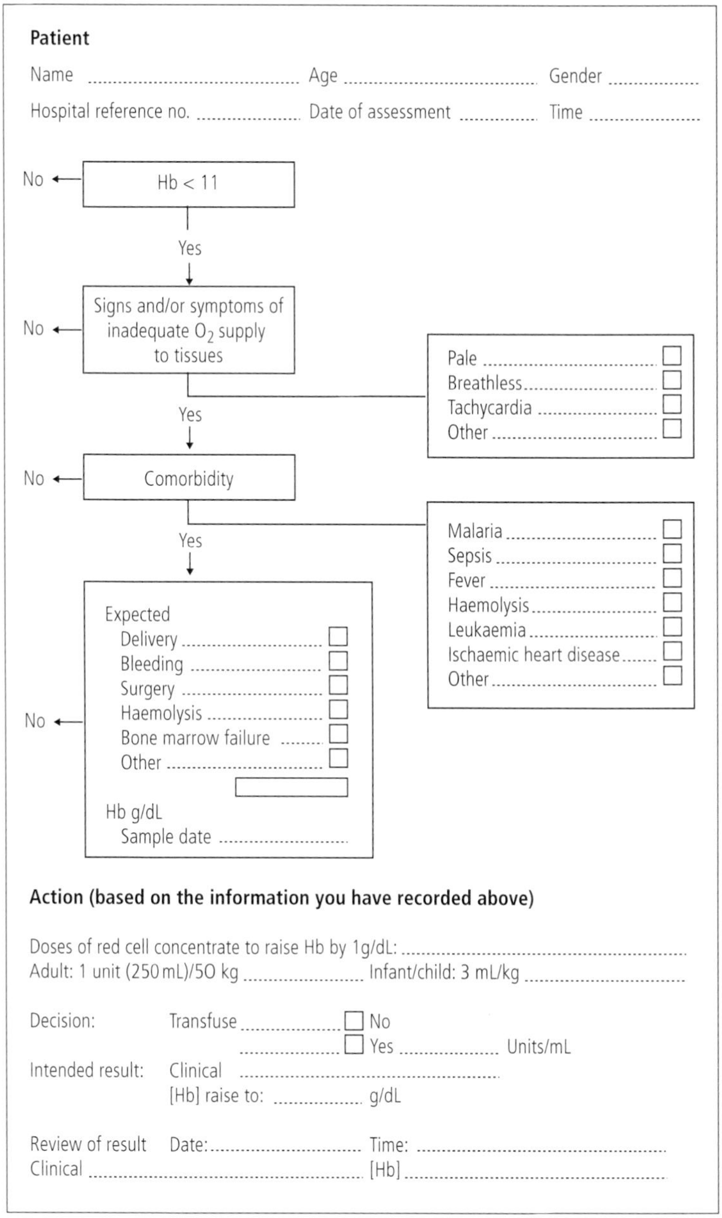

Patient

Name .... Age .... Gender ....

Hospital reference no. .... Date of assessment .... Time ....

No ← | Hb < 11 |

Yes

No ← | Signs and/or symptoms of inadequate O_2 supply to tissues |

Pale .... ☐
Breathless............................ ☐
Tachycardia .... ☐
Other .... ☐

Yes

No ← | Comorbidity |

Malaria .... ☐
Sepsis .... ☐
Fever .... ☐
Haemolysis .... ☐
Leukaemia .... ☐
Ischaemic heart disease........ ☐
Other.................................. ☐

Yes

Expected
  Delivery .... ☐
  Bleeding .... ☐
  Surgery .... ☐
No ← Haemolysis .... ☐
  Bone marrow failure .... ☐
  Other .... ☐

Hb g/dL
  Sample date ....

Action (based on the information you have recorded above)

Doses of red cell concentrate to raise Hb by 1g/dL: ....
Adult: 1 unit (250 mL)/50 kg .... Infant/child: 3 mL/kg ....

Decision: Transfuse .... ☐ No
                              .... ☐ Yes .... Units/mL
Intended result: Clinical ....
                   [Hb] raise to: .... g/dL

Review of result   Date:............................ Time: ....
Clinical .... [Hb] ....

Figure 25.2   Example of a transfusion decision chart.

UK donors, and while this concern persists it would preclude the use of whole blood.

Fresh or stored red cells for transfusion?

There are biologically plausible reasons why stored red cells may be less effective in restoring oxygen-carrying capacity than fresh red cells. A widely quoted clinical study suggested that transfusion of stored red cells could actually impair regional oxygenation. The clinical trial summarised in Table 25.1 suggested that some ICU patients maintained at a lower Hb concentration, and so receiving less

Table 25.6 Whole blood or red cell concentrates?

Whole blood concentrates	Red cell concentrates
Contains plasma	Minimal plasma content
Replaces fibrinogen and other stable coagulation factors	Does not replace coagulation factors
Volume-expanding effect of plasma may be an advantage in a hypovolaemic patient	If colloid volume expansion is shown to be harmful, the absence of plasma could be a benefit
Red cells and plasma from the same donor	If both red cells and plasma are required, the patient is exposed to more donors
Colloid volume expansion effect could cause volume overload	Less volume load per dose of red cells, so safer if the patient is normovolaemic
Does not produce plasma	Provides plasma (FFP is likely to be used inappropriately if available!)
Does not contain platelets or factor VIII	
In the UK and some other countries, supplied as leucocyte-depleted	
There is little or no good clinical trial evidence to compare the effectiveness of whole blood vs. red cell concentrates	
Whole blood is intrinsically simpler and cheaper to prepare. This may be extremely important in countries with restricted health budgets.	

FFP, fresh frozen plasma.

transfusion, may have improved outcomes. One interpretation of this observation is that this could be associated with some adverse effect of transfusing stored red cells. This could not be confirmed in a recent blinded randomised controlled study comparing the effect of fresh versus stored leucocyte-depleted red cells on systemic and regional oxygenation in ICU patients. Another study of the effect of acute anaemia on cognitive function in healthy subjects detected no difference in the response when haemoglobin concentrations were restored with fresh or stored autologous red cells. Conversely, several large uncontrolled studies have found associations between transfusing older stored red cells and fresher red cells, even after adjusting for other potentially important factors. The current evidence does not provide a clear answer regarding the clinical importance of red cell storage, especially with leucodepleted blood. Therefore, although there are strong beliefs in the superiority of fresh red cells, there is no clear evidence to support the selection of fresh red cells for critically ill patients.

Fresh frozen plasma (Table 25.7)

Worldwide, the largest avoidable risk to patients from transfusion is probably due to the transfusion of fresh frozen plasma (FFP) for unproven clinical indications. Plasma is just as likely as whole blood to transmit viral infections (other than those that are strictly cell associated). In any area where blood safety testing may be unreliable, transfusion of FFP can be an important source of transmission of these infections. A recent systematic review suggests that there are few well-supported indications for transfusing FFP, and this is reflected in the recent UK clinical guideline.

FFP should be used only to replace rare clotting factor deficiencies for which no virus-safe fractionated plasma product is available or when there is a multifactor deficiency due to severe bleeding and DIC. Other indications for FFP (Chapter 30) are the management of thrombotic thrombocytopenic purpura (TTP) and haemolytic uraemic syndrome (HUS), in which plasma infusion or plasma exchange with FFP is effective. A recent systematic review concludes that

Table 25.7 Use of fresh frozen plasma (FFP) and cryoprecipitate.

Replacement of plasma coagulation factors if a suitable
  licenced virus-inactivated product is not available
Some special indications, e.g. thrombotic
  thrombocytopenia purpura: infusion of plasma or
  plasma exchange with FFP (see Chapter 12)
Contraindications
To replace circulatory fluid volume
To raise plasma albumin level
As an alternative to TPN
Example of clinical quality assurance indicator – FFP prescription

Indicator	Observed* Pre-transfusion (%)	Post-transfusion (%)
Prothrombin ratio recorded	94	94
Prothrombin ratio >2	68	11

*19 FFP transfusion episodes in 12 consecutive patients (unpublished local audit report).

there is little sound evidence for other uses of FFP.

Does fresh frozen plasma have to be used immediately after thawing?

After thawing, the level of factor VIII falls rapidly. Factor V also falls, but levels of fibrinogen and the other haemostatic proteins are maintained. UK guidelines permit the use of plasma that has been stored in the blood bank for up to 24 hours after thawing. This has the advantage that plasma can be released quickly when required for urgent management of massive bleeding.

Minimising vCJD risk in the UK

In the UK, because of concerns about possible risks of transmitting vCJD (Chapter 15), the Departments of Health have recommended that plasma imported from countries not affected by BSE be used for all patients born after 1 January 1996 for whom FFP is indicated. To safeguard against viral infections undetected by testing, this plasma is treated to reduce any risk of infectivity and is termed pathogen-reduced plasma. This additional processing causes reduced levels of plasma proteins, including procoagulants such as fibrinogen and anticoagulants such as Protein S. In one product, in which pooled plasma was treated with solvent and detergent, there were reports that reduced levels of natural anticoagulant proteins may cause an increased risk of thrombosis in some patients receiving large doses of FFP

Fibrinogen replacement (Table 25.7)

Cryoprecipitate is generally only indicated as a source of fibrinogen in management of DIC, e.g. in obstetric haemorrhage. If no virus-inactivated plasma fraction is available, cryoprecipitate is used to replace factor VIII in haemophilia A and von Willebrand's disease (vWD) (Chapter 30). Pathogen-reduced cryoprecipitate from non-UK plasma should be used for patients born after 1996 according to Departments of Health guidance. An alternative is the use of a virus-inactivated fibrinogen concentrate, but the only such product currently available in UK is not currently licenced for use in haemorrhage.

Platelets (Table 25.8)

Use of platelet transfusions has increased over many years. Audit against current guidelines may reveal possible ways of reducing prescribing within current guidelines. A brief summary of indications for platelet transfusion follows (and see Chapter 27).

Table 25.8 Use of platelets (platelet concentrate).

Treat bleeding due to thrombocytopenia, e.g.
   Platelet below 10×10^9/L due to bone marrow failure
   Platelet count below 50×10^9/L prior to surgery in critical area (head and neck)
      or invasive procedure (see Chapter 27)
   In management of haemorrhage ('massive transfusion')
   During/after surgery on cardiopulmonary bypass, where 'pump' damages
      platelets (see Chapters 27 and 30)
Example of clinical quality assurance indicator – platelet prescription

Indicator Platelet count recorded	Observed[*] (%) % of transfusion episodes
Within guideline	70
Pre-transfusion	89
Post-transfusion	85
Increased by at least 20×10^9/L	70

[*]1701 episodes of platelet transfusion in 138 patients (unpublished local audit report).

Prophylaxis of bleeding due to bone marrow failure with thrombocytopenia

Recent studies indicate that the clinically stable patient is unlikely to benefit from prophylactic platelet transfusion if the platelet count is greater than 10×10^9/L. A higher threshold for transfusion is appropriate with sepsis and other complications (see Chapter 28).

Surgery in the thrombocytopenic patient

UK guidelines provide recommendations to minimise the risks due to bleeding in critical surgical sites such as head, neck and spinal canal (see Chapter 27).

Urgent and emergency transfusion – major bleeding

Examples of clinical scenarios in which transfusion may be needed are summarised in Table 25.9 and discussed in detail in other chapters.

This section concludes by reviewing some of the issues that arise in clinical situations where there is acute haemorrhage, or the expectation of it, so that blood is required very rapidly. There is little or no systematic evidence for the effectiveness of the measures suggested, and trials to evaluate them

are required although these trials will be extremely difficult to perform.

Clinical and blood bank experience and a recent report from France on anaesthetic-related deaths indicate that delays in providing blood in a life-threatening emergency (or failure to detect and respond promptly to severe anaemia) can put patients at risk. Consistent use of a simple, agreed terminology and for urgent contacts between, for example the labour ward and the blood bank may avoid delays in blood supply and save lives.

Hospital major haemorrhage protocol

The use of a hospital major haemorrhage protocol communicated effectively to all relevant staff is a sensible measure to improve responses, and occasional 'fire drills' to familarise staff and test the protocol have been found useful by staff in at least one large teaching hospital. Analysis by national haemovigilance schemes of delays in supplying blood in emergencies would be a valuable way of sharing experience and building knowledge of effective strategies for providing blood safely in emergencies.

Table 25.9 Some clinical situations where component transfusion may be needed.

Situation	Factors that may influence the decision to transfuse or not
Emergencies	
Obstetric haemorrhage	Clinical assessment during resuscitation
Trauma	
Ruptured aortic aneurysm	
Upper GI bleeding	
Elective surgery	
Cardiac	Previously fit patient
Orthopaedic	Elderly, cardiovascular disease
Solid tumours	Liver disease
	Other comorbidity
	Pre-existing anaemia
	Bleeding tendency
	Jehovah's Witness
Bone marrow failure	
Malignant	Stable
Myelodysplastic	Fever
Drugs or chemicals	Splenomegaly
Infective	Platelet count
	Stage of treatment
The ITU patient	
Postoperative recovery	Oxygenation measurements
Sepsis syndrome	Hb
	Platelet count
Inherited Hb disorders	
Infections	
Malaria	Age
HIV	Pregnancy, delivery
	Surgery
Immunological disorders	
Immune haemolysis	
Immune cytopenias	
Neonatal problems	
HDN, blood sampling	

Dealing with emergency casualties

A single patient with catastrophic bleeding is a major challenge for the clinical team. Road traffic accidents and other less common disasters may bring several desperately ill patients in quick succession, adding the risks that can result from uncertainties in patient identification. These are situations when it is vital for all the team to know and use the established local emergency procedures for:

- requesting blood;
- completing request forms and labelling samples;
- communicating precisely with the transfusion laboratory; and
- checking blood components before collection and transfusion.

It is extremely important to have clear communications between clinicians and the blood bank, and essential to have a simple standard procedure, such as that described below. All staff (medical, nursing, laboratory and transport) play a very important part, and should be trained in the use of this procedure, including an understanding of the importance of their role.

Emergency transfusion procedures

An example of a hospital protocol for major haemorrhage is given in Table 25.10.

1 In an emergency, insert at least two large bore intravenous cannulae, use one to take the blood sample for cross-matching and other blood tests, set up the intravenous infusion and get the blood sample and blood request form to the blood bank as quickly as possible.

2 Make sure yourself that the blood bank staff know when the blood is required and why.

3 For each patient, the cross-match sample tube and the blood request form must be clearly labelled. If the patient is unidentified, some form of emergency admission number should be used. Use the patient's name only if you are sure you have correct information.

4 If another request for blood is needed for the same patient within a short period, use the same identifiers as on the first request form and blood sample so that the blood bank staff will know it is the same patient.

5 If there are several staff working with emergency cases, one person should take charge of ordering blood and communicating with the blood bank about the incident. This is especially important if several injured patients are involved at the same time.

6 If there is a special stock of 'emergency O negative' blood, e.g. in the labour ward, use this first in an emergency. *Do not wait for cross-matched blood if the patient is exsanguinating.*

Table 25.10 Example of a hospital policy for massive blood loss.

Immediate actions	Key points	Other considerations
Arrest bleeding	Early surgical or obstetric intervention Upper gastrointestinal tract procedures Interventional radiology	
Contact key personnel	Most appropriate surgical team Duty anaesthetist Blood transfusion laboratory	
Restore circulating volume	Insert wide-bore peripheral cannulae	Blood loss is often underestimated
NB: In patients with major vessel or cardiac injury, it may be appropriate to restrict volume replacement after discussion with surgical team	Give adequate volumes of crystalloid/blood	Refer to local guidelines for the resuscitation of trauma patients and for red cell transfusion
	Aim to maintain normal blood pressure and urine output >30 mL/h in adults (0.5 mL/kg per h)	Monitor CVP if haemodynamically unstable
Request laboratory investigations	FBC, PT, APTT, fibrinogen; blood bank sample, biochemical profile, blood gases	Take samples at earliest opportunity as results may be affected by colloid infusion
	Ensure correct sample identity and use of red label for transfusion samples	Misidentification is commonest transfusion risk
	Repeat FBC, PT, APTT, fibrinogen every 4 h, or after one-third blood volume replacement, or after infusion of FFP	May need to give FFP and platelets before the FBC and coagulation results available
Request suitable red cells NB: All red cells are now leucocyte depleted. Volume is provided on each pack, and is in the range 190–420 mL	*Blood needed immediately*	Contact blood transfusion laboratory or on-call laboratory scientist and provide relevant details
	Use 'emergency stock' group O RhD negative	
	Blood needed in 15–60 min	Collect sample for group and cross-match before using emergency stock
	Un-cross-matched ABO group specific will be provided when blood group known (15–60 min from receipt of sample in laboratory)	Emergency use of RhD-positive blood is acceptable if patient is male or postmenopausal female
	Blood needed in 60 min or longer	Blood warmer indicated if large volumes are transfused rapidly
	Fully cross-matched blood will be provided	Consider use of cell salvage
Consider use of platelets	Anticipate platelet count < 50 × 10^9/L after 1.5–2 × blood volume replacement	Target platelet count >100 × 10^9/L for multiple/CNS trauma, > 50 × 10^9/L for other situations

(*Continued*)

Table 25.10 (*Continued*)

Immediate actions	Key points	Other considerations
	Dose: 10 mL/kg body weight for a neonate or small child, otherwise one 'adult therapeutic dose' (one pack)	May need to use platelets before laboratory results available: take FBC sample before platelets transfused
Consider use of FFP	Anticipate coagulation factor deficiency after blood loss of 1.5 × blood volume	PT/APTT >1.5 × mean control correlates with increased surgical bleeding
	Aim for PT/APTT < 1.5 × mean control	May need to use FFP before laboratory results available: take sample for PT, APTT, fibrinogen before FFP transfused
	Allow for 30-min thawing time Dose: 12–15 mL/kg body weight (1 L or 4 units for an adult)	
Consider use of cryoprecipitate	To replace fibrinogen and factor VIII	Fibrinogen < 0.5 g/L strongly associated with microvascular bleeding
	Aim for fibrinogen > 1.0 g/L Allow for 30 min thawing time Dose: 1 pack/10 kg body weight	
Suspect DIC	Treat underlying cause if possible	Shock, hypothermia, acidosis: increased risk of DIC
	Mortality of DIC is high	

APTT, activated partial thromboplastin time; CNS, central nervous system; CVP, central venous pressure; DIC, disseminated intravascular coagulation; FBC, full blood count; FFP, fresh frozen plasma; PT, prothrombin time.
Adapted from Stainsby D, MacLennan S, Thomas D, Isaac J & Hamilton PJ. Guidelines on the management of massive blood loss. British Committee for Standards in Haematology 2000. with permission.

7 Tell the blood bank how quickly the blood is needed for each patient. Communicate using words that have been previously agreed with the blood bank to explain how urgently blood is needed.

8 Do not ask for 'cross-matched blood' in an emergency. Ask the blood bank to supply what can be provided most quickly with reasonable safety according to the local policy.

Step 1: Ask the patient to tell you their full name and date of birth

Step 2: Check these details against the patient's wristband

Step 3: Check the hospital ID number on the patient's wristband against documentation, e.g. patient case notes or request form

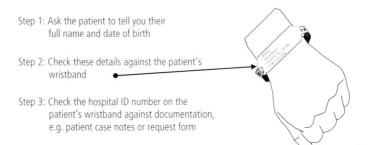

Figure 25.3   Hospital procedures for safe transfusion. (a) Collection of blood sample for pretransfusion testing. Be extra vigilant when checking the identity of the unconscious/compromised patient.

(a)

Step 1: Complete the blood collection form (or follow the
local collection procedure) with the following information:

- Forename
- Surname
- Date of birth
- Hospital number

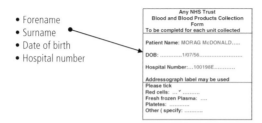

For each blood component collected

Step 2: Check patient ID details
against compatibility label
attached to the blood
component

Step 3: Document removal of
unit on blood fridge
register or electronic
release system

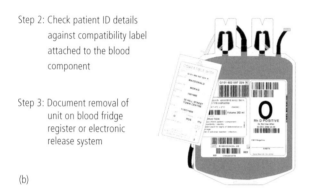

(b)

Step 1: Check the blood component has been prescribed
Step 2: Undertake baseline observations
Step 3: Before approaching the patient check the component for:

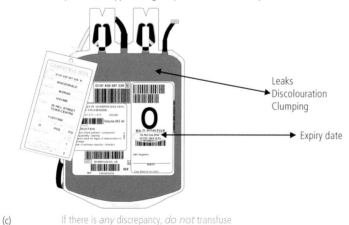

Leaks
Discolouration
Clumping

Expiry date

(c)   If there is *any* discrepancy, *do not* transfuse

Figure 25.3 (*Continued*) (b) Procedure for
collection of blood from the blood
refrigerator. NB Follow procedure for each
blood component collected. (c) Procedure
for the administration of blood.

Step1: Ask the patient to tell you their full name and date of birth (where possible)
Step2: Check ID details against the patient's wristband and compatibility label

Compatibility label

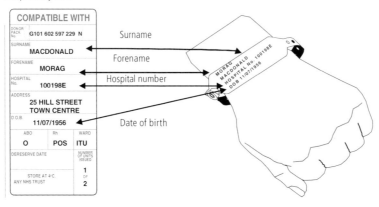

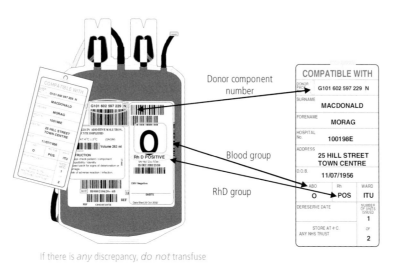

If there is *any* discrepancy, *do not* transfuse   (d)

Figure 25.3 (*Continued*) (d) Identification checks at the bedside before transfusion. Be extra vigilant when checking the identity of the unconscious/compromised patient.

9 Make sure that both you and the blood bank staff know:
  ○ who is going to bring the blood to the patient; and
  ○ where the patient will be, for example if your patient is about to be transferred to an-

other part of the hospital for an X-ray, make sure the blood will be delivered to the X-ray room.

10 The blood bank may send group O (and possibly RhD negative) blood, especially if there is any risk of errors in patient identification. In an

Example compatibility report
form

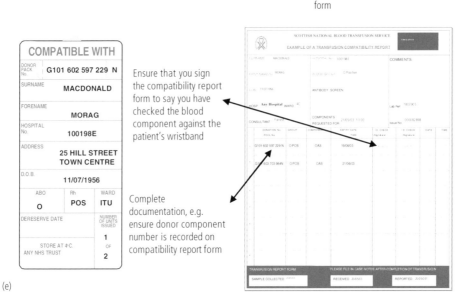

Figure 25.3 (*Continued*) (e) Documenting the transfusion on the compatibility report form.

emergency, this may be the safest way to avoid a serious mismatched transfusion.

Resuscitation and management of massive blood loss are dealt with in Chapters 29 and 29, and more information about hospital transfusion procedures can be found in Chapter 23.

Avoiding the biggest risks of transfusion

A full review of transfusion risks is given in Part 2 of this book. This section deals with risks that are common and which the clinical staff can prevent by adhering to simple procedures. The first is the risk of patients receiving a blood component that was intended for someone else, and the second is that of a special requirement – such as gamma-irradiated or CMV seronegative blood – which is not specified when blood is ordered. Following the simple rules shown below and in Figure 25.3 will go a long way in preventing avoidable harm to patients.

• When completing the blood request form, make sure the need for the transfusion and any special product, such as CMV seronegative or gamma-irradiated blood components, is clearly stated.

• Record your decision to prescribe and administer a transfusion. There are two important reasons for writing in the patient's notes the reason for giving a transfusion. It concentrates the mind to have to write down and sign a permanent record of the basis of your clinical decision.

• Should the patient have a problem related to the transfusion, such as developing hepatitis in the future, the record of the clinical decision may prove to be important medicolegal evidence. A record that the patient has been given information about the transfusion (see above) may equally be an important medicolegal evidence, as doctors have been criticised for alleged past failures to inform patients about the risks of blood products.

Key points

It may be helpful when considering risks and benefits to think of a transfusion as a transplant of human tissue, and not as a drug, or when you are uncertain if transfusion is likely to offer a useful benefit to the patient.

Before ordering blood in preparation for planned surgery

1 Can I reduce this patient's need for transfusion by correcting anaemia, stopping warfarin or aspirin, checking for a coagulation disorder or arranging in advance for intraoperative cell salvage to be available in theatre?

Before prescribing blood or blood products

2 What improvement in the patient's clinical condition am I aiming to achieve?

3 Are there any other treatments I should give before making the decision to transfuse, such as intravenous replacement fluids or oxygen?

4 What are the specific clinical or laboratory indications for transfusion for this patient?

5 Do the benefits of transfusion outweigh the risks for this particular patient?

6 What other options are there if no blood is available in time?

7 Will a trained person monitor this patient and respond immediately if any acute transfusion reactions occur?

8 Have I recorded my decision and reasons for transfusion on the patient's chart and the blood request form?

9 Finally, ask yourself. If this were myself, my child or my partner, would I agree to the transfusion?

Further reading

Websites

www.learnbloodtransfusion.org.uk. E learning programmes for safe blood transfusion, information about blood components etc. Accessed at January 2009.

www.transfusionguidelines.org.uk. *Free access to UK Handbook of Transfusion Medicine*, 4th edn 2007, Better Blood Transfusion Toolkit, UK standards for blood components. Links to BCSH Guidelines, Cochrane library etc. Accessed at January 2009.

Systematic reviews

Carless PA, Henry DA, Moxey AJ, O'Connell DL, Brown T & Fergusson DA. Cell salvage for minimising perioperative allogeneic blood transfusion. *Cochrane Database Syst Rev* 2006;(4):CD001888.

Carson JL, Hill S, Carless P, Hebert P & Henry D. Transfusion triggers: a systematic review of the literature. *Transfus Med Rev* 2002;16:187–199.

Hill SR, Carless PA, Henry DA *et al.* Transfusion thresholds and other strategies for guiding allogeneic red blood cell transfusion. *Cochrane Database Syst Rev* 2000;(1):CD002042.

Stanworth SJ, Brunskill SJ, Hyde CJ, McClelland DB & Murphy MF. Is fresh frozen plasma clinically effective? A systematic review of randomised controlled trials. *Br J Haematol* 2004;126:139–152.

Stanworth SJ, Brunskill SJ, Hyde CJ, Murphy MF & McClelland DBL. Appraisal of the evidence for the clinical use of FFP and plasma fractions. *Best Pract Res Clin Haematol* 2006;19:67–82.

Stanworth SJ, Hyde C, Brunskill S & Murphy M. Platelet transfusion prophylaxis for patients with haematological malignancies: where to now? *Br J Haematol* 2005;131:588–595.

Stanworth SJ, Hyde C, Heddle N, Rebulla P, Brunskill S & Murphy MF. Prophylactic platelet transfusion for haemorrhage after chemotherapy and stem cell transplantation. *Cochrane Database Syst Rev* 2004;(4):CD004269.

Wilson J, Yao GL, Raftery J *et al.* A systematic review and economic evaluation of epoetin alfa, epoetin beta and darbepoetin alfa in anaemia associated with cancer, especially that attributable to cancer treatment. *Health Technol Assess* 2007;11:1–220.

Original papers

Auroy Y, Lienhart A, Péquignot F & Benhamou D. Complications related to blood transfusion in surgical patients: data from the French national survey on anesthesia-related deaths. *Transfusion* 2007;47(Suppl 2):184S–189S.

Carson JL, Terrin ML, Magaziner J *et al.*, FOCUS Investigators. Transfusion trigger trial for functional outcomes in cardiovascular patients undergoing surgical hip fracture repair (FOCUS). *Transfusion* 2006;46:2192–2206.

Finfer S, Bellomo R, Boyce N, French J, Myburgh J & Norton R, SAFE Study Investigators. A comparison of albumin and saline for fluid resuscitation in the intensive care unit. *N Engl J Med* 2004;350:2247–2256.

Hébert PC, Wells G, Blajchman MA *et al.* With the Transfusion Requirements in Critical Care Investigators for the Canadian Critical Care Trials Group. A multicentre, randomized controlled clinical trial of transfusion requirements in critical care. *N Engl J Med* 1999;340:409–417.

Kirpalani H, Whyte RK, Andersen C *et al.* The Premature Infants in Need of Transfusion (PINT) study: a randomized, controlled trial of a restrictive (low) versus liberal (high) transfusion threshold for extremely low birth weight infants. *J Pediatr* 2006;149:301–307.

Lienhart A, Auroy Y, Péquignot F *et al.* Survey of anesthesia-related mortality in France. *Anesthesiology* 2006;105:1087–1097.

Mangano DT, Miao Y, Vuylsteke A *et al.* Investigators of The Multicenter Study of Perioperative Ischemia Research Group; Ischemia Research and Education Foundation. Mortality associated with aprotinin during 5 years following coronary artery bypass graft surgery. *JAMA* 2007;297:471–479.

McLellan SA, Walsh TS & McClelland DBL. Should we demand fresh red blood cells for perioperative and critically ill patients? *Br J Anaesth* 2002;89:537–540. (Editorial)

Rao SV, Jollis JG, Harrington RA *et al.* Relationship of blood transfusion and clinical outcomes in patients with acute coronary syndromes. *JAMA* 2004;292:1555–1562.

Sanguis Study Group. Use of blood products for elective surgery in 43 European hospitals. *Transfus Med* 1994;4:251–268.

Walsh TS, McArdle F, McLellan SA *et al.* Does the storage time of transfused red blood cells influence regional or global indexes of tissue oxygenation in anemic critically ill patients? *Crit Care Med* 2004;32:364–371.

Weiskopf RB, Feiner J, Hopf H *et al.* Fresh blood and aged stored blood are equally efficacious in immediately reversing anemia-induced brain oxygenation deficits in humans. *Anesthesiology* 2006;104:911–920.

CHAPTER 26

Prenatal and childhood transfusions

Irene Roberts

Departments of Haematology and Paediatrics, Imperial College London, London, UK

Obstetrics: transfusion during pregnancy

One of the most important aspects of transfusion medicine in obstetrics is the prevention, recognition and treatment of haemolytic disease of the newborn (HDN), which causes at least 50 neonatal deaths per year in the UK. This is considered in detail in this chapter. Other topics covered include:
- aspects of maternal platelet and white cell disorders relevant to transfusion;
- maternal haemorrhagic disorders, including major obstetric haemorrhage; and
- transfusion requirements during pregnancy of patients with major haemoglobinopathies.

Antenatal red cell antibody testing

The three factors essential in the pathogenesis of HDN are:
- maternal red cell alloantibodies which cross the placenta;
- fetal red blood cells which express antigens against which the antibodies are directed; and
- antibodies which are able to mediate red cell destruction.

Clinically relevant alloantibodies are almost always immunoglobulin G (IgG) and are reactive at 37°C. Women develop these antibodies as a result of previous transfusions, previous pregnancies or

Practical Transfusion Medicine, 3rd edition. Edited by Michael F. Murphy and Derwood H. Pamphilon. © 2009 Blackwell Publishing, ISBN: 978-1-4051-8196-9.

both. Identification of such antibodies is the main goal of antenatal screening.

Objectives of red cell antibody testing in pregnancy are:
- to identify red cell alloantibodies that are present at booking or develop during pregnancy;
- to identify the pregnancy at risk of fetal or neonatal HDN as a result of antibodies;
- to identify the fetus requiring treatment in utero or in the neonatal period;
- to identify RhD-negative women who require anti-D prophylaxis (around 16% women are RhD negative); and
- to ensure swift provision of compatible blood for obstetric emergencies.

Red cell serology at the booking visit

At the booking visit, which should take place before the 16th week of pregnancy, all women should have their ABO and RhD group determined and should be screened for red cell alloantibodies. If red cell antibodies are detected at the booking visit and/or if there is a history of HDN, the antibodies should be identified, quantified and monitored as outlined below. It is particularly important to monitor women with anti-D, anti-c and anti-K since these antibodies may be associated with severe HDN. If no red cell alloantibodies are detected at booking, all pregnant women should be retested at 28 weeks' gestation. Further testing of women without detectable antibodies is unnecessary since immunisation later in pregnancy is unlikely to result in antibody levels sufficient to cause HDN requiring treatment.

Partial D and weak D

D^u (weak D) individuals, rather than having 10,000–100,000 RhD proteins on the surface of each red cell as is usually the case, have 50–5,000 per red cell. This low antigen density may be difficult to detect, but as they have minimal or no structural RhD abnormality they are regarded as RhD positive, do not form immune anti-D and therefore do not require prophylaxis with anti-D. Individuals who have significant structural abnormalities of the RhD antigen with part of the protein missing are described as having partial D status, e.g. D^{VI}. Partial D individuals can make anti-D against the epitopes of RhD that they lack if they are exposed to normal RhD antigens, and they should therefore receive anti-D prophylaxis and RhD-negative red cell transfusions as if they were RhD negative. It is important that reagents for RhD grouping do not detect D^{VI} (so that these individuals group as RhD negative).

ABO antibodies

There is no need to test for ABO immune antibodies in antenatal samples as their presence is not predictive of HDN and such antibodies very rarely cause significant haemolysis in utero.

Samples at delivery

At the time of delivery a maternal and a cord blood sample should be collected from all pregnancies in RhD-negative women. A direct antiglobulin test (DAT) should be performed on the cord blood: a positive DAT is a good predictor of HDN.

Women with no previously detected anti-D should have prophylactic anti-D administered if the infant is RhD positive. A Kleihauer test should also be carried out on all such women to assess the requirement for additional anti-D. In women who have had prophylactic anti-D during pregnancy, the anti-D remains detectable in serum for up to 12 weeks, and may cause confusing serological results in the mother and a positive DAT in the baby in the absence of HDN.

In the case of women with other clinically significant red cell alloantibodies (see below), a DAT should be carried out on cord blood. If it is positive, a red cell eluate may help identify the red cell antibody. Infants born to mothers with clinically significant antibodies should be monitored for 48–72 hours for the presence of haemolytic disease.

Clinically relevant red cell alloantibodies

Main antibodies implicated in HDN:

- Rh group- D, c, C, e, E, Ce and Cw;
- Kell group- K1, K2 and Kp^a;
- Duffy group- Fy^a; and
- Kidd group- Jk^a.

The antibodies most commonly implicated in severe-to-moderate HDN are anti-D, anti-c and anti-K.

Anti-D is the commonest cause of HDN (approximately 40% of cases in the UK). This is because anti-D is highly immunogenic and a high proportion of women are RhD negative (16%). Most anti-D antibodies are IgG1 or IgG1 plus IgG3. The presence of IgG3 alone, which has 100 times the destructive ability of IgG1, is uncommon and rarely associated with HDN in utero, but can cause severe postnatal manifestations of HDN.

Anti-c is found most commonly in women with the R_1R_1 genotype (CDe/CDe) which occurs in 20% of pregnant women. Such women also have the propensity to make anti-E. HDN due to anti-E is both less common and less severe. However, anti-E and anti-c in combination cause more severe HDN than either antibody alone. Note that in such cases only the anti-E is detectable in eluates from cord blood red cells.

Anti-K1 is the most common red cell alloantibody outside the ABO and Rh system. K1 is the principal antigen of the Kell blood group system and is highly immunogenic; 5% of K1-negative individuals will produce anti-K1 if transfused with K1-positive blood. K1 has around twice the potency of c and E and 20 times the potency of Fy^a. Anti-K1 often causes severe HDN; the haemolytic anaemia is compounded by suppression of erythropoiesis by anti-K1 inhibiting the growth of erythroid progenitor cells. Anti-K titres can be an unreliable predictor of the severity of HDN. Therefore, it is important to identify the fetuses at risk of HDN by determining the fetal Kell genotype in all mothers with anti-K1 whose partners are heterozygous for K1 (since only 50% of such fetuses will be K1-positive). Moderate-to-severe HDN may also be caused by anti-K2 (anti-cellano) and anti-Kp[a].

A number of other red cell alloantibodies have also been reported to cause HDN of variable severity, e.g. anti-U. These are initially present with a positive indirect antiglobulin test (IAT) in maternal serum; therefore, all women with a positive IAT should have further investigation to try and identify any clinically relevant red cell alloantibodies.

Red cell alloantibodies not implicated in HDN

These are as follows:
- anti-Le[a] and anti Le[b];
- anti-Lu[a];
- anti-P;
- anti-N;
- anti-Xg[a]; and
- anti-Gerbish.

Management of pregnant women with red cell alloantibodies

Anti-D

- Women with anti-D should have their anti-D titres monitored monthly until 28 weeks' gestation and then every 2 weeks.
- All samples should be checked in parallel with the previous sample.
- An increase in anti-D by 50% or more compared with the previous sample is a significant increase irrespective of gestation (it is important to note that titres of anti-D do not always correlate closely with the development of HDN).
- The paternal Rhesus genotype should be ascertained to determine the risk to the fetus of haemolysis due to anti-D (100% of fetuses of RhD homozygous fathers and 50% of fetuses of RhD heterozygous fathers are at risk, whereas fetuses of RhD-negative fathers are not at risk).
- The fetal genotype should be determined where the father is RhD heterozygous (non-invasive fe-

tal Rhesus genotyping on maternal blood samples is now reliable and available in most centres).
- All women with affected pregnancies should be referred early to specialist fetal medicine units for fetal assessment (Doppler ultrasonography of the fetal middle cerebral artery to assess fetal anaemia has largely superceded amniocentesis and fetal blood sampling for monitoring of the fetus in recent years).

Anti-c

- Women with anti-c should have their anti-c titres monitored monthly until 28 weeks' gestation and then every 2 weeks.
- All samples should be checked in parallel with the previous sample.
- An increase in anti-c by 50% or more compared with the previous sample is a significant increase irrespective of gestation.
- Anti-c titres of >10 IU/mL are associated with a moderate risk of HDN and may require intrauterine transfusion (IUT).
- Fetal Rhesus c typing on maternal blood is now reliable and should be performed where the father is c heterozygous.
- All women with anti-c should be referred to a specialist fetal medicine unit early in pregnancy.

Anti-Kell

- Women with anti-K1 should have their anti-K titre monitored monthly until 28 weeks' gestation and then every 2 weeks.
- Anti-K titres may not accurately reflect the degree of fetal anaemia
- Fetal K typing on maternal blood is now reliable and should be performed where the father is heterozygous for K1.
- Fetal growth, fetal anaemia and the presence of hydrops should be monitored by serial ultrasound scans and Dopplers and anaemia confirmed by fetal blood sampling as indicated.
- Amniocentesis is not a good indicator of the severity of fetal anaemia since anaemia due to anti-K results from a combination of haemolysis and red cell hypoplasia.
- All women with anti-K should be referred to a specialist fetal medicine unit early in pregnancy.

Other red cell alloantibodies

The main points to note are:

• If the antibody is likely to cause problems with the provision of blood to cover an obstetric emergency, it is important to inform the obstetrician in charge of the case and the transfusion laboratory in the hospital, and efforts should be made to ensure that appropriate blood products can be supplied.

• Any babies born to mothers with an IAT-reacting antibody must be assessed at birth for evidence of HDN.

Blood transfusion support for mother and baby

Mother

• Red cell components of the same ABO and RhD group must be selected.

• Group O blood may be used in emergencies, provided it is plasma depleted and does not contain high-titre agglutinins.

• Note that in pregnancy, immunisation following a transfusion is most likely to occur in the third trimester.

• Samples used for pre-transfusion testing should ideally be taken immediately before transfusion and must never be more than 7–10 days old (see Table 26.1).

The fetus and neonate: cross-matching and general considerations

Management of the fetus and neonate at risk of HDN is discussed in detail below. The general principles for transfusion are summarized here.

• Prior to the first transfusion, samples should be obtained from the mother for ABO, RhD grouping and antibody screening and from the fetus/neonate for ABO, RhD and DAT (plus an antibody screen if no maternal sample is available).

• In the fetus/neonate, the ABO group is determined on the cells only (as reverse grouping can detect passive maternal antibodies).

• For red cells which are ABO compatible with maternal and neonatal plasma, RhD negative (or RhD identical with neonate) should be used. (*Note*: if exchange or 'top up' transfusion is required for HDN due to ABO incompatibility, group O red cells with low-titre anti-A and -B or group O red cells suspended in AB plasma should be used.)

• Group O blood is acceptable; units with high-titre anti-A/anti-B must be excluded.

• If the mother's blood group is unknown, blood for the fetus/neonate should be cross-matched against the baby's serum.

• If no atypical antibodies are present in the maternal (or infant) sample, and if the DAT of the infant is negative, cross-matching is not necessary for the first 4 months of postnatal life.

• If the antibody screen or DAT is positive, full serological investigation and compatibility testing are necessary.

• An electronic cross-match is not advisable unless an appropriate algorithm has been created, as ABO-identical adult blood transfused to an infant with maternal anti-A or -B may haemolyse even if the pre-transfusion DAT is negative, due to stronger ABO antigen expression on adult cells.

• Red cells (and platelets if given) should be cytomegalovirus (CMV) and leucocyte reduced.

• Note that alloantibody formation is rare in the fetus and neonate and is usually associated with massive transfusion or with the use of fresh or whole blood.

• Gamma-irradiation of cellular blood components to reduce the risk of transfusion-associated graft-versus-host disease (TA-GVHD) is recommended for:

  ◦ all IUTs;

  ◦ all transfusions to neonates previously transfused in utero;

  ◦ exchange transfusions as long as gamma-irradiation would not result in a delay in transfusion;

  ◦ all transfusions from a family member;

Table 26.1 Pre-transfusion testing of maternal samples.

Timing of last transfusion	Timing of pre-transfusion sample
3–14 days before	24 h before transfusion
14–28 days before	72 h before transfusion
28 days to 3 months	1 week before transfusion

○ all neonates with known inherited immune deficiencies (e.g. severe combined immunodeficiency).

These precautions are due to the immaturity of the fetal and neonatal immune system which may lead to a reduced ability to reject transfused allogeneic lymphocytes, immune tolerance and the persistence of donor lymphocytes for up to 6–8 weeks after exchange transfusion.

HDN: guidelines for prevention

The introduction of anti-D prophylaxis for recently delivered RhD-negative women in 1969 led to a reduction in new immunisations against anti-D from 17% of pregnancies in RhD-negative women to 1.5% in the UK. Every year in the UK 80,000 RhD-negative women have an RhD-positive infant, and despite national guidelines sensitisation still occurs, largely due to non-compliance with the guidelines. A dose of anti-D of 125 IU (25 mg) suppresses immunisation by 1 mL of RhD-positive red cells (i.e. 2 mL of whole blood). (Note that in the UK the dose of anti-D is given in IU whereas in other countries it is expressed in milligrams.) While anti-D is extremely effective as prophylaxis, it cannot reverse immunisation once it has occurred and has no effect on the development of non-D antibodies.

Indications for anti-D immunoglobulin (see Table 26.2)

Anti-D should be given to all RhD-negative women without anti-D antibodies after the following sensitising events:
- abortion (see below);
- CVS;
- ectopic pregnancy;
- amniocentesis;
- external cephalic version;
- abdominal trauma;
- antepartum haemorrhage;
- premature labour;
- pre-eclampsia; and
- intrauterine death (associated with chronic foetomaternal haemorrhage).

Anti-D should be administered following all abortions after 12 weeks, both spontaneous and induced, and following abortion at any gestation following surgical or medical treatment, including the use of abortifacients. Anti-D should also be administered in cases of threatened abortion if there is any bleeding after 12 weeks' gestation. Current UK guidelines also recommend the administration of anti-D immunoglobulin as antenatal prophylaxis since foetomaternal bleeding can happen at any gestation; in the UK, this is usually given as two 500 IU doses of anti-D at 28 and 34 weeks (see below).

Dose and schedule of administration of anti-D during the antenatal period

Therapeutic anti-D immunoglobulin to prevent the development of immune anti-D after sensitising events should be given within 72 hours of the sensitising event. However, anti-D may still be worthwhile up to 10 days after the event. In threatened abortion continuing to term, it is important to repeat the dose every 6 weeks (or use higher doses – see Table 26.2) since low antibody levels can augment the antibody response.

Table 26.2 Antenatal and postnatal prophylaxis with anti-D.

Indications for anti-D	Dose and schedule of administration
Sensitising event <26 weeks' gestation	250 IU (50 mg) IM
Threatened abortion continuing to term	500 IU every 6 weeks until term or 1250 IU every 10 weeks until term
RhD-negative women without anti-D or sensitising event	500 IU at 28 weeks and 34 weeks
Standard postnatal prophylaxis	500 IU (1500 IU in US and some European countries)

The dose of anti-D is:

- sensitising event <26 weeks' gestation: 250 IU (50 mg) intramuscularly;
- threatened abortion continuing to term: 500 IU (100 mg) every 6 weeks or 1250 IU (250 mg) every 10 weeks until term; and
- it is now recommended in the UK that routine antenatal prophylaxis is provided in RhD-negative women without anti-D in the absence of a sensitising event: 500 IU (100 mg) at 28 weeks and 34 weeks (no antibody screen is necessary before the dose at 34 weeks or at delivery).

Dose and schedule of administration of anti-D in the postnatal period

Therapeutic anti-D immunoglobulin to prevent the development of immune anti-D should be given within 72 hours of delivery; however, anti-D may still be worthwhile up to 10 days after the event.

The dose of anti-D is:

- 500 IU (100 mg) is the standard dose to cover a foetomaternal bleed of ≤4 mL.
- Quantitation of foetomaternal haemorrhage using flow cytometry or the Kleihauer test should always be performed to detect larger bleeds (bleeds >4 mL occur in 0.8% and of >15 mL in 0.3% of deliveries) so that an additional dose of anti-D (125 IU/mL blood loss) can be given.
- The standard dose of anti-D in the US and some European countries is higher (1500 IU).

It takes 48 hours following an intramuscular dose of anti-D to reach a good level and 72 hours for clearance of sensitised red cells. If clearance of the RhD-positive cells is not complete, further anti-D must be given until RhD-positive cells can no longer be detected in maternal blood.

Kleihauer test

This simple and inexpensive test is used to detect whether there has been a foetomaternal haemorrhage and its size. The Kleihauer test correlates well with enumeration of fetal haemoglobin (HbF)-containing fetal red cells by flow cytometry which is quicker but requires expensive specialised equipment. The principle and method for the Kleihauer test is as follows:

- HbF-containing fetal red cells resist acid elution and therefore stain dark pink in comparison to HbA-containing cells which appear as unstained 'ghost' cells (Plate 26.1).
- To quantitate foetomaternal haemorrhage, the numbers of pink-staining HbF-containing cells in each single low-power field are counted; using this method a count of ≤ 200 HbF-containing cells in 50 low-power fields is equivalent to a foetomaternal haemorrhage of ≤4 mL.
- Samples of maternal blood for the Kleihauer test must be taken within 2 hours of administration of anti-D to avoid a falsely low estimate of the size of the foetomaternal bleed.
- Maternal hereditary persistence of fetal haemoglobin may cause a false-positive Kleihauer to maternal HbF-containing red cells.

Large foetomaternal bleeds

Larger bleeds (>4 mL) may be measured using the Kleihauer test or flow cytometry. Larger foetomaternal bleeds are associated with:

- amniocentesis;
- abdominal trauma;
- antepartum haemorrhage;
- stillbirth;
- twin pregnancy; and
- manual removal of the placenta.

For any foetomaternal haemorrhage >4 mL, an appropriate supplementary dose of anti-D must be given immediately and *a repeat test for fetal cells and free anti-D should be carried out on the mother 48 hours after the initial anti-D injection.* A further appropriate dose of IgG anti-D should be given to the mother:

- if fetal cells are no longer present but there is no residual free anti-D detectable (to make sure there is sufficient anti-D to eliminate small numbers of fetal cells below the limits of detection); and
- if fetal cells are still present but there is no detectable anti-D.

Note that if fetal cells are still present after 48 hours but there is still detectable anti-D, a repeat test for fetal cells and free anti-D should be carried out after a further 48 hours to determine whether more anti-D IgG should be given to the mother.

Anti-D immunoglobulin is not indicated in the following circumstances:

- patients who are already sensitised;
- those classified as weak D (e.g. D^u);
- if the infant is RhD negative;
- for women not capable of child-bearing (following transfusion of RhD-positive blood); and
- for complete abortions <12 weeks' gestation if there has been no surgical treatment.

Preparation of anti-D immunoglobulin

Anti-D is a polyclonal antibody prepared by plasmapheresis of hyperimmunised donors, 95% of whom are women who have been sensitised during pregnancy. Anti-D is now prepared using US donor plasma because of concerns about transmission of variant Creutzfeldt–Jakob disease (vCJD). Work continues on the development of monoclonal anti-D for clinical use (Chapter 30).

Platelet and white cell disorders in pregnant women

Differential diagnosis of thrombocytopenia in pregnancy

The most common causes of maternal thrombocytopenia are:
- gestational;
- pregnancy induced (pre-eclampsia; eclampsia; HELLP syndrome, **h**aemolysis with **e**levation of **l**iver enzymes and **l**ow **p**latelets);
- immune: immune thrombocytopenia (ITP) and systemic lupus erythematosus (SLE); and
- virus associated (e.g. HIV).

Less common causes of maternal thrombocytopenia are:
- antiphospholipid syndrome (APS);
- thrombotic thrombocytopenic purpura (TTP);
- disseminated intravascular coagulation (DIC);
- type IIb von Willebrand disease (vWD);
- congenital bone marrow failure (e.g. Fanconi anaemia);
- heparin-induced thrombocytopenia (HIT);
- folate/B12 deficiency; and
- myelodysplasia/acute leukaemia.

It may be difficult to distinguish between gestational, pregnancy-induced and immune thrombocytopenia in pregnancy. ITP is more likely if the platelet count was subnormal prior to or in the first trimester of pregnancy. Further investigation depends on careful evaluation of the blood film and marrow smear, which may reveal characteristic changes (e.g. acute leukaemia). The disorders of particular relevance to transfusion medicine are ITP, HELLP and type IIb vWD.

Management of maternal ITP

ITP usually presents either in an otherwise well mother with or without a previous history of ITP or, less commonly, SLE. In those without a previous history, the diagnosis may be difficult, and platelet antibody studies are of limited value since they may be positive even in the absence of ITP.

The management of the mother with active ITP and who is thrombocytopenic should be as conservative as possible. The most common approach to therapy is with intravenous immunoglobulin (IVIG; 0.3–0.5 mg/kg/day) for 3–5 days. However, prednisolone (1 mg/kg) can also be used. The indications for treatment of maternal ITP are:
- platelets <20 × 10^9/L in the first, second or early third trimester;
- aim to have platelets >80 × 10^9/L in the late third trimester;
- avoid epidural or spinal anaesthesia if the platelet count is <80 × 10^9/L;
- platelet transfusion is very rarely indicated;
- splenectomy should be postponed until after delivery if possible; and
- fetal blood sampling and elective Caesarean section for maternal ITP are unnecessary since significant fetal thrombocytopenia is uncommon (12%) and intracranial haemorrhage is even less common (1%).

The fetal platelet count cannot be predicted from maternal platelet counts nor from platelet serology. The most important factor predicting the presence and severity of fetal thrombocytopenia is a history of maternal ITP prior to pregnancy. In this higher risk group, 10–30% of babies will have significant thrombocytopenia (<50 × 10^9/L).

Pre-eclampsia and HELLP syndrome

In pre-eclampsia thrombocytopenia is usually moderate, not severe. Fulminant pre-eclampsia precipitating early delivery may be associated with

DIC and require treatment with platelet transfusion and fresh frozen plasma (FFP) (with or without cryoprecipitate). Thrombocytopenia in HELLP syndrome is more often severe and platelet transfusion may be indicated, particularly at delivery, which is usually by urgent Caesarean section, and postpartum.

Type IIb vWD

This is characterised by:
- low factor VIII and von Willebrand Factor (vWF);
- thrombocytopenia due to platelet activation/consumption;
- reduced high-molecular-weight vWF multimers; and
- the need for prophylactic treatment at delivery with vWF or factor VIII.

Leukaemia in pregnancy

When chemotherapy is administered during an ongoing pregnancy, both the mother and fetus may develop pancytopenia. Platelet transfusion for the mother should be given according to the usual guidelines, aiming to have a platelet count $>80 \times 10^9$/L at delivery and for the first few days postpartum. The fetus should be monitored and fetal blood sampling with or without blood/platelet transfusion of irradiated blood products may be indicated on rare occasions.

Maternal haemorrhagic problems

Guidelines for the investigation and management of haemorrhagic disorders in pregnancy have been published by the British Committee for Standards in Haematology (BCSH) Haemostasis and Thrombosis Task Force (1994), with more recent updates for vWD and the rare disorders (2004), and are summarized here.

Inherited disorders

The most common inherited coagulation disorder is vWD. The prevalence of vWD is around 1% but many are only mildly affected. There are three main types of vWD: type I is the commonest (75%); type IIa occurs in 10%; type IIb in 7% and may be accompanied by severe thrombocytopenia; and type III is the most severe. Most women with vWD have increased factor VIII and vWF during pregnancy and do not bleed excessively.

Bleeding in pregnant women with vWD, when it does occur, usually causes problems:
- during invasive procedures in the first trimester (e.g. CVS); and
- after birth, particularly after surgical delivery and/or perineal damage.

Management of vWD in pregnancy can be summarized as follows:
- For first-trimester procedures, factor VIIIC activity should be raised to 50 IU/dL.
- At delivery, operative procedures should be avoided except for obstetric indications and trauma should be minimised.
- Type I vWD: for vaginal delivery no blood product support is necessary if the factor VIIIC is >40 IU/dL; if <40 IU/dL or if Caesarean section is planned factor VIIIC should be given to raise the level to at least 50 IU/dL.
- Type II and type III vWD: prophylactic factor VIIIC should be started at the onset of labour in all type III patients, most type IIa patients and some type IIb patients; the aim should be to raise the level of factor VIIIC to >40 IU/dL; products with large amounts of large vWF multimers should be used (e.g. 8Y, intermediate purity factor VIII concentrate containing vWF); for Caesarean section factor VIIIC should be raised to >50 IU/dL.

Acquired disorders

The most common acquired disorder is DIC. This occurs secondary to:
- severe eclampsia/pre-eclampsia;
- intrauterine death;
- placental abruption;
- amniotic fluid embolism; and
- hydatidiform mole (chronic DIC).

Haemorrhage may be severe. Treatment is as for DIC in non-pregnant patients except that the use of heparin is not recommended. Women who develop HELLP syndrome with associated hepatic failure may also develop severe DIC with low fibrinogen and extremely low antithrombin levels. Maternal mortality approaches 30%; fetal mortality is around 50%.

Major obstetric haemorrhage protocol

Severe bleeding is an obstetric emergency. It is essential to establish a major obstetric emergency haemorrhage protocol in any hospital where pregnant women are likely to deliver (see Chapters 24 and 28). This protocol must be agreed by haematologists, including the haematology and transfusion laboratory staff, obstetricians and midwives, and those responsible for transporting urgent specimens and blood products.

The most important points include the following:
• If the blood group is known and there are no atypical antibodies, ABO- and RhD-group-compatible red cells (6 units) should be issued.
• If there are atypical antibodies, phenotyped red cells should be issued whenever possible.
• If the blood group is unknown, group O RhD-negative blood (6 units) should be issued.
• Samples should be obtained from the patient as soon as possible for blood group, full blood count and coagulation screen.
• Once results are available further units of red cells, FFP, cryoprecipitate and/or platelets should be issued as indicated.
• An antibody screen and retrospective cross-match should be performed on the units issued as soon as time allows.
• Recombinant factor VIIa may be considered as a treatment for life-threatening haemorrhage, but should not be considered as a substitute for, nor should it delay, the performance of a life-saving procedure such as embolisation or surgery, nor transfer to a referring centre.

Management of the major haemoglobinopathies during pregnancy

Sickle cell disease

The frequency of maternal complications related to sickle cell disease, particularly vaso-occlusive crises, is not particularly increased during pregnancy. However, pregnant sickle cell disease patients do have an increased risk of:
• placental insufficiency causing intrauterine growth restriction;
• eclampsia/pre-eclampsia;
• preterm delivery;
• stillbirth and neonatal death;
• urinary tract infection (sickle cell disease); and
• pulmonary thromboembolism (particularly HbSC disease).

Indications for red cell transfusion in pregnant women with sickle cell disease:
• Exchange transfusion should be carried out prior to planned operative delivery.
• Exchange transfusion should be continued in any patients already on a regular exchange programme (e.g. for prevention of recurrent stroke).
• Exchange transfusion should be considered for severe, prolonged vaso-occlusive crises during pregnancy.
• 'Top up' transfusion should be considered for severe anaemia if symptomatic.
• Regular prophylactic transfusion therapy during pregnancy does not reduce pregnancy-related complications or improve outcome.
• Red cells should be phenotyped (for Rh, Kell, Duffy, Kidd and MNS) to reduce the risk of alloimmunisation, and red cells from sickle trait donors should not be used.

Thalassaemia major and intermedia

Both maternal and fetal morbidity are higher in pregnant women with thalassaemia major and intermedia. In the mother the degree of anaemia, the cardiovascular changes associated with pregnancy and pre-existing cardiac damage may aggravate the multiorgan damage secondary to iron overload. For the fetus, most reports suggest an increase in intrauterine growth restriction and preterm delivery. The rate of Caesarean section is increased possibly because of cephalopelvic disproportion. Management is complex requiring close liaison between haematologists and obstetricians.

Management guidelines for pregnant women with thalassaemia major or intermedia:
• Haemoglobin should be maintained above 10–12 g/dL to optimise fetal outcome.
• Transfusion requirements usually increase during pregnancy.
• Iron chelation is usually avoided during the first trimester and used with caution in the second and

third trimesters if iron overload is a significant clinical problem.

Fetal and neonatal transfusion

Causes of fetal and neonatal anaemia

The principal causes of fetal and neonatal anaemia are shown in Table 26.3. The commonest causes of fetal anaemia in the UK are parvovirus infection, HDN and twin-to-twin transfusion and the commonest causes of neonatal anaemia are iatrogenic blood loss and anaemia of prematurity.

Table 26.3 Principal causes of fetal and neonatal anaemia.

Impaired red cell production
- Diamond–Blackfan anaemia
- *Congenital infection, e.g. parvovirus, CMV*
- Congenital dyserythropoietic anaemia
- Pearson's syndrome

Haemolytic anaemias
- *All-immune: haemolytic disease of the newborn (Rh, ABO, Kell, others)*
- Autoimmune, e.g. maternal autoimmune haemolysis
- Red cell membrane disorders, e.g. hereditary spherocytosis
- Red cell enzyme deficiencies, e.g. pyruvate kinase deficiency
- Some haemoglobinopathies, e.g. α *thalassaemia major*, HbH disease
- Infection, e.g. bacterial, syphilis, malaria, CMV, toxoplasma, Herpes simplex

Anaemia due to haemorrhage
- Occult haemorrhage before or around birth, e.g. *twin-to-twin*, foetomaternal
- Internal haemorrhage, e.g. intracranial, cephalhaematoma
- Iatrogenic: due to frequent blood sampling

Anaemia of prematurity
- Due to impaired red cell production, impaired RhEpo production and reduced red cell lifespan
- Hb nadir usually 6.5–9 g/dL

Causes in italics commonly present in the fetus; other causes may present during fetal life but neonatal presentation is more common.

Management of neonatal anaemia

(HDN is discussed in the next section)
The only available treatment of neonatal anaemia is red cell transfusion. Prevention or amelioration of anaemia sufficient to reduce red cell transfusion requirements may be achieved by using recombinant RhEpo but this is not useful in the acute setting due to the 2-week delay in increasing haemoglobin in response to RhEpo.

Indications for 'top up' transfusion

Guidelines for 'top up' transfusion have been devised by committees in a number of countries, including the UK, Canada and the US. Since there is almost no objective evidence, these guidelines are based on clinical experience and represent consensus views. Table 26.4 summarises the indications for 'top up' transfusions agreed by the BCSH (2003) and used in many UK neonatal intensive care units.

Hazards of transfusion in neonates

Transfusion of neonates is becoming safer, especially with the more widespread use of satellite packs. The most important hazards of transfusion in neonates are:
- infection: bacterial or viral;
- hypocalcaemia (more common in neonates than in infants or children);
- volume overload;
- citrate toxicity;
- rebound hypoglycaemia (high glucose levels from blood additives);

Table 26.4 Indications for neonatal 'top up' transfusions.

Clinical situation	Transfuse at
• Anaemia in the first 24 h	Hb < 12 g/dL
• Neonate receiving mechanical ventilation	Hb < 12 g/dL
• Acute blood loss	10% blood volume lost
• Oxygen dependency (not ventilated)	Hb < 8–10 g/dL
• Late anaemia, stable patient (off oxygen)	Hb 7 g/dL

- thrombocytopenia (after exchange transfusion); and
- TA-GVHD (if non-irradiated products given to those at risk: see above).

Strategies to minimise transfusion risk in neonates

The following strategies have been shown to reduce the need for red cell transfusion and/or donor exposure in neonates:
- development and implementation of local transfusion guidelines for each neonatal unit;
- minimising iatrogenic blood sampling;
- prevention and treatment of haematinic deficiencies (iron and folic acid);
- use of dedicated satellite packs ('paedipacks');
- improved antimicrobial screening;
- judicious use of RhEpo (see below); and
- autologous cord blood transfusion: delayed clamping of the cord at delivery.

Neonatal 'top up' transfusions: product specification

- Small-volume 'top up' transfusions can be given without further testing provided that there are no atypical maternal antibodies in maternal/infant serum and the infant's DAT is negative.
- The red cells should be ≤ 35 days old (if in SAG-M or similar additive system) or ≤ 28 days old (if in CPD).
- 'Paedipacks' (aliquotted donations from a single unit) should be used wherever possible for repeated transfusions to minimise donor exposure.
- The recommended haematocrit for red cells for neonatal 'top up' transfusion is 0.5–0.7.
- The volume of a neonatal 'top up' transfusion is usually 10–20 mL/kg.

T antigen activation

Severe haemolytic transfusion reactions are occasionally seen in neonates or young children transfused with adult blood or FFP containing anti-T antibodies. This may be due to exposure or 'activation' of the T antigen on neonatal red cells, usually as a result of infection with clostridia, streptococci or pneumococci and/or in association with necrotising enterocolitis (NEC). Up to 25% of infants with NEC have T antigen activation but so do many healthy neonates, and haemolysis is extremely rare. Therefore, although there remains some controversy, majority of centres worldwide consider that no special provision for neonates with NEC is necessary, and screening of neither neonates for T activation nor donors for high-titre anti-T.

Role of RhEpo in reducing neonatal red cell transfusion

There have been numerous clinical trials of RhEpo for the prevention or amelioration of neonatal anaemia, particularly anaemia of prematurity, since endogenous RhEpo production is low in preterm babies for the first 6–8 weeks of life. These trials show that RhEpo (250 units/kg/day 3 times per week for the first 6 weeks of life) can reduce red cell transfusions in well preterm babies but has a negligible effect on transfusion requirements of sick preterm babies, particularly those of less than 26 weeks' gestation at birth. In practice, this means that RhEpo has a limited role in neonates as it works best in those that need it least.

Therefore, most neonatal units no longer use RhEpo routinely. The situations in which RhEpo can be useful are:
- in neonates whose parents refuse permission to use blood products; and
- to prevent 'late anaemia' in babies with HDN.

Management of HDN in the fetus

Fetal monitoring of 'at-risk' pregnancies

The aims are to prevent hydrops developing in utero and to time delivery so that the baby has the best chance of survival. Fetal monitoring includes the following:
- Weekly Doppler ultrasonography of the fetal middle cerebral artery to identify fetal anaemia; this is reliable up to 36 weeks' gestation.
- Regular ultrasound scans for fetal growth, hepatosplenomegaly and/or hydrops.
- Where expertise for fetal Doppler ultrasonography is unavailable, amniocentesis may be used to measure amniotic fluid bilirubin as an

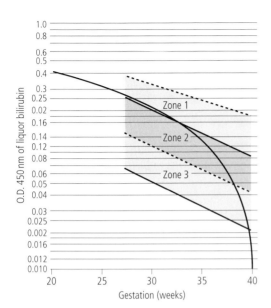

Figure 26.1 Whitfield's (1970) curved action line is superimposed on Liley zones of severity of fetal haemolysis based on estimations of amniotic fluid bilirubin concentrations. This gives guidelines for appropriate management related to gestation, i.e. intrauterine transfusion or, if the fetus is viable, delivery and exchange transfusion. (Adapted from Hann *et al.* 1991.)

indirect measure of fetal haemolysis (not reliable before 25 weeks' and after 34 weeks' gestation); the bilirubin is plotted on a graph of Liley zones modified by Whitfield (Figure 26.1) in order to predict the severity of HDN and plan management.

• Fetal blood sampling if severe HDN before 24 weeks' gestation is suspected, if there is a rapid rise in maternal antibody or if there has been a previous intrauterine death due to HDN (note that fetal blood sampling carries a 1–3% fetal loss rate and may cause foetomaternal haemorrhage with further sensitisation).

• IUT if anaemia is severe and delivery is not possible due to extreme prematurity.

Intrauterine transfusion (IUT)

The aims of IUT are:

• to prevent or treat fetal hydrops before the fetus can be delivered;

• to enable the pregnancy to advance to a gestational age that will ensure survival of the neonate (in practice, up to 36–37 weeks) with as few invasive procedures as possible (because of the risk of fetal loss).

These are achieved by starting the transfusion programme as late as safely possible but before hydrops develops and maximising the intervals between transfusions by transfusing as large a volume of red cells as is considered safe. Transfusions may be intravascular, intraperitoneal or intracardiac. All transfusions are carried out with ultrasound guidance (Figure 26.2). During transfusion the point of the needle and fetal heart should be watched closely for signs of needle displacement, cardiac tamponade and bradycardia. The fetal loss rate associated with IUT is usually around 5% but is higher when the fetus is hydropic. IUT is generally indicated when the haematocrit falls to below 0.25 between 18 and 26 weeks' gestation or to less than 0.3 after 26 weeks' gestation. The aim of the transfusion is to raise the haematocrit to 0.45 and repeat transfusion is often necessary after 2–3 weeks.

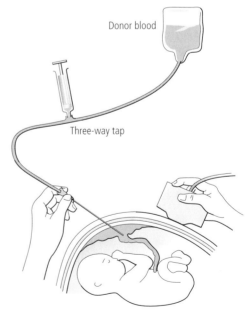

Figure 26.2 Intrauterine transfusion. (Adapted from Alter 1989.)

Intrauterine transfusion: product specification

• Plasma-reduced red cells with a haematocrit of 0.7–0.85 should be used.
• The red cells should be 5 days old or less, in CPD anticoagulant and sickle screen negative.
• The red cells should be group O (low-titre haemolysin) or ABO identical with the fetus (if known) and RhD negative (unless the HDN is due to anti-c, in which case RhD-positive, c-negative blood should be used). K-negative blood is recommended to reduce additional maternal alloimmunisation risks.
• An IAT-cross-match compatible with maternal serum and negative for the relevant antigen(s) determined by maternal antibody status should be carried out.
• Red cells for IUT should always be irradiated because of the risk of TA-GVHD.
• Red cells for IUT should be warmed to $37°C$ immediately prior to transfusion and transfused at a rate of 5–10 mL/min.

Management of HDN in the neonate

The severity of HDN varies considerably from a hydropic infant with gross hepatosplenomegaly who needs immediate exchange transfusion to mild jaundice with or without anaemia.

The following tests should be carried out at delivery from all suspected cases:
• ABO and RhD group;
• DAT;
• serum bilirubin; and
• full blood count, reticulocyte count and blood film.

Affected babies should be monitored by checking their bilirubin and haemoglobin every 3–4 hours. A rising bilirubin level may require treatment with exchange transfusion and/or phototherapy depending upon gestational age, postnatal age and birth weight (action charts are available for guidance). Phototherapy should be given from birth to all Rh-alloimmunised infants with haemolysis as the bilirubin can rise steeply after birth and this expectant approach will prevent the need for exchange transfusion in some infants. 'Late' anaemia presents at a few weeks of age in some babies with milder haemolytic disease who do not require exchange transfusion and in babies who have had earlier exchange transfusion; 'top up' transfusion may be required. The blood film shows evidence of ongoing haemolysis and the anaemia is aggravated by the normal postnatal suppression of erythropoiesis.

Exchange transfusion in neonates with HDN

Exchange transfusion is used to treat severe anaemia at birth, particularly in the presence of heart failure, and severe hyperbilirubinaemia. The aim is to remove both antibody-coated red cells and excess bilirubin. Exchange transfusion is a specialist procedure and should be undertaken only by experienced staff. Double volume exchange (160–200 mL/kg) gives the best reduction in bilirubin (50%) and removes 90% of the infant's circulating RhD-positive cells. The pH of whole blood or plasma-reduced red cells used in exchange transfusion is around 7.0, which does not cause acidosis in the infant. Some studies have shown that administration of IVIG to neonates with HDN reduces the need for exchange transfusion; IVIG is not currently recommended for HDN in the UK.

Indications for exchange transfusion

• Cord haemoglobin less than 8 g/dL.
• Cord bilirubin more than 100 μmol/L.
• Rapidly rising bilirubin.

Exchange transfusion in the neonate: product specification

• Plasma-reduced red cells with a haematocrit of 0.5–0.6 should be used as packed cells may have a haematocrit up to 0.75 and cause a very high post-exchange haematocrit.
• The red cells should be less than 5 days old, collected into CPD anticoagulant and sickle screen negative.
• The most recent BCSH guidelines (2003) state that red cells for neonatal exchange transfusion should be gamma-irradiated (and transfused within 24 hours of irradiation); gamma-irradiation is essential in the case of neonates who have previously received IUT and in all other cases is advisable unless to do so would lead to clinically relevant delay.

• Red cells for exchange should be warmed to 37°C immediately prior to transfusion.

Special features of HDN due to ABO antibodies

• ABO haemolytic disease occurs only in offspring of women of blood group O and is confined to the 1% of women who have high-titre IgG antibodies.
• Haemolysis due to anti-A is more common (1 in 150 births) than anti-B.
• Jaundice may be severe but anaemia is usually mild.
• The blood film shows very large numbers of spherocytes with little or no increase in nucleated red cells.
• The DAT is usually, but not always, positive.
• Severe HDN requiring exchange transfusion occurs in only 1 in 3000 births.
• If an exchange transfusion is required, this should be with group O red cells, with low-titre anti-A and B or with group O red cells suspended in AB plasma.

Neonatal thrombocytopenia

Thrombocytopenia occurs in 1–4% of neonates. It is much more common in sick preterm infants, 30–40% of whom will develop thrombocytopenia in the first 4 weeks of life. Causes of neonatal thrombocytopenia are shown in Table 26.5. The most common cause presenting in the first few days of life is that associated with intrauterine growth restriction or maternal hypertension; however, the most important cause of severe thrombocytopenia (platelets $<50 \times 10^9$/L) at birth is neonatal alloimmune thrombocytopenia (NAITP).

Investigation of neonatal thrombocytopenia

In most cases the following tests will identify the diagnosis.
• Full blood count and film: the combination of mild neutropenia and large numbers of nucleated red cells together with moderate thrombocytopenia suggests that the cause is intrauterine growth restriction and/or maternal hypertension. The presence of neutrophil left shift and toxic granulation with more severe thrombocytopenia suggests that the cause is bacterial infection with or without DIC.

Table 26.5 Causes of neonatal thrombocytopenia.

Early onset (<72 h after birth)
Placental insufficiency (PET, IUGR, diabetes)
NAITP
Birth asphyxia
Peri-natal infection (Group B *Streptococcus*, *Escherichia coli*, *Listeria*)
Congenital infection (CMV, toxoplasmosis, rubella)
Maternal autoimmune (ITP, SLE)
Severe Rhesus HDN
Thrombosis (renal vein, aortic)
Aneuploidy (Trisomy – 21, 18, 13)
Congenital/inherited (TAR, Wiskott–Aldrich)

Late onset (>72 h after birth)
Bacterial and fungal sepsis
Necrotising enterocolitis
Congenital infection (CMV, toxoplasmosis, rubella)
Maternal autoimmune (ITP, SLE)
Congenital/Inherited (TAR, Wiskott-Aldrich)

The most common causes are in bold type.
PET, pre-eclampsia; IUGR, intrauterine growth restriction; NAITP, neonatal alloimmune thrombocytopenia; CMV, cytomegalovirus; ITP, idiopathic thrombocytopenic purpura; SLE, systemic lupus erythematosus; HDN, haemolytic disease of the newborn; TAR, thrombocytopenia with absent radii.

• Congenital infection screen: the most common congenital infection associated with neonatal thrombocytopenia is CMV.
• Screening for NAITP (see below) should be carried out in any case of severe thrombocytopenia (platelets $<50 \times 10^9$/L) presenting in the first week of life unless there is very clear evidence of acute infection.

Neonatal alloimmune thrombocytopenia (NAITP)

• NAITP is analogous to HDN: maternal alloantibodies to antigens present on fetal platelets cause immune destruction of platelets in utero.
• The 5 principal human platelet antigens (HPA1–5) show biallelic autosomal inheritance.
• Alloantibodies to HPA-1a, HPA-5b and HPA-3a account for almost all cases of NAITP, the commonest being anti-HPA-1a (80–90% of cases of NAITP).

- NAITP affects around 1:1000 pregnancies and occurs in the first pregnancy in almost 50% of the cases.
- Thrombocytopenia is frequently severe (platelets $<30 \times 10^9$/L) and may present prenatally (as early as 20 weeks' gestation) or at birth.
- The ability of an HPA-1a-negative woman to form anti-HPA-1a is controlled by the HLA DRB3*0101 allele: HLA DRB3*0101-positive women are 140 times more likely to make anti-HPA-1a than HLA DRB3*0101-negative women.
- The main clinical problem in NAITP is intracranial haemorrhage; this occurs in 10% of the cases with long-term neurodevelopmental sequelae in 20% of survivors.
- The diagnosis of NAITP is made by demonstrating platelet antigen incompatibility between mother and baby serologically or by PCR (polymerase chain reaction) and is carried out in reference transfusion labs (see Chapter 4).

Management of NAITP

- In all suspected cases the platelet count must be monitored for at least 72 hours after birth as it may continue to fall during this time.
- Severely thrombocytopenic babies (platelets $<30 \times 10^9$/L) should be transfused with HPA-compatible platelets (available 'off the shelf' from transfusion centres).
- Babies with an intracranial haemorrhage in association with NAITP should have their platelet count maintained above 50×10^9/L with HPA-compatible platelets.
- If there is ongoing severe thrombocytopenia and/or haemorrhage despite HPA-compatible platelets, intravenous IgG (total dose 2 g/kg over 2–5 days) is often useful until spontaneous recovery occurs 1–6 weeks after birth.
- All babies with severe thrombocytopenia due to NAITP should have a cranial ultrasound to look for evidence of intracranial haemorrhage (Figure 26.3).

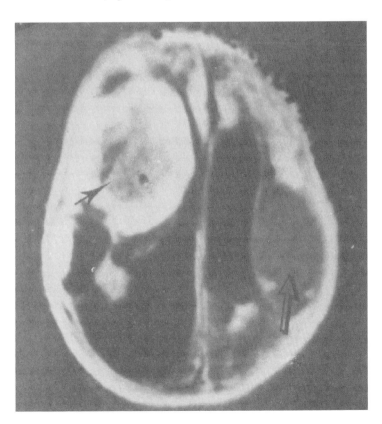

Figure 26.3 MRI studies: inversion recovery sequence (IR 1800/600/33) showing subacute haematoma (black arrow) and chronic haematoma (open arrow). (Adapted from de Vries *et al.* 1988.)

Management of pregnancies at risk for NAITP
(see also Chapter 4)

• Prenatal management of NAITP remains controversial and all pregnancies should be monitored in a specialist fetal medicine centre with experience of NAITP.

• The principal options that have been used are an invasive approach using fetal transfusion with HPA-compatible platelets or a non-invasive approach relying on the treatment of the mother with intravenous IgG and/or steroids. The latter approach is now recommended because of the risks associated with fetal blood sampling and transfusion.

• Paternal HPA genotyping is helpful since all fetuses fathered by men homozygous for HPA-1a (HPA-1a/1a) will be HPA-1a-positive and therefore at high risk of developing severe thrombocytopenia, whereas only 50% of fetuses will be at risk if the father is heterozygous for HPA-1a (HPA-1a/1b).

There is no clear correlation between the titre of maternal anti-HPA antibodies and the severity of fetal thrombocytopenia and/or the development of intracranial haemorrhage.

Neonatal thrombocytopenia due to maternal ITP

• Around 10% of infants of mothers with ITP or SLE develop neonatal thrombocytopenia secondary to transplacental passage of maternal platelet autoantibodies.

• The thrombocytopenia is usually mild and intracranial haemorrhage occurs in less than 1% of at-risk babies.

• The platelet count of babies born to mothers with ITP or SLE should be checked at birth and monitored daily for 2–3 days if below 200×10^9/L at birth.

• If the baby is well, treatment is unnecessary unless the platelet count falls below 20×10^9/L.

• If the baby has severe thrombocytopenia (platelets $<20 \times 10^9$/L), treatment with intravenous IgG (0.4–1 g/kg per day, total dose 2–4 g/kg) is usually effective.

• Cranial ultrasound to look for intracranial haemorrhage should be performed in all neonates with severe thrombocytopenia.

Table 26.6 Guidelines for platelet transfusion in neonatal thrombocytopenia.

• Platelet count $<30 \times 10^9$/L in otherwise well infants, including NAITP if no evidence of bleeding and no family history of intracranial haemorrhage
• Platelet count $<50 \times 10^9$/L in infants with: clinical instability
    concurrent coagulopathy
    birthweight <1000 g and age <1 week
    previous major bleeding (e.g. GMH-IVH)
    current minor bleeding (e.g. petechiae)
    planned surgery or exchange transfusion
    platelet count falling and likely to fall below 30
    NAITP if previous affected sibling with ICH
• Platelet count $<100 \times 10^9$/L in infants with major bleeding

---

• Platelet transfusion is reserved for life-threatening haemorrhage and should be given in conjunction with intravenous IgG.

Indications for platelet transfusion in neonates

Published guidelines for neonatal platelet transfusion acknowledge the lack of evidence on which to base recommendations and aim for a safe approach. Suggested guidelines based on clinical experience are shown in Table 26.6. There is some evidence to suggest that prophylactic platelet transfusions are not required for healthy neonates until the platelet count falls to 2030×10^9/L. However, a higher trigger level (50×10^9/L) should be used for babies with the greatest risk of haemorrhage, especially extremely low birth weight neonates (<1000 g) in the first week of life.

Neonatal platelet transfusion: product specification

• ABO identical or compatible;
• RhD identical or compatible;
• HPA compatible in infants with NAITP;
• Produced by standard techniques without further concentration;
• Irradiated if appropriate; and
• Volume transfused usually 10–20 mL/kg.

Neonatal neutropenia

Normal neutrophil levels vary with postnatal age, falling in healthy babies from around $5{-}10 \times 10^9/L$ at birth to $2{-}6 \times 10^9/L$ by the end of the first week of lie. Neutropenia is therefore variably defined depending on postnatal age: less than $2.0 \times 10^9/L$ at birth and less than $1.0 \times 10^9/L$ from 1 week of age. The most common causes are neutropenia secondary to intrauterine growth restriction or maternal hypertension and neutropenia secondary to severe sepsis. The presence of neutrophil left shift and toxic granulation in a neutropenic neonate suggests acute bacterial infection.

Alloimmune neonatal neutropenia (see Chapter 5)

- This is analogous to HDN: there is maternal sensitisation to fetal neutrophil antigens during pregnancy.
- The most common implicated antibodies are anti-NA1 and anti-NA2.
- The estimated incidence of neonatal alloimmune neutropenia is 3% of live births, but most cases are mild and asymptomatic and the diagnosis may be missed.
- Infants with severe neonatal alloimmune neutropenia develop severe cutaneous, respiratory or urinary tract infection.
- Treatment is with antibiotics and, if necessary, granulocyte colony-stimulating factor.

Granulocyte transfusions in neonates

There is no good evidence of the benefit of granulocyte transfusions for the treatment of neonatal infection. Both granulocyte colony-stimulating factor and granulocyte-macrophage colony-stimulating factor can be used to increase the neutrophil count in neutropenic neonates but there is no clear evidence that this improves outcome.

Coagulation problems in the newborn

Causes of haemorrhage in the newborn

In well infants, the most common causes of bleeding are:
- vitamin K deficiency (haemorrhagic disease of the newborn);

- inherited disorders, particularly haemophilias; and
- NAITP.

In sick infants the most common causes are:
- DIC – secondary to perinatal asphyxia, necrotising enterocolitis or, less commonly, sepsis; and
- liver disease.

Vitamin K deficiency

Vitamin K deficiency remains a clinical problem largely because of the controversy in recent years surrounding the possible carcinogenic effects of intramuscular vitamin K administered to newborn infants to prevent haemorrhagic disease of the newborn. Vitamin K is necessary for the post-translational carboxylation of coagulation factors II, VII, IX and X and, of the natural anticoagulants protein C and protein S. Levels of vitamin K and of all of these factors are physiologically low at birth. This physiological deficiency can be exacerbated by breast-feeding, prematurity and liver disease, resulting in haemorrhagic disease of the newborn, often now referred to as vitamin K-dependent bleeding (VKDB).

There are three patterns of VKDB:
- Early VKDB presents in the first 24 hours of life usually with severe haemorrhage, including gastrointestinal bleeding and intracranial haemorrhage. It is caused by severe vitamin K deficiency in utero usually as a result of maternal medication that interferes with vitamin K, e.g. anticonvulsants (phenobarbitone, phenytoin), anti-tuberculous therapy and oral anticoagulants.
- Classical VKDB presents at 2–7 days old in babies who have not received prophylactic vitamin K at birth. The risk is increased in breast-fed babies and in those with poor oral intake. The incidence in babies not receiving vitamin K supplementation is 0.25–1.7%. Classical VKDB can be prevented by a single intramuscular dose of vitamin K at birth.
- Late VKDB occurs 2–8 weeks after birth. It usually presents with sudden intracranial haemorrhage in an otherwise well, breast-fed term baby or in babies with liver disease. Late VKDB in healthy breast-fed babies can be prevented either by a single intramuscular dose of vitamin K or by repeated oral doses of vitamin K over the first 6 weeks of life;

babies with chronic liver disease or malabsorption, including critically ill term and preterm neonates, require prolonged vitamin K supplementation.

• Diagnosis of VKDB is based on clotting studies which show a prolonged PT with normal platelets and fibrinogen; in severe deficiency the APTT may also be prolonged.

• Treatment of VKDB depends on the severity of the bleeding. Mild cases should be given vitamin K (1 mg) intravenously or subcutaneously, as this increases the levels of active vitamin K-dependent coagulation factors within a few hours; where there is significant bleeding, FFP may be given in addition to vitamin K.

Vitamin K prophylaxis

Guidelines for the prevention of early VKDB are to give a single intramuscular injection of vitamin K at birth together with antenatal administration of oral vitamin K to the mother during the last 4 weeks of pregnancy. For classical and late VKDB there are several options because although intramuscular vitamin K at birth prevents classical and late VKDB, some studies have suggested a link between intramuscular vitamin K at birth and later childhood malignancies. Although other studies have not confirmed the link with malignancy, the controversy is unlikely to be resolved unequivocally in the short term. There is no link between oral vitamin K and malignancy. Both the American Academy of Pediatrics and the Royal College of Paediatrics and Child Health recommend vitamin K supplementation at birth. In healthy babies the choice of which route of administration is left to parents who have to balance a possible risk of leukaemia (odds ratio between 1.06 (CI 0.89–1.25) and 1.16 (CI 0.97–1.39)) with intramuscular vitamin K against the slightly higher risk of VKDB (2.7/100,000) in infants given 3 doses of 1 mg vitamin K orally at birth, 1 week and 1 month of age.

Use of FFP, cryoprecipitate and human albumin solution in neonates

Guidelines for the use of FFP, cryoprecipitate and albumin in neonates have been published by national committees in a number of countries. The guidelines aim to minimise their risks in the newborn both by the use of pathogen-inactivated (PI) products and by recommending their use for a small number of clinical indications.

The only indications for FFP in neonates recommended in the recent BCSH guidelines (2003) and supported by evidence are DIC, VKDB and inherited deficiencies of coagulation factors.

Prophylactic FFP administered to preterm neonates at birth does not prevent intraventricular haemorrhage or improve outcome at 2 years of life. Similarly, FFP is not superior to other colloid or crystalloid solutions as a volume replacement solution in standard neonatal practice, and there is no evidence to support its use to 'correct' the results of abnormal coagulation screens.

Product specifications

• The current BCSH guidelines state that FFP for transfusion to neonates should be group AB (since this contains neither anti-A nor anti-B) or the same ABO group as the neonate.

• The volume transfused is usually 10–20 mL/kg with the larger dose given if possible in order to limit donor exposure where repeated dosing is likely.

• FFP may be standard or PI. In England at the present time the Department of Health has indicated that single-unit methylene blue-treated FFP should be used for all neonates and children under 16 years. FFP for this group is sourced from plasma from the US. It carries a small residual risk of transmitting transfusion-transmissible viruses (with the exception of CMV). Coagulation factor levels are 20–25% lower in PI-FFP than untreated FFP.

Human albumin solution (HAS) is associated with excess mortality in adults receiving intensive care, but data about the risks of HAS in neonates are not available. Current studies suggest that there is no good indication for the use of HAS in standard neonatal practice.

Transfusion in children

General points

Although most children never require blood transfusion, there are several groups who are

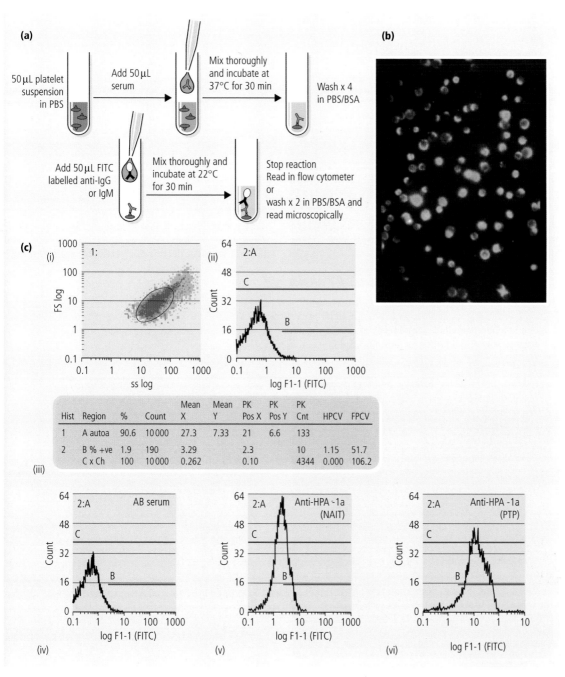

Hist	Region	%	Count	Mean X	Mean Y	PK Pos X	PK Pos Y	PK Cnt	HPCV	FPCV
1	A autoa	90.6	10000	27.3	7.33	21	6.6	133		
2	B % +ve	1.9	190	3.29		2.3		10	1.15	51.7
	C x Ch	100	10000	0.262		0.10		4344	0.000	106.2

Plate 5.1 Indirect platelet immunofluorescence test.
(**a**) Outline of assay. (**b**) Results of microscopic analysis of PIFT showing a strongly positive reaction. (**c**) Results of flow cytometric analysis of PIFT. (i) The platelet population is identified from forward/side scatter characteristics and the population gated for analysis. Figures (ii) to (iv) show plots of fluorescence intensity versus number of events for (ii) a negative sample, (iii) a sample containing weak anti-HPA-1a and (iv) a potent anti-HPA-1a.

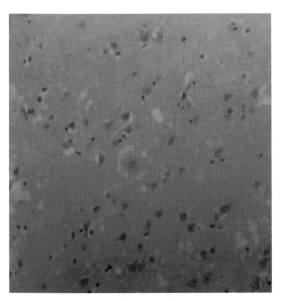

Plate 15.1 Section through the brain of a patient with CJD demonstrating spongiform degeneration of neuronal tissue and a florid amyloid plaque (centre). (Reproduced with the permission of Professor James Ironside.)

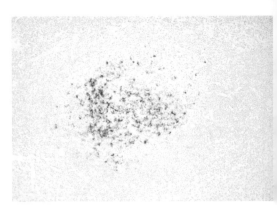

Plate 15.3 Section through the lymphoid tissue of a patient with variant CJD with immunohistochemical staining for PrP demonstrating abnormal accumulation of PrP^{Sc} in follicular dendritic cells. (Reproduced with the permission of Professor James Ironside.)

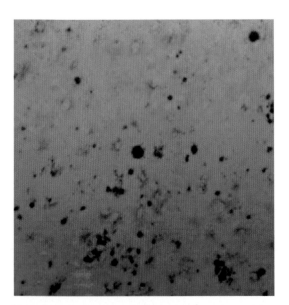

Plate 15.2 Section through the brain of a patient with variant CJD with immunohistochemical staining for PrP demonstrating abnormal accumulation of PrP^{Sc} throughout the brain. (Reproduced with the permission of Professor James Ironside.)

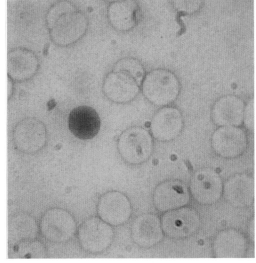

Plate 26.1 Acid elution technique (Kleihauer test) for haemoglobin F containing cells; the blood specimen was taken from a postpartum woman and shows that a foetomaternal haemorrhage had occurred. A single stained foetal cell is seen against a background of ghosts of maternal cells. (Adapted from Bain 1995.)

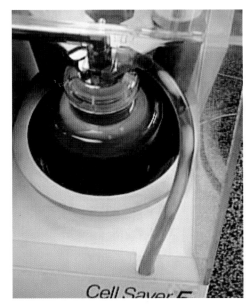

Plate 34.1 Centrifuge bowl within an apheresis machine showing the dense red cell layer towards the outside of the bowl and separation from the buffy coat and plasma layers.

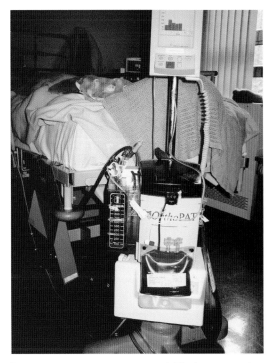

Plate 34.3 Equipment is now available that can wash salvaged blood in the ward environment.

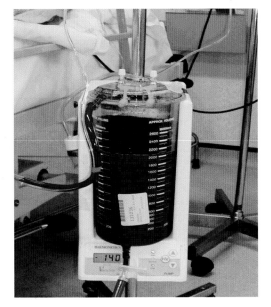

Plate 34.2 Collection reservoir which may be used either operatively or postoperatively to collect the spilt blood or wound drainage.

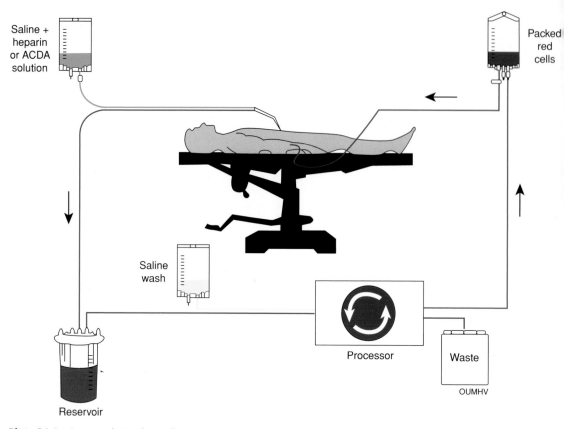

Plate 34.4 Diagram of complete cell saver set-up (provided by the UK Cell Salvage Action Group).

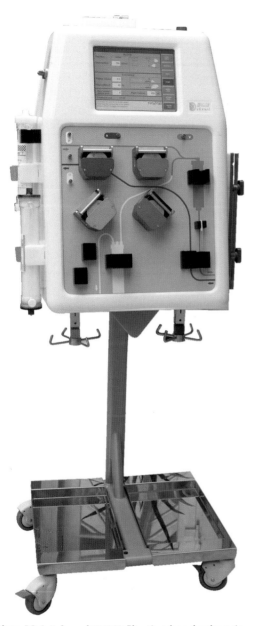

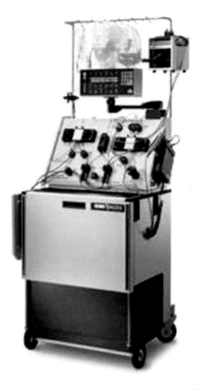

Plate 38.2 COBE Spectra continuous-flow centrifugal apheresis systems.

Plate 38.1 Infomed HF440 filtration-based apheresis system.

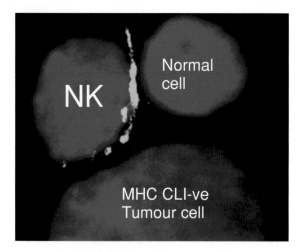

Plate 42.1 Capping of KIR molecules on NK cell. Anti-KIR antibody (green) shows co-localisation of KIR and MHC class I molecules at the synapse between the NK and autologous normal cell. In contrast, the MHC-negative tumour cell fails to initiate capping of the KIR molecules.

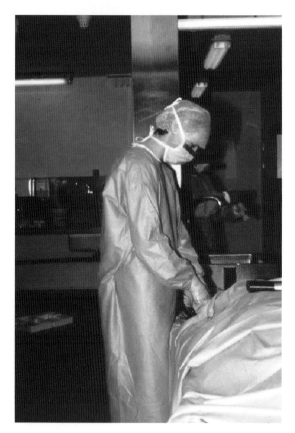

Plate 44.1 Tissue retrieval. (Reproduced with permission from NHSBT Tissue Services.)

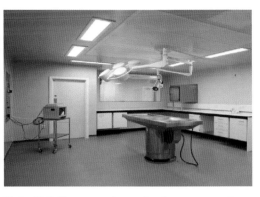
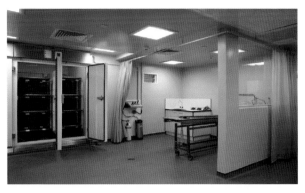

Plate 44.2 Tissue recovery suite, donor preparation and storage room. (Reproduced with permission from NHSBT Tissue Services.)

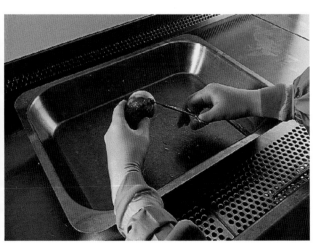
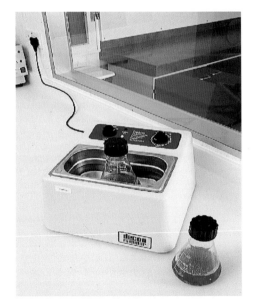

Plate 44.3 Processing of bone in NHSBT processing facility in Edgware, London. (Reproduced with permission from NHSBT Tissue Services.)

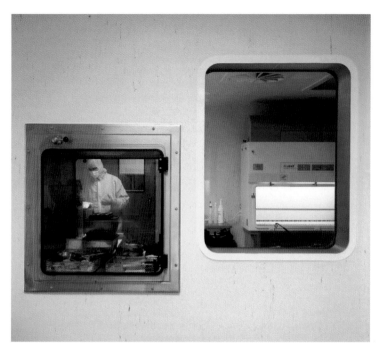

Plate 44.4 Clean rooms in NHSBT, Tissue Services, Liverpool Blood Centre. (Reproduced with permission from NHSBT Tissue Services.)

frequently transfused, including those with inherited transfusion-dependent disorders, such as thalassaemia major, and those undergoing intensive chemotherapy for haematological malignancies. For many of those patients, including those with thalassaemia major and sickle cell disease, bone marrow transplantation (BMT) or cord blood transplantation is a possible future treatment. Therefore, all such children for whom BMT is a possible option should receive CMV-negative blood components. All children on regular transfusions should be vaccinated against hepatitis B as early as possible. Those on chronic transfusion therapy particularly those with haemoglobinopathies, but also those with congenital dyserythropoietic anaemia, aplastic anaemia and other bone marrow failure syndromes, should have an extended red cell phenotype (see below) performed prior to, or as soon as possible after, commencing regular transfusions.

Formula for calculating red cell transfusion volume in children

Several different formulae for calculating transfusion volume in children are in widespread use. Most formulae are based on the increase in Hb or haematocrit required and a 'transfusion factor'. The transfusion factor used varies from 3 to 5. There is a lack of evidence from prospective randomised trials to show which transfusion factor best predicts the rise in Hb/haematocrit and whether the same factor should be applied to all groups of children. Some recent retrospective studies suggest that a transfusion factor of 5 better predicts the Hb/haematocrit in critically ill children but transfusion factors of 3 or 4 appear satisfactory for most children on long-term red cell transfusion. An example using a transfusion factor of 3 is shown here:

Desired Hb (g/dL) – actual Hb (g/dL) × weight (kg) × 3*

*3 represents 3 mL of red cells which has been calculated to raise the haemoglobin by 1 g/dL. The normal rate of red cell transfusion is around 5 mL/kg/h.

Transfusion support for children with haemoglobinopathies (see also Chapter 27)

Thalassaemia major

By definition all patients with thalassemia major are transfusion dependent. Transfusion therapy is determined by the degree of anaemia and evidence of failure to thrive. Most children start transfusion when their haemoglobin drops below 6 g/dL.

Current BCSH and Thalassaemia International Federation guidelines recommend:
- Maintaining an *average* Hb of 12 g/dL.
- Maintaining a *pre-transfusion* Hb of 9–10 g/dL.
- That transfusion should prevent marrow hyperplasia, skeletal changes and organomegaly;
- extended red cell phenotyping should be carried out before starting transfusions (for Rh and Kell antigens).
- Red cell requirements should be adjusted to accommodate growth.
- Splenectomy may be considered if hypersplenism develops and causes a sustained increase in red cell requirements.
- Iron chelation therapy should be considered after 10 transfusions and started once the ferritin is >1000 ng/mL (if possible starting after the age of 2 years because of desferrioxamine toxicity).
- Since BMT and cord blood transplantation are the only cure, families should be offered HLA typing of siblings as possible bone marrow donors and/or cryopreservation of HLA-matched sibling cord blood.

Sickle cell disease

Red cell transfusion in children with sickle cell disease should not be routine but reserved for specific indications (Table 26.7). Extended red cell phenotyping before the first transfusion is very important because up to 50% of patients otherwise develop red cell alloimmunisation and may be very difficult to cross-match. The majority of antibodies are in the Rh or Kell systems and may be transient and very difficult to detect, leading to a risk of delayed transfusion reactions.

Table 26.7 Indications for transfusion in sickle cell disease.

'Top-up'	Splenic sequestration*
	Hepatic sequestration*
	Aplastic crises*
Exchange transfusion	Chest syndrome*
	Stroke*
	Priapism
	Mesenteric syndrome
Hypertransfusion	Stroke (to prevent recurrence)*
	Primary stroke prevention (raised TCD velocity)*
	Renal failure (to prevent/delay deterioration)
	Chronic sickle lung disease
Surgery	Selected patients preoperatively (e.g. joint replacement)

* Proven value.
TCD, transcranial Doppler.

Indications for 'top-up' transfusion in sickle cell disease

Indications include splenic or hepatic sequestration and aplastic crisis. The aim is to raise the haemoglobin to the child's normal steady state (the haemoglobin should never be raised acutely to >10 g/dL since this is likely to cause an increase in blood viscosity).

Indications for exchange transfusion in sickle cell disease

- Acute chest syndrome;
- Mesenteric (abdominal) syndrome;
- Stroke;
- Selected patients preoperatively; and
- Priapism (occasionally).

The aim is to reduce sickling and increase oxygen carriage without an increase in viscosity.

Indications for hypertransfusion in sickle cell disease

- To prevent recurrence of stroke (i.e. secondary prevention of stroke).
- To prevent the development of stroke in children with sickle cell disease with Doppler evidence of cerebrovascular infarction/haemorrhage in the absence of clinical evidence of stroke (i.e. primary prevention of stroke).
- To delay or prevent deterioration in end organ failure (e.g. chronic sickle lung).

The aims are to maintain the percentage of HbS below 25% and the Hb between 10 and 14.5 g/dL. After 3 years a less intensive regimen maintaining the HbS at 50% or less may be sufficient for stroke prevention.

Indications for preoperative transfusion in sickle cell disease

The BCSH guidelines are based on observational studies and one large randomised controlled study, as there are no other available data. These guidelines state that:

- top up transfusion (Hb 8–10 g/dL) is as effective as exchange transfusion and may be safer;
- minor and straightforward procedures (e.g. tonsillectomy, possibly cholecystectomy) can be safely undertaken without transfusion in most patients; and
- exchange transfusion should be performed preoperatively for major procedures such as hip/knee replacement, organ transplantation and eye surgery, and also considered for major abdominal surgery.

Practical aspects of transfusion in sickle cell disease

- Extended red cell phenotyping (for Rh K, Fy, Jk and MNS) should be carried out; this should be done before the first transfusion and may be usefully arranged at outpatient clinic follow-up during the first year of life.
- In particular patients should be typed for U.
- The R_0 blood group (cDe/cDe) is common in patients of African or Caribbean origin: all R_0 patients should receive C-negative or E-negative blood (i.e. rr or R_0).
- The use of sickle trait-positive blood should be avoided by testing for HbS in blood centres or hospitals.
- During exchange transfusion in the acute situation, a total exchange of 1.5–2 times their blood volume is required to achieve an HbS level of 20%

or less; this may take 2–3 procedures if carried out manually. Automated exchange using a cell separator allows the exchange to be completed as a single procedure. The volume of packed cells (in ml) for each exchange is: weight (kg) × 30.
• Normal saline (not FFP or albumin) should be used as volume replacement at the beginning of the exchange prior to starting venesection to avoid dropping the circulating blood volume.

Leukaemia, chemotherapy and BMT

All children being treated with high-dose chemotherapy/radiotherapy or with aplastic anaemia may at some time be candidates for future BMT. While components leucocyte-reduced to less than 5×10^6/unit are widely considered to be CMV-safe, not all BMT centres agree.

Gamma-irradiation of blood components is not necessary for most children receiving chemotherapy for leukaemia or solid tumours, but there are several important situations where irradiation of blood products (25 Gy) is necessary.

Gamma-irradiated blood components should be given to the following children:
• For 2 weeks before allogeneic haemopoietic stem cell transplant (SCT) and during conditioning for all types of SCT until at least 6 months post-SCT or until all immunosuppressive agents have been discontinued, whichever is later.
• For 2 weeks before autologous SCT irradiation and during conditioning until 3 months post-SCT (6 months if total body irradiation given).
• For SCT in children with severe combined immunodeficiency irradiation should continue for at least a year following SCT or until normal immune function has been achieved.
• For 7 days prior to harvesting of autologous bone marrow or peripheral blood stem cells.
• For children with Hodgkin's disease during treatment and thereafter (susceptibility to TA-GVHD is now considered to be life-long).
• During treatment with fludarabine and other purine analogues, and for at least a further 2 years or until full recovery of cellular immune function.
• Where blood products from relatives are being used.

Transfusions for children undergoing blood group-mismatched BMT:
• Major incompatibility arises when the recipient has antibodies to the donor cells (e.g. patient group O, donor group A).
• Minor incompatibility arises when the donor has antibodies to recipient cells (e.g. patient group A, donor group A).
• Current BCSH and European Blood and Bone Marrow Transplantation Group guidelines recommend that in ABO-incompatible SCT, group O red cells should be given (irrespective of the ABO group) until ABO antibodies to the donor ABO type are undetectable and the DAT is negative; thereafter red cells of the donor group are given (high-titre ani-A/anti-B donor units must be excluded).
• RhD-negative red cells are given if the patient is RhD negative and/or the donor is RhD negative.
• After an ABO-incompatible SCT, platelets of the recipient's ABO group should be given until there is conversion to the donor ABO group and ABO antibodies to the donor ABO group are undetectable; thereafter platelets of the donor group should be given.
• After an ABO-incompatible SCT, FFP of the recipient's ABO group should be given. If there is both a major and minor mismatch, group AB should be given.

Platelet transfusion in children undergoing chemotherapy or BMT:
• Indications for platelet transfusion in children are consensus based; those developed by the BCSH are shown in Table 26.8; in general, in non-infected, well children a platelet count of 10×10^9/L can be used as a transfusion trigger, but higher thresholds are used for children who are sick and/or bleeding.
• Platelets should be ABO-compatible where possible because of the risk of haemolysis (see above for ABO-incompatible SCT patients).
• Platelets should be RhD compatible and RhD-negative girls must receive RhD-negative platelets because of the risk of sensitisation by contaminating red cells.
• A transfusion of 10–20 mL/kg is given to children under 15 kg and an apheresis unit for children over 15 kg.

Table 26.8 Indications for platelet transfusion in children with thrombocytopenia.

Platelet count $<10 \times 10^9/L$
Platelet count $<20 \times 10^9/L$ and one or more of the following:
Severe mucositis
DIC
Anticoagulant therapy
Platelets likely to fall $<10 \times 10^9/L$ before next evaluation
Risk of bleeding due to a local tumour infiltration
Platelet count $20\text{–}40 \times 10^9/L$ and one or more of the following:
DIC in association with induction therapy for leukaemia
Extreme hyperleucocytosis
Prior to lumbar puncture or central venous line insertion

DIC, disseminated intravascular coagulation.

Granulocyte transfusion in children undergoing chemotherapy or BMT:
• There is no evidence to support the use of prophylactic granulocyte transfusions.
• Empirical data from some studies support their use where there is severe bacterial or fungal infection in neutropenic children, including SCT, but they increase the risk of platelet refractoriness.
• Granulocytes for transfusion should be ABO and RhD compatible.
• Granulocytes for all recipients should always be irradiated.
Haemopoietic stem cell donors:
• Children who act as bone marrow donors for their sibling(s) usually require blood transfusion to cover blood lost during the procedure; allogeneic blood transfused to the donor during the bone marrow harvest should always be irradiated and CMV-seronegative unless both the patient and the donor are known to be CMV-IgG.
• In older children (>25 kg and more than 8 years old) autologous blood donation should be considered around 2 weeks prior to marrow/peripheral blood stem cell donation.
• For autologous donation children should have no unstable cardiovascular or pulmonary problems and a Hb of more than 11 g/dL. The maximum collected at each donation should be 12% of the estimated blood volume and the amount of citrate anticoagulant in the pack should be adjusted to maintain the appropriate ratio of blood to anticoagulant.

Key points

1 All pregnant women should have ABO and RhD group determined and red cell alloantibody screening done before 16 weeks to identify those at risk of HDN and those requiring anti-D prophylaxis.
2 Antibodies commonly implicated in severe HDN are anti-D, anti-c and anti-K.
3 Anti-D should be given to all RhD-negative women without anti-D antibodies at 28 and 34 weeks' gestation and after all sensitising events during pregnancy and at delivery.
4 The most important factor predicting severity of fetal thrombocytopenia due to maternal ITP is a history of maternal ITP before pregnancy.
5 The most important cause of severe neonatal thrombocytopenia is NAITP.

Further reading

Alcock GS & Liley H. Immunoglobulin infusion for isoimmune haemolytic jaundice in neonates. *Cochrane Database Syst Rev* 2002;3:CD003313.

BCSH Blood Transfusion and Haematology Task Forces. The estimation of fetomaternal haemorrhage. *Transfus Med* 1999;9:87–92.

Bolton-Maggs PHB, Perry DJ, Chalmers EA *et al*. The rare coagulation disorders – review with guidelines for management from the United Kingdom Haemophilia centre Doctors' Organization. *Haemophilia* 2004;10:593–628.

Boralessa H, Modi N, Cockburn H *et al*. RBC T activation and hemolysis in a neonatal intensive care population: implications for transfusion practice. *Transfusion* 2002;42:1428–1434.

British Committee for Standards in Haematology Haemostasis and Thrombosis Task Force. The investigation and management of neonatal haemostasis and thrombosis. *Br J Haematol* 2002;119:295–309.

British Committee for Standards in Haematology Transfusion Task Force: transfusion guidelines for neonates and older children. Available at www.bcshguidelines.com. Accessed 7 December 2005.

Bruce M, Chapman JF, Duguid J *et al*. Addendum for guidelines for blood grouping and red cell antibody testing during pregnancy. BCSH Transfusion Task Force. *Transfus Med* 1999;9:99.

Bussel JB & Primiani A. Fetal and neonatal alloimmune thrombocytopenia: progress and ongoing debates. *Blood Rev* 2008;22:33–52.

Bussel JB, Zacharoulis S, Kramer K, McFarland JG, Pauliny J, Kaplan C, for Neonatal Alloimmune Thrombocytopenia Registry Group. Clinical and diagnostic comparison of neonatal alloimmune thrombocytopenia to non-immune cases of thrombocytopenia. *Pediatr Blood Cancer* 2005;45:176–183.

Kelton JG. Idiopathic thrombocytopenic purpura complicating pregnancy. *Blood Rev* 2002;16:43–46.

Kumar S & Regan F. Management of pregnancies with RhD alloimmunisation. *Br Med J* 2005;330:1255–1258.

Laffan M, Brown SA, Collins PW *et al.* The diagnosis of von Willebrand disease: a guideline from the UK Haemophilia Centre Doctors' Organization. *Haemophilia* 2004;10:199–217.

Meyer MP, Sharma E & Carsons M. Recombinant erythropoietin and blood transfusion in selected preterm infants. *Arch Dis Child Fetal Neonatal Ed* 2003;88:F41–F45.

Murray NA, Howarth LJ, McMcloy M, Letsky EA & Roberts IAG. Platelet transfusion in the management of severe thrombocytopenia in neonatal intensive care unit (NICU) patients. *Transfus Med* 2002;12:35–41.

Murray NA & Roberts IAG. Haemolytic disease of the newborn. *Arch Dis Child* 2007;92:83–88.

National Institute for Clinical Excellence (NICE). Guidelines on the use of routine antenatal anti-D prophylaxis for RhD-negative women. Technology Appraisal Guidance No 41, 2002. Available at www.nice.org.uk/pdf/prophylaxisFinalguidance.pdf.

Patra K, Storfer-Isser A, Siner B, Moore J & Hack M. Adverse events associated with neonatal exchange transfusion in the 1990s. *J Pediatr* 2004;144:626–631.

Puckett RM & Offringa M. Prophylactic vitamin K for vitamin K deficiency bleeding in neonates. *Cochrane Database Syst Rev* 4: CD002776, 2000.

Thompson J. Haemolytic disease of the newborn: the new NICE guidelines. *J Fam Health Care* 2002;12:133–136.

Wee LY & Fisk NM. The twin–twin transfusion syndrome. *Semin Neonatol* 2002;7:187–202.

Zuppa AA, Maragliano G, Scapillati ME *et al.* Recombinant erythropoietin in the prevention of late anaemia in intrauterine transfused neonates with Rh-haemolytic disease. *Fetal Diagn Ther* 1999;14:270–465.

CHAPTER 27

Haematological disease

Michael F. Murphy[1] *& Simon J. Stanworth*[2]

[1]University of Oxford; NHS Blood and Transplant and Department of Haematology, John Radcliffe Hospital, Oxford, UK
[2]NHS Blood and Transplant, John Radcliffe Hospital, Oxford, UK

Background

Patients with haematological diseases are major users of blood products. Haematological diseases requiring transfusion support cover a whole spectrum of clinical disorders: foetal, neonatal and paediatric practice (Chapter 26), haemoglobinopathies (Chapter 28), haemophilia (Chapter 30), immune disorders and bone marrow failure syndromes, in addition to haematological malignancies. Although over 15% of all red cell units are transfused to patients with haematological disease, most are to patients with malignant disorders. The requirement for blood transfusions in this group is related to both the underlying condition itself and the myelosuppressive/myeloablative effects of the specific treatments used.

This chapter considers the following topics:
• the *indications* for red cell, platelet and granulocyte transfusions in haematology patients; and
• the approaches to the management and prevention of *complications* associated with transfusions in haematology patients, including the use of special types of blood components.

In any discussion of transfusion support for patients with haematological disease, it should be recalled that the haemopoietic system has a dramatic capacity for increasing the production of mature blood cells, but this capability varies between different diseases. The scenario of anaemia related to marrow ablation following chemotherapy is very different to anaemia in an individual with a well-compensated chronic haemolytic process. While much of the current impetus in transfusion practice is aimed at reducing inappropriate transfusions, there is now some evidence indicating a risk of 'under-transfusing' certain groups of patients, for example those with coexisting cardiac disease, and therefore general recommendations should be applied according to individual patients' needs.

Red cell transfusions

The ready availability of red cell concentrates means that anaemia in haematology patients can be easily treated. There are some specific considerations in the management of anaemia in haematology patients:

• Its cause should be established, and treatment other than blood transfusion should be used where appropriate, for example in patients with iron deficiency or megaloblastic or autoimmune haemolytic anaemia (AIHA). Anaemia of malignancy may be due to a number of causes including the effects of marrow infiltration or therapy and 'inhibitory' cytokine-mediated influences (or cytokine dysregulation – Chapter 43) leading to the secondary anaemias (of chronic disorders) or low RhEpo.

• There is no universal 'trigger' for red cell transfusions in haematology patients, i.e. a given level of haemoglobin at which red cell transfusion is

Practical Transfusion Medicine, 3rd edition. Edited by Michael F. Murphy and Derwood H. Pamphilon. © 2009 Blackwell Publishing, ISBN: 978-1-4051-8196-9.

appropriate for all patients. Clinical judgement balancing factors such as quality-of-life indices plays an important role in the decision to transfuse red cells or not.

Patients receiving intensive myelosuppressive/myeloablative treatment

There are specific considerations relating to the use of red cell transfusions in patients receiving intensive myelosuppressive/myeloablative treatment, including the need to provide a 'reserve' in case of severe infection or haemorrhage, and the convenience of having a standard policy for red cell transfusion in the setting of an acute haematology service, even if this may result in some patients being over-transfused.

The level of haemoglobin concentration used as the 'trigger' for transfusion varies from centre to centre but is usually in the range 8–10 g/dL. There are no definite data to support the use of a higher level, although studies in animal models of thrombocytopenia and in uraemic patients suggest that correction of anaemia also results in correction of prolonged bleeding times.

The clinical use of recombinant RhEpo might be considered in some situations, e.g. delayed erythroid engraftment after allogeneic bone marrow/peripheral blood progenitor cell transplantation, the treatment of anaemia in patients with myeloma or myelodysplasia, and in the management of Jehovah's Witnesses with haematological disorders. Evidence supports an association between increases in haemoglobin concentration, reduced red cell transfusion requirements and possibly improvement in quality-of-life indices with RhEpo therapy, although the findings concerning quality-of-life measures are more difficult to compare between studies. However, as discussed in Chapter 43, recent systematic reviews have raised concerns about adverse events in patients treated with RhEpo.

Uncertainties also remain about the factors predicting responsiveness, since a number of individuals fail to show adequate responses to RhEpo. Finally, overall cost-effectiveness studies have not documented a major cost–benefit for RhEpo, but this balance could change in the light of changes to the supply and costs of donor blood.

Red cell transfusions and chronic anaemias

In patients with chronic anaemia requiring regular transfusions, red cell transfusions should be used to maintain the haemoglobin level just above the lowest level not associated with symptoms of anaemia. There is considerable variation in this level depending on the patient's age, level of activity and coexisting medical problems, such as cardiovascular and respiratory disease; for example, some young patients are asymptomatic with a haemoglobin concentration below 8 g/dL, while some elderly patients are symptomatic even at haemoglobin concentrations above 10 g/dL. Special considerations apply to patients with haemoglobinpathies, and these are considered in Chapter 28.

Immune blood disorders

In immune haemolytic anaemia, antibodies bind to red blood cell surface antigens and initiate destruction via the complement system and/or the macrophage system. Immune haemolytic anaemia may be alloimmune, autoimmune or drug induced.

Alloimmune haemolytic anaemia occurs in haemolytic disease of the newborn (see Chapter 26), haemolytic transfusion reactions and after allogeneic bone marrow, renal, liver or cardiac transplantation when donor lymphocytes transferred in the allograft ('passenger lymphocytes') may produce red cell antibodies against the recipient and cause haemolytic anaemia (see Chapter 7).

AIHAs are uncommon, with estimates of the incidence at 1–3 per 100,000 of the population per year. They are characterised by the production of antibodies directed against high-frequency red cell antigens and often exhibit reactivity against donor red cells. The degree of haemolysis depends on a number of factors, including the characteristics of the bound antibody (e.g. class, quantity, specificity, thermal amplitude), the target antigen (e.g. density, expression), and other host-related genetic factors (e.g. markers of macrophage activity). The antibody class in turn will affect the degree of classical complement activation (IgM) or binding to splenic and other tissue macrophages via Fc receptors (IgG1 and IgG3 antibodies). AIHA is divided into 'warm' and 'cold' types, depending on whether the antibody attaches better to red cells at body temperature (37°C) or at lower temperatures.

In warm antibody AIHA, IgG antibodies predominate and the direct antiglobulin test is positive with IgG alone (20%), IgG and complement (67%), or complement only (13%); the red cell autoantibodies usually have Rh specificity. In cold AIHA, the antibodies are usually IgM. They easily elute off red cells, leaving complement, which is detected as C3d.

The cause of warm antibody AIHA remains unknown in more than 30% of cases, but may be associated with lymphoid malignancies or diseases such as rheumatoid arthritis and systemic lupus erythematosus or certain drugs. Therapy of warm antibody AIHA depends on the severity of the haemolysis. Treatment is usually required once symptomatic anaemia develops. Steroids are the first-line treatment (e.g. prednisolone in doses of 1 g/kg daily) and are effective in inducing a remission in about 80% of patients. Steroids reduce both production of the red cell autoantibody and destruction of antibody-coated cells. Splenectomy may be necessary if there is no response to steroids or if remission is not maintained when the dose of prednisolone is reduced. Other immunosuppressive drugs, such as azathioprine and cyclophosphamide, may be effective in patients who fail to respond to steroids and splenectomy. Ciclosporin and rituximab may also be effective in patients' refractory to all treatment.

Blood transfusion may be required if there is fulminant haemolytic anaemia or severe anaemia not responding to steroids or other therapy. The presence of red cell autoantibodies on the patient's red cells and in the plasma can cause problems in the identification of compatible blood. It is important to exclude the presence of red cell alloantibodies and autoabsorption of autoantibodies in the plasma using enzyme treatment of the patient's red cells may be necessary to permit the investigation of the plasma for alloantibodies (see Chapter 23).

Cold antibody AIHA is usually due to IgM antibodies. Normally, low titres of IgM cold agglutinins reacting at 4°C are present in plasma and are harmless. At low temperatures these antibodies can attach to red cells and cause their agglutination in the cold peripheries of the body. In addition, activation of complement may cause intravascular haemolysis when the cells return to the higher temperatures in the core of the body. After certain infections, e.g. *Mycoplasma*, cytomegalovirus (CMV) and Epstein–Barr virus (EBV), there is increased synthesis of polyclonal cold agglutinins, producing a mild-to-moderate transient haemolysis.

Chronic cold haemagglutinin disease usually occurs in the elderly, with a gradual onset of haemolytic anaemia owing to the production of monoclonal IgM cold agglutinins, usually with anti-I specificity. After exposure to cold the patient develops an acrocyanosis similar to Raynaud's disease as a result of red cell autoagglutination. The underlying cause should be treated, if possible, and patients should avoid exposure to cold. Treatment with steroids, alkylating agents and splenectomy is usually ineffective. Rituximab is increasingly used as a well-tolerated and effective treatment, producing remission in about 50% of patients. Regular blood transfusion is occasionally required to prevent symptoms of anaemia.

Paroxysmal cold haemoglobinuria is a rare condition more commonly associated with childhood infections, such as measles, mumps and chickenpox, but was originally described in association with syphilis. Intravascular haemolysis is associated with polyclonal IgG complement-fixing antibodies. These antibodies are biphasic, reacting with red cells in the cold in the peripheral circulation, with lysis occurring due to complement activation when the cells return to the central circulation. The antibodies have specificity for the P red cell antigen. The lytic reaction is demonstrated in vitro by incubating the patient's red cells and serum at 4°C and then warming the mixture to 37°C (Donath–Landsteiner test). Haemolysis is self-limiting, but supportive transfusions may be necessary. P-negative blood should be considered if there is no sustained response to transfusion of P-positive cross-match compatible blood.

The issue of whether it is necessary to use an in-line blood warmer when transfusing patients with cold antibody AIHA is controversial. It is logical to keep the patient warm and a common practice to use a blood warmer if the patient has florid haemolytic anaemia.

Platelet transfusions

In general, platelet transfusions are indicated for the prevention and treatment of haemorrhage in patients with thrombocytopenia or platelet function defects. The cause of the thrombocytopenia should be established before platelet transfusions are used because they are not always appropriate treatment for thrombocytopenic patients, and in some instances are contraindicated, for example in thrombotic thrombocytopenic purpura, haemolytic–uraemic syndrome, and heparin-induced thrombocytopenia.

Bone marrow failure

Therapeutic platelet transfusions are established as effective treatment for patients who are bleeding. However, the issue of the benefit of *prophylactic* platelet transfusions for the prevention of haemorrhage in chronically thrombocytopenic patients with bone marrow failure remains more *controversial*. Guidelines for platelet transfusion in many countries recommend that the platelet transfusion trigger for prophylaxis is 10×10^9/L. A critical question is whether the combined trials that have been published evaluating different triggers have sufficient power to demonstrate equivalence in terms of the safety of a threshold of 10×10^9/L rather than 20×10^9/L. There have been no recent randomised trials comparing the frequencies of bleeding events and patient survival in patients receiving either prophylactic *or therapeutic platelet transfusions*, and much of the historical literature supporting prophylaxis may not be applicable to current practice.

A strategy of transfusing platelets only for therapeutic indications in the context of clinical bleeding is appropriate for some patients with *chronic* persisting thrombocytopenia due to bone marrow failure syndromes.

Prophylaxis for invasive procedures depends on the type of procedure:
• No increase in platelet count required: bone marrow aspiration and biopsy.
• Platelet count should be raised to 50×10^9/L: lumbar puncture, epidural anaesthesia, insertion of intravascular lines, transbronchial and liver biopsy, and laparotomy.
• Platelet count should be raised to more than 100×10^9/L: surgery in critical sites such as the brain or the eyes.

Immune thrombocytopenias

• Autoimmune thrombocytopenias: platelet transfusions should be used only in patients with major haemorrhage.
• Post-transfusion purpura: platelet transfusions are usually ineffective in raising the platelet count, but may be needed in large doses to control severe bleeding in the acute phase (see Chapter 12).
• Neonatal alloimmune thrombocytopenia: human platelet antigen (HPA)-matched platelet concentrates are the most appropriate treatment for this condition (see Chapter 26).

Massive blood transfusion

• Clinically significant dilutional thrombocytopenia only occurs with the transfusion of more than 1.5 times the blood volume of the recipient.
• The platelet count should be maintained above 50×10^9/L in patients receiving transfusions for massive acute blood loss (see Chapter 29).

Disseminated intravascular coagulation

• In acute disseminated intravascular coagulation (DIC), where there is bleeding associated with severe thrombocytopenia, platelet transfusions should be given in addition to coagulation factor replacement (see Chapter 30).
• In chronic DIC, or in the absence of bleeding, platelet transfusions are not indicated.

Cardiopulmonary bypass surgery

• Platelet function defects and some degree of thrombocytopenia frequently occur after cardiac bypass surgery, but prophylactic platelet transfusions are not indicated.
• Platelet transfusions should be reserved for patients with bleeding not due to surgically correctable causes.

Granulocyte transfusions

Severe persisting neutropenia is the principal limiting factor in the use of intensive treatment of patients with haematological malignancies. It may last for 2 weeks or more after chemotherapy or bone marrow/peripheral blood progenitor cell transplantation, and during this period the patient is at risk of life-threatening bacterial and fungal infections. The use of haemopoietic growth factors, such as granulocyte colony-stimulating factor (G-CSF), may reduce the duration and severity of severe neutropenia, but they are only effective if the patient has sufficient numbers of haemopoietic precursors. Moreover, the time to response may be several days. Supportive treatment with granulocyte transfusions is a logical approach, although a number of factors have limited its application:

• Difficulties in the collection of neutrophils, which are present in low numbers in normal individuals and which are difficult to separate from red cells because of their similar densities (commercially available long-chain starch solutions now facilitate this separation).

• The short half-life of neutrophils after transfusion, coupled with short storage times and negative effects on function of prolonged storage.

• The frequent occurrence of adverse effects such as febrile reactions, including occasional severe pulmonary reactions and human leucocyte antigen (HLA) alloimmunisation causing platelet refractoriness.

Various methods have been used in the past to increase the number of neutrophils collected, including obtaining granulocytes from patients with chronic myeloid leukaemia, treating donors with steroids, and using hydroxyethyl starch to promote sedimentation of red cells. However, a number of clinical trials of granulocyte transfusions in the 1970s and 1980s suggested they had limited efficacy in adults, and interest in their usage declined. Some centres continued to use granulocyte transfusions for small children and neonates because concentrates collected from adult donors produced a relatively much greater dose per recipient weight, and sometimes appeared to be clinically effective.

There has recently been a resurgence of interest in granulocyte transfusions because of the accumulating evidence that G-CSFs can be safely administered to normal individuals. Much larger doses of granulocytes can be collected from donors using regimens including G-CSF administered 12–

16 hours prior to apheresis, together with oral steroids such as dexamethasone to further improve the yields. Further evidence of the safety of this approach for donors, and the efficacy of granulocyte transfusions collected in this way, are required before granulocyte transfusion therapy becomes accepted in the care of patients with severe neutropenia and fungal infection, in conjunction with other potential approaches such as improved diagnostic strategies and organism-targeted antimicrobials. Trials to evaluate evidence of survival benefit following granulocyte transfusions are clearly needed, but their design is complicated by several issues including the numbers of patients required to power a trial and the methodological difficulties related to incorporating blinding in such studies.

High-dose granulocyte transfusions collected using donors treated with G-CSFs might therefore be considered as indicated in patients of any age with severe neutropenia due to bone marrow failure under the following circumstances:

• Proven bacterial or fungal infection unresponsive to antimicrobial therapy, or probable bacterial or fungal infection unresponsive to appropriate blind antimicrobial therapy.

• Neutrophil recovery not expected for 5–7 days.

• Children and lighter adults might be expected to show better incremental responses to granulocyte transfusions.

Granulocyte transfusions might be considered inappropriate for:

• patients with haematological disease resistant to treatment;

• ventilated patients; and

• patients with known HLA alloimmunisation.

Approach to complications associated with blood transfusion in haematology patients

Transfusion-transmitted CMV infection

Clinical features and risk factors

CMV infection may cause significant morbidity and mortality in immunocompromised patients, mainly due to pneumonia. Patients who have never been exposed to CMV are at risk for primary infection transmitted by blood components prepared from blood donors who have previously had CMV infection and still carry the virus.

Patients who have been previously exposed to CMV and are CMV seropositive are at risk of reactivation of CMV during a period of immunosuppression. The extent to which CMV-seropositive patients are at risk from reinfection with different strains of CMV remains unknown, but this risk is generally considered to be low. The patients at risk of transfusion-transmitted CMV infection are shown in Table 27.1, and the generally accepted indications for the use of CMV-seronegative blood components are shown in Table 27.2.

Prevention

The use of CMV-seronegative blood components has been shown to reduce the incidence of CMV infection in groups at risk for transfusion-transmitted

Table 27.1 Patients at risk for transfusion-transmitted cytomegalovirus (CMV) infection.

Risk well established
CMV-seronegative recipients of allogeneic bone marrow/peripheral blood progenitor cell transplants from CMV-seronegative donors
CMV-seronegative pregnant women
Premature infants (<1.2 kg) born to CMV-seronegative women
CMV-seronegative patients with HIV infection

Risk less well established
CMV-seronegative patients receiving autologous bone marrow/peripheral blood progenitor cell transplants
CMV-seronegative patients who are potential recipients of allogeneic or autologous bone marrow/peripheral blood progenitor cell transplants
CMV-seronegative patients receiving solid organ (kidney, heart, lung liver) transplants from CMV-seronegative donors

Risk not established
CMV-seronegative recipients of allogeneic bone marrow/peripheral blood progenitor cell transplants from CMV-seropositive donors
CMV-seropositive recipients of bone marrow/peripheral blood progenitor cell transplants
CMV-seropositive recipients of solid organ transplants

Table 27.2 Indications for the use of cytomegalovirus (CMV)-seronegative blood components.

Transfusions in pregnancy
Intrauterine transfusions
Transfusions to neonates and to infants in the first year of life
Transfusions to the following groups of CMV-seronegative patients
    After allogeneic bone marrow/peripheral blood progenitor cell transplants where the donor is also CMV seronegative
    After autologous bone marrow/peripheral blood progenitor cell transplants
    Potential recipients of allogeneic bone marrow/peripheral blood progenitor cell transplants
    Patients with HIV infection

CMV infection to 1–3%. This incomplete prevention may be due to:

• occasional failure to detect low-level CMV antibodies;
• loss of antibodies in previously infected blood donors; and
• transfusion of blood components prepared from recently infected donors.

CMV is transmitted by leucocytes, and a number of studies have found that leucocyte reduction of blood components is as effective as the use of CMV-seronegative blood components in the prevention of transfusion-transmitted CMV infection in neonates, patients undergoing remission induction therapy for acute leukaemia and after bone marrow transplantation (the only prospective randomised trial was conducted in transplant recipients using bedside filtration, which cannot be adequately quality controlled). These data suggest that leucocyte-reduced blood components can be accepted as a substitute for CMV-seronegative blood components for patients at risk of transfusion-transmitted CMV infection when CMV-seronegative blood components are not available. Further information about the effectiveness of leucocyte reduction of blood components in the prevention of transfusion-transmitted CMV infection in different patient groups is required before CMV-seronegative blood components can be discontinued. A consensus conference in Canada recommended that where universal leucocyte re-duction had been implemented, both leucocyte-reduced and CMV-seronegative blood should be used for CMV-seronegative pregnant women, in-trauterine transfusions, and CMV-seronegative al-logeneic haemopoietic cell transplant recipients.

Transfusion-associated graft-versus-host disease

Pathogenesis and clincal features

Transfusion-associated graft-versus-host disease (TA-GVHD) is a rare but serious complication of blood transfusion. As discussed in Chapter 11, there is engraftment and proliferation of donor T lymphocytes, and interaction with recipient cells expressing HLA antigens causing cellular damage particularly to the skin, gastrointestinal tract, liver and spleen, and the bone marrow. Clinical manifestations usually occur 1–2 weeks after blood transfusion, and early features include fever, maculopapular skin rash, diarrhoea and hepatitis. At-risk transfused haematology patients are those who are undergoing transplantation, have Hodgkin's disease, or have received therapy with certain drugs, e.g. purine analogues.

Prevention

The dose of donor lymphocytes sufficient to cause TA-GVHD is unknown, but may be lower than is achievable by current techniques for leucocyte reduction of blood components. However, there have been no case reports of TA-GVHD in the UK since 2001 following the implementation of universal leucocyte-reduction of blood in the UK in 1999. Gamma-irradiation to remove the prolif-erative capability of donor lymphocytes remains the usual method of choice to prevent TA-GVHD (see Chapter 11), although it is a radioactive source and requires regular recalibration. An alternative to gamma-irradiation is X-ray irradiation, which is used in several European countries. Key con-siderations in the assessment of methods for the prevention of TA-GVHD are their effectiveness, and the avoidance of excessive damage to red cells and platelets. The currently recommended

Table 27.3 Indications for gamma-irradiation of blood components in haematology patients.

Indications

Acute leukaemia: only for HLA-matched platelets or donations from first- or second-degree relatives

Allogeneic bone marrow/peripheral blood progenitor cell transplantation: from the time of initiation of conditioning therapy and continuing while the patient remains on GVHD prophylaxis (usually 6 mo) or until lymphocytes are greater than 1×10^9/L. It may be necessary to irradiate blood components for SCID patients for up to 2 yr, and for patients with chronic GVHD if there is evidence of immunosuppression

Donors of allogeneic bone marrow: to prevent TA-GVHD mediated by lymphocytes in donor blood transfused before or during the harvest

Autologous bone marrow/peripheral blood progenitor cell transplantation: during and 7 days before the harvest of haemopoietic cells, and then from the initiation of conditioning therapy until 3 mo post-transplant (6 mo if total body irradiation is used)

Hodgkin's disease

Patients treated with purine analogues

Non-indications

Aplastic anaemia (even if treated with antilymphocyte globulin)

Non-Hodgkin's lymphoma (although this may be reviewed following some recent reports of TA-GVHD in patients with B-cell non-Hodgkin's lymphoma)

HIV infection

SCID, severe combined immunodeficiency; TA-GVHD, transfusion-associated graft-versus-host disease.

indications for the use of gamma-irrradiated blood for haematology patients are shown in Table 27.3.

How to ensure that patients receive the correct 'special' blood?

An important issue for haematology departments and hospital blood banks is how to ensure that pa-tients receive special blood components (e.g. CMV-seronegative, gamma-irradiated) when they are in-dicated and that standard blood components are not transfused as this may have devastating con-sequences.

Each hospital needs to establish its own proce-dures so that patients receive the correct special blood components, where they are indicated. These should include the following:

• Education of ward medical and nursing staff about the indications for special blood components, and the importance of receiving the correct type of blood component.

• Requests for blood components to include the patient's diagnosis and any requirement for special blood components.

• Storing of individual patient's requirements for special blood components in the blood bank computer.

• The prescription for blood components should include any requirement for special blood components, enabling the ward staff to check that the blood component to be transfused complies with these requirements.

• Providing patients with cards indicating their special blood requirements, particularly for those patients receiving shared care between two hospitals and those with a long-term requirement for gamma-irradiated blood, e.g. patients with Hodgkin's disease.

HLA alloimmunisation and refractoriness to platelet transfusions

Platelet refractoriness is the repeated failure to obtain satisfactory responses to platelet transfusions, and occurs in more than 50% of patients receiving multiple transfusions.

Various methods are used to assess response to platelet transfusions. If the patient is bleeding, the clinical response is an important indication of the effectiveness of the transfusion. The response to a prophylactic platelet transfusion is assessed by measuring the increase in platelet count after the transfusion. Various formulas have been used to correct for the variation in response dependent on the patient's size and the number of platelets transfused; these include platelet recovery and corrected count increment. However, in practice, a (non-sustained) increase in the patient's platelet count of less than 5×10^9/L at 20–24 hours after the transfusion can be used as a simple measure of a poor response.

Causes

Many causes of platelet refractoriness have been described, and they can be subdivided into immune mechanisms, most importantly HLA alloim-

Table 27.4 Causes of platelet refractoriness.

Immune
Platelet alloantibodies
   HLA
   HPA
   ABO
Other antibodies
   Platelet autoantibodies
   Drug-dependent platelet antibodies
Immune complexes

Non-immune
Infection and its treatment, especially amphotericin B
Splenomegaly
Disseminated intravascular coagulation
Fever
Bleeding

munisation, and non-immune mechanisms involving platelet consumption (Table 27.4). Platelet consumption is the most frequent mechanism of platelet refractoriness, usually associated with sepsis. However, immune-mediated platelet destruction remains an important cause of platelet refractoriness; HLA antibodies are the commonest immune cause, and the other immune causes are rare.

The precise mechanism of HLA alloimmunisation remains uncertain, but primary HLA alloimmunisation appears to be initiated by intact cells expressing both HLA class I and class II antigens such as lymphocytes and antigen-presenting cells. Platelets only express HLA class I antigens, and leucocyte-reduced blood components will not cause primary HLA alloimunisation. However, secondary HLA alloimmunisation does not require the presence of HLA class II antigens, and may occur in patients who have been pregnant or previously transfused with non-leucocyte-reduced blood components.

Investigation and management

If platelet refractoriness occurs, the following algorithm can be used for investigation and management (Figure 27.1).

1 A clinical assessment should be made for clinical factors likely to be associated with non-immune platelet consumption.

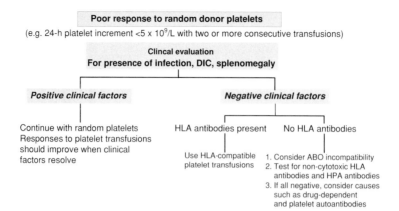

Figure 27.1 Algorithm for the investigation and management of patients with platelet refractoriness. DIC, disseminated intravascular coagulation.

2 If non-immune platelet consumption appears likely, an attempt should be made to correct the clinical factors responsible, where possible, and platelet transfusions from random donors should be continued. If poor response to random donor platelet transfusions persists, the patient should be tested for HLA antibodies.

3 If non-immune platelet consumption appears to be unlikely, an immune mechanism should be suspected, and the patient's serum should be tested for HLA antibodies. If HLA antibodies are present, the specificity of the antibodies should be determined as this may help in the selection of HLA-compatible donors. However, HLA antibodies stimulated by repeated transfusions are often 'multispecific', and it is not possible to determine their specificity.

4 Platelet transfusions from HLA-matched donors (matched for the HLA-A, -B antigens of the patient) should be used for patients with apparent immune refractoriness, and the response to further transfusions should be observed carefully. Figure 27.2 shows improved responses to HLA-matched platelet transfusions in a patient with platelet refractoriness due to HLA alloimmunisation. If responses to HLA-matched transfusions are not improved, the reason should be sought, and platelet cross-matching of the patient's serum against the lymphocytes and platelets of one of the HLA-matched donors may be helpful in determining the cause, and the selection of compatible donors for future transfusions.

5 If there are no factors for non-immune platelet consumption and HLA antibodies are not detected, consideration should be given to less frequent causes of immune platelet refractoriness.

(a) High-titre ABO antibodies in the recipient. This is an unusual cause of platelet refractoriness, and can be excluded by switching to ABO-compatible platelet transfusions, if

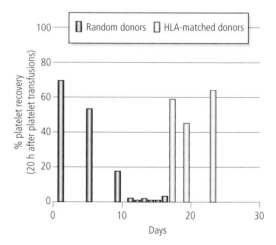

Figure 27.2 Responses to platelet transfusions in a female patient with acute myeloblastic leukaemia undergoing remission induction therapy. There were poor responses to the initial platelet transfusions, and the patient was found to have HLA antibodies. There were improved responses to platelet transfusions from HLA-matched donors.

ABO-incompatible transfusions have been used for previous transfusions.

(b) HPA antibodies, which usually occur in combination with HLA antibodies, but sometimes occur in isolation.

(c) Drug-dependent platelet antibodies, which may be underestimated as a cause for platelet refractoriness.

Alloimmunisation to red cell antigens

Incidence

Alloimmunisation to red cell antigens is another important consequence of repeated transfusions in haematology patients. The incidence of red cell alloimmunisation in adult haematology patients is in the range of 10–15% and is similar to other groups of multitransfused patients, e.g. patients with renal failure. However, a higher proportion of children requiring long-term transfusion support develop red cell alloimmunisation. In sickle cell disease, the incidence is in the range of 20–30%. The implications of these observations include the following.
• Patients with sickle cell disease should be phenotyped for Rh, Kell, Fy, Jk and MNS antigens before the first transfusion, and patients with thalassaemia and other children requiring chronic transfusion support should be phenotyped for Rh and Kell antigens.
• Blood for transfusion to children requiring long-term transfusion support, including patients with haemoglobinopathies, should be matched for Rh and Kell antigens to prevent alloimmunisation.
• Phenotyping and antigen matching to prevent red cell alloimmunisation is not required for other groups of patients requiring repeated transfusions.

Timing of sample collection for compatibility testing

In patients with haematological disorders receiving repeated transfusions, an important issue is the timing of blood sample collection in relation to the previous transfusion.
• Where the patient is receiving very frequent transfusion, e.g. daily, it is only necessary to request a new sample every 72 hours.

• Where the previous transfusion was 3–14 days earlier, the sample should ideally be taken within 24 hours of the start of the transfusion, although some laboratories stretch this to 48 hours for patients who have been repeatedly transfused without developing antibodies.
• Where the previous transfusion was 14–28 days earlier, the sample should be taken within 72 hours of the start of the transfusion.
• Where the previous transfusion was more than 28 days ago, the sample should be taken within 1 week of the planned transfusion.

ABO-incompatible bone marrow/peripheral blood progenitor cell transplants

ABO-incompatible bone marrow/peripheral blood progenitor cell transplants present particular problems (Table 27.5). The transplant may provide a new A and/or B antigen from the donor (major

Table 27.5 Problems associated with ABO-incompatible bone marrow/peripheral blood progenitor transplants.

Major ABO incompatibility (e.g. recipient O, donor A)
Failure of engraftment: risk not increased in ABO-incompatible transplants
Acute haemolysis at the time of reinfusion: avoided by processing donor bone marrow/peripheral blood progenitor cells
Haemolysis of donor-type red cells: avoid by using red cells of recipient type in the early post-transplant period
Delayed erythropoiesis: may be due to persistence of anti-A in the recipient, but minimise transfusion of anti-A by using platelets and plasma from group A donors
Delayed haemolysis due to persistence of recipient anti-A: only switch to donor red cells when recipient anti-A undetectable and direct antiglobulin test undetectable

Minor ABO incompatibility (e.g. recipient A, donor O)
Graft-versus-host disease: risk not increased in ABO-incompatible transplants
Acute haemolysis at the time of reinfusion: avoid by removing donor plasma if the donor anti-A titre is high
Delayed haemolysis of recipient cells due to anti-A produced by donor lymphocytes (passenger lymphocyte syndrome): maximum haemolysis usually occurs between days 9 and 16 post-transplant, and occasionally there is severe intravascular haemolysis

---

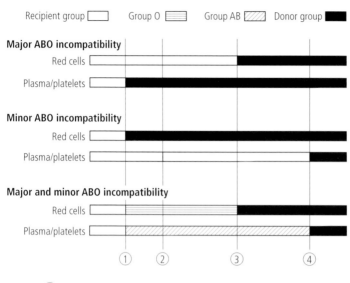

Recipient group ☐   Group O ☰   Group AB ▨   Donor group ■

Major ABO incompatibility
Red cells
Plasma/platelets

Minor ABO incompatibility
Red cells
Plasma/platelets

Major and minor ABO incompatibility
Red cells
Plasma/platelets

① ② ③ ④

① Begin pre-transplant chemotherapy
② Bone marrow transplant
③ ABO antibodies to donor RBC not detected. Direct antiglobulin test negative
④ RBC of recipient group no longer detected

Figure 27.3 Recommendations for ABO type of blood components in ABO-incompatible bone marrow/peripheral blood progenitor cell transplants. (Adapted from Warkentin 1983, with permission.)

mismatch) or a new A and/or B antibody (minor mismatch). Recommendations for the use of donor blood components are given in Figure 27.3, and can be briefly summarised as follows.

• Major ABO mismatch: use red cells of patient's ABO type until recipient ABO antibodies are undetectable and the direct antiglobulin test is negative, and platelets and plasma from donors of recipient's ABO type.

• Minor ABO mismatch: use red cells of donor ABO type throughout, and plasma and platelets of recipient type until recipient-type red cells are no longer detectable.

• Major and minor ABO mismatch: use group O red cells until recipient ABO antibodies are undetectable, and then switch to donor-type red cells. Use group AB plasma and platelets until recipient-type red cells are undetectable.

RhD-incompatible transplants can also cause difficulties. It is recommended that RhD-negative blood components should be used for RhD-positive recipients with RhD-negative donors. However, no cases of immunisation have been reported when RhD-negative recipients have received RhD-

positive transplants, and RhD-positive blood components may be used.

Iron overload

A major adverse consequence of repeated red cell transfusions over a long period in patients with haemoglobinopathies or myelodysplastic syndromes is iron overload. This important complication is described in detail in Chapter 28.

Key points

1 Specialist transfusion support and advice is required for many patients with haematological disorders.

2 The need for transfusion, as in other groups of patients, is determined by assessment of individual patient's symptoms and blood counts and guided by national and local recommendations for the use of blood.

3 Special blood components are frequently needed to avoid complications such as TA-GvHD and

transfusion transmission of CMV in haematology patients susceptible to these complications.

4 Responses to platelet transfusions should be carefully monitored to identify patients having poor responses which require clinical and laboratory investigation to determine the most likely cause and the best approach to management.

5 Further work is needed to define the optimal thresholds for red cell and platelet transfusion in patients with haematological malignancies and the role of granulocyte transfusions.

Further reading

British Committee for Standards in Haematology. Guidelines on gamma irradiation of blood components for the prevention of graft-versus-host disease. *Transfus Med* 1996;6:261–271.

British Committee for Standards in Haematology. Guidelines on the clinical use of red cell transfusions. *Br J Haematol* 2001;113:24–31.

British Committee for Standards in Haematology. Guidelines for platelet transfusions. *Br J Haematol* 2003; 122:10–23.

Campell-Lee SA. The future of red cell alloimmunisation. *Transfusion* 2007;47:1959–1960.

Cohen AR. New Advances in iron chelation therapy. *Hematology Am Soc Hematol Educ Program* 2006:42–47.

Drew WL & Roback JD. Prevention of transfusion-transmitted cytomegalovirus: reactivation of the debate? *Transfusion* 2007;47:1955–1958.

Dzik S. How I do it: platelet support for refractory patients. *Transfusion* 2007;47(3):374–378.

Laupacis A, Brown J, Costello B *et al*. Prevention of post-transfusion CMV in the era of universal WBC reduction: a consensus statement. *Transfusion* 2001;41:560–569.

Price TH. Granulocyte transfusion: current status. *Semin Hematol* 2007;44:15–23.

Silberstein LE & Cunningham MJ. Autoimmune hemolytic Anemias. In: Hillyer CD, Silberstein LE, Ness PM, Anderson KC, Roback JD. (eds), *Blood Banking and Transfusion Medicine: Basic Principles & Practice*, 2nd edn. Philadelphia: Churchill Livingstone, 2007.

Stanworth SJ, Hyde C, Brunskill S & Murphy M. Platelet transfusion prophylaxis for patients with haematological maligancies: where to now? *Br J Haematol* 2005;131:588–595.

Wilson J, Yao GL, Raftery J *et al*. A systematic review and economic evaluation of epoetin alfa, epoetin beta and darbepoetin alfa in anaemia associated with cancer, especially that attributable to cancer treatment. *Health Technol Assess* 2007;11(13):1–220.

CHAPTER 28

Blood transfusion in the management of patients with haemoglobinopathies

David Rees

Department of Haematological Medicine, King's College Hospital, Denmark Hill, London, UK

Introduction

Haemoglobinopathies are inherited disorders caused by mutations in the globin genes. The α-globin family is on chromosome 16 and the β-globin family on chromosome 11. Together with haem, they produce haemoglobin, which is a tetramer of two α-like and two β-like globins. Two different α-globins and four different β-globins are produced, resulting in a variety of haemoglobins (Table 28.1). At birth there is a gradual switch from fetal to adult haemoglobin, which is largely complete in a year. Quantitative defects in globin chain synthesis cause thalassaemia, whereas qualitative defects result in haemoglobin variants; the most important haemoglobin variant is haemoglobin S (HbS, $β^6$ Glu-Val), causing sickle cell disease (SCD). Blood transfusion is important in haemoglobinopathies, allowing correction of anaemia, suppression of abnormal erythropoiesis and replacement of abnormal erythrocytes.

α-Thalassaemia syndromes

Most people have four α-globin genes, and the common types of α-thalassaemia are due to large

deletions. Deletion of both α-globin genes on a chromosome can occur, although this is only common in Southeast Asia and the eastern Mediterranean. There are three main α-thalassaemia syndromes.

α-Thalassaemia trait

This is usually due to the deletion of one or two α-globin genes. The haemoglobin is normal with mild hypochromia. Blood transfusion is never needed to treat the condition itself.

HbH disease

This usually occurs when there is only one functional α-globin gene. It is typically a mild condition, with haemoglobin of 7–10 g/dL, and HbH (tetramers of β-globin) inclusion bodies in erythrocytes. The spleen is moderately enlarged. Blood transfusion is unusual, but may be necessary following Parvovirus B19 infection.

Hb Bart's hydrops fetalis

A complete or near-complete absence of functional α-globin genes results in progressive fetal anaemia from the 10th week of gestation. Without intervention this results in a hydropic fetus and miscarriage at 30–40 weeks, reflecting the importance of α-globin in forming HbF. Occasionally fetal anaemia has been detected and the pregnancy maintained until term with regular intrauterine transfusions. The resulting babies are transfusion dependent and

Practical Transfusion Medicine, 3rd edition. Edited by Michael F. Murphy and Derwood H. Pamphilon. © 2009 Blackwell Publishing, ISBN: 978-1-4051-8196-9.

Table 28.1 Normal haemoglobins.

Structure	Name	Predominant expression
$\zeta_2\varepsilon_2$	Hb Gower 1	0–10th-week gestation
$\alpha_2\varepsilon_2$	Hb Gower 2	5th–10th-week gestation
$\zeta_2\gamma_2$	Hb Portland	5th–10th-week gestation
$\alpha_2{}^G\gamma_2$	HbF	12th-week gestation – 4th month
$\alpha_2{}^A\gamma_2$	HbF	12th-week gestation – 4th month
$\alpha_2\beta_2$	HbA	4th month – death
$\alpha_2\delta_2$	HbA$_2$	4th month – death

Table 28.2 Causes of β-thalassaemia intermedia.

Factors lessening severity of predicted β-thalassaemia major
Mild β-thalassaemia mutations, e.g. HbE/β-thalassaemia
Coinheritance of α-thalassaemia
Coinheritance of increased capacity to make HbF
Unexplained

Factors worsening severity of predicted β-thalassaemia trait
Coinheritance of triplicated α-globin gene
Dominant β-thalassaemia mutation
Unexplained

usually are seriously handicapped. This may either result from the effects of fetal anaemia or be caused by large deletions on chromosome 16. If fetal anaemia is found to be due to Hb Bart's hydrops fetalis, the likelihood of serious handicap should be discussed with the parents prior to starting intrauterine transfusions.

β-Thalassaemia syndromes

β-Thalassaemia results from a deficiency of β-globin synthesis, and much of the pathology arises from the resulting excess of α-globin. β-Globin is not part of fetal haemoglobin and there are no adverse fetal or neonatal effects. In contrast to α-thalassaemia, most cases of β-thalassaemia are caused by small mutations or deletions in the β-globin gene. More than 200 different mutations have been identified, and the many different combinations result in a phenotypic continuum from asymptomatic to transfusion dependence.

β-Thalassaemia trait
This results from the inheritance of one mutated β-globin gene. There is minimal anaemia, with hypochromia and microcytosis. Anaemia becomes more marked during pregnancy, and occasionally blood transfusion is necessary, although regular or frequent blood transfusions have no role.

β-Thalassaemia intermedia
This is a clinical term referring to a range of conditions characterised by significant anaemia, splenomegaly and increased iron absorption. Pa-

tients typically grow and develop normally without the need for regular blood transfusions. Many different combinations of β-globin mutation cause thalassaemia intermedia (Table 28.2). Anaemia may increase during infection or illness and intermittent transfusions may be necessary. The trigger for blood transfusion is based on clinical signs and symptoms rather than any specific haemoglobin level. Acute symptoms suggesting that transfusion may be beneficial include dyspnoea and fatigue. It can be difficult to decide if someone with severe thalassaemia intermedia would benefit from regular blood transfusions and treatment as for thalassaemia major. In children this is suggested by poor growth, recurrent illness or marked bony expansion. Sometimes children require regular blood transfusions to progress through puberty or older adults increasingly develop symptoms that convert to thalassaemia major. The decision to start regular transfusions is clinical, not based on a particular genotype or haemoglobin level. Once regular transfusions start they should be continued long term. Iron overload can be a problem in thalassaemia intermedia even in the absence of regular transfusions, and iron stores should be monitored regularly, and chelation started as necessary.

β-Thalassaemia major
Thalassaemia major is the term used when a patient with β-thalassaemia is treated with regular blood transfusions. Without transfusions, the patient either dies or is seriously ill, with poor growth, bony deformity or a poor quality of life. It is usually

due to the coinheritance of severe β-thalassaemia mutations (β° mutations) from both parents but can be caused by combinations of less severe mutations (β⁺-thalassaemia) with exacerbation from epigenetic and environmental factors. The clinical problems result from excess α-globin chains, damaging the developing erythroid cells in the marrow such that they fail to mature into circulating red cells (ineffective erythropoiesis). This causes:

- severe anaemia;
- bone marrow expansion with bony deformity and osteopenial;
- hypersplenism and hypermetabolism; and
- increased iron absorption.

Before starting a transfusion programme, children should be vaccinated against hepatitis B. An extended red cell phenotype should be performed (C, c, D, E, e, K, k, Jka, Jkb, Fya, Fyb, Kpa, Kpb, MNS, Lewis). The risk of alloimmunisation can be reduced by transfusing blood matched for Rh and Kell groups and transfused blood should be leucocyte reduced. With regular blood transfusion from an early age, the expectation is that children will grow and develop normally, with near normal quality of life. With adequate iron chelation, life expectancy should approach the normal range, although chelation failure means that median life expectancy is shortened; patients in developed countries born in the 1960s had a median survival of 30 years, but this has progressively increased.

Blood transfusion in β-thalassaemia major

The aim of a blood transfusion programme in thalassaemia major is to:

- reduce or eliminate symptoms of anaemia;
- suppress ineffective erythropoiesis to prevent bony deformity;
- prevent the development of significant hypersplenism; and
- suppress extramedullary haemopoiesis.

Studies measuring soluble transferrin receptor have shown that erythropoiesis is suppressed by maintaining pre-transfusion haemoglobin greater than 9.5 g/dL, and it is recommended to keep the post-transfusion haemoglobin below 15 g/dL. In practice this is achieved by regular, simple transfu-

sions given every 2–5 weeks, the frequency being determined by local resources and pre-transfusion symptoms. Occasionally, more intensive transfusion is used to support cardio-respiratory problems or suppress extramedullary haemopoiesis. Automated exchange transfusions are also used, and typically patients have a full-volume exchange every 6 weeks. This has the advantages of decreasing iron loading and less frequent hospital attendances, although it involves more donor exposure with increased risk of alloimmunisation and infection; good vascular access is also important, and the procedure is more difficult in young children. It is more expensive than simple transfusion and unavailable in many parts of the world. The insertion of semi-permanent venous access devices is sometimes necessary if venous access is difficult.

Sickle cell disease

SCD includes a group of conditions in which the mutated sickle haemoglobin (HbS, β⁶ Glu-Val) occurs (Table 28.3). The two main pathological processes are:

- Vaso-occlusion: Deoxygenated HbS polymerises and damages the red cell membrane, causing cellular dehydration, and abnormal expression of adhesion molecules on the erythrocyte. This causes red cells to block small blood vessels, resulting in acute and chronic hypoxic damage. Typical vaso-occlusive syndromes include hyposplenism, acute

Table 28.3 Types of SCD.

Severe SCD
HbSS (sickle cell anaemia)
HbS β-thalassaemia
HbS O^Arab
HbS D^Punjab
Mild SCD
HbSC
HbS β⁺-thalassaemia
HbS Lepore
Very mild SCD
HbSE
HbS/hereditary persistence of fetal haemoglobin

pain, acute chest syndrome, acute abdominal pain and chronic restrictive lung defects.

• Haemolysis: The premature destruction of red cells results in chronic anaemia. Intravascular haemolysis causes increased plasma haemoglobin, which binds avidly to and causes a functional deficiency of nitric oxide. This is thought to cause vasculopathy and lead to the complications of stroke, pulmonary hypertension, priapism and leg ulcers.

Blood transfusion plays an important role in reversing both these processes by reducing the number of cells able to cause vaso-occlusion in the blood, and decreasing the rate of haemolysis. Increasing the haemoglobin too much is potentially harmful as it increases blood viscosity, particularly in small blood vessels and so can precipitate vaso-occlusion. When planning a transfusion in SCD, it is important to decide what the target haemoglobin and HbS percentages are, and then decide how best to achieve this. This can be through either a simple top-up transfusion or an exchange transfusion of some sort, in which blood is also removed. In SCD, there is not thought to be any benefit from exchange per se, and it is a way of decreasing the HbS percentage without increasing the haematocrit excessively.

Indications for transfusions in acute complications of SCD

• Acute anaemia: the need for transfusion is dependent on symptoms rather than on haemoglobin level, but is usually necessary when the haemoglobin falls below 5 g/dL. A single, simple transfusion aiming to increase the haemoglobin to 7–8 g/dL is typically used. Specific causes of acute anaemia include:
  ○ Parvovirus B19 infection – low reticulocyte count, viral symptoms;
  ○ acute splenic/hepatic sequestration – high reticulocyte count, enlarging spleen/liver;
  ○ acute pain – occasionally the haemoglobin falls significantly (>2 g/dL) during an episode of acute pain, and transfusion may be necessary to correct the anaemia.
• Acute chest syndrome: This is defined as new pulmonary shadowing on a chest X-ray in someone with SCD and is typically accompanied by chest pain, tachypnoea, hypoxia and increasing anaemia. Many cases recover with oxygen and antibiotics, although 5–10% cases deteriorate and require respiratory support. Blood transfusion has an important role in managing severe cases. Increasing anaemia often accompanies deterioration, and a simple transfusion to haemoglobin of 10 g/dL can often result in 50% or less HbS and marked clinical improvement. In general, the target haemoglobin should not be greater than 10 g/dL, as there is a danger of precipitating cerebrovascular complications. If deterioration is rapid or mechanical ventilation necessary, the HbS should be reduced to less than 30% with a haemoglobin of 10 g/dL, which will often involve an exchange.

• Stroke: If acute neurological symptoms are likely to be due to a stroke, urgent blood transfusion should be arranged, with the aim of reducing the HbS to less than 30% and increasing the haemoglobin to about 11 g/dL. This will usually require an exchange transfusion, and a retrospective study suggested that outcome was better if an exchange transfusion was used initially rather than a top-up.

• Multiorgan failure: This can occur following severe sepsis or acute chest syndrome, and often patients will have been fully exchanged as part of the prodrome to this often agonal event.

• There is no evidence to support the use of blood transfusions in the treatment of acute pain, priapism or osteomyelitis. In some cases these may be accompanied by significant anaemia and so benefit from transfusion, or surgery may be necessary and transfusion used preoperatively.

Indications for regular transfusion in SCD

• Secondary stroke prevention: Following a stroke there is a 90% chance of further episodes. Retrospective studies suggest that the risk of recurrence is reduced by up to 90% by regular blood transfusion to keep the HbS less than 30 or 50%. This requires regular exchange or top-up transfusions, with evidence suggesting that the high risk of stroke returns once the transfusions stop.

• Primary stroke prevention in children with abnormal transcranial Doppler (TCD) scans – children with narrowed intracerebral blood vessels, as detected by TCD, are at high risk of acute stroke. A randomised controlled trial showed that keeping HbS less than 30% with regular transfusions reduced stroke risk by 90%.

- Recurrent acute chest syndrome: Hydroxyurea is effective at stopping recurrent acute chest syndrome in 80% cases; if hydroxyurea fails, regular blood transfusions may help prevent further episodes.
- Progressive organ failure: Hepatic, renal, cardiovascular and pulmonary failure are problems in older SCD patients, and regular transfusions can help support organ function or prevent further deterioration.
- Other indications: Regular transfusions may have a role in preventing frequent episodes of acute pain, chronic pain, avascular joint necrosis, leg ulcers, pulmonary hypertension, acute pain in pregnancy and recurrent splenic sequestration, depending on individual circumstances.

An extended red cell phenotype should be performed prior to starting transfusions, as for thalassaemia major. Similarly, transfused blood should be matched for Kell and all Rh groups.

Preoperative blood transfusion in SCD

Perioperative complications are increased in SCD, including the development of pain and acute chest syndrome. In cardiac, brain and other major surgery, it is accepted that preoperatively the HbS should be less than 30% with minimal anaemia. This will usually involve an exchange transfusion. For other surgery, the need for transfusion is less clear. Studies suggest no advantage of exchange over top-up transfusion, unless the patient has significant organ damage, cerebrovascular disease or had previous severe complications. In practice, most people with haemoglobin less than 7 g/dL are transfused preoperatively.

Complications of transfusions in haemoglobinopathies

All the routine complications of blood transfusion can occur. Particular problems include:

- Alloimmunisation: Rates vary from 10 to 20% depending on the similarity between the ethnicities of donor and recipient populations, and the extent of blood group matching.
- Autoantibody formation: This typically accompanies the development of alloantibodies and occurs in up to 25% of thalassaemia major patients. It is associated with non-leucocyte-reduced transfusions and splenectomy. This can result in hyperhaemolysis, in which both transfused and non-transfused cells are destroyed, causing severe anaemia. Management includes avoiding further blood transfusion if at all possible, with a possible role for corticosteroids and intravenous immunoglobulin.
- Infection: The prevalence of transfusion-transmitted infections varies widely but is rare in most developed countries. Prion infection is an increasing concern.
- Iron overload.

Iron chelation

Regular blood transfusions inevitably cause iron overload. Each unit of transfused blood contains about 200 mg iron, and typically iron chelation is started after 12 months of regular transfusions, or when the ferritin exceeds 1000 μg/L. Without treatment, iron accumulates in and damages the liver, heart and endocrine organs. In thalassaemia, iron-related heart disease is the major cause of death. Cardiac iron deposition is unusual in SCD.

It is important to assess iron stores accurately to monitor chelation therapy (Table 28.4). Iron chelation techniques include:

- Venesection rapidly removes excess iron, although clearly this is not possible in transfusion-dependent patients. Venesection is useful in haemoglobinopathies post-bone marrow transplantation.
- Desferrioxamine: this has been used for more than 30 years. Good compliance has been shown to improve survival. Side effects are few but include growth impairment, retinal and cochlear toxicity. Side effects become increasingly common as iron

Table 28.4 Assessment of iron overload.

	Description	Advantages	Disadvantages
Monitoring transfused volume	Annual review of volume of transfused blood	Accurate measure of iron input; cheap	Does not assess iron loss through chelation or other means
Serum ferritin	Simple blood test	Cheap, widely available; monitors trends in hepatic iron	Increased by inflammation. Variable correlation with liver iron
Liver biopsy	Chemical measurement of liver iron in tissue sample	Accurate quantitation. Also shows liver histology	Invasive. Only small sample of liver analysed
Magnetic susceptrometry	Magnetic assessment of liver iron	Non-invasive. Accurate	Very few calibrated machines in world
T2* MRI	Assessment of liver and heart iron using MRI	Technology widely available. Assesses heart iron. Accurate	Variable results from different scanners. Young children need anaesthesia
R2 MRI	Assessment of liver iron using MRI	Widely available. Approved in US and EU. Results similar between scanners	Cannot assess cardiac iron. Young children need anaesthesia

stores approach normal. Negative iron balance is typically achieved in a transfusion-dependent patient at a dose of 40 mg/kg 5 nights per week. The main problem is that it has to be given parenterally, typically by overnight subcutaneous infusions. Adherence to desferrioxamine treatment is poor and this results in toxic iron accumulation. In heart failure secondary to iron overload, continuous intravenous desferrioxamine has been shown to be effective.

• Deferiprone (L1): This oral iron chelator was developed in the 1980s. Side effects include neutropenia and arthritis. The drug is licensed as a second-line chelator in Europe but is not available in North America. Recent studies suggest that it is particularly effective at removing cardiac iron, and various regimes in combination with desferrioxamine have been devised.

• Deferasirox: This oral iron chelator has recently been licensed as first-line treatment for transfusional iron overload around the world. It seems to be as effective as desferrioxamine with relatively few side effects. The main toxicity involves increases in serum creatinine, which in general have been non-progressive and reversible. There is emerging evidence that it also removes cardiac iron.

Key points

1 Regular intrauterine transfusions should not be used in fetuses with Hb Bart's hydrops fetalis until the risk of severe handicap has been discussed with the parents.

2 Transfusions should be started in severe β-thalassaemia syndromes on the basis of symptoms rather than a particular haemoglobin level or genotype.

3 Blood transfused to haemoglobinopathy patients should be fully matched for Rh and Kell blood groups.

4 Regular transfusions are important in children with sickle cell disease as primary and secondary stroke prevention.

5 Iron chelation should be actively considered after 10–12 blood transfusions.

Further reading

Adams RJ, McKie VC, Hsu L et al. Prevention of a first stroke by transfusions in children with sickle cell anemia and abnormal results on transcranial Doppler ultrasonography. *N Engl J Med* 1998;339: 5–11.

Guidelines for the Clinical Management of Thalassaemia, 2nd edn. Thalassaemia International Federation, 2007. Available at www.thalassaemia.org.cy.

Koshy M, Weiner SJ, Miller ST et al. Surgery and anesthesia in sickle cell disease. Cooperative Study of Sickle Cell Diseases. *Blood* 1995;86:3676–3684.

Olivieri NF & Brittenham GM. Iron-chelating therapy and the treatment of thalassemia. *Blood* 1997;89:739–761.

Serjeant GR & Serjeant BE. *Sickle Cell Disease,* 3rd edn. Oxford UK: Oxford University Press, 2001.

Singer ST, Wu V, Mignacca R *et al.* Alloimmunization and erythrocyte autoimmunization in transfusion-dependent thalassemia patients of predominantly Asian descent. *Blood* 2000;96:3369–3373.

Stuart MJ & Nagel RL. Sickle-cell disease. *Lancet* 2004;364:1343–1360.

Vichinsky E. Clinical application of deferasirox: practical patient management. *Am J Hematol* 2007;83:398–402.

Vichinsky EP, Earles A, Johnson RA *et al.* Alloimmunization in sickle cell anemia and transfusion of racially unmatched blood. *N Engl J Med* 1990;322:1617–1621.

Weatherall DJ & Clegg JB. *The Thalassaemia Syndromes,* 4th edn. Oxford, UK: Blackwell Scientific Publications, 2001.

CHAPTER 29

Massive blood loss

Beverley J. Hunt

Thrombosis & Haemostasis, King's College and Departments of Haematology, Pathology and Rheumatology, Guy's and St Thomas' NHS Foundation Trust, London, UK

Definition and burden of massive blood loss

Massive blood loss is arbitrarily defined as the replacement of the patient's total blood volume in less than 24 hours. It is the major cause of death in the developing world through injury and obstetric haemorrhage. Indeed injury is the leading cause of death worldwide among those aged 5–44 years. In the US, it is the leading cause of death in the 1–44-year age group and the third leading cause of death overall. Of the early deaths, 30–50% are due to exsanguination.

Obstetric haemorrhage remains the leading cause of maternal mortality worldwide:
• One woman dies from obstetric haemorrhage every 4 minutes, that is 140,000–160,000 each year.
• The latest Confidential Enquiries into Maternal Deaths in the UK, 2003–2005 'Saving Mothers' Lives', indicates that obstetric haemorrhage accounts for 11% of all maternal deaths, with almost three-fifths of those who died received less than optimal care.
• The European Project on Haemorrhage Reduction (EUPHRATES) observed considerable variation between the 14 participant European countries in the medical policies for immediate management of obstetric haemorrhage.

Practical Transfusion Medicine, 3rd edition. Edited by Michael F. Murphy and Derwood H. Pamphilon. © 2009 Blackwell Publishing. ISBN: 978-1-4051-8196-9.

Massive blood loss in some situations such as liver transplantation can be predicted, and thus sophisticated monitoring and management protocols can be employed. Best practice in managing massive blood loss as shown by 'Saving Lives' is not always followed. This seems, in part, to be due to poor understanding in the appropriate use of blood components and pharmacological agents.

Management is aimed at preventing tissue hypoxia by maintaining an adequate circulating volume of red cells. This requires a multidisciplinary approach including control of the relevant physiological parameters, rapid control of bleeding, maintenance of tissue perfusion, temperature control and blood component or pharmacological treatment to support coagulation. This chapter aims to concentrate on the appropriate use of blood components, the use of pharmacological agents is covered in Chapter 36. It is important to recognise that the evidence base to support current management guidelines is poor.

Physiological response of coagulation to blood loss

During traumatic, surgical and obstetric haemorrhage, as well as blood loss depleting blood components, massive tissue factor exposure may result in intensive early fibrin clot formation. This loss and activation of coagulation factors and subsequent fibrinolysis will consume and deplete haemostatic factors. Haemostasis is also strongly influenced by the body temperature. In hypothermia, a coagulation screen, which is performed at 37°C, will underestimate the extent of any coagulopathy. Furthermore, coagulation disorders are aggravated by acidosis. Metabolic acidosis due to high lactate levels usually reflects the degree of tissue hypoxia and persistent elevation is associated with poor outcome. Early abnormalities of coagulation in massive blood loss due to trauma are independent predictors of mortality. Key factors in the development of coagulopathy include:

- the severity of the injury;
- hypothermia;
- hypocalcaemia;
- acidosis;
- bleeding;
- haemorrhagic shock;
- haemodilution as a result of fluids given during resuscitation;
- consumption of clotting factors; and
- hyperfibrinolysis.

These factors combine to form a vicious cycle. If the lethal triad of hypothermia, acidosis and coagulopathy are present, surgical control of bleeding alone is unlikely to be successful and a disseminated intravascular coagulation may occur and mortality rates are high.

Management of bleeding

The general principles are to achieve rapid control of bleeding and volume resuscitation with fluids and blood products. Adequate analgesia is necessary to control pain and prevent tachycardia secondary to pain, being misinterpreted as a sign of hypovolaemia.

Heart rate, blood pressure and urine output are useful but non-reliable parameters for the initial assessment of the degree of blood loss. A heart rate >100 bpm or decrease in urine output are probably the earliest signs of hypovolaemia and can be detected with blood loss of around 15% (750 mL in a person of 70 kg). Systolic blood pressure below 90 mmHg generally requires a greater blood loss of approximately 20–30% of blood volume, but it

should be remembered that young patients might maintain an adequate blood pressure until blood loss is even greater.

The clinical symptoms of shock are the 'three windows to the microcirculation':

(a) Mental status/level of consciousness (cerebral perfusion) – agitation, confusion, somnolence or lethargy.

(b) Peripheral perfusion – cold and clammy skin, delayed capillary refilling, tachycardia.

(c) Renal perfusion – urine output (<0.5 mL/kg/h).

These clinical findings help to differentiate whether a patient is 'haemodynamically normal' or just 'apparently haemodynamically stable' but in compensated shock. Arterial blood gas can indicate lactate levels, and base deficit represents highly sensitive parameters for recognition of metabolic acidosis reflecting 'hidden shock'.

Fluid management

Fluids used are isotonic and hypertonic crystalloids, colloids (mainly gelatins and starch solutions) and blood products. Crystalloids are not associated with anaphylaxis and are inexpensive, safe and easy to store. However, the disadvantages include the need to use large volumes, the short duration of effect, the resultant oedema and occasional metabolic disturbances. Colloids are efficient volume expanders, have rapid activity, improve colloid osmotic pressure, and cause less pulmonary impairment than crystalloids. Yet they are expensive compared with crystalloids and they carry a risk of anaphylactic response. Moreover, meta-analyses have shown an increased risk of death in patients treated with colloids except for the most recent Cochrane review.

The SAFE study compared 4% albumin with 0.9% sodium chloride in nearly 7000 ICU patients and showed no significant differences in outcomes, but a trend towards higher mortality in the trauma subgroup that received albumin. Promising results have been obtained with hypertonic solutions and a meta-analysis showed improved survival with hypertonic saline group in resuscitation[23].

Traditional guidelines generally employ early and aggressive fluid administration to restore the blood volume. Some studies have shown increased mortality rates with rapid infusion of fluids compared with standard infusion, and with immediate compared with delayed resuscitation. The concept of low-volume fluid resuscitation or 'permissive hypotension' avoids the detrimental effects of early aggressive resuscitation, while maintaining a level of tissue perfusion that, although decreased from normal, is adequate for short periods. This approach is contraindicated in brain and spinal injuries and its effectiveness still needs to be confirmed in randomised clinical trials.

Volume expanders may produce other haemostatic hazards, apart from dilution. Dextrans, and to a lesser extent hydroxylethyl starch, have a fibrinoplastic effect: they accelerate the action of thrombin in converting fibrinogen to fibrin, which makes clots more amenable to fibrinolysis. Both are absorbed on to the platelet surfaces and von Willebrand factor, causing decreased platelet function and an acquired von Willebrand syndrome. Gelatins produce few problems, although they decrease plasma fibronectin activity.

Prevention of hypothermia and strategies for re-warming

In general, the greater the degree of hypothermia, the greater is the risk of uncontrolled bleeding. When hypothermia is associated with severe injury, mortality rates up to 100% have been reported. The effects of hypothermia include altered platelet function, impaired coagulation factor function (a 1°C drop in temperature is associated with a 10% drop in function), enzyme inhibition and fibrinolysis. Preventive measures include covering the patient to avoid additional heat loss, increasing the ambient temperature, forced air warming, giving warm fluid therapy and, in extreme cases, extracorporeal re-warming devices.

Blood component use

A coagulation screen and full blood count should be performed as soon as possible to guide the use of blood components with frequent repeat testing determined by the rate of blood loss. The results may be misleading if the patient is hypothermic. Near-patient haemostatic monitoring such as thromboelastography may be a future alternative, but currently there are no satisfactory management algorithms that are evidence based.

High infusion rates of blood products containing citrate can decrease calcium concentrations, particularly in patients with hypothermia or liver failure (who are unable to metabolise the citrate), so monitoring of serum calcium may be required.

Use of RBC transfusion in trauma

RBC transfusion is recommended to maintain Hb above 8 g/dL. No prospective randomised trial comparing restrictive and liberal transfusion regimens in massive blood loss exists. However, 203 trauma patients from the Transfusion Requirements in Critical Care (TRICC) trial were recently re-analysed. A restrictive transfusion regimen (Hb transfusion trigger <7.0 g/dL) resulted in fewer transfusions as compared with the liberal transfusion regimen (Hb transfusion trigger <10 g/dL) and appeared to be safe. However, it cannot be excluded that the number of RBC units transfused merely reflects the severity of injury, and thus later multiorgan failure (MOF) may simply reflect a correlation between the severity of injury and MOF. Adequately powered studies similar to the TRICC trial are therefore needed in massive blood loss.

A prospective observational study in 15,534 trauma patients, of whom 1703 received RBC transfusion with a mean of 6.8 ± 6.7 units, showed that after controlling for severity of shock, RBC transfusion within the first 24 hours was associated with increased mortality, admission to the intensive care unit (ICU), and length of ICU and hospital stays. Blood products are linked to MOF and an increased incidence of infections and there is a strong dose–response relationship between early RBC transfusion and the development of MOF. Reducing the number of RBC units transfused may thus decrease the risk and severity of MOF. Moreover, the age of transfused RBC units has been shown to be an independent risk factor for post-injury MOF. It is thought that tissue damage and hypoxia caused by injury and blood loss prime the inflammatory system; subsequent transfusions of stored RBCs containing bioreactive lipids activate systemic inflammatory response resulting in MOF [35].

There are no evidence-based guidelines for RBC transfusion in obstetric haemorrhage. In the Netherlands a prospective randomised multicentre trial, the 'Wellbeing of Obstetric patients on minimal blood transfusions' (WOMB) study, is currently ongoing in ten hospitals in the Netherlands, aiming to develop a new transfusion policy.

Platelets

Platelets are recommended by all guidelines in the management of massive blood loss when the platelet counts fall below 50×10^9/L. A higher target level of $\geq 100 \times 10^9$/L is for those with multiple injury undergoing surgery or high-risk invasive procedures. In the UK one platelet apheresis concentrate will increase the platelet count by 50×10^9/L in adults. The platelet count should be checked 10–15 minutes after platelet infusion to ensure the adequacy of therapy. A poor increment of less than 20×10^9/L after 15 minutes may be indicative of antiplatelet antibodies, usually human leucocyte antigen (HLA) antibodies (see Chapter 27).

Fresh frozen plasma (FFP)

The indication for use of FFP in massive transfusion and disseminated intravascular coagulation with significant bleeding is an INR or APTT ratio >1.5. There is no evidence base for the dose that should be used. However, 15 mL/kg is widely accepted for the initial dose. For the acute reversal of the effects of warfarin, the best practice is to use prothrombin complex concentrate (PCC). However, if this is not available, a similar effect can be produced with an FFP dose of 15 mL/kg.

Fibrinogen and cryoprecipitate

Cryoprecipitate or fibrinogen is indicated when fibrinogen levels are <1 g/L with bleeding. Ten units of cryoprecipitate increases the plasma fibrinogen level by approximately 1.0 g/L. Although ABO blood group compatibility is not required with cryoprecipitate, it is preferred because of the 10–20 mL of plasma in each unit. Indications for the use of fibrinogen concentrate are the same as for cryoprecipitate, but this product is not licensed for this indication in the UK.

Other coagulation factors

Coagulation factor concentrates have been used in treating severe bleeding but their clinical efficacy is unproven.

In patients receiving vitamin K antagonists, the recommendations for serious bleeding at any elevation of the INR is to withhold the vitamin K antagonist therapy and to give vitamin K_1 supplemented with FFP or prothrombin complex concentrate; the latter has just been licensed for this indication.

Summary of practical haematological management of a bleeding patient

• Send blood sample to blood transfusion laboratory for ABO group and RhD group and phone the laboratory indicating the need for blood. If possible, wait for ABO and RhD compatible blood. In emergency cases. In emergency cases use group O RhD-negative red cells until patients' ABO and RhD groups are known. Switch to blood of the same ABO and RhD groups as the patient as soon as possible to avoid inappropriate use of group O Rh-negative red cells.
• Send baseline sample for FBC, coagulation screen and urea and electrolytes.
• When a fast rate of transfusion is required, a presser or infuser or pump and a blood warmer should be used.
• Haemostasis. An early coagulation screen and platelet count or thromboelastography will provide a guide to the use of blood components. It is important to appreciate that at least 1.5 blood volumes (i.e. 7–8 L in adults) must be transfused before the platelet count falls below 50×10^9/L in an average healthy individual. Transfusion of replacement blood components should be given as necessary according to the results of the screening coagulation tests, aiming to keep:

   (a) platelet count >50×10^9/L;

(b) PT and APTT ratios less than 1.5 times the control value by giving FFP 15 mL/kg;

(c) fibrinogen >1 g/L with cryoprecipitate; and

(d) be mindful of other possible complications of blood transfusion:

- Hypocalcaemia. Calcium gluconate (2 mL of 10% solution per unit of blood) when calcium concentration is low or there are clinical signs or ECG changes.
- Hyperkalaemia may occur due to its high concentration (approximately 40 mmol/L) in stored blood. This is usually only a problem in those with hepatic or renal disease.
- Acid–base disturbances. Despite the presence of lactic acid in transfused blood fluid resuscitation, this usually improves acidosis in shocked patients. Furthermore, transfused citrate produces an alkalosis once it is metabolised.
- Hypothermia. Warm patient and blood.

Organisation of transfusion for patients with trauma and for major accidents

In a major accident large numbers of people may be injured within a short space of time. This requires a coordinated approach from the rescue services and the hospital. A 'major accident procedure' is a necessity within every hospital and should be tested periodically by holding a 'major accident exercise'.

The following must be incorporated into the procedure:

- The telephone numbers of those who 'need to know' held by the hospital switchboard.
- Suspend the issue of blood for non-emergency cases.
- Increase the stocks to a predefined level by arranging deliveries from the nearest transfusion centre and maintain the stocks throughout the emergency. The blood transfusion laboratory must have a dedicated telephone line to arrange this, as the main hospital switchboard may be blocked with other calls.
- The risk of clinical clerical errors can be high in this emergency situation, so special care must be taken in the identification of casualties, and in labelling blood samples. In the emergency department, every attempt to maintain good clinical practice should be made. Full identification details of each patient should be given on blood request forms and sample bottles, wherever possible, and at least the hospital record number of the patient and their sex.

- The practice of issuing blood in a major disaster is best not changed from routine practice, i.e. compatibility testing should be carried out wherever possible. If this is not possible, every effort should be made to ensure that blood is ABO and RhD specific so that blood issued is ABO and RhD group matched. When the recipients blood group is not known Group O RhD negative blood should be given to girls and women in the reproductive age, unless there is life-threatening bleeding and O RhD-negative blood is not available. O RhD-positive blood can be given to males with unknown blood groups.

- Blood components such as FFP and platelets need to be available quickly for those who are receiving massive transfusion.

- Dealing with requests to donate blood. Following a major accident, there may be calls from the public, offering to donate blood. These potential donors should be given the telephone number of the nearest blood centre so that they can attend one of the routine donor clinics.

The future

Current guidelines advise the use of haemostatic components after a review of coagulation profiles. However, a recent review of 246 patients in the US army suffering from massive blood loss ($\geq$10 units of RBCs in 24 hours) after combat-related trauma showed that the plasma-to-red cell ratio was independently associated with survival. The authors of the study recommended that for practical purposes, massive transfusion should utilise a 1:1 ratio of plasma to RBCs for all patients who are hypocoagulable with traumatic injuries. These findings need to be followed up with further studies.

Conclusions

The management of bleeding and coagulopathy in massive blood loss is an area that has not received the attention necessary to answer the many questions that remain. It is clear that the priority during initial treatment must be the maintenance of tissue oxygenation through appropriate use of fluid and blood components. Coagulation may be supported by controlling temperature and blood pH and by correcting coagulopathic deficiencies.

Key points

1 Massive transfusion is the loss of more than one blood volume within 24 hours.
2 The aim of immediate resuscitation is to maintain adequate tissue oxygenation through adequate numbers of circulating red cells.
3 Check the full blood count and coagulation screen regularly.
4 Maintain haemoglobin >8 g/dL.
5 Maintain INR and APTT ration <1.5 with fresh frozen plasma at 15 mL/kg.
6 Maintain platelet count >50 × 10^9/L with platelet transfusion.
7 Maintain fibrinogen >1 g/L with cryoprecipitate.
8 Consider tranexamic acid 2–3 g.

Further reading

Ansell J, Hirsh J, Poller L, Bussey H, Jacobson A & Hylek E. The pharmacology and management of the vitamin K antagonists: the Seventh ACCP Conference on Antithrombotic and Thrombolytic Therapy. *Chest* 2004;126(Suppl 3):204S–233S.

Borgman MA, Spinella PC, Perkins JG *et al.* The ratio of blood products transfused affects mortality in patients receiving massive transfusions at a combat support patients. *J Trauma* 2007;63:805–813.

British Committee for Standards in Haematology Blood Transfusion Task Force. Guidelines for the use of platelet transfusions. *Br J Haematol* 2003;122(1):10–23.

Hébert PC, Wells G, Blajchman MA *et al.* A multicenter, randomized, controlled clinical trial of transfusion requirements in critical care. Transfusion Requirements in Critical Care Investigators, Canadian Critical Care Trials Group. *N Engl J Med* 1999;340(6):409–417.

Khan KS, Wojdyla D, Say L, Gülmezoglu AM & Van Look PFA. WHO analysis of causes of maternal death: a systemic review. *Lancet* 2006;367:1066–1074.

Krug EG, Sharma GK & Lozano R. The global burden of injuries. *Am J Public Health* 2000;90(4):523–526. The data on bleeding as a major cause of global death.

Lewis G. (ed). The Confidential Enquiry into Maternal and Child Health. (CEMACH). Saving Mothers; Lives: reviewing maternal deaths to make motherhood safer-2003–2005. The Seventh Report on Confidential Enquiries into Maternal Deaths in the United Kingdom. London: CEMACH, 2007.

O'Shaughnessy DF, Atterbury C, Bolton Maggs P *et al.* Guidelines for the use of fresh-frozen plasma, cryoprecipitate and cryosupernatant. *Br J Haematol* 2004;126(1):11–28.

Roberts I, Alderson P, Bunn F, Chinnock P, Ker K & Schierhout G. Colloids versus crystalloids for fluid resuscitation in critically ill patients. *Cochrane Database Syst Rev* 2004(4):CD000567.

Spahn DR, Cerny V, Coats TJ *et al.*, for Task Force for Advanced Bleeding Care in Trauma. Management of bleeding following major trauma: a European guideline. *Crit Care* 2007;11(1):R17.

Winter C, Macfarlane A, Deneux-Tharaux C *et al.* The European project on haemorrhage reduction: attitudes, trial and early warning system (EUPHRATES). *BJOG* 2007;114(7):845–854.

CHAPTER 30

Inherited and acquired coagulation disorders

Vickie McDonald[1], J. Kim Ryland[1], Joanne E. Joseph[2] & Samuel J. Machin[1]

[1]Haemostasis Research Unit, Department of Haematology, University College London, London, UK
[2]Department of Haematology and Stem Cell Transplantation, St Vincent's Hospital, Darlinghurst, New South Wales, Australia

Normal haemostasis

Haemostasis is a complex process involving the interaction of many components – blood vessels, platelets, coagulation factors, coagulation factor inhibitors and fibrinolytic enzymes.

The procoagulant cascade (shown in Figure 30.1) is activated when tissue factor (TF) expressed on damaged or stimulated cells (vascular cells or monocytes) comes in contact with circulating factor VII and VIIa (which accounts for approximately 1–2% of circulating plasma factor VII). This TF/factor VIIa complex activates limited quantities of factors IX and X. Newly generated factor IXa forms a complex with factor VIIIa (activated by traces of thrombin generated slowly by factor Xa) in the presence of calcium and membrane phospholipid. This complex subsequently also activates factor X to Xa, and is known as tenase. Factor Xa binds to factor Va (again activated by thrombin), which with calcium and phospholipid rapidly converts prothrombin to thrombin.

The initial TF-VIIa complex is quickly inhibited by tissue factor pathway inhibitor; however, by this time, the thrombin that has already been produced activates factor XI as well as factors V

and VIII, therefore augmenting the formation of factor Xa and ultimately the production of more thrombin. Factor XI can also be activated by factor XIIa formed from the HMWK-prekallikrein complex on endothelial cells; however, this contribution to physiological haemostasis is minimal. The ultimate function of thrombin is to cleave fibrinogen to fibrin and activate factor XIII that results in the cross-linked stable clot.

Fibrinolysis is also part of the normal haemostatic response. Circulating plasminogen is activated to form the serine protease plasmin, which digests cross-linked fibrin to form D-dimers and other fibrinogen fragments.

Investigation of abnormal haemostasis

A careful clinical history and physical examination should be undertaken – this aims to differentiate between bleeding caused by a local factor and that due to an underlying haemostatic defect. Continued oozing from venepuncture and injection sites or from wound drains suggests the possibility of generalised haemostatic failure.

Initially, some simple 'screening' laboratory tests (listed in Table 30.1) that are easy to perform and give quick, reliable results should be undertaken. If one/more of these tests suggest an abnormality,

Practical Transfusion Medicine, 3rd edition. Edited by Michael F. Murphy and Derwood H. Pamphilon. © 2009 Blackwell Publishing, ISBN: 978-1-4051-8196-9.

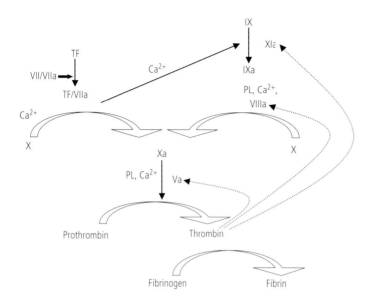

Figure 30.1 The procoagulant pathway.

then further specialised investigations (such as specific coagulation factor assays) should be performed in order to define precisely the defect and its severity.

In high dependency units, the availability of near patient testing devices to rapidly assess coagulation (PT and APTT) and overall global haemostasis (thromboelastogram) potentially allows rapid treatment decisions to be made without sending a citrated sample to the laboratory.

It is important to note that in some disorders (such as mild forms of haemophilia or von Willebrand disease (vWD)), 'screening' tests such as the APTT may not be overly prolonged, and hence if a bleeding disorder is strongly suspected from the patients history and clinical picture, specific factor assays and/or immunological tests should be performed regardless of the 'screening' test result.

Transfusion support for patients with acquired haemostatic defects

Disseminated intravascular coagulation (DIC)

This is a disorder resulting from inappropriate and excessive activation of the haemostatic system that can be manifested by both thrombotic and haemorrhagic pathology. DIC may be acute (uncompensated) with decreased levels of haemostatic components or chronic (compensated) with normal or sometimes elevated levels of coagulation factors.

The main triggering mechanism for DIC is the exposure of blood to a source of tissue factor (TF) that initiates coagulation. This can occur as a result of:

Table 30.1 Simple laboratory haemostasis screening tests.

System	Test
Coagulation	PT
	APTT
	INR – only in patients receiving oral anticoagulation.
	TT
	Fibrinogen assay
Platelets	Platelet count
	Blood film inspection
	Platelet function (using PFA-100™ which measures in vitro 'high shear' bleeding time)
Fibrinolysis	D-dimers
	Euglobulin clot lysis time
Global haemostasis	Thromboelastogram

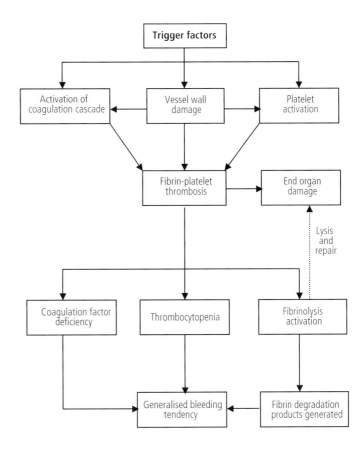

Figure 30.2   Pathogenesis of acute DIC.

• synthesis of TF on surface of endothelial cells or monocytes stimulated by endotoxins and cytokines as a result of sepsis;

• release or exposure of TF as a result of direct tissue injury (as in placental abruption, cerebral trauma) or from malignant cells; and

• snake venoms may cause DIC as a result of direct activation of coagulation factors such as FX or prothrombin.

The final consequence of coagulation activation is thrombin generation and fibrin formation, which may result in microthrombus formation (e.g. gangrene of fingers, toes, and renal failure). Following intravascular thrombosis, secondary activation of the fibrinolytic pathway occurs with subsequent lysis of fibrin, and the formation of cross-linked complexes such as D-dimers, which can be detected by a number of assays. Raised levels of these fibrin degradation products further add to the

bleeding diathesis as they inhibit the action of thrombin and also inhibit platelet function by binding to the platelet membrane.

Due to ongoing activation of the coagulation cascade, hepatic synthesis of coagulation factors is unable to fully compensate for their consumption, so there is a reduction in levels of all coagulation factors, but particularly factors V, VIII, XIII and fibrinogen. The bone marrow is unable to maintain a normal platelet count, and thrombocytopenia develops. This combination of coagulation factor deficiency, thrombocytopenia and the inhibitory actions of raised fibrin degradation products causes the generalised and continued bleeding tendency characteristic of DIC. These events are summarised in Figure 30.2.

The main causes of DIC are listed in Table 30.2.

Laboratory abnormalities that are seen in DIC include:

Condition	Examples
Infection	Septicaemia, viraemia
Malignancy	Leukaemia (especially acute promyelocytic)
	Metastatic carcinomas
Obstetric disorders	Septic abortion
	Placenta praevia and abruptio placentae
	Eclampsia
	Amniotic fluid embolism
Trauma	Extensive surgical trauma
	Fat embolism
Shock	Burns
	Heat stroke
Liver disease	Acute hepatic necrosis
Transplantation	Tissue rejection
Extracorporeal circulation	Cardiac bypass surgery
Extensive intravascular haemolysis	ABO-incompatible transfusion
Certain snake bites	
Vascular abnormalities	Kasabach–Merrit syndrome

Table 30.2 Main causes of DIC.

• prolonged thrombin time (TT), variably prolonged prothrombin time (PT) and activated partial thromboplastin time (APTT);
• reduction of fibrinogen levels, increased levels of D-dimers;
• thrombocytopenia; and
• anaemia, fragmented red cells, raised reticulocyte count.

The most important aspect of management is removal or alleviation of the triggering event or underlying cause, as well as treatment of any associated infection, hypovolaemia, etc. Obstetric emergencies should be attended to immediately. In the presence of widespread bleeding, specific replacement therapy should be given which includes:
• fresh frozen plasma (FFP) – almost all procoagulant factors and inhibitors are contained within FFP. An initial dose of 12–15 mL/kg should be given (approximately 1 L for an adult);
• cryoprecipitate – contains fibrinogen in a 'concentrated' form and two pooled packs (adult therapeutic doses) should be infused to adults if fibrinogen levels are critically low (<1.0 g/L);
• platelet concentrates – approximately 1–2 adult therapeutic doses;

• fibrinogen concentrates (Hemocomplettan®, CSL Behring) – virally inactivated plasma-derived preparations which also have the advantage of being highly concentrated. The recommended initial adult dose is 1–2 g which can be given up to 4 times per day; and
• following initial replacement therapy, laboratory tests should be repeated and any further treatment guided by both the clinical and laboratory response. The British Committee for Standards in Haematology (BCSH) recommend targets for these laboratory tests in order to act as a guide for replacement therapy: platelets $>75 \times 10^9$/L, fibrinogen >1.0 g/L and the maintenance of the PT and APTT <1.5 times the mean control.

Heparin anticoagulation may also be useful in situations where initial replacement therapy has failed to control excessive bleeding or when DIC is complicated by microvascular thrombosis or large vessel thrombosis. Low-dose continuous intravenous therapy (500–1000 IU/h) is one suggested regimen.

Specific clotting factor inhibitor concentrates (including antithrombin and activated protein C) may have a role in the management of certain groups of patients (e.g. those who do not respond to simple replacement therapy, overwhelming sepsis, and meningococcaemia).

Liver disease

All coagulation factors (except von Willebrand factor (vWF)) and protease inhibitors are synthesised by hepatocytes. The liver also serves to remove activated intermediates of coagulation from the blood stream.

In liver disease, coagulopathy may result from a number of mechanisms – reduced synthesis of coagulation factors; cholestasis and subsequent malabsorption resulting in vitamin K deficiency; and an acquired 'dysfibrinogenaemia'. The platelet count is often reduced due to hypersplenism.

Laboratory abnormalities seen in liver disease include:
- prolonged PT and APTT;
- prolonged TT: this may result from low fibrinogen concentration or dysfibrinogenaemia. A prolonged reptilase time in spite of a normal fibrinogen concentration implies a dysfibrinogenaemia; and
- elevated D-dimers.

It is important to note that abnormal coagulation tests are not always associated with bleeding, and in such cases, patients do not require replacement therapy. However, if there is active bleeding, then replacement of clotting factors with FFP and platelet transfusions to maintain a platelet count above 50×10^9/L should be instituted. Vitamin K in doses of 10–20 mg may produce some improvement in the coagulation abnormalities. Prothrombin complex concentrates which contain factors II, VII, IX and X may sometimes be used in severe cases, but if so, with great caution, as they may precipitate DIC.

Complications of anticoagulant and thrombolytic drugs

Oral anticoagulants

Coumarin and phenindione derivatives act by blocking the γ-carboxylation of glutamic acid residues of vitamin K-dependent coagulation factors, resulting in decreased biological activity of factors II, VII, IX and X, as well as Proteins C and S.

Table 30.3 Conditions associated with increased risk of bleeding during anticoagulation.

Age (possible)
Uncontrolled hypertension
Alcoholism
Liver disease
Poor drug or clinic visit compliance
Active major bleeding
Previous intracranial bleeding
Potential bleeding lesion (e.g. aneurysm, internal ulcer)
Thrombocytopenia
Platelet dysfunction (e.g. use of aspirin)

The INR monitors their effect on the haemostatic system. Some clinical situations may be associated with an increased risk of bleeding during anticoagulation and these are listed in Table 30.3.

Management of excessive anticoagulation depends on the INR level and whether there is minor or major bleeding. It should be noted that the risk of major bleeding on warfarin is around 2% per year, with a case fatality of 20%. Therefore, in the event of major bleeding, prompt appropriate action is required. In the absence of haemorrhage, warfarin should be stopped for a few days and recommenced when the INR falls into the desired range. Small doses of vitamin K (1–2.5 mg) may be given intravenously/orally if the INR >5.0, as there is a significantly greater risk of serious haemorrhage at this level.

If the patient is bleeding, then the anticoagulant effect should be reversed. Vitamin K 5–10 mg should be given intravenously and will have an initial onset of action after 4–6 hours. The action of vitamin K is, however, not maximal for at least 24 hour and therefore additional measures are required.
- Prothrombin complex concentrates (PCCs) – Beriplex®, CSL Behring; Octaplex®, Octapharma – which contain variable amounts of factors II, VII, IX and XI, are now recommended as first line for warfarin reversal when available. Ideal dosing is however unclear. Two regimens are currently in use: either dosing calculated on 50 IU FIX/kg body weight, or alternatively fixed dosing regimens giving either 500 IU or 1000 IU. Whilst a dose of

50 IU FIX/kg will effectively reverse anticoagulation, it should be remembered that clinical assessment still remains paramount as INR correction is quickly achieved by the correction of FVII levels alone. The disadvantage of these concentrates is that they carry the potential risk of inducing thromboembolism as they often contain activated coagulation components. Therefore, when using these products, caution should be exercised especially in high-risk groups.

• In the absence of PCCs, FFP (12–15 mL/kg) will immediately supply the necessary coagulation factors. However, there are some potential problems with this type of therapy. Very large amounts of plasma (1–2 L) may need to be infused in order to correct the coagulopathy; and even though the INR may correct into the normal range, this is misleading since it is not sensitive to factor IX – the concentration of which is only minimally increased by treatment with FFP. The levels of individual clotting factors will typically remain <20% after FFP infusion.

Haemorrhage occurring in a warfarinised patient with an INR in the therapeutic range should be managed as above, and repeat dosing may be required due to the short duration of action of both PCC and FFP. Red cell and platelet transfusion may become necessary if major bleeding occurs. Additional investigations to exclude any underlying local lesions should also be remembered.

Thrombolytic agents

These agents generally cause a state of systemic lysis. However, the degree to which this is affected varies according to the particular drug used. Streptokinase has a greater effect on the laboratory markers of systemic lysis than does tissue plasminogen activator, but this does not appear to correlate with the incidence of bleeding.

Laboratory tests such as the thrombin time and fibrinogen levels will detect the presence of a systemic lytic state, but they do not predict the likelihood of haemorrhage, and nowadays most protocols use fixed-dose schedules.

Haemorrhage complicating these agents is most commonly local (e.g. at the site of catheterisation in the groin); however, intracranial or gastrointestinal bleeding may occur. Measures such as pressure packs will often control local bleeding; more serious bleeding usually necessitates discontinuing thrombolysis. Most agents have a short half-life (minutes) and so the fibrinolytic state will reverse within a few hours of drug cessation. The exception to this is APSAC (acylated plasminogen-streptokinase activator complex), which has a half-life of 90 minutes. In the case of life-threatening haemorrhage, infusions of cryoprecipitate or FFP can be given to reverse the hypocoagulable state. Antifibrinolytic drugs such as epsilon-aminocaproic acid may/may not provide some additional benefit.

Uraemia

Bleeding is a relatively common complication of renal failure – the major cause is that of platelet dysfunction as well as a defect in platelet–vessel wall interaction. Deficiencies of coagulation factors are not a common feature, unless there is complicating liver disease or DIC.

Many qualitative platelet defects can be demonstrated in vitro, including impaired aggregation in response to agonists as well as storage pool defects. However, these abnormalities do not appear to correlate well with clinical bleeding. It is also thought that plasma from uraemic patients contains an inhibitor that interferes with normal vWF–platelet interaction.

Dialysis is useful in reversing the haemostatic defects in uraemia – although this may not correct them entirely. Anaemia (particularly when PCV <20%) should be corrected by either blood transfusion or RhEpo as this improves platelet function and shortens bleeding time. Infusions of 1-deamino-8-D-arginine vasopressin (DDAVP) (0.4 μg/kg) have been used successfully to provide short-term correction of the bleeding time and decreased symptoms of bleeding.

Massive transfusion

Massive blood loss is arbitrarily defined as the loss of one blood volume within a 24-hour period although other, more convenient, definitions include 50% blood volume loss within 3 hours or a rate of loss of 150 mL/h. This degree of blood loss may be associated with significant coagulation abnormalities. Thrombocytopenia can occur reasonably quickly and usually results from dilution, but increased consumption of platelets may also occur. The use of plasma-reduced red cell concentrates can result in significant dilution of coagulation factors.

The management of ongoing bleeding requires both clinical and laboratory input. The inability of standard laboratory tests to keep pace with the clinical picture is well recognised; nonetheless, patients receiving massive transfusions should have routine tests of haemostasis performed early in order to define precise abnormalities.

Whilst there is no clear evidence to support transfusion triggers, guidelines do exist in order to prevent the indiscriminate use of component therapy. The British Committee for Standards in Haematology recommends the following:

- Maintain Hb>8 g/dL.
- Keep platelets $>75 \times 10^9$/L – microvascular bleeding and general oozing from wounds or venepuncture sites are particularly likely when the platelet count falls below 50×10^9/L.
- Maintain PT & APTT <1.5 × mean control – administer FFP 12–15 mg/kg. Anticipate need for replacement after 1–1.5 × blood volume replacement.
- Maintain fibrinogen >1.0 g/L – if not corrected by FFP, give two pooled packs of cryoprecipitate or fibrinogen concentrate.
- The need for ongoing haemostatic treatment should be guided by the patient's clinical response and results of repeated laboratory tests.

In recent years, recombinant FVIIa (NovoSeven®) has been used for patients with uncontrollable, life-threatening haemorrhage. This product was originally developed for use in haemophilia patients with inhibitors to FVIII or rIX. In the setting of massive blood loss, the evidence for rVIIa use is limited and anecdotal but is increasing. A recent systematic review concluded that the application of rVIIa in severe bleeding is promising and relatively safe with a 1–2% incidence of thrombotic complications. Due to its expense, its use is generally limited to 'rescue' therapy for massively transfused patients with persistent bleeding despite appropriate blood component transfusion,

haemostatic and pharmacological measures and surgical intervention. A dosing schedule of 300 μg/kg followed by further doses of 100 μg/kg at 1 and 3 hours as required is suggested – as the half-life is relatively short, repeat doses may be needed to decrease bleeding significantly. The decision to use this product should generally be made in consultation with a haematologist.

Transfusion support for patients with inherited haemostatic defects

Haemophilia A

This disorder results in reduced or absent levels of coagulation factor VIII. It is usually sex-linked recessive although it may also arise from a spontaneous mutation in up to one-third cases.

The clinical features vary according to the factor VIII level and patients can be classified into mild, moderate or severe according to their factor VIII coagulant activity (Table 30.4). The severity and type of bleeding is related to the absolute level of factor VIII. The minimal effective level for haemostasis is generally about 25–30%.

Investigations

Laboratory abnormalities seen in haemophilia A include:

- prolonged APTT;
- reduction of factor VIII coagulant activity;
- normal vWF activity (it is important to measure vWF activity in order to exclude vWD, which will also give low factor VIII levels).

Management

The mainstay of treatment is to raise the concentration of factor VIII sufficiently to arrest spontaneous and traumatic bleeds or to cover surgery. There are a number of products currently available which can be used to treat this condition, including:

- recombinant factor VIII preparations;
- plasma-derived factor VIII concentrates (which may vary in degree of purity);
- DDAVP (for mild disease only – baseline factor VIII above 15%).

Table 30.4 Clinical manifestations in haemophilia A.

Factor VIII level (% normal)	Clinical manifestation
<1% (severe disease)	Usual age of onset <1 yr
	Spontaneous bleeding common (haemarthrosis, muscle haematoma, haematuria)
	Bleeding post-surgery and dental extraction
	Post-traumatic bleeding
	Crippling joint deformity if inadequate treatment
1–5% (moderate disease)	Usual age of onset <2 yr
	Occasional spontaneous bleeding
	Bleeding post-surgery and dental extraction
	Post-traumatic bleeding
6–40% (mild disease)	Usual age of onset >2 yr
	Bleeding post-surgery and dental extraction
	Post-traumatic bleeding

Recombinant products are recommended as the initial product of choice for prophylaxis to prevent spontaneous joint bleeding for children with severe haemophilia, as well as replacement therapy for previously untreated patients because of the lack of risk of transmission of infection. The choice of which recombinant product to use is determined by cost and availability. There has been concern that patients treated with recombinant factor VIII products have a higher incidence of inhibitor development than those treated with plasma-derived factor concentrates. The current evidence is conflicting and at present recombinant products are recommended first line for previously untreated patients to reduce transmission of infectious agents.

Plasma-derived clotting factor concentrates are currently considered to be 'safe' in terms of HIV and hepatitis viruses due to effective donor screening and specific double viral inactivation procedures. However, transmission of some viruses, such as human parvovirus B19, and new emerging infections such as prion disease remain a theoretical risk.

Mild haemophilia A should be treated with DDAVP (with or without tranexamic acid) rather than coagulation factor concentrates where possible. DDAVP (0.3 μg/kg body weight) is given intravenously, subcutaneously or alternatively a 300 μg dose (for adults) can be administered via intranasal spray. This dose typically increases the levels of factor VIII and vWF 3–5 times above baseline.

Hyponatraemia and water intoxication are side effects of this drug, and hence it is not recommended for patients with cardiac failure or children under 2 years of age. It is also thought to have thrombogenic potential and should be used with caution in the elderly or those with known vascular disease. The response to DDAVP should be assessed in all patients with the initial dose to ensure that an adequate increase in factor VIII levels is achieved prior to its use to treat bleeding or cover invasive procedures.

Tranexamic acid reduces fibrinloysis and is of particular use in patients with bleeding from mucosal surfaces, such as epistaxis, oral bleeding or menorrhagia. It is given as an adjunct to DDAVP to reduce bleeding. It should be avoided in patients with haematuria to avoid the complication of clot retention.

Patients with moderate/severe haemophilia will require treatment with recombinant or plasma-derived factor VIII concentrates for bleeding, prior to invasive procedures, surgery, etc. It is known that 1 unit factor VIII/kg body weight will result in an increase in plasma factor VIII level by 2%. The level of factor VIII concentrate required to achieve adequate haemostasis will depend on the type of bleeding, but can be calculated according to the formula:

Units of factor VIII required = weight (kg) × desired level (%) × 0.5

The plasma half-life of factor VIII is 8–12 hours, and thus repeated doses at 12-hourly intervals are usually needed. Alternatively, a continuous infusion of factor VIII can be given. For major soft tissue bleeds, levels above 50% are generally sufficient; however, for major surgery, a preoperative level of 100% is necessary and thereafter levels of 50–100% are sufficient for adequate wound healing. Factor VIII coagulant activity can be measured before and after doses of concentrate to ensure appropriate levels have been achieved.

The choice of product for previously treated patients will depend on factors such as previous response to treatment, a history of inhibitor development and whether they have been previously exposed to plasma products.

Haemophilia B

This sex-linked recessive disorder results in a deficiency of factor IX. The clinical features are identical to those of haemophilia A.

Investigations

Laboratory abnormalities seen in haemophilia B include:
- prolonged APTT; and
- reduction of factor IX coagulant activity.

Management

The main types of products that are currently used for treatment include:
- recombinant factor IX products; and
- high purity factor IX concentrates.

The product of choice for prophylaxis, treatment of bleeding or cover for surgical procedures in previously untreated patients is recombinant factor IX. If unavailable then high purity plasma-derived factor IX concentrates should be used. Prothrombin complex concentrate (PCC), containing factors II, VII, IX and X, have been used in the past but are not recommended now due to their prothrombotic effects.

The dosage of factor IX required can be calculated according to the formula:

Units of factor IX required = weight (kg) ×

desired level (%) × 1.0

The plasma half-life of factor IX is 18–30 hours, and therefore if repeated doses are needed, they should be given every 12–24 hours or by continuous infusion.

The choice of product for patients who have required previous treatment with factor concentrates depends on the history of inhibitor development and response to treatment. There is some evidence to suggest that plasma-derived products have different pharmacokinetic properties to recombinant products; therefore, the response to treatment should be monitored closely if switching from one product to another.

Treatment of patients with inhibitors

Patients with haemophilia can develop inhibitor antibodies to factors VIII or IX, sometimes making their treatment quite difficult. Inhibitors are most common in patients with severe haemophilia A and in patients with large gene deletions. Inhibitor development is often heralded by increased frequency of bleeding or loss of response to factor VIII. It is diagnosed by measuring factor VIII coagulant activity levels before and after a dose of factor VIII concentrate and by a Bethesda inhibitor assay.

For patients with haemophilia A:
- If the inhibitor is of low titre (i.e. <10 Bethesda units), then bleeding episodes can be treated with higher than normal doses of human factor VIII.
- If the inhibitor is of high titre (i.e. >10 Bethesda units), human factor VIII is ineffective to control bleeding, and the use of recombinant factor VIIa or FEIBA® (Boxten) is recommended. For major haemorrhage, recombinant factor VIIa (dose of 70–90 μg/kg initially every 2 hours) is generally recommended as first-line therapy (if available). Eradication of inhibitors with 'immune tolerance induction' using factor VIII concentrates alone or together with immunosuppression is considered the best long-term treatment option for these patients.

For patients with haemophilia B:

The prevalence of inhibitors in patients with haemophilia B is reported to be around 1–3%. Up to 50% of haemophilia B patients who develop an inhibitor have anaphylaxis or severe allergic reactions to factor IX concentrates.

Table 30.5 Variants of von Willebrand disease.

Type 1	Autosomal dominant inheritance
	Partial quantitative deficiency of vWF
	Normal vWF multimers
	Mild bleeding disorder which decreases during pregnancy, elderly
Type 2	Autosomal dominant inheritance
	Qualitative deficiency of vWF
	Numerous subtypes
	Abnormal vWF multimers
	Generally mild bleeding disorder
Type 3	Autosomal recessive inheritance
	Severe quantitative deficiency of vWF
	Severe haemophilia-like bleeding disorder

• Recombinant factor VIIa should be used for bleeding.

• Immune tolerance using factor IX concentrates can be attempted, although this is more difficult than in haemophilia A patients.

von Willebrand disease (vWD)

This is the most common of the inherited bleeding disorders and is due to a quantitative and/or qualitative defect in the vWF protein. vWF has two main functions – firstly, it promotes the adhesion of platelets to the subendothelium by binding to the platelet receptor glycoprotein Ib; secondly it protects factor VIII:c from proteolytic degradation by forming a noncovalent association.

vWD is a heterogeneous group of disorders and is classified into three different types (Table 30.5). Depending on the type of vWD, some patients may be asymptomatic whereas others will have haemophilia-like bleeding.

Laboratory abnormalities seen in vWD include:
• prolonged PFA-100™ closure time (an in vitro 'high shear' bleeding time device);
• reduction of vWF antigen (vWF:Ag);
• reduction of vWF ristocetin cofactor activity (vWF:RiCoF);
• reduction of factor VIII coagulant activity (which can cause prolonged APTT); and
• abnormal vWF multimers in some subtypes.

The goal of therapy in patients with vWD is to correct the dual defect of haemostasis, i.e. the abnormal platelet adhesion and the abnormal coagulation due to low FVIII levels. It is important to distinguish between the various types of vWD as treatment will differ:

• For patients with type 1 disease, DDAVP is the treatment of choice and a dose of 0.3 μg/kg body weight is usually given intravenously or subcutaneously. Intranasal doses (300 μg for adults or 150 μg for children) can also be given. These doses give a two- to fivefold increase in vWF and factor VIII levels. The choice of route of administration depends on the patient and the nature of the bleeding or surgery. It is important to first test an individual patient's response to DDAVP prior to using it to 'cover' procedures. Tranexamic acid is often given in vWD, either alone for minor bleeding or in conjunction with DDAVP/ vWF for more severe bleeding and to cover surgery.

• For patients with types 2 and 3 diseases, vWF 'replacement therapy' is generally required. At present there are no recombinant vWF concentrates available, so all products are plasma derived. Either a factor VIII concentrate rich in vWF or a purified vWF concentrate is the treatment of choice. One problem with factor VIII concentrates is that they rarely contain the highest molecular weight multimers of vWF, which are very important for adequate haemostasis. Similarly, the very low content of FVIII in purified vWF concentrates may make it necessary (in the event of acute bleeding or emergency surgery) to infuse vWD patients with a single first dose of purified FVIII concentrate to ensure immediate correction of the low FVIII levels.

In the past, cryoprecipitate was used to treat patients with vWD; however, it is now unacceptable to use such untreated plasma derivatives when there are 'safer' alternatives available.

Other inherited disorders

Hereditary deficiencies of other coagulation factors are rare. Factor XI deficiency is particularly common amongst Ashkenazi Jews and is transmitted as an autosomal recessive trait. There is a poor correlation between factor XI levels and bleeding tendency, which usually presents following surgery or dental procedures. If available, plasma-derived factor XI concentrates should be given to treat bleeding; if not, then FFP should be administered. There have been concerns about the potential thrombogenicity of factor XI concentrates, so peak levels should ideally not exceed 70 IU/dL.

Deficiencies of factors II, V, VII, X, XIII and fibrinogen can all be treated with FFP; if there are more specific therapies available then they should be used. Currently, there are specific factor concentrates for factors VII, XIII and fibrinogen, although these may not always be available. Cryoprecipitate can be used for fibrinogen deficiency/dysfibrinogenaemias, but fibrinogen concentrates should be used in preference if they are available because fibrinogen concentrates undergo additional viral inactivation steps; PCCs can be given to patients with factors II or X deficiency (although thromboembolic risks should be considered). Factor V-deficient patients are treated with FFP and it is recommended that virally inactivated plasma is used.

Patients with deficiencies of 'contact factors' (factor XII, prekallikrein, and high-molecular-weight kininogen) do not bleed excessively and do not require any treatment.

Appropriate and inappropriate use of FFP, cryoprecipitate and coagulation factor concentrates

FFP

FFP is obtained from either single donations or plasmapheresis collections and is prepared by freezing plasma to a temperature of $-30\,^{\circ}$C or less within 6 hours of collection, in order to preserve the activity of coagulation factors. Each unit contains all of the coagulation factors and has a volume of approximately 200 mL. When ready for use, it must be thawed at $37\,^{\circ}$C and ideally it should be infused within 2 hours of thawing. It can be stored at $4\,^{\circ}$C for up to 24 hours as long as factor VIII replacement is not required.

The dose of FFP required will depend on the clinical indication; however, an initial dose of 12–15 mL/kg body weight is usually given. As this is an empirical dose, laboratory tests should be used to monitor its efficacy, and results of these tests as well as the patient's clinical response should guide any further dosing requirements.

ABO-compatible FFP should be used. Group O FFP should only be given to Group O individuals, and in the case of other groups, FFP of the patient's group should be the first choice. If not possible, FFP of a different group may be given as long as it is not 'high-titre' anti-A or anti-B. In case of an emergency when the patient's blood group is not known, group AB plasma may be safely given. It is not necessary to provide RhD-negative FFP for RhD-negative patients even though FFP contains small amounts of red cell stroma. No anti-D prophylaxis is required if RhD-negative patients receive RhD-positive FFP.

Single-unit FFP is not a virally inactivated product. Other alternatives include light or methylene blue-treated FFP (MBFFP), or solvent–detergent (SD)-treated pooled plasma. All of these products have been shown to be clinically effective, although SD plasma lacks the high-molecular-weight forms of vWF. In the UK, virally inactivated FFP from BSE-free countries is recommended by the Department of Health for children born after 1 January 1996; the viral inactivation will be carried out by methylene blue treatment method. Virus inactivated FFP sourced from non-UK untransfused male donors is the safest product for the UK to avoid the risks of transfusion-related acute lung injury (TRALI – see Chapter 9), and vCJD (see Chapter 15). There are obvious difficulties in establishing a year of patient birth after which only the safest available FFP must be used, especially if many patients (such as adults) are excluded. Although extending the use of virus-inactivated FFP sourced from non-UK donors to all recipients remains under consideration, the main constraint is cost.

While the use of FFP has become widespread, it may be transfused inappropriately. There are a limited number of situations where the use of FFP is indicated:

Acute DIC

In acute DIC, activation of the coagulation and fibrinolytic systems results in depletion of platelets and coagulation factors (especially factors V, VIII and fibrinogen). Treatment is always aimed at removing the underlying cause. In cases of haemorrhage associated with laboratory abnormalities, replacement therapy with FFP, cryoprecipitate and platelet concentrates is indicated. If there is no bleeding, then replacement therapy should not be given in an attempt to correct the coagulopathy.

Immediate reversal of overdosing with oral anticoagulant

In the event of serious or life-threatening bleeding requiring immediate reversal of the anticoagulant effect, PCC is regarded as the treatment of choice. FFP is an alternative if PCCs are not available, using a dose of 12–15 mL/kg body weight. Further doses of PCC or FFP should be given according to laboratory results and patient's clinical state.

Vitamin K deficiency

Conditions that impair Vitamin K absorption (e.g. biliary tract obstruction) as well as haemorrhagic disease of the newborn can result in a coagulopathy similar to that seen with warfarin overdosage. Any serious/life-threatening bleeding should be treated in the same manner as described above.

Thrombotic thrombocytopenic purpura

Patients with acute thrombotic thrombocytopenic purpura (TTP) require plasma exchange with FFP to achieve remission. Large daily doses of FFP are needed, usually in the order of 3 L/day. Because large volumes of plasma are given, solvent–detergent plasma should be used if available to reduce the risk of virus transmission. In some series, the supernatant portion formed during the preparation of cryoprecipitate (cryosupernatant)

has been shown to be more effective than standard FFP when used as the replacement fluid. Cryosupernatant plasma is depleted in factor VIII and fibrinogen (but whereas the factor VIII concentration may only be about 0.11 IU/mL up to 70% fibrinogen may remain). FFP contains ADAMTS13, the metalloproteinase enzyme which is deficient or inhibited in TTP. ADAMTS13 degrades ultra-large multimers of vWF that cause the excessive platelet activation and consumption in this condition. The reduced activity of protein S in SD-treated FFP has been associated with the development of venous thromboembolism in patients with TTP; this risk is small and SD plasma should still be used in preference to standard FFP. Methylene blue-treated plasma is not recommended because it has been shown to be less effective than solvent–detergent plasma in these patients. Patients with acute idiopathic TTP often require immunosuppression to maintain remission. Rituximab is increasingly being used in TTP and may reduce the total amount of plasma received by patients by reducing the number of relapses.

Replacement of single factor deficiencies

As more specific factor concentrates become increasingly available, FFP should only be used as replacement when specific/combined factor concentrates are unavailable.

Inherited deficiencies of inhibitors of coagulation

Previously, FFP has been used as a source of antithrombin, protein C and protein S for patients with inherited deficiencies of these inhibitors who may be receiving heparin therapy for spontaneous thrombosis or who are undergoing surgery. Now that specific concentrates are being manufactured (antithrombin and protein C), FFP should be used only when these are not available.

There are several other circumstances where FFP may be used appropriately to treat bleeding in the presence of abnormal coagulation. These include the following:

Liver disease

Coagulation abnormalities occur quite frequently in patients with severe liver disease. Bleeding is often precipitated by an event such as surgery or liver biopsy and is rarely attributable to the haemostatic defect alone. If there is bleeding (or a very strong possibility that bleeding will occur), then FFP is indicated. Large volumes are often required to control the bleeding/correct the defect, and this can be problematic in patients who may already have an expanded plasma volume. Complete normalisation of a prolonged PT is often not possible, and the use of PCCs may be considered. However, one must be aware of the potential risks of inducing thrombosis or DIC in these patients, particularly since they already suffer from impaired clearance of activated clotting factors and reduced levels of antithrombin. Since thrombocytopenia and platelet function defects are also a feature of hepatic disease, platelet concentrates may also need to be given.

Massive transfusion

This is defined as the replacement of a patient's total blood volume within 24 hours. Coagulation abnormalities seen in this setting are more closely related to the clinical condition necessitating the transfusion rather than the volume of blood transfused. Prophylactic 'replacement' regimens with FFP are not indicated. Instead, treatment with both FFP and cryoprecipitate should be guided by the patient's clinical status as well as the results of laboratory tests (if available). Thrombocytopenia is a frequent occurrence and should be treated with platelet concentrates if necessary (usually when the platelet count falls below 75×10^9/L). More recently, recombinant FVIIa (NovoSeven®) has been used for massively transfused patients with persistent bleeding despite appropriate blood component transfusion, haemostatic and pharmacological measures and surgical intervention.

Cardiopulmonary bypass

Haemostatic disturbances that occur during cardiopulmonary bypass are usually due to platelet dysfunction. If there is persistent bleeding (despite adequate platelet transfusion) and a coagulopathy other than that caused by heparin has been demonstrated, then FFP should be used.

Special paediatric conditions

FFP can be used in the treatment of neonatal DIC, and is also sometimes used in newborn/premature infants with severe sepsis, although FFP should be avoided in neonates with T-antigen activation (see Chapter 26). Special paediatric packs of FFP that contain smaller volumes than standard FFP should be used.

The use of FFP is inappropriate in the following conditions:

- hypovolaemia;
- routine plasma exchange;
- part of a 'predetermined' replacement protocol; and
- treatment of immunodeficiency or protein-losing states.

Cryoprecipitate

Cryoprecipitate is prepared from plasma that is frozen quickly and then thawed slowly at 1–6°C, leaving behind a small amount of precipitated protein. The cryoprecipitate protein is then resuspended in a small volume of residual supernatant plasma. It contains factor VIII, fibrinogen, vWF, factor XIII and fibronectin in higher concentrations than they are found in plasma.

In the UK, cryoprecipitate is pooled in to adult therapeutic doses of 150–200 mL containing 3.2–4 g fibrinogen. It can be used appropriately in cases of hypofibrinogenaemia such as DIC, reversal of fibrinolytic agents and advanced liver disease. Plasma levels of fibrinogen >1.0 g/L are generally considered as adequate for haemostasis. When using cryoprecipitate, it is usual to thaw approximately two adult therapeutic doses for infusion; however, the dose will vary according to the clinical condition and the patient's fibrinogen level. In the past, cryoprecipitate was used to treat vWD and haemophilia A, but with the advent of drugs such as DDAVP and the availability of specific factor concentrates, it should no longer be used for the treatment of these disorders. Cryoprecipitate exposes the patient to multiple donors and there is an alternative in the form of fibrinogen concentrate (as mentioned previously) although this is not yet licenced in the UK.

Cryoprecipitate has more recently been used for the production of fibrin surgical adhesive ('glue'), which can be used in various surgical procedures and can be prepared from autologous donors.

Coagulation factor concentrates

Both specific and non-specific coagulation factor concentrates are prepared from plasma using a number of different techniques in an attempt to produce a 'purified' product that has undergone viral inactivation.

Specific factor concentrates for many of the coagulation factors have now been developed and are in clinical use as replacement therapy for inherited deficiencies. Their use has been discussed previously in the treatment of inherited haemostatic defects.

Non-specific factor concentrates such as PCCs generally contain factors II, IX and X together with variable amounts of factor VII. They are generally used in conditions associated with deficiencies of one/more of these factors (e.g. treatment of overdosage with warfarin). However, since they often contain 'activated' forms of coagulation factors, they have thrombogenic potential, which can limit their use.

Key points

1 Basic initial screening tests for haemostasis include the platelet count, prothrombin time, activated partial thromboplastin time, and fibrinogen level
2 PCCs should be the first choice for reversal of oral anticoagulation. FFP may be used if PCCs are contraindicated or unavailable.
3 The mainstay of treatment of DIC remains management of the underlying cause. In bleeding patients, prompt administration of FFP and cryo-

precipitate with regular laboratory monitoring is required.
4 Appropriate guidelines (e.g. those provided by the BCSH) should be followed when managing major haemorrhage, aiming for the following parameters: Hb>8 g/dL; platelets $>75 \times 10^9$/L; PT & APTT $<1.5 \times$ mean control; fibrinogen >1.0 g/L.
5 In inherited bleeding disorders, recombinant products should be used where available.
6 Patients with TTP should receive plasma exchange with solvent–detergent plasma, or standard FFP if not available. Methylene blue treated plasma should not be used.

Further reading

Bolton-Maggs PHB, Perry DJ & Chalmers EA. The rare coagulation disorders – review with guidelines for management from the United Kingdom Haemophilia Centre Doctors' Organisation. *Haemophilia* 2004;10:593–628.

British Committee for Standards in Haematology. Guidelines for the use of fresh frozen plasma, Cryoprecipitate and Cryosupernatant. *Br J Haematol* 2004;126:11–28.

British Committee for Standards in Haematology. Guidelines on oral anticoagulation (warfarin): third edition – 2005 update. *Br J Haematol* 2005;132:277–285.

British Committee for Standards in Haematology. Guidelines on the management of massive blood loss. *Br J Haematol* 2006;135:634–641.

Keeling D, Tait C & Makris M. Guideline on the selection and use of therapeutic products to treat haemophilia and other hereditary bleeding disorders. *Haemophilia* 2008:1–14.

Nash MJ, Cohen H, Liesner R et al. Acquired coagulation disorders and vascular bleeding. In: Hoffbrand AV, Catovsky D & Tuddenham EGD. eds, *Postgraduate Haematology*. Oxford: Blackwell Publishing, 2005, pp. 859–875.

Pasi KJ, Collins PW, Keeling DM et al. Management of von Willebrand disease: a guideline from the UK Haemophilia Centre Doctors' Organization. *Haemophilia* 2004;10:218–231.

CHAPTER 31

Recombinant proteins in diagnosis and therapy

Marion Scott
NHS Blood and Transplant, Bristol, UK

Introduction

Many potentially useful human proteins for therapeutic, diagnostic and research use are expressed in the body at very low concentrations, and it is difficult, if not impossible, to isolate them by conventional biochemical methods. Other proteins, such as antibodies of a particular specificity, are difficult to purify from a complex mixture of very similar proteins. However, once the gene encoding a protein has been cloned and sequenced, it becomes possible to express the protein at high concentrations, using virally derived expression vectors that are designed to produce full-length proteins at high levels in various different in vitro culture 'host' cell systems. Some blood proteins, such as the coagulation factors to treat haemophilia, have been efficiently purified by fractionation of pooled human plasma, but have been shown to have the potential of transmitting diseases, such as HIV and HCV. The cloning and expression of these proteins has led to the availability of recombinant coagulation factors for the treatment of haemophilia, with reduced risk of infection. As the recombinant coagulation factors are grown in vitro, there is also the advantage of an unlimited supply of constant guaranteed product. Similar drivers have led researchers to try

and develop recombinant replacements for specific immunoglobulins currently fractionated from high-titre blood donations, such as anti-D. Some concern has been expressed about the safety of such recombinant products, as they may potentially contain viruses or other infectious agents arising from the host cells used to express the protein, or the culture medium components used to grow the host cells. Increasing awareness of the risks from pooled polyclonal blood products have been heightened by concerns about variant Creutzfeldt–Jakob disease (vCJD) in the UK. Are the potential risks from such biotechnology products any worse than the risks from blood products derived from pooled human plasma?

Apart from cloning and expressing such naturally occurring proteins, it is possible using recombinant DNA technology to produce modified forms of the proteins that do not occur naturally and that might have desired therapeutic effects or diagnostic advantages.

General methods for recombinant protein expression

The choice of the host cell system to use for recombinant protein expression relies on several factors. Bacterial expression systems, such as *Escherichia coli*, are the cheapest, simplest and most effective, but cannot be used for many types of human

Practical Transfusion Medicine, 3rd edition. Edited by Michael F. Murphy and Derwood H. Pamphilon. © 2009 Blackwell Publishing, ISBN: 978-1-4051-8196-9.

Table 31.1 Production systems for recombinant mammalian proteins.

System	Cost	Production timescale	Scale-up capacity	Product quality	Glycosylation	Contamination risks
Bacteria	Low	Short	High	Low	None	Endotoxins
Yeast	Medium	Medium	High	Medium	Incorrect	Low risk
Plants	Low	Long	High	High	Some differences	Low risk, but environmental concerns
Insect cells	Medium	Medium	High	Medium	Incorrect	Low risk
Mammalian cells	High	Long	Low	Very high	Correct	Animal viruses
Transgenic animals	High	Very long	Low	Very high	Correct	Animal viruses

proteins that require eukaryotic post-translational modifications for biological activity, e.g. glycosylation, since prokaryotes lack the enzymes that catalyse many of the post-translational modifications found on eukaryotic proteins. Proteins produced in prokaryotes may not be folded properly, and/or can be insoluble, forming inclusion bodies. Genetically modified strains of yeast which have human glycosylation pathways have been produced for the efficient production of human glycoforms of recombinant proteins. Insect cells have also been used for recombinant protein expression, using baculoviral vectors. Transgenic animals have also been produced, with targeted production of recombinant proteins in milk.

A comparison of different production systems for recombinant proteins is shown in Table 31.1.

For many types of human proteins, expression in a mammalian system is the best option, as this is the approach most likely to yield soluble, biologically active proteins, although it is considerably more expensive than expression in *E. coli*, yeast or insect cells. Cell lines commonly used are NS0 (mouse myeloma), CHO (Chinese hamster ovary) and COS-7 (African green monkey fibroblast).

A number of techniques have been developed for rapid, one-stage purification of recombinant proteins. Epitope tags are short amino acid sequences for which commercial monoclonal antibodies are available, and can be placed anywhere within the protein where it will not disrupt the protein's function. It is also common to create fusion proteins, i.e. to create a single open reading frame that encodes a well-characterised protein such as glutathione-*S*-transferase (GST) together with the sequence of the

protein of interest. When the tag protein is produced, the protein of interest is produced as well, as one fusion protein. Fusion proteins are useful because they enable rapid purification by affinity chromatography, and the fused tag can be removed after purification using a specific protease.

Plasmids used for expression commonly contain a viral promoter sequence, an antibiotic resistance gene, a fusion tag sequence and a restriction endonuclease site for insertion of the coding sequence of interest (Figure 31.1). cDNA coding for the protein sequence of interest is normally derived by reverse transcriptase polymerase chain reaction (RT-PCR) from cells expressing the protein, using sequence specific primers to amplify the region required. This cDNA is then inserted into the expression vector and used to transfect a mammalian cell line. Growth in medium containing the antibiotic to which the vector codes resistance results in selection of transfected cells only. Production of the fusion protein can then be detected using antibodies to the fusion tag sequence, and the fusion protein purified and characterised. Some expression vectors do not insert into the host cell nuclear material and give rise to transient expression. Other vectors insert into the host cell DNA and give rise to stable expression.

Recombinant antibodies

Limitations of rodent monoclonal antibodies

Conventional monoclonal antibody technology uses immunisation of mice or rats with antigen

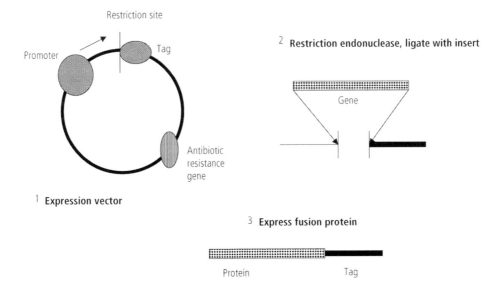

Figure 31.1 Production of recombinant fusion proteins.

to yield hyperimmunised spleen cells, which are then fused with non-secreting myeloma cell lines to yield hybridoma cell lines that can be grown in vitro to produce monoclonal antibodies. Effectively the fusion process inserts the DNA from the spleen cells into the myeloma cells. Whilst many such conventional monoclonal antibodies were very successfully developed into diagnostic reagents (such as the high avidity anti-A and anti-B now used routinely world-wide for blood grouping), it was not possible to produce antibodies of certain specificities in rodents, and attempts to use rodent monoclonal antibodies in man as therapeutics rapidly ran into problems, as the recipients developed a strong human anti-rodent response, which rapidly cleared the antibodies from the body.

Humanising rodent monoclonals

The early promise of monoclonal antibodies as therapeutics was not realised, and many became disillusioned with the concept of the 'magic bullet'. The success rate of rodent monoclonal antibodies that entered clinical trials was only 9% over the 20 years from 1980 to 2000. However, when the possibility of making recombinant antibodies became available in 1986, things rapidly changed. Using recombinant DNA technology, it was possi-

ble to replace the mouse constant domains of antibodies with corresponding human domains and express these chimeric recombinant immunoglobulin molecules in cell lines. Further engineering work also allowed the replacement of the framework regions of the mouse variable domains with human framework regions, resulting in virtually fully humanised antibodies.

Human recombinant antibodies

Human circulating B cells can be selected from immune individuals and transformed into cell lines that can be grown in culture by transformation with Epstein–Barr virus (EBV). The cDNA coding for the antibodies can then be derived from these cells using RT-PCR, ligated into expression vectors and expressed in a suitable mammalian host cell line.

Alternatively phage display technology can be used (Figures 31.2 and 31.3). Bacteriophages that infect *E. coli* are modified such that they carry the cDNA encoding for antibody variable domains, whilst at the same time they express the antibody protein on their surface. This permits in vitro selection of antibodies of the required specificity,

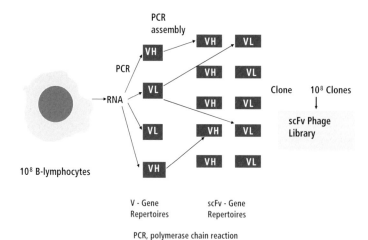

V - Gene   scFv - Gene
Repertoires   Repertoires

Figure 31.2 Generation of sc-Fv phage libraries.

PCR, polymerase chain reaction

and then expansion in *E. coli*. RT-PCR is used to amplify all of the heavy and light chain variable domains in a buffy coat sample. PCR is then used to assemble these randomly into VH and VL pairs, by inclusion of DNA encoding for a flexible linker chain between the heavy and light chain domains. A 'tag' sequence is also included to aid detection and purification. These linked heavy and light chain domains are known as single-chain Fv (scFv). The scFv constructs are then ligated into a phage display vector. The scFv domain is ligated into the vector next to regions that code for the PIII phage coat protein. The recombinant phage then expresses the scFv protein alongside their PIII coat protein at the tip of the phage. Phage libraries can be panned against antigens, and those phage selected that are displaying scFv that bind to the antigen. Selected phage are eluted from the antigen, expanded by culture in *E. coli* and then repanned against antigen. Selected human scFv can then removed from the phage vector and can be ligated to cloned human IgG constant domains to express full-length human recombinant antibody molecules. One large advantage of this approach is that antibodies can be derived from phage display libraries made from non-immunised individuals, and that normally restricted antibodies (e.g. anti-self) can be derived.

Using these approaches, many recombinant antibodies are now successfully licenced for clinical use in a variety of applications with many more in the pipeline, and they are now amongst the most commercially successful biotech drugs.

Human recombinant monoclonal anti-D

Despite the overall success in the production of rodent monoclonal antibodies to human ABO blood group antigens, no such monoclonal antibodies have been produced to the Rh antigens. Various different approaches have been developed to produce human monoclonal antibodies specific for RhD.

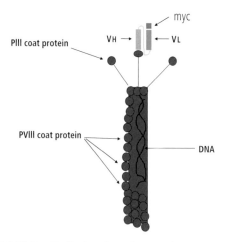

Figure 31.3 scFv displayed on phage surface.

Early work used the immortalisation of human B cells by infection with EBV. Improvements in the stability of human cell lines have been achieved by back-crossing human anti-D secreting EBV lines to a mouse–human heterohybridoma line or to a mouse myeloma line. Use of these approaches has enabled the production of a large number of blood group-specific human anti-Rh monoclonal antibodies. The cDNA coding for these antibodies has then been expressed in suitable mammalian host cell lines to produce recombinant anti-D suitable for therapeutic use (i.e. free from EBV).

More recently, the single-chain human Fv technique has been used to produce recombinant human antibodies with Rh specificity.

Candidate monoclonal anti-D's for immunoprophylaxis are selected, firstly, on their ability to bind to the RhD antigen via the Fv part of the molecule, and secondly on their ability to interact with Fc receptors via the Fc part of the molecule to bring about immunomodulation. The exact mechanism of immunosuppression by anti-D is not known, but it is clear that it involves interaction of anti-D with Fc receptors. To be effective, prophylactic antibody must be capable of not only binding to the RhD antigen on the red cells via its Fv regions, but also interacting with the effector cells of the immune system via its Fc region. Selection of recombinant monoclonal anti-D for therapeutic use therefore depends on not only the antigen specificity and avidity of the monoclonal antibody but also its functional activity in interacting with effector cells. To suppress immunisation, IgG-coated RBC need to be rapidly cleared from the maternal circulation and localised in the spleen. It has been suggested that D antigen specific B cells in the spleen are then deactivated by the simultaneous binding of the Fc region of the anti-D to $Fc\gamma RIIb$ together with binding of the B cell receptor to the D antigen. Interactions of anti-D with $Fc\gamma RI$, $Fc\gamma RIIb$ and $Fc\gamma RIIIa$ may thus all be required for effective immunosuppression.

IgG monoclonal anti-D antibodies have been evaluated in various in vitro systems to test how effective the antibodies are at interacting with immune system effector cells. Each assay tests efficacy at binding to different Fc receptors. Rosette formation of sensitised cells with monocytes and phagocytes, adherence of sensitised cells to monocyte monolayers and chemiluminescent measurements of the oxidative burst caused when monocytes react with sensitised red cell are all in vitro measures of interaction with $Fc\gamma RI$. Antibody-dependent cellular cytotoxicity measurements by radiolabelled chromium release from natural killer cells measures interaction with $Fc\gamma RIIIa$. It is not clear at present how well performance in these various in vitro assays will predict in vivo efficacy.

Two monoclonal anti-D antibodies, BRAD-3 and BRAD-5 were selected for clinical study because of their high activity in in vitro functional assays, high avidity and specificity for the immunodominant epitope region of the RhD antigen and initial studies in D negative male volunteers showed expected half-lives and pharmacokinetics after injection. Further studies on the antibodies administered with ^{51}Cr-labelled D-positive red cells demonstrated accelerated red cell clearance in all subjects and provided preliminary evidence for protection from immunisation.

It is clear from the clinical trials to date that recombinant anti-D has the potential to replace polyclonal prophylactic anti-D. There is a case for universal antenatal prophylaxis if sufficient supplies of anti-D are available. How quickly recombinant anti-D becomes available will largely be determined by commercial investment and regulatory procedures.

Anti-prion recombinant antibodies

A range of monoclonal antibodies to human recombinant prion proteins has been produced by immunising prion knockout mice. Selected antibodies have been developed into a diagnostic test for bovine spongiform encephalopathy using homogenised bovine brain post-mortem. Work is currently underway to try and increase the sensitivity of the assay to make it suitable for screening human blood for vCJD. It has been shown that these mouse monoclonal antibodies can prevent the spread of vCJD prion disease in a mouse model. Currently efforts aim to engineer human chimeric and humanised versions of these mouse antibodies to progress this work into clinical trials for the potential treatment of vCJD.

Anti-HPA-1a recombinant antibodies

scFv specific for the human platelet antigen HPA-1a have been derived from a phage display library and ligated to scFv specific for the RhD antigen on red blood cells, and the novel bispecific recombinant antibody can be used in a mixed passive haem-agglutination test for the HPA-1a antigen on platelets. The scFv has also been expressed as a full-length human IgG antibody by ligation to the constant domains of human IgG1, and this antibody had been used either fluorescently labelled or enzyme labelled in other diagnostic tests for the HPA-1a antigen on platelets.

'Null' recombinant antibodies

Using site directed mutagenesis, the Fc domains of human IgG antibodies have been mutated to have as little biological function as possible. Recombinant anti-D and anti-HPA-1a antibodies have been produced with this 'null' Fc region. In vitro studies have shown that these 'null' antibodies can effectively compete with clinically significant antibodies and prevent them, causing immune destruction of red cells and platelets, respectively. A clinical trial in male volunteers showed that the 'null' anti-D protected D-positive red cells from clearance by anti-D in vivo. The aim is to see if the 'null' anti-HPA-1a antibody can be administered to HPA-1a-negative pregnant women who are carrying HPA-1a-positive fetuses and prevent neonatal alloimmune thrombocytopaenia by crossing the placenta and competing with maternal anti-HPA-1a that can cause destruction of fetal platelets (see also Chapter 5).

Recombinant phenotyping reagents

Many monoclonal human IgG antibodies have been produced that react with blood group antigens, but these must be used in enzyme or antiglobulin techniques that are not suited to high-throughput, automated blood grouping machines. By cloning the variable regions of these antibodies, it is possible to ligate them to the constant domains of human IgM antibodies and express hybrid recombinant molecules in myeloma cells. These antibodies are highly potent because they combine the high affinity of the affinity-matured IgG antibodies with the polymeric structure of IgM. They are very potent direct agglutinins that can readily be used in automated blood grouping machines.

Recombinant antigens

Blood group antigens

Detection and identification of clinically significant blood group, platelet and granulocyte antibodies currently relies on the availability of high-quality antibody screening and identification cells that cover all clinically significant antigens and carry them in combinations such that the specificity of antibodies can be deduced. The quality of these panels of cells is critical, and their variability has been shown in UK National External Quality Assessment Scheme exercises to be the main cause of error in the detection and identification of antibodies. Quantitation of antibodies during pregnancy is carried out using titration or autoanalyzer technology, both of which show high levels of variation, such that it is difficult to set levels at which clinical action is required.

Most of the relevant antigens have been sequenced and cloned. Some have been inserted in expression vectors and expressed in the membranes of in vitro cultured cells, e.g. expression of the Rh protein in K562 human erythroleukaemia cells. For some antigens it is possible to amplify just the extracellular domain of the protein that carries the antigen and express a soluble recombinant protein that carries antigenic activity. This has been demonstrated for the Kell, Lutheran, Duffy, MNSs, and Cartwright red cell antigens, HPA-1a and HPA-1b platelet antigens and HNA-1 and HNA-2 granulocyte antigens.

The target of this work is to be able to produce microarrays of recombinant antigens which could then be used for high-throughput antibody screening, identification, sub-class determination and quantitation of antibodies in transfusion recipients and pregnant women.

Microbial antigens

In a similar way, recombinant microbial antigens have been produced to test blood donor plasma for the presence of anti-microbial antibodies, and thus exposure to transfusion transmitted diseases. Viral antigens and tests have been produced in this way, and more recently tests for parasites, such as those causing malaria (*Plasmodium falciparum* and *P. vivax*) and Chagas (*Trypanosoma cruzi*), have produced and shown to have good specificity and sensitivity for screening blood donors.

Recombinant enzymes

It has long been known that it is possible to treat group A, B or AB red cells with glycosidase enzymes, and convert them to group O, such that they would theoretically be a safe blood transfusion product for any ABO blood group recipient. However, the naturally occurring enzymes have poor kinetic properties and difficult-to-achieve pH optima, such that the process was not economically viable or able to pass rigorous quality assurance requirements for clinical use. New recombinant enzymes have now been produced from bacterial glycosidases with remarkably improved kinetic properties, such that the enzymes reproducibly cleave the A and B antigens with low enzyme protein consumption, short incubation times and at neutral pH. Clinical trials evaluating the safety and efficacy of such recombinant enzyme-treated red cells are looking promising.

Recombinant coagulation factors

Recombinant coagulation factors have been successfully used for the treatment of haemophilia for several years. Recombinant protein technology has virtually eliminated transmissible disease risk from these products, such that the recombinant products are the products of choice for haemophiliacs. In the UK, most patients with severe haemophilia now receive recombinant factor VIII and factor IX. Recom-binant factor VIIa was originally developed for the treatment of haemophilia patients who had developed inhibitory alloantibodies to factors VIII and IX, and is licenced for this application. Reports indicate that it can be effective in treating haemorrhage in trauma, surgery or obstetric cases (see Chapter 36).

Recombinant haemoglobin and cytokines are considered elsewhere, in Chapters 35 and 42, respectively.

Conclusions

Recombinant protein technology has rapidly advanced over the last 25 years, and we are now starting to see the routine use of recombinant proteins in transfusion medicine. Recombinant proteins will probably totally replace coagulation factors and specific immunoglobulins that are currently produced from fractionated pooled plasma. However, it is unlikely that recombinant products will replace intravenous immunoglobulin or albumin. Intravenous immunoglobulin works because of its broad specificity – it would be very difficult/impossible to mimic this successfully with a recombinant product. Albumin could be produced as a recombinant protein, but this is unlikely to be economically viable, compared to the ease of production from plasma. Only evidence of disease transmission by plasma-derived albumin could drive the production of recombinant albumin.

Further specific recombinant immunoglobulins are being produced that are not currently available as blood products – anti-HCV and anti-vCJD, and the efficacy of these needs to be investigated in clinical trials. Blood group antigens are now available as recombinant molecules, such that there may no longer be a need to use red cells, platelets and granulocytes for antibody screening, identification and quantitation.

Key points

1 Proteins expressed at low levels naturally can be cloned and expressed as recombinant proteins at high levels.

2 The sequence of recombinant proteins can be altered to give properties not found in naturally occurring proteins.

3 Human recombinant antibodies can be produced from non-immune donors.

4 Murine monoclonal antibodies can be humanised for clinical use.

5 Recombinant antibodies with inactive Fc regions can be produced as blocking antibodies.

6 Recombinant antigens can be used for screening, identification and quantification of clinically significant antibodies.

7 Recombinant coagulation factors have largely replaced those derived from pooled plasma.

Further reading

Chang CD, Cheng KY, Jiang LX et al. Evaluation of a prototype Trypanosoma cruzi antibody assay with recombinant antigens on a fully automated chemiluminescence analyzer for blood donor screening. *Transfusion* 2006;46:1737–1744.

Corwin HL. The role of erythropoietin therapy in the care of the critically ill. *Transfus Med Rev* 2006;20:27–33.

Goodnough LT & Shander AS. Recombinant factor VIIa: safety and efficacy. *Curr Opin Hematol* 2007;14:504–509.

Jefferis R. Antibody therapeutics: isotype and glycoform selection. *Expert Opin Biol Ther* 2007;7:1401–1413.

Kitchen AD, Lowe PH, Lalloo K & Chiodini PL. Evaluation of a malarial antibody assay for use in the screening of blood and tissue products for clinical use. *Vox Sang* 2004;87:150–155.

Mondon P, Dubreuil O, Bouyadi K & Kharrat H. Human antibody libraries. *Front Biosci* 2008;13:1117–1129.

Olsson ML & Clausen H. Modifying the red cell surface: towards an ABO-universal blood supply. *Br J Haematol* 2008;140:3–12.

Rasmussen SK, Rasmussen LK, Weilgunny D & Tolstrup AB. Manufacture of recombinant polyclonal antibodies. *Biotechnol Lett* 2007;29:845–852.

Ridgwell K, Dixey J & Scott ML. Production of soluble recombinant proteins with Kell, Duffy and Lutheran blood group activity, and their use in screening human sera for Kell, Duffy and Lutheran antibodies. *Transfus Med* 2007;5:384–394.

Spencer KA, Osorio FA & Hiscox JA. Recombinant viral proteins for use in diagnostic ELISAa to detect virus infection. *Vaccine* 2007;25:5653–5659.

Stanworth SJ, Birchall J, Doree CJ & Hyde C. Recombinant factor VIIa for the prevention and treatment of bleeding in patients without haemophilia. *Cochrane Database Syst Rev* 2007;CD005011.

Tsai CH, Fang TY, Ho NT & Ho C. Novel recombinant hemoglobin, rHb (beta N108Q), with low oxygen affinity, high co-operativity and stability against autooxidation. *Biochemistry* 2000;39:13719–13729.

Wilson J, Yao GL, Raftery J et al. A systematic review and economic evaluation of epoetin alpha, epoetin beta and darbepoetin alpha. *Health Technol Assess* 2007;11:1–202.

CHAPTER 32

Immunodeficiency and immunoglobulin therapy

Siraj A. Misbah
Oxford Radcliffe Hospitals, University of Oxford, Oxford, UK

Immunodeficiency and immunoglobulin therapy

The increasing awareness of immunodeficiency and the rapid pace of genetic discovery have helped to ensure that immunodeficiency disorders are no longer viewed as arcane rarities by both clinical immunologists and non-immunologists. In haematology, alongside the major changes in practice that have been driven by advances in fundamental immunology, haematologists are also likely to encounter patients with primary immunodeficiency disease because of the frequency of haematological complications associated with this group of disorders. Given that most haematologists will be familiar with the consequences of secondary immunodeficiency, either iatrogenic or associated with lymphoproliferative disease, this chapter will focus primarily on primary immunodeficiency disorders followed by a separate section on immunoglobulin therapy.

Primary immunodeficiency disorders

Many primary immunodeficiency disorders associated with single gene mutations have been

aptly called experiments of nature in view of the unique insights that these diseases have provided in unravelling complex immunological functions. Currently, the World Health Organization – International Union of Immunological Societies (WHO/IUIS) committee on primary immunodeficiency diseases recognises over 120 primary immunodeficiencies for which the underlying molecular basis has been elucidated. Although primary immunodeficiencies can affect any part of the immune system, in practice patients with predominant defects of B-cell function and combined B- and T-cell defects constitute the bulk of a clinical immunologist's workload.

The immunopathogenesis of antibody deficiency disorders and combined B- and T-lymphocyte deficiency is best understood within the context of B- and T-lymphocyte development. Whilst a detailed discussion of B- and T-cell development is outside the scope of this chapter, the schematic diagrams set out in Figures 32.1 and 32.2 summarise the major events in B- and T-cell development and the points at which developmental arrest leads to immunodeficiency.

Predominant B-cell deficiency disorders

Common variable immunodeficiency

Of the 20 antibody deficiency disorders currently recognised, common variable immunodeficiency

Practical Transfusion Medicine, 3rd edition. Edited by Michael F. Murphy and Derwood H. Pamphilon. © 2009 Blackwell Publishing. ISBN: 978-1-4051-8196-9.

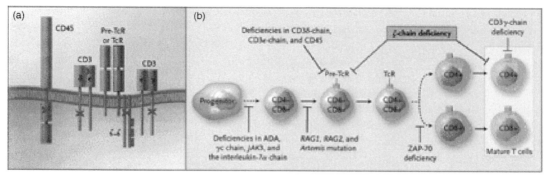

Figure 32.1 Mutations in multiple proteins, including the CD3 and ζ chains, that cause T-cell immunodeficiencies. The pre-T-cell receptor (pre-TcR) and mature TcR complexes consist of a receptor dimer associated with CD3 chains γ, δ, and ε and a ζ-chain dimer (Panel (a)). The pre-TcR complex differs from the mature complex owing to the presence of a surrogate chain (indicated by a dotted line) in the pre-TcR dimer. The CD3 and ζ chains facilitate the expression of the complex on the cell surface and send intracellular signals. Mutations in the receptor complexes that have been linked to T-cell immunodeficiencies are indicated with a red X. T-cell differentiation (Panel (b)) entails the progression from a progenitor cell to a CD4−CD8−

thymocyte that expresses a pre-TcR, followed by differentiation into a CD4+CD8+ thymocyte expressing the mature TcR. This cell develops into a single CD4+CD− or CD4−CD+ thymocyte and, finally, into a CD4+CD8− or CD4−CD8+ mature T cell. Dashed lines indicate that intervening steps occur that are not shown. The stages of differentiation affected by mutations and deficiencies of different proteins are shown by T bars. Red bars indicate a partial effect. ADA, adenosine deaminase; JAK3, Janus kinase 3; RAG, recombination-activating gene; and ZAP-70, zeta-chain-associated protein of 70 kDa. (Reproduced with permission from Rudd CE. *N Engl J Med* 2006;354:1874; Copyright 2006 Massachusetts Medical Society. All rights reserved.)

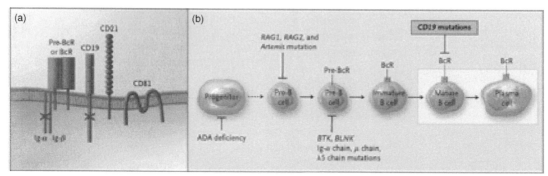

Figure 32.2 Mutations in multiple proteins, including pre-B-cell receptor (Pre-BcR) and CD19, that cause B-cell immunodeficiencies. The pre-BcR and mature BcR complexes consist of an immunoglobulin dimer associated with the lg-α and lg-β subunits that generate intracellular signals (Panel (a)). The pre-BcR differs from the mature complex owing to the presence of a surrogate light chain (indicated by a dotted line) in the pre-BcR dimer. Further associated with the BcR are CD19, CD21, CD81 (TAPA-1), and CD225 (Leu-13, not shown), which act as coreceptors to modulate the threshold of signalling. Mutations in the receptor complexes that have been linked to B-cell immunodeficiencies are indicated with a

red X. B-cell differentiation (Panel (b)) entails a progression from a progenitor stem cell to a pro-B cell to a pre-B cell to an immature B cell and, finally, to a mature B cell. The dashed line indicates that intervening steps occur that are not shown. The pre-BcR provides signals for Pre-B-cell differentiation. The stages of B-cell differentiation affected by mutations and deficiencies of different proteins are shown by T bars. ADA, adenosine deaminase; RAG, recombination-activating gene; BTK, Bruton's tyrosine kinase; and BLNK, mutated B-cell-linked protein. (Reproduced with permission from Rudd CE. *N Engl J Med* 2006;354:1875; Copyright 2006 Massachusetts Medical Society. All rights reserved.)

(CVID) is the commonest acquired primary immunodeficiency that is likely to be encountered by haematologists. As its name implies, CVID is characterised by a severe reduction in at least two serum immunoglobulin isotypes associated with low or normal B-cell numbers. In contrast, antibody deficiency disorders associated with severe reduction of all serum immunoglobulin isotypes with absent circulating B cells is a feature of diseases associated with mutations which interrupt B-cell development (Figure 32.2).

The term *CVID* embraces a heterogeneous group of disorders all of which are characterised by late-onset hypogammaglobulinaemia as the unifying theme. The commonest infective manifestation of antibody deficiency is recurrent infection with encapsulated bacteria, particularly *Streptococcus pneumoniae* and to a lesser extent with unencapsulated *Haemophilus influenzae*. Many patients develop frank bronchiectasis as a consequence of recurrent chest infections. Despite their inability to mount effective antibody responses to exogenous pathogens many patients with CVID mount paradoxical immune responses to self-antigens leading to autoimmune disease. In a haematological context, the most frequent of these autoimmune complications are immune thrombocytopenic purpura and autoimmune haemolytic anaemia.

A whole host of other organ-specific and systemic autoimmune diseases may also occur ranging from Addison's disease to systemic lupus erythematosus. Other non-infective complications associated with CVID include a curious predisposition to granulomatous disease, lymphoid interstitial pneumonitis and a 100-fold increase in the risk of lymphoma. Although the latter may occasionally be driven by Epstein–Barr virus (EBV), in the majority of cases no underlying infection is evident raising the possibility that lymphoproliferative disease in these patients is a manifestation of defective immunoregulation.

Despite the inability of B cells in CVID to produce antibodies, recovery of antibody production has been documented following infection with hepatitis C virus and HIV, respectively. This observation supports the concept that defective immunoregulation is contributing to poor B-cell function in these patients.

Given the range of infective and non-infective complications associated with CVID, many attempts have been made to produce a clinically useful disease classification based on immunological indices. Recent evidence suggests that a deficiency of switched IgM$^-$ IgD$^-$ CD27$^+$ memory B cells may well correlate with the development of bronchiectasis, autoimmunity and reactive splenomegaly in CVID. The molecular basis for some of the diseases previously included under the umbrella of CVID has recently been elucidated by the detection of mutations in a number of genes associated with B-cell function (Table 32.1). In addition to the molecular defects listed in Table 32.1, there are rare patients with mutations in certain X-linked genes (Bruton tyrosine kinase, CD40 ligand and signalling lymphocyte activation – associated protein) who may present with a clinical phenotype resembling CVID.

The management of CVID revolves around regular immunoglobulin replacement optimised to ensure a trough IgG level well within the normal range for effective prophylaxis against bacterial infections. Early diagnosis and therapeutic intervention with immunoglobulin therapy significantly minimises the risk of permanent bronchiectatic lung damage.

Table 32.1 Known molecular defects which present with a CVID-like clinical picture.

- Inducible costimulatory receptor (ICOS) deficiency
- CD19 deficiency
- Mutations in the transmembrane activator and calcium-modulator and cyclophilin ligand interactor (TACI) receptor
- Mutations in the receptor for B-cell activating factor of the TNF family (BAFF)

X-linked agammaglobulinaemia

X-linked agammaglobulinaemia (XLA) was one of the earliest primary immunodeficiencies to be clinically characterised in the 1950s. Its molecular basis was only elucidated in the 1990s with the discovery of mutations in a protein tyrosine kinase gene, named Bruton's tyrosine kinase (Btk).

The Btk gene is located on the long arm of the X-chromosome and encodes for a cytoplasmic tyrosine kinase which is essential for B-cell signal transduction. Btk mutations are associated with B-cell developmental arrest in the bone marrow. The consequent disappearance of circulating B cells in association with severe panhypogammaglobulinaemia and poorly developed lymphoid tissue constitutes the cardinal immunological features of XLA. Over 400 different mutations in the Btk gene have been recorded to date but there are no significant correlations between genotype and clinical phenotype.

Most boys with XLA present with a history of recurrent sinopulmonary infections on a background of panhypogammaglobulinaemia after the age of 6 months, once the protective effect of transplacentally acquired maternal IgG has waned. As with CVID, delayed diagnosis of XLA and consequent failure to institute adequate immunoglobulin replacement is associated with a high risk of bronchiectasis.

In keeping with the absence of a T-cell defect in XLA, infection with intracellular pathogens is generally not a problem. The major exception to this rule is the predisposition to chronic enteroviral infections, including echovirus meningoencephalitis and vaccine-induced poliomyelitis. A clinical phenotype identical to XLA may be caused by mutations in the μ-immunoglobulin heavy-chain gene and other components of the B-cell receptor.

Severe combined immunodeficiency

Severe combined immunodeficiency (SCID) refers to a group of genetically determined disorders characterised by arrested T-cell development accompanied by impaired B-cell function. The incidence of SCID is estimated to be between 1:50,000 and 1:100,000 live births.

Babies with SCID present with recurrent infections associated with lymphopenia. Amongst the range of pathogens responsible for infection in SCID, *Pneumocystis jiroveci* (*carinii*), aspergillus species and cytomegalovirus predominate in keeping with the profound T-cell deficiency seen in these babies.

To date, 11 distinct molecular defects which cause the SCID phenotype have been identified (Table 32.2). Whilst lymphopenia is characteristic of all forms of SCID (Figure 32.3), the circulating lymphocyte surface marker profile (Table 32.2) provides a useful clue as to the underlying genetic defect. For example, deficiency of adenosine deaminase, a key purine enzyme results in severe lymphopenia affecting T, B and NK cells leading to its characterisation as T− B− NK− SCID.

Given the profound impairment in T-cell immunity, babies with SCID are at risk of iatrogenic

Table 32.2 Classification of severe combined immunodeficiency.

Affected gene	Inheritance	Circulating lymphocyte phenotype
Adenosine deaminase (ADA)	AR	T− B− NK−
Common cytokine γ-chain (γc)	X-linked	T− B+ NK−
Jak-3	AR	T− B+ NK−
IL-7α	AR	T− B+ NK+
Recombination activating gene 1,2 (RAG1/RAG2)	AR	T− B− NK+
Artemis	AR	T− B− NK+
CD3 δ, ζ, ε	AR	T− B+ NK+
CD45	AR	T− B+ NK+

AR, autosomal recessive.

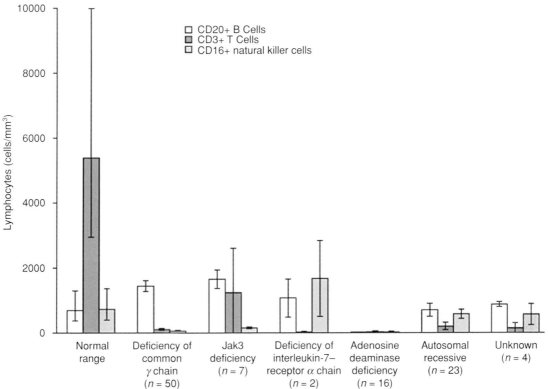

Figure 32.3 Mean (± SE) numbers of CD20+ B cells, CD3+ T cells and CD16+ natural killer cells at presentation in 102 patients with severe combined immunodeficiency, according to the cause of the disorder. The lymphopenia characteristic of all forms of severe combined immunodeficiency is apparent, as are the differences in the lymphocyte phenotypes in the various forms of the syndrome. The normal ranges at the author's institution are shown for comparison. Jak3 denotes Janus kinase 3. 'Autosomal recessive' refers to 23 patients with autosomal recessive severe combined immunodeficiency in whom the molecular defect has not been identified. (Reproduced with permission from Buckley RH. *N Engl J Med* 2000;343:1314; Copyright 2000 Massachusetts Medical Society. All rights reserved.)

disease with live vaccines and transfusion-associated graft-versus-host disease. For these reasons, immunisation with live vaccines should be regarded as absolutely contraindicated in these babies. Equally, any baby with SCID should only receive irradiated and cytomegalovirus-seronegative blood.

The severity of disease and the urgency with which curative haemopoietic stem cell transplantation (HSCT) should be undertaken has led SCID to be regarded as a paediatric emergency. The results of HSCT have improved significantly with early diagnosis and aggressive management of infections and nutritional problems seen in these babies at the time of diagnosis. At present, HSCT from an HLA-matched sibling donor offers an 80% chance of cure whilst a fully HLA-matched unrelated transplant offers a 70% chance of cure (Figure 32.4).

In view of the single gene defects underlying SCID, gene therapy is an attractive option. Whilst offering great promise, the results of gene therapy to date have been mixed. Gene therapy has been successful in some children with ADA and common cytokine γ-chain deficiency, respectively, with evidence of T-, B- and NK-cell reconstitution in the former and T- and NK-cell reconstitution in the latter. However, the occurrence of insertional mutagenesis leading to T-cell lymphoproliferative disease in some children with common γ-chain SCID

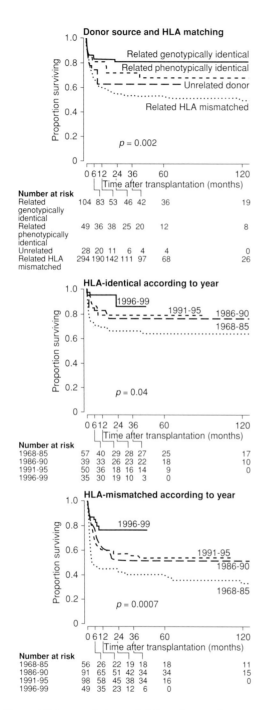

Figure 32.4 Cumulative probability of survival in SCID patients, according to donor source (related or unrelated donor) and HLA matching, and year of transplantation. (Reproduced with permission from Antoine C *et al. Lancet* 2003;361:556.)

is an important reminder of the obstacles associated with this ground-breaking therapy.

Investigation of suspected immunodeficiency

Although a few patients may have distinctive clues on examination pointing towards an immunodeficiency, most patients have no physical signs that would specifically point to an immunodeficiency disorder. Conversely, it follows that a normal physical examination does not exclude immunodeficiency disease.

Immunodeficiency should be included in the differential diagnosis of any patient with severe, prolonged or recurrent infection with common pathogens or even a single episode of infection with an unusual pathogen. The type of pathogen involved provides important clues as to which component of the immune system may be defective and consequently guides the selection of relevant immunological tests (Table 32.3). Although this chapter is primarily devoted to primary immunodeficiency, it is essential to consider and exclude the possibility of HIV infection as a driver for immunodeficiency in many of these clinical scenarios.

In view of the complexity of many immunological tests it is essential that immunological investigations are performed under the guidance of a clinical immunologist to enable appropriate test selection, interpretation and advice on clinical management.

Management

Infections in any immunodeficient patient should be treated aggressively with appropriate antimicrobial therapy. In patients with antibody deficiency, lifelong immunoglobulin replacement remains the cornerstone of management. For children with SCID, HSCT remains the main curative option with the prospect of gene therapy for some forms of SCID. Patients with complement deficiency should be fully immunised with the full range of available vaccines against neisserial, pneumococcal and haemophilus infections. However, it is vital to avoid the use of live vaccines in any patient with immunodeficiency in view of the real risks of vaccine-associated disease as exemplified by vaccine-induced poliomyelitis in XLA and BCG-induced mycobacterial disease in SCID.

Table 32.3 Patterns of infection as a guide to selection of immunological tests in suspected immune deficiency.

Type of pathogen	Consider	Relevant immunological tests
A – Encapsulated pathogens	Antibody deficiency Complement deficiency	Serum immunoglobulins, specific antibodies to polysaccharide and protein antigens Haemolytic complement activity
B – Viruses and intracellular pathogens	T-cell defect	Lymphocyte surface marker analysis Lymphocyte transformation
C – Combination of encapsulated pathogens and viruses and other intracellular pathogens	Combined B- + T-cell defect	As for A and B
D – Recurrent neisserial infection	Complement deficiency	Haemolytic complement activity
E – Recurrent staphylococcal abscesses and/or invasive fungal infections	Phagocyte defect	Neutrophil respiratory burst Leucocyte adhesion molecule expression (selected cases)

Immunoglobulin therapy

Therapeutic immunoglobulin is a blood product prepared from the plasma of 10,000–15,000 donors. The broad spectrum of antibody specificities contained in pooled plasma is an essential ingredient underpinning the success of intravenous (IVIg), and more recently, subcutaneous immunoglobulin in infection prophylaxis in patients with antibody deficiency. In addition to its role in straightforward antibody replacement, the success of high-dose IVIg in the treatment of immune thrombocytopenic purpura (ITP) has led to a veritable explosion in its use as a therapeutic immunomodulator in many autoimmune diseases spanning multiple specialties (Table 32.4).

The mechanisms of action of high-dose IVIg in autoimmune disease are complex and reflect the potent immunological actions of the different regions of an IgG molecule. It is helpful conceptually, to consider the potential mechanisms of action in relation to the variable regions of IgG (F(ab')2), the Fc region and the presence in IVIg of other potent immunomodulatory substances other than antibody (Figure 32.5). In ITP, the traditional view of Fc-receptor blockade as the predominant mechanism by which IVIg is effective has recently been complemented by evidence from murine studies showing that IVIg-mediated amelioration of ITP is crucially dependent on interactions with the inhibitory FcγRIIB as well as the activating receptor, FcγRIII.

Immunoglobulin replacement in secondary antibody deficiency

IVIg replacement is beneficial in prophylaxis against infection in selected patients with secondary antibody deficiency associated with B-cell lymphoproliferative disease and myeloma. The predictors of response to IVIg are the presence of hypogammaglobulinaemia accompanied by low concentrations of pneumococcal antibodies and a failure to respond to test immunisation with pneumococcal polysaccharide (Pneumovax). Whilst IVIg is clinically efficacious in patients fulfilling the above criteria, questions remain regarding its overall cost-effectiveness. For this reason, IVIg replacement should be reserved for those patients who have failed a trial of prolonged antibody prophylaxis. Despite evidence supporting the use of IVIg in secondary antibody deficiency, in practice its use has not been widespread due to the advent of more immunogenic pneumococcal conjugate vaccines coupled with improved overall management of these haematological malignancies.

Adverse effects of intravenous immunoglobulin therapy

Immediate infusion-related adverse effects

Minor to moderate immediate infusion-related adverse effects in the form of headaches, chills,

Disorder	Comments
Neurology	
Guillain–Barre syndrome	Treatment of choice and as efficacious as plasmapheresis (RCT, CR)
Multifocal motor neuropathy	Treatment of choice (RCT)
Chronic inflammatory demyelinating polyneuropathy	As an alternative to steroids (RCT)
Dermatomyositis	As an adjunct to immunosuppressive therapy (RCT)
Myasthenia gravis	For myasthenic crises (RCT)
Lambert–Eaton syndrome	For non-cancer-associated cases which have failed to respond to standard therapy (RCT)
Stiff-person syndrome	For severe cases unresponsive to standard therapy (RCT)
Haematology	
Immune thrombocytopenic purpura	Selected cases unresponsive to standard treatment (RCT)
Parvovirus-associated pure red cell aplasia	Selected cases
Paediatrics	
Kawasaki disease	Treatment of choice (RCT)
Dermatology	
Toxic epidermal necrolysis	Open studies/case series suggest benefit
Autoimmune blistering disorders	Open studies/case series suggest benefit
Streptococcal toxic shock syndrome	Open studies/case series suggest benefit

Table 32.4 Use of IVIg as an immunomodulatory agent.

The list of indications is not exhaustive but covers those disorders where IVIg is frequently used. RCT – evidence from randomised controlled trials. CR – evidence from Cochrane review.

rigors and backache occur in approximately 1% of patients irrespective of the therapeutic dose of immunoglobulin. These adverse effects are largely related to the rate of infusion and/or the presence of underlying infection in the recipient and respond to a combination of a reduction in infusion rate coupled with simple analgesia. Very rarely, some patients with total IgA deficiency and pre-existing anti-IgA antibodies may develop anaphylaxis on exposure to IVIg preparations containing IgA. This risk is greatly minimised by the use of an IgA-depleted IVIg preparation in such patients.

Dose-related adverse effects

The increasing use of IVIg for therapeutic immunomodulation has been associated with the development of a range of haematological, neurological, nephrological and dermatological adverse effects that are directly linked to the high doses (2 g/kg) required for autoimmune disease in contrast to the low doses (0.4 g/kg) used for antibody replacement.

Haematological

High-dose IVIg causes a dose-dependent increase in plasma viscosity which is sufficient to precipitate

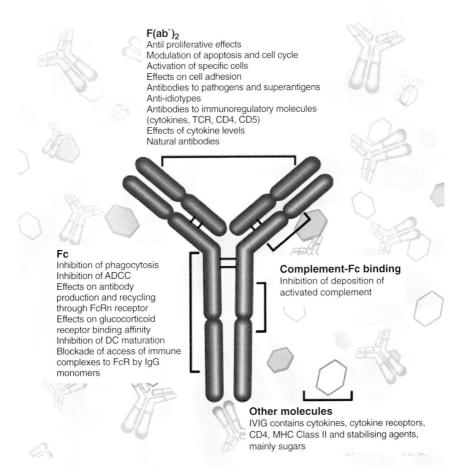

F(ab´)₂
Antil proliferative effects
Modulation of apoptosis and cell cycle
Activation of specific cells
Effects on cell adhesion
Antibodies to pathogens and superantigens
Anti-idiotypes
Antibodies to immunoregulatory molecules
(cytokines, TCR, CD4, CD5)
Effects of cytokine levels
Natural antibodies

Fc
Inhibition of phagocytosis
Inhibition of ADCC
Effects on antibody
production and recycling
through FcRn receptor
Effects on glucocorticoid
receptor binding affinity
Inhibition of DC maturation
Blockade of access of immune
complexes to FcR by IgG
monomers

Complement-Fc binding
Inhibition of deposition of
activated complement

Other molecules
IVIG contains cytokines, cytokine receptors,
CD4, MHC Class II and stabilising agents,
mainly sugars

Figure 32.5 Immunomodulatory actions of intravenous immunoglobulin. (Reproduced with permission from Jolles S, Sewell WAC & Misbah SA. *Clin Exp Immunol* 2005;142:3.)

serious arterial and venous thrombosis in patients with pre-existing thrombophilia, paraproteinaemia, severe polyclonal hypergammaglobulinaemia and atheromatous cardiovascular disease.

The risk of IVIg-associated acute haemolysis due to passive transmission of anti-blood group antibodies has been greatly minimised by the institution of rigorous quality control measures designed to ensure that the titre of anti-blood group antibodies in IVIg does not exceed 1:8.

Neurological

High-dose IVIg is associated with the development of self-limiting acute aseptic meningitis in a minor-ity of patients (<5%). Patients with background migraine are at higher risk raising the possibility that meningeal irritation may be due to the interaction of exogenous IgG with meningeal endothelium.

Renal

Nephrotoxicity due to high-dose IVIg is a particular risk associated with sucrose-containing preparations which trigger osmotic tubular injury leading to extensive vacuolar changes suggestive of historical cases of sucrose-induced nephropathy. The risk of renal damage is greatly minimised by avoiding the use of sucrose-containing IVIg preparations in patients with pre-existing diabetes and renal disease.

IVIg should also be avoided or used with caution in patients with mixed cryoglobulinaemia because of the real risk of the IgM component of cryoglobulin, containing rheumatoid factor reactivity complexing with infused exogenous IgG to cause acute immune-complex-mediated renal injury.

Dermatological

A variety of cutaneous adverse effects including eczema, erythema multiforme, urticaria and cutaneous vasculitis may be triggered by high-dose IVIg. The relatively small number of cases reported to date does not enable any useful analysis which might help in minimising the development of dermatological adverse reactions.

Risks of viral transmission

Viral transmission is a risk with both low- and high-dose IVIg therapy. However, the increasingly stringent screening of donors coupled with the introduction of additional anti-viral steps during plasma fractionation has greatly reduced but not eliminated the risk of hepatitis C virus transmission with IVIg. For this reason, patients on maintenance IVIg should have their liver function monitored along with regular testing for hepatitis C. The lack of any outbreaks of IVIg-associated hepatitis C transmission since the last outbreak in 1993 attests to the success of current viral safety measures. Unlike hepatitis C, HIV and hepatitis B have never been transmitted by IVIg since the process of Cohn-ethanol fractionation specifically inactivates both of these viruses.

Whilst recent reports of the development of new variant Creutzfeldt–Jakob disease in recipients of blood from donors with asymptomatic disease have raised concerns of the possibility of prion transmission by blood products, this risk remains largely theoretical with IVIg. Leucocyte reduction and the use of plasma from countries free of bovine spongiform encephalopathy are measures designed to minimise this risk in the UK (see Chapter 15).

Practical aspects of immunoglobulin therapy – product selection and safe use

The availability of several different preparations of IVIg (at least six in the UK at present) has raised the question of whether IVIg should be considered to be a generic product. For the purposes of antibody replacement, it is reasonable to consider the different products equally efficacious since each product is required to fulfil the stringent criteria laid down by the World Health Organization for therapeutic immunoglobulin. With regard to the use of high-dose IVIg as an immunomodulator, the only study comparing the efficacy of different products was in Kawasaki disease which showed no difference. Nonetheless, because differences in the manufacturing process affect opsonic activity, Fc-receptor function and complement fixation, it is best not to consider IVIg as a generic product. In view of this and the potential difficulty in tracking any future outbreak of IVIg-associated viral transmission, it is prudent to maintain patients requiring long-term treatment on the same IVIg product, irrespective of whether IVIg is being used for antibody deficiency or immunomodulation.

Table 32.5 provides a useful checklist for the safe use of high-dose IVIg, including advice on product selection. Advice on individual products should be sought from a clinical immunologist.

Key points

1 Over 120 primary immunodeficiency disorders are currently recognised.
2 Common variable immunodeficiency is the commonest acquired treatable immunodeficiency.
3 IVIg is the mainstay of treatment for patients with antibody deficiency.
4 Haemopoietic stem cell transplantation remains the main curative option for children with SCID.
5 High-dose IVIg is widely used as a therapeutic immunomodulator in a range of autoimmune diseases.

Table 32.5 Checklist for the use of high-dose IVIg.

1 Prior to first infusion:

Check renal and liver function, full blood count, viscosity, serum C-reactive protein, serum immunoglobulins and electrophoresis. Take blood for hepatitis C serology (not necessary to delay treatment whilst awaiting result) and save aliquot of frozen serum.

Normal renal and liver function and serum IgA	Impaired renal function	Total IgA deficiency (<0.05 g/L)	Partial IgA deficiency	IgM/IgG paraprotein	Patients at risk of hyperviscosity: >4 cp (i.e. serum IgG >50 g/L or with serum IgM >30 g/L) or with background arterial disease
Proceed with any IVIg product	Avoid sucrose-containing IVIg and exercise caution; suggest using 0.4 g/kg/daily for 5 days and slower rate of infusion (suggest halving rate). Check creatinine daily before repeat dose is given	Use IVIg product containing low IgA content Check anti-IgA antibodies	Proceed with any IVIg product	Consider possibility of mixed cryoglobulinaemia. Seek immunological advice before proceeding with IVIg	Exercise caution: use slower rate of infusion (suggest halving rate) and check viscosity at end of course

2 Adhere to the manufacturer's recommendations regarding reconstitution and rate of infusion.

3 Record batch number of product.

Reproduced with permission from Association of British Neurologists. Guidelines on IVIg in neurological diseases. www.abn.org.

Further reading

Caligaris-Cappio F. How immunology is reshaping clinical disciplines: the example of haematology. *Lancet* 2001;358:49–55.

Castigli E & Geha RS. Molecular basis of common variable immunodeficiency. *J Allergy Clin Immunol* 2006;117:740–746.

Cavazzano-Calvo M & Fischer A. Gene therapy for severe combined immunodeficiency: are we there yet? *J Clin Invest* 2007;117:1456–1465.

Geha RS, Notarangelo LD, Casanova JL *et al.* Primary immunodeficiency diseases: an update from the International Union of Immunological Societies Primary Immunodeficiency Diseases Classification Committee. *J Allergy Clin Immunol* 2007;120:776–794.

Jolles S, Sewell WAC & Misbah SA. Clinical uses of intravenous immunoglobulin. *Clin Exp Immunol* 2005;142:1–11.

Plebani A, Soresina A, Rondelli R *et al.* Clinical, immunological and molecular analysis in a large cohort of patients with X-linked agammaglobulinaemia. *Clin Immunol* 2002;104:221–230.

PART 5
Alternatives to transfusion

CHAPTER 33

The principles of bloodless medicine and surgery

Aryeh Shander[1] *& Lawrence Tim Goodnough*[2]

[1]Department of Anesthesiology, Critical Care and Hyperbaric Medicine, Englewood Hospital and Medical Center, Englewood; Mount Sinai School of Medicine, New Jersey, USA
[2]Department of Pathology, Stanford University School of Medicine, Stanford, California, USA

Introduction

Concerns about risks and complications of allogeneic blood transfusions (see Part 2 of this book) and the rising costs associated with obtaining, processing and administering blood components (see Part 3), and managing its consequences are fundamentally changing transfusion practice. Blood components should no longer be viewed as readily available commodities, but rather, highly processed products with limited availability and less-than-impeccable safety records, to be used sparingly.

'Blood management' or 'blood conservation' is defined as the appropriate use of blood components with the goal of minimising or avoiding their use. On the other hand, the term 'bloodless medicine and surgery' has been reserved to describe similar strategies used to avoid allogeneic transfusions altogether for either religious reasons or personal preferences. Although these terms are frequently used interchangeably (as in this chapter), readers should be aware of their significant differences.

Despite its primary roots in providing care for patients who object to transfusion for religious reasons (e.g. Jehovah's Witnesses), the scope of bloodless medicine goes beyond this single issue. For example, in trauma, combat injuries and disasters where massive transfusions are needed and available blood products may become quickly exhausted, bloodless medicine and surgery where available, offers a life-saving option. The same rule applies to patients who are alloimmunised to red blood cells (RBCs) and patients with autoimmune haemolytic anaemia in whom allogeneic transfusions are undesirable.

In major disasters, the blood supply can easily be affected due to interruption of any of the numerous links of its complicated chain (donation, screening, processing, storage, transportation etc.). Transfusion demand, however, is expected to increase to manage trauma and non-elective surgical cases. How does the blood transfusion laboratory respond with an empty inventory? Bloodless medicine and surgery can be the answer to the paradox of increased demand and diminished supply in this context. This example clearly highlights the importance of global and adequate training in blood management as part of crisis preparedness.

Currently in the US and much of the developed world, blood supply is considered to be safe. This safety, however, has been achieved with increasing expense of more complex screening procedures which have added to the costs and limited the supply of major blood components. Quite surprisingly

Practical Transfusion Medicine, 3rd edition. Edited by Michael F. Murphy and Derwood H. Pamphilon. © 2009 Blackwell Publishing, ISBN: 978-1-4051-8196-9.

and in spite of widespread use of allogeneic transfusions, evidence supporting that blood transfusions are efficacious is lacking. On the other hand, increasing number of studies have linked transfusions to undesirable outcomes (Table 33.1). For instance, a landmark multicenter study has shown that critically ill anaemic patients managed with a restrictive transfusion trigger of 7.0 g/dL haemoglobin concentration had an overall similar mortality rate compared with patients managed with a liberal transfusion trigger of 10 g/dL haemoglobin. In the subgroup analysis, it was noted that mortality rates were actually lower in restrictive transfusion group among patients who were less acutely ill and among younger patients, but not among those with cardiac disease (Hebert *et al.*, 1999). While the search for the minimum acceptable haemoglobin levels and proper transfusion indications in various patient populations is still ongoing, the studies shown in Table 33.1 suggest that not only limiting the allogeneic RBC transfusions is safe and practical, but it can also be beneficial to many patients. As a result, we are witnessing a paradigm shift in the use of transfusion in management of bleeding and anaemia, favouring restrictive transfusion strategies.

General principles of blood conservation

Exposure of patients to allogeneic blood can be minimised by the systematic use of blood management strategies. These strategies routinely include a combination of medications and devices as well as medical and/or surgical techniques applied via an interdisciplinary team approach. The general principles of blood conservation can be summarised as follows:

• A plan of care to avoid and minimise blood loss should be tailored according to clinical management and anticipated procedures of each patient.

• A multidisciplinary treatment approach using a combination of interventions should be utilised.

• Anaemia should be screened for and if present, promptly diagnosed and appropriately treated, preferably preoperatively.

• The lead clinician should be proactive in managing the patient and readily anticipate and address complications.

• Routine practice should be modified as per clinical judgement when required.

• A 'watch and wait' approach to the bleeding patient should be avoided.

• Specialists experienced in blood conservation should be consulted at an early stage in case of deterioration or complications.

• If necessary, transferring stabilised patient to a major centre before further deterioration of condition should be considered.

• Blood sampling for laboratory tests should be restricted.

• A restrictive transfusion strategy based on tolerance of anaemia should be implemented.

• Before the surgery, the amount of blood loss that can be tolerated by the patient, and the lowest acceptable haemoglobin should be estimated.

• Use of anticoagulant and antiplatelet agents should be reassessed pre- and postoperatively.

• For emergencies, a management plan for rapid location and control of haemorrhage and transfer to the appropriate centre, if necessary, should be established in advance.

Implementation of a comprehensive blood conservation strategy begins well ahead of the scheduled day of surgery and continues into the postoperative period. Some key measures throughout this period are screening for and treatment of anaemia, minimising iatrogenic blood loss, and restricting transfusion based on valid 'triggers'. Figure 33.1 depicts an overview of the blood conservation techniques to be considered in the perioperative period. Autologous transfusions and pharmacological agents useful in blood conservation are discussed in details in Chapters 34 and 36, respectively. While many of these strategies apply to specific periods of care, some (including anaemia management and restrictive transfusion) are applicable throughout the care and will be discussed first.

Management of anaemia

As many as 75% of patients undergoing elective surgery may have anaemia, and low preoperative

Table 33.1 Outcomes of transfused versus not transfused patients in various settings.

Study	Studied population	Outcome
Hebert *et al.* (1999)	Critically ill patients (*n* = 838)	30-day mortality: Overall: 18.7% (RS) vs. 23.3% (LS); $p = 0.11$ Less acutely ill subset: 8.7% (RS) vs. 16.1% (LS); $p = 0.03$ Cardiac disease: 22.2% (RS) vs. 22.9% (LS); $p = 0.69$ Mortality during hospitalisation: 22.2% (RS) vs. 28.1% (LS); $p = 0.05$
Leal-Noval *et al.* (2001)	Cardiac surgery patients (*n* = 738)	Mortality 13.3% (T) vs. 8.9% (NT); $p < 0.01$ ICU stay 6.1 days (T) vs. 3.7 days (NT); $p < 0.01$
Wu *et al.* (2001)	Elderly (≥65 years old) Medicare patients with MI (*n* = 78,974)	ORs and their 95% CI for 30-day mortality in T vs. NT stratified by Hct on hospital admission: Hct 5.0–24.0%, 0.22 (0.11–0.45); Hct 24.1–27.0%, 0.48 (0.34–0.69); Hct 27.1–30.0%, 0.60 (0.47–0.76); Hct 30.1–33.0%, 0.69 (0.53–0.89); Hct 33.1–36.0%, 1.13 (0.89–1.44); Hct 36.1–39.0%, 1.38 (1.05–1.80); Hct 39.1–48.0%, 1.46 (1.18–1.81)
Engoren *et al.* (2002)	Cardiac surgery (*n* = 1915)	Mortality after 5 years: RR for T vs. NT: 1.7 (95% CI 1.4–2.0; $p = 0.001$) Does-dependent association of T with serious postoperative infection
Vincent *et al.* (2002)	Critically ill patients (*n* = 3534)	14-day mortality: Overall: 29.0% (T) vs. 14.9% (NT); $p < 0.001$ ICU: 18.5% (T) vs. 10.1% (NT); $p < 0.001$ 28-day mortality matched by propensity score: 22.7% (T) vs. 17.1% (NT); $p = 0.05$
Malone *et al.* (2003)	Trauma patients (*n* = 15,534)	Mortality OR for T vs. NT: 2.83 (95% CI 1.83–4.40; $p < 0.001$) ICU admission OR for T vs. NT: 3.27 (95% CI 2.69–3.99; $p < 0.001$) ICU and hospital lengths of stay were also longer in T vs. NT ($p < 0.001$)
Corwin *et al.* (2004)	Critically ill patients (*n* = 4892)	Transfusion and number of units were independently associated with longer length of stay Mortality rate: 10% in NT vs. 25% in T, adjusted mortality ratio, 1.65; 95% CI 1.35–2.03 for T vs. NT ($p < 0.002$) Transfused cases had more total number of complications and were more likely to experience a complication
Dunne *et al.* (2004)	Trauma patients (*n* = 9539)	Mortality OR for T vs. NT: 4.23 (95% CI 3.07–5.84; $p < 0.0001$) ICU admission OR for T vs. NT: 4.62 (95% CI 3.84–5.55; $p < 0.0001$) SIRS OR for T vs. NT: 2.43 (95% CI 1.99–2.95; $p < 0.0001$)
Innerhofer *et al.* (2005)	Orthopaedic surgical patients (*n* = 308)	Transfusion of allogeneic WBC-filtered RBC was an independent predictor of infection: OR 23.7 (95% CI 1.3–422.1; $p = 0.02$)
Silverboard *et al.* (2005)	Trauma patients (*n* = 102)	ARDS developed in 21% of patients receiving 0–5 units (group I); 31% of patients receiving 6–10 units (group II); 57% of patients receiving over 10 units (group III); $p = 0.007$ Mortality higher in patients receiving more T in first 24 h; $p = 0.03$
Weber *et al.* (2005)	Orthopaedic surgery patients (*n* = 695)	Compared with NT patients, T patients had longer time to ambulation (3.8 vs. 3.1 days; $p < 0.001$) and longer length of stay (12.0 vs. 10.2 days; $p < 0.001$)
Koch *et al.* (2006)	Cardiac surgery (*n* = 5841)	AF higher in T: OR per unit transfused 1.18 (95% CI 1.14–1.23, $p < 0.0001$) In propensity-matched pairs, new-onset AF was more frequent in T (46%) vs. NT (38%) ($p < 0.001$)

(Continued)

Table 33.1 (*Continued*)

Study	Studied population	Outcome
Koch *et al.* (2006)	Cardiac surgery ($n = 11,963$)	Postoperative morbidity and mortality was higher in T: mortality OR 1.77 (95% CI 1.67–1.87; $p < 0.0001$); renal failure OR 2.06 (95% CI 1.87–2.27; $p < 0.0001$); prolonged ventilatory support OR 1.79 (95% CI 1.72–1.86; $p < 0.0001$); serious infection OR 1.76 (95% CI 1.68–1.84; $p < 0.0001$); cardiac complications OR 1.55 (95% CI 1.47–1.63; $p < 0.0001$); neurologic events OR 1.37 (95% CI 1.30–1.44; $p < 0.0001$)
Lacroix *et al.* (2007)	Critically ill anaemic children ($n = 637$)	Same rates of mortality, multiple-organ dysfunction and adverse events in RS vs. LS cases
Murphy *et al.* (2007)	Cardiac surgery ($n = 8598$)	Adjusted OR for composite infection and ischaemic outcomes for T vs. NT: 3.38 (95% CI 2.6–4.4) and 3.35 (95% CI 2.68–4.35), respectively Any transfusion was associated with increased relative cost of admission (1.42 times (95% CI 1.37–1.46)) HR of being discharged from hospital on any time after operation for T vs. NT: 0.63 (95% CI 0.6–0.67) HR of death within 30 days in T vs. NT: 6.69 (95% CI 3.66–15.1)

AF, atrial fibrillation; ARDS, acute respiratory distress syndrome; CI, confidence interval; Hct, haematocrit; HR, hazard ratio; LS, liberal transfusion; NT, not transfused; OR, odds ratio; RR, risk ratio; RS, restrictive transfusion; SIRS, systemic inflammatory response syndrome; T, transfused.

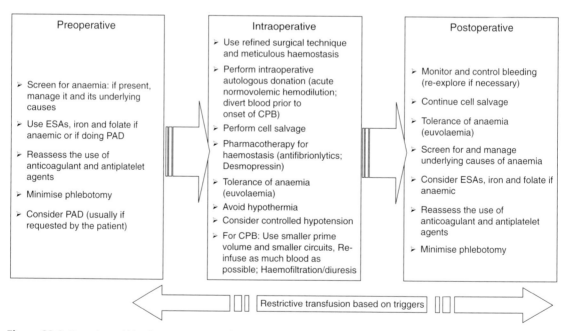

Figure 33.1 Overview of blood conservation techniques and strategies in general and cardiac surgery. CPB, cardiopulmonary bypass; ESA, erythropoiesis-stimulating agent; PAD, preoperative autologous donation. (Modified from Shander A, Goodnough LT. Objectives and limitations of bloodless medical care. *Curr Opin Hematol* 2006;13:462–470.)

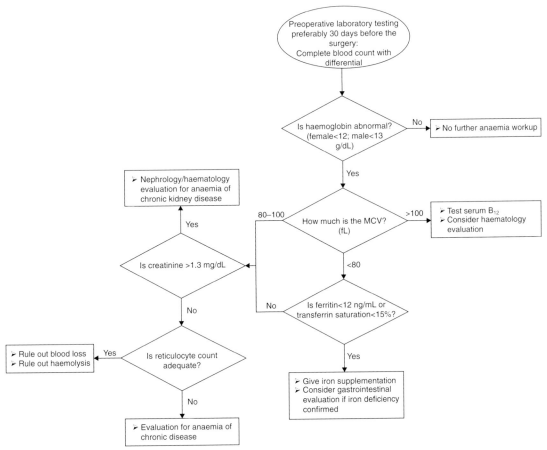

Figure 33.2 Evaluation and management of anaemia in patients undergoing elective surgery. MCV, mean corpuscular volume. (Modified from Goodnough *et al*. Detection, evaluation and management of anemia in the elective surgical patient. *Anesth Analg*. 2005;109(6):1858–1861.)

haemoglobin is associated with a greater risk of being transfused. Moreover, anaemia is an independent predictor of morbidity and mortality and it has been linked to decreased quality of life. Finally, anaemia can be a sign of underlying diseases, many of which, potentially fatal (e.g. colorectal carcinoma and renal disorders). Therefore, it is recommended to perform anaemia screening on patients undergoing elective surgery in a timely manner (30 days prior to surgery) to allow enough time for diagnosis and management of anaemia and the underlying cause (Figure 33.2).

Restrictive transfusion practice

For many years, a haemoglobin (haematocrit) value of 10 g/dL (30%) was regarded as the thresh-

old below which, a transfusion was required prior to the inception of surgery (the so-called 10/30 rule). As previously discussed, many studies have shown that a restrictive transfusion strategy is beneficial to many patients (Table 33.1). Most investigators agree that transfusions are usually required in patients with haemoglobin levels below 6 g/dL, and they are almost never required in patients with haemoglobin levels above 10 g/dL. Yet, the lowest permissible haemoglobin level varies among individual patients, depending on their physiopathological status, and thus, physiologic parameters (triggers) should be given precedence over haemoglobin level alone when making transfusion decisions (Table 33.2). In general, patients with known coronary artery disease might be more

Table 33.2 Physiologic transfusion triggers in anaemic patients.

Parameter	Intraoperatively or in the ICU	Postoperatively or in the ward
Physiologic transfusion trigger		
Relative hypotension (MAP <70–80% of baseline or 60 mm Hg)	Consider transfusion	Consider transfusion
Relative tachycardia (rate >120–130% of baseline or 110–130 beats/min)	Consider transfusion	Consider transfusion
New ST-segment depression >0.1 mV	Consider transfusion	Consider transfusion
New ST-segment elevation >0.2 mV	Consider transfusion	Consider transfusion
New wall motion abnormality in transesophageal/transthoracic echocardiography	Consider transfusion	Consider transfusion
Mixed venous oxygen partial pressure (PvO_2) <32 mm Hg	Consider transfusion	Not applicable
Oxygen extraction rate > 40%	Consider transfusion	Not applicable
Mixed venous oxygen saturation (SvO_2) <60%	Consider transfusion	Not applicable
Decrease in oxygen consumption (VO_2) >10%	Consider transfusion	Not applicable

These triggers are based upon assumption that (a) normovolaemia is maintained and (b) anaemia is the only probable cause of the abnormal reading. Modified from Madjdpour & Spahn (2007) and Madjdpour *et al.* (2006).

susceptible to anaemia, and transfusion is considered if signs of myocardial ischaemia persist in spite of proper medication and volume replenishment. Importantly, tachycardia (due to hypovolaemia) can be extremely detrimental in these patients and should be avoided. Other at risk patients include those of extreme age and febrile/hypermetabolic patients. Table 33.2 summarises suggested physiologic parameters to be used perioperatively, as well as in the intensive care units and wards.

Preoperative period

Advance planning is essential for successful blood conservation. Preoperative assessment begins with thorough history taking, with emphasis on personal/family history of bleeding disorders. As discussed before, anaemia screening should be done well ahead of the surgery. Patients with low haemoglobin should undergo adequate work-up, and their red cell mass should be increased preoperatively to minimise their risk of perioperative transfusion (Figure 33.2). This can be achieved through preoperative use of erythropoiesis-stimulating agents (ESAs). It should

be remembered that patients' iron storage or release may not be sufficient to support the increased haemopoiesis following ESA administration, resulting in 'relative' iron deficiency (with apparently normal or even elevated iron levels in blood tests) and therefore, these patients should receive iron, folate and vitamin B_{12} supplementation as well. This therapy can yield equivalents of one and five blood units over a course of 7- and 28-day, respectively. However, benefits of ESAs should be carefully weighed against their risks (thrombotic events, hypertension and possibly, tumour progression) and they should not be used at doses higher than indicated or in patients with haemoglobin levels exceeding 12 g/dL. ESAs are discussed in more detail in Chapter 43.

Restricting diagnostic blood sampling is a simple yet effective measure of blood conservation in the perioperative period. Careful management and reassessment of anticoagulants and agents affecting coagulation (such as aspirin, non-steroidal anti-inflammatory drugs and antiplatelet medications) is another effective measure.

Preoperative autologous donation (PAD) is occasionally considered as an alternative to allogeneic blood transfusion in patients undergoing elective

surgery. PAD is a procedure in which patients donate a unit of their blood per week for 4 weeks before surgery to be stored and reinfused back to them if required during the surgery or immediate postoperative period. PAD faces several limitations:
• It involves significant costs and inconvenience to the patients (multiple trips back and forth to hospital prior to the surgery).
• To avoid becoming anaemic due to the required aggressive phlebotomies, many patients require ESA and iron, folate and vitamin B_{12} supplementation.
• Since patient's autologous blood is stored in blood bank, PAD suffers from the same risk of clerical error as well as the issue of 'storage lesion' (decreased 2,3,DPG and ATP resulting in reduced life span of the RBCs) similar to stored allogeneic blood.
• As many as 50% of patients undergoing PAD will be anaemic on the day of surgery, and thus, may eventually become even more at risk of receiving allogeneic transfusions.
• Many units of PAD blood are not eventually used and are discarded, further shadowing the cost-effectiveness of this procedure.

As a result, PAD is not usually recommended, unless absolutely necessary, or requested by the patient, in which case it should be combined with other blood conservation techniques with adequate anaemia prophylaxis/management.

Intraoperative period

During surgery, every effort should be made to minimise blood loss and collect and reinfuse any shed blood. Minimally invasive surgical techniques directly translate into less blood loss as well as a quicker recovery course and should be considered whenever possible. In all procedures, a meticulous surgical technique with emphasis on minimising bleeding can significantly reduce transfusion requirement. Examples of such techniques include:
• Control of potential bleeding sources using electrocautery and its newer variants (e.g. argon-beam coagulation) and various sutures and clamps.
• Use of heparin-coated tubing in lieu of systemic heparinisation.

• Local infusion of vasoconstrictor and haemostatic agents.
• Topical application of tissue sealants and adhesives (containing extracellular matrix components and coagulation factors such as purified fibrinogen and thrombin).
• Avoidance of unnecessary hypothermia (which can adversely affect platelet aggregation).

Meticulous planning is another way of streamlining the surgical procedure and avoiding unnecessary blood loss. In cardiopulmonary bypass (CPB), removing and saving a portion of patient's blood prior to CPB onset (through acute normovolaemic haemodilution (ANH) – see below) and using a smaller prime volume and smaller circuits can reduce the adverse effects on coagulation.

Positioning the patient during the surgery to elevate the surgical site and use of tourniquets are other simple yet effective measures for decreasing arterial blood pressure and reducing the blood loss. The same concept applies to the use of controlled hypotension although this approach is not without controversy, due to the potential risk of inadequate blood supply to vital organs. Finally and as mentioned earlier, every effort should be made to maintain normovolaemia (and the heart rate within the normal range) with proper administration of fluids.

ANH is a simple, low-cost blood conservation technique, especially effective in surgeries with high expected blood loss. In this procedure, a pre-calculated volume of patient's blood is removed and replaced by crystalloid or colloid solutions before or after the induction of anaesthesia to achieve a predetermined target haematocrit while maintaining the patient normovolaemic. During surgery, patients bleed a 'diluted' blood and therefore the lost blood contains fewer cells and factors, effectively reducing the actual amount of blood loss. Collected blood is kept in the operating room and it is transfused to patients at wound closure, or if a transfusion trigger is reached.

Compared to PAD, ANH has several advantages. It does not involve any extensive preoperative arrangements or any inconveniences to the patients and it can be done in both elective and urgent procedures. Moreover, since ANH blood is stored at patient's bedside, there is no storage and processing cost and risk of clerical errors as is the case with the PAD. While studies have shown conflicting results on the efficacy of ANH in reducing allogeneic transfusions, it is generally accepted that it can be effective in surgical procedures with significant blood loss. Given its low cost and the acceptable safety profile, ANH remains an appealing blood conservation technique.

Intraoperative autotransfusion (cell salvage) involves recovery of patient's shed blood from the surgical field and sponges. This blood is then washed, filtered and reinfused back to patient. Similar to ANH, cell salvage is most effective in procedures with significant blood loss. Controversy exists on the potential link between intraoperative cell salvage and loss of coagulation factors (if washed), haemolysis and increased risk of infection, amniotic fluid infusion and tumour cell reintroduction. Use of leucocyte depletion filters in cell salvage devices appears to be an effective measure to remove the tumour cells or amniotic fluid and should be considered in cancer surgery and obstetrics. Intraoperative cell salvage devices are widely used in cardiovascular, orthopaedics and trauma surgery and current evidence shows that they are safe and effective in reducing allogeneic transfusion, especially in procedures characterised with extensive blood loss. Autologous transfusion techniques are discussed in more detail in Chapter 34.

Better understanding of coagulation pathways is expected to provide us with more specific and effective tools to manipulate coagulation in the desired direction. Currently, antifibrinolytic and haemostatic agents such as lysine analogues (ε-aminocaproic acid (EACA) and tranexamic acid (TXA)) and aprotinin are widely available and used in surgeries to reduce bleeding. As the name implies, these agents are effective when fibrinolysis is contributing to bleeding. Lysine analogues inhibit plasminogen and plasmin-mediated fibrinolysis. They are low cost and they have been used successfully in many surgical settings (with TXA usually being more effective than EACA). Aprotinin is a serine protease inhibitor that neutralises plasmin and a host of other enzymes. It has been shown to be more effective than lysine analogues in reducing

bleeding and transfusion requirement. However, it is more expensive, and there are concerns regarding its safety (anaphylaxis) and possibly, links with renal and cardiac adverse events, and marketing of this drug has recently been stopped because of initial data safety report of increased all-cause mortality in cardiac surgery patients compared with the other two antifibrinolytic drugs. Desmopressin and recombinant activated factor VII (rFVIIa) are pharmacologic agents with very narrow indications, but their use to control bleeding and in blood conservation has been generally successful in a variety of clinical scenarios. Despite these reports, current evidence is not sufficient to declare their routine use for blood conservation. Pharmacologic agents used in blood conservation are discussed in detail in Chapter 36.

Postoperative period

Following the surgery, patients should be closely monitored for bleeding, and if present, it should be immediately controlled. A low threshold for re-exploration is advisable. Postoperative cell salvage of the washed shed blood is another effective way of minimising allogeneic transfusion where large volumes of blood are being lost. Adequate oxygenation, restricted phlebotomies, haemostatic pharmacologic therapy, control of hypertension, adequate analgesia, maintenance of normovolaemia and normal body temperature and careful re-evaluation of anticoagulant and antiplatelet drugs are other simple and effective blood conservation strategies in the postoperative period. Finally, pre-existing or new-onset anaemia should be managed (using ESAs, iron, folate and vitamin B_{12} supplementation alone or in combination when appropriate) to avoid transfusions in the postoperative period and to ensure optimum recovery.

Blood conservation in practice

When managed properly and in combination, blood conservation techniques can achieve

Table 33.3 Some recommendations for a multimodality blood conservation approach to cardiac surgery.

Recommended	Not recommended
Preoperative identification of high-risk patients (old age, preoperative anaemia, small body size, or urgent operation, preoperative antithrombotic drugs, acquired or congenital coagulation/clotting abnormalities and multiple patient co-morbidities) and performing all available preoperative and perioperative measures of blood conservation in this group as they account for the majority of blood products transfused.	Dipyridamole to reduce postoperative bleeding or to prevent graft occlusion after coronary artery bypass grafting. It may increase bleeding risk unnecessarily. Leucocyte filters on the CPB circuit for leucocyte-depletion for perioperative blood conservation. It may actually activate leucocytes during CPB.
High-dose aprotinin to reduce the number of patients requiring blood transfusion, to reduce total blood loss, and to limit re-exploration in high-risk patients undergoing cardiac operations. Benefits of use should be balanced against the increased risk of renal dysfunction.	Direct reinfusion of shed mediastinal blood from postoperative chest tube drainage as a means of blood conservation. Routine use of ultrafiltration during or immediately after CPB in adult cardiac operations.
Low-dose aprotinin to reduce the number of patients requiring blood transfusion and to reduce the total blood loss in patients having cardiac procedures.	Transfusion when the haemoglobin concentration is greater than 10 g/dL since it is unlikely to improve oxygen transport.
Lysine analogues to reduce the number of patients who require blood transfusion and to reduce total blood loss after cardiac operations (less potent compared to aprotinin).	Routine prophylactic use of desmopressin acetate (DDAVP) to reduce bleeding or blood transfusion after cardiac operations using CPB.
Routine use of red-cell salvage in cardiac operations using CPB, except in patients with infection or malignancy.	Preoperative screening of the intrinsic coagulation system, unless there is a clinical history of bleeding diathesis.
Preoperative measurement of haematocrit and platelet count for risk prediction.	Routine use of intraoperative platelet or plasmapheresis for blood conservation during cardiac operations using CPB.
A multimodality approach involving multiple stakeholders, institutional support, enforceable transfusion algorithms supplemented with point-of-care testing, and other efficacious blood conservation interventions to limit blood transfusion and to provide optimal blood conservation for cardiac operations.	Topical haemostatic agents that employ bovine thrombin during CPB (not helpful and may be potentially harmful). Use of prophylactic positive end-expiratory pressure (PEEP) to reduce bleeding postoperatively.

Modified from Society of Thoracic Surgeons Blood Conservation Guideline Task Force *et al.* (2007).

excellent results. Every drop of patient's blood produced or saved can effectively prevent transfusion of a drop of allogeneic blood. A combination of strategies most appropriate for each patient and setting should be selected and applied. Table 33.3 lists some of the recommendations of the Society of Thoracic Surgeons Blood Conservation Guideline Task Force and the Society of Cardiovascular Anaesthesiologists Special Task Force on Blood Transfusion for the cardiac surgery cases. Approximate amounts of blood saved by some blood conservation techniques are listed in Table 33.4. While some of the discussed blood conservation techniques are not free of costs or potential risks, the outcomes in terms of avoidance of exposure to allogeneic blood and its risks, complications and costs are enormous. Interestingly, measures as simple as limited phlebotomies, restrictive transfusion and timely use of relatively inexpensive and readily available medications such as iron,

Option	Number of units of blood saved
Preoperative	
Tolerance of anaemia/restrictive transfusion	1–2
Increased preoperative RBC mass	2
Preoperative autologous donation (PAD)	1–2
Intraoperative	
Meticulous haemostasis and operative technique	1 or more
Acute normovolaemic haemodilution (ANH)	1–2
Blood salvage	1 or more
Postoperative	
Restricted phlebotomy	1
Blood salvage	1

Table 33.4 Estimated contribution of selected blood conservation techniques in terms of equivalent unit blood saved in surgical patients. Reproduced with permission from Goodnough *et al. Transfusion*. 2003;43(5):668–676.

folate and vitamin B_{12} can yield impressive results compared with some more complex and costly techniques.

Similar to every other practices, blood conservation is not free of risk and certainly, not free of controversies. Recent concerns on the safety of ESAs and aprotinin are valid and require further investigation. It has also been argued that the effect of blood conservation modalities in reducing morbidity and mortality is undetermined. While most of the blood conservation studies have focused on transfusion outcomes as opposed to morbidity and mortality, and many have been essentially underpowered to detect differences in latter outcomes, one should remember the well-established (and growing) risks of transfusions, their outcomes (Table 33.1) as well as their increasing costs. For example, while the effect of storage on RBC function and viability has been scrutinised in various studies comparing fresh with old blood units, recent data suggest that RBC functions are adversely affected soon after collection, and thus, even 'fresh' blood units might not be offering the optimum functionality. Additionally, while the cost of procuring and administering transfusions is generally underestimated and on the rise, receiving transfusions itself is shown to be associated with increased cost of admission beyond the cost of transfusion alone. On the other hand, many blood conservation strategies have been demonstrated to be associated with little (if any) risk and modest cost. More importantly,

blood conservation should be viewed as an assortment of various techniques and as this field progresses, we are bound to find some of these techniques no longer risk/cost-beneficial to be recommended (e.g. PAD), to be replaced by newer alternatives.

Blood conservation is an ever-evolving field. Advances in our understanding of circulation system in physiological and pathological conditions, oxygen demand of organs, tolerance of anaemia and adaptive measures and coagulation as well as more refined surgical techniques and more specific pharmacologic agents have revolutionised our approach to transfusion. The trend is only expected to escalate in the years to come, with many more blood conservation modalities becoming available. One example is the development of haemoglobin-based oxygen carriers and artificial blood. Blood substitutes are reviewed in Chapter 35. With all these exciting developments in mind, one should not forget that in all cases, having the right attitude towards value of blood and importance of its conservation is the first (and perhaps the biggest) step towards achieving global blood conservation.

Key points

1 Blood conservation is defined as the appropriate use of blood components with the goal of minimising their use.

2 It requires a multidisciplinary team approach and an individual plan of care tailored to each patient's condition.

3 It spans pre-, intra- and postoperative periods.

4 Key strategies include management of anaemia and restrictive transfusion.

5 Limited phlebotomies, readjustment of anticoagulants/antiplatelets, meticulous haemostasis and surgical technique, maintenance of normovolaemia, ANH, blood salvage and use of pharmacological agents are other effective strategies.

6 When done properly and in combination, these techniques can significantly reduce the risk of exposure to allogeneic blood.

Acknowledgements

The authors would like to thank Dr Mazyar Javidroozi for his help in producing this chapter.

Further reading

Bennett-Guerrero E, Veldman TH, Doctor A *et al.* Evolution of adverse changes in stored RBCs. *Proc Natl Acad Sci U S A* 2007;104(43):17063–17068.

Carson JL, Noveck H, Berlin JA & Gould SA. Mortality and morbidity in patients with very low postoperative Hb levels who decline blood transfusion. *Transfusion* 2002;42(7):812–818.

Catling S. Blood conservation techniques in obstetrics: a UK perspective. *Int J Obstet Anesth* 2007;16(3):241–249.

FDA Alert. Information for Healthcare Professionals: Erythropoiesis Stimulating Agents (ESA) [Aranesp (darbepoetin), Epogen (epoetin alfa), and Procrit (epoetin alfa)]. Rockville, MD: Food and Drug Administration, 9 March 2007. Available at http://www.fda.gov/cder/drug/InfoSheets/HCP/RHE2007HCP.htm.

Forgie MA, Wells PS, Laupacis A & Fergusson D, for International Study of Perioperative Transfusion (ISPOT) Investigators. Preoperative autologous donation decreases allogeneic transfusion but increases exposure to all red blood cell transfusion: results of a meta-analysis. *Arch Intern Med* 1998;158(6):610–616.

Franchini M. The use of desmopressin as a hemostatic agent: a concise review. *Am J Hematol* 2007;82(8):731–735.

Goodnough LT. Erythropoietin and iron-restricted erythropoiesis. *Exp Hematol* 2007;35(4, Suppl 1):167–172.

Goodnough LT, Price TH, Rudnick S & Soegiarso RW. Preoperative red cell production in patients undergoing aggressive autologous blood phlebotomy with and without erythropoietin therapy. *Transfusion* 1992;32(5):441–445.

Goodnough LT & Shander A. Blood management. *Arch Pathol Lab Med* 2007;131(5):695–701.

Goodnough LT, Shander A & Brecher ME. Transfusion medicine: looking to the future. *Lancet* 2003;361(9352):161–169.

Goodnough LT, Shander A & Spence R. Bloodless medicine: clinical care without allogeneic blood transfusion. *Transfusion* 2003;43(5):668–676.

Hebert PC, Wells G, Blajchman MA et al., for Transfusion Requirements in Critical Care Investigators, Canadian Critical Care Trials Group. A multicentre, randomized, controlled clinical trial of transfusion requirements in critical care. *N Engl J Med* 1999;340(6):409–417.

Karkouti K & McCluskey SA. Perioperative blood conservation – the experts, the elephants, the clinicians, and the gauntlet. *Can J Anaesth* 2007;54(11):861–867.

Madjdpour C & Spahn DR. Allogeneic red blood cell transfusion: physiology of oxygen transport. *Best Pract Res Clin Anaesthesiol* 2007;21:163–171.

Madjdpour C, Spahn DR & Weiskopf RB. Anaemia and perioperative red blood cell transfusion: a matter of tolerance. *Crit Care Med* 2006;34(5, Suppl):S102–S108.

Murphy GJ, Reeves BC, Rogers CA, Rizvi SI, Culliford L & Angelini GD. Increased mortality, postoperative morbidity, and cost after red blood cell transfusion in patients having cardiac surgery. *Circulation* 2007;116(22):2544–2552.

Preoperative red cell transfusion. *Natl Inst Health Consens Dev Conf Consens Statement* 1988;7(4):1–19.

Segal JB, Blasco-Colmenares E, Norris EJ & Guallar E. Preoperative acute normovolemic haemodilution: a meta-analysis. *Transfusion* 2004;44(5):632–644.

Shander A. Surgery without blood. *Crit Care Med* 2003;31(12, Suppl):S708–S714.

Shander A & Goodnough LT. Objectives and limitations of bloodless medical care. *Curr Opin Hematol* 2006;13:462–470.

Shander A, Hofmann A, Gombotz H, Theusinger OM & Spahn DR. Estimating the cost of blood: past, present, and future directions. *Best Pract Res Clin Anaesthesiol* 2007;21(2):271–289.

Shander A, Moskowitz D & Rijhwani TS. The safety and efficacy of 'bloodless' cardiac surgery. *Semin Cardiothorac Vasc Anesth* 2005;9(1):53–63.

Society for Advancement of Blood Management (SABM) [www.sabm.org]. Available at http://www.sabm.org/professionals/faqlist.php?question=15.

Society of Thoracic Surgeons Blood Conservation Guideline Task Force, Society of Cardiovascular Anesthesiologists Special Task Force on Blood Transfusion. Perioperative blood transfusion and blood conservation in cardiac surgery: the Society of Thoracic Surgeons and the Society of Cardiovascular Anesthesiologists clinical practice guideline. *Ann Thorac Surg* 2007;83(5, Suppl):S27–S86.

Waters JH. Indications and contraindications of cell salvage. *Transfusion* 2004;44(12, Suppl):40S–44S.

Zumberg MS, Procter JL, Lottenberg R, Kitchens CS & Klein HG. Autoantibody formation in the alloimmunized red blood cell recipient: clinical and laboratory implications. *Arch Intern Med* 2001;161(2):285–290.

CHAPTER 34

Autologous transfusion

Dafydd Thomas[1] & John Thompson[2]

[1]Welsh Blood Implementation Group, Morriston Hospital, Swansea, Wales
[2]Royal Devon and Exeter Hospitals, Exeter, UK

Autologous blood transfusion has come full circle. The salvage and reinfusion of blood lost during an amputation was first reported by Dr John Duncan in 1885. The development of blood storage, banking and understanding of serology then led to safe and effective transfusion support for medicine, surgery and obstetrics using donor blood. However, the increased cost of blood products, decreasing numbers of blood donors and successive threats of bacterial, viral and prion infection changed our emphasis at the end of the last century. Perhaps the major driver was a medicolegal one, with a new benchmark, namely 'The public has a legitimate expectation of receiving blood that is 100 per cent safe'. As a result of haemovigilance, several successful measures were introduced to improve blood safety and the various techniques for the provision of autologous blood have been refined, studied scientifically and audited.

The 'Appropriate Use of Blood' subcommittee was established by NHS Blood Transplant in England to discuss and investigate strategies for blood conservation. It came to the conclusion that an integrated programme was more successful than piecemeal implementation and that autologous blood transfusion should be part of a total quality management approach based on four strands (Table 34.1):

Practical Transfusion Medicine, 3rd edition. Edited by Michael F. Murphy and Derwood H. Pamphilon. © 2009 Blackwell Publishing, ISBN: 978-1-4051-8196-9.

- preoperative identification of patients at increased risk of bleeding and optimisation before surgery (e.g. correction of anaemia);
- perioperative blood salvage (collection of blood that would otherwise be lost in the surgical field or in postoperative drains);
- blood sparing methods such as drugs and surgical technique; and
- a strict postoperative transfusion protocol.

Reasons to consider autologous transfusion

Clinical transfusion practice should reduce the risks involved in blood transfusion. Extensive testing of blood to decrease the risk of transfusion-transmitted infection has reassured clinicians and maintained demand for donor blood. Blood conservation strategies should minimise the use of donor blood by withholding transfusion until strictly clinically necessary, and employing techniques such as autologous transfusion. In some situations, autologous transfusion is definitely indicated, such as in patients with rare blood groups or complex red cell antibodies for whom it is difficult to find compatible blood. Autologous transfusion should also be used instead of, or to supplement the use of donor blood, in situations where it has been shown to be effective and safe. It has been suggested that more than 20% of surgical demand can be met by autologous transfusion. Certain procedures can be undertaken with virtually no donor blood support

Table 34.1 An approach to blood conservation and the reduction of risk associated with blood transfusion in patients having elective surgery.

- Check the blood count well in advance of surgery and correct any treatable anaemia
- Ask about antiplatelet or anticoagulant drugs the patient is taking and consider if any should be stopped
- Check antibody status and blood group so group-specific blood can be used in an emergency
- Consider whether patient has a hereditary or acquired bleeding tendency and investigate/treat as appropriate
- During surgery consider technical methods to reduce bleeding
- Postoperatively, consider whether blood transfusion is clinically indicated (transfusion trigger) and, if it is, consider how many units are required to achieve the desired Hb (transfusion target)
- If operation would normally require blood transfusion, consider the option of autologous blood transfusion. The options are listed below:

Technique	Situations in which it might be considered
Intraoperative cell salvage	Any patient with estimated blood loss >0.5 L; especially suitable for massive blood loss
Postoperative cell salvage	Patients with postoperative drain loss from a clean site

Some principles apply to other situations where blood transfusion is being considered.

(see Chapter 33), conserving supplies for areas of medicine where there are few alternatives such as haematological oncology.

Blood conservation strategies

Since the second edition of *Practical Transfusion Medicine*, there has been considerable research, audit and re-evaluation of blood sparing strategies with the result that several are no longer used in clinical practice.

Pre-deposit autologous donation

This technique was much vaunted as a means of donating and reserving one's own blood prior to elective surgery. Several observational (but very few randomised) studies were published. The problems were as follows:

- Patients were chronically anaemic at the time of surgery, with little reserve for bleeding and so they were subsequently transfused more frequently.
- Anaemia increases the bleeding time.
- The practical difficulties were significant.
- Cancelled operations meant that blood could go out of date.
- Prospective randomised trials showed comparatively modest savings in donor blood transfusion.

- Careful blood transfusion protocols in the control groups seriously reduced overall transfusion and surgical teams began to introduce other more effective techniques to reduce blood loss, because they knew they were being observed.
- There was a lower threshold for transfusing the pre-deposited blood (because it was there), but there was still the potential for clerical or other errors.

Pre-deposit may be useful in certain special situations, such as in paediatric surgery, where there is a great incentive to avoid transfusion-associated infection. In such cases, it can be assisted by boosting the patient's haemoglobin (Hb) concentration in red cell mass with recombinant erythropoietin and iron (usually parenterally). Directed pre-deposit from relatives was abandoned for ethical reasons as it would place relatives under pressure to reveal lifestyle choices that they might want to keep private.

Acute normovolaemic haemodilution

Acute normovolaemic haemodilution (ANH) seemed to have great promise but is seldom practiced outside special areas. Blood is withdrawn at the beginning of surgery and replaced with a balance of colloid (usually complexed starch) and clear fluid to maintain normovolaemia. The patient consequently bleeds dilute blood during the procedure, so decreasing red cell loss. After surgical blood loss ceases, the fresh autologous blood is returned. The problems are as follows:

• There is no level 1 scientific evidence (from a properly powered randomised controlled trial) to show that ANH actually reduces donor blood exposure.

• ANH takes on average 20 minutes to perform and theatre time is precious.

• Haemodilution may increase bleeding by reducing the haematocrit and diluting clotting factors.

• Haemodilution may precipitate cardiac ischaemia and even myocardial infarction.

Most studies of ANH were not randomised, or used ANH in conjunction with other methods, so it was difficult to ascribe benefit to one or the other. In addition, although theoretical formulas could be used to determine exactly how much blood could be withdrawn, in clinical practice most authors reported comparatively modest volumes of ANH. There may be circumstances where high volume ANH could be employed in fit patients at low risk of myocardial ischaemia, particularly paediatric spinal surgery. Pilot studies have been successful and randomised trials in niche areas are awaited.

Other techniques that have been abandoned

• Routine preoperative coagulation tests (unless there is a positive personal or family history of bleeding).

• Transfusion if Hb > 10 g/dL (accepted as unnecessary).

• Aprotinin (withdrawn by manufacturer because of renal failure and decreased survival).

• Ultrafiltration to remove excess water after cardiac bypass.

• Leucocyte filters in bypass circuits (may activate white cells).

• Platelet-rich plasmapheresis (no benefit).

• Unwashed mediastinal blood (may lead to coagulopathy).

• DDAVP (unless there is an established platelet defect such as uraemia or von Willebrand's disease).

• Bovine thrombin-derived haemostats in cardiac surgery (can provoke antibody response and allergy).

Effective methods for blood conservation

The following techniques are accepted and should be part of a hospital's blood conservation strategy:

• total quality management (continuous audit and improvement of the process of blood transfusion in the perioperative setting) (see Chapters 25 and 33);

• intraoperate cell salvage (ICS);

• postoperative cell salvage (PCS) from wound drain;

• *appropriate* transfusion and acceptance of the very low risk of viral and other risk;

• transfusion if Hb < 7 g/dL postoperatively;

• stopping drugs associated with increased bleeding such as aspirin (unless high cardiac risk) or clopidogrel (unless drug eluting coronary stent inserted in last 6 months);

• blood component therapy if active oozing and supported by abnormal tests and possibly thromboelastography;

• near patient testing; and

• limited sampling in intensive care (reduced volume, near patient testing).

Before surgery: optimising Hb and haemostasis

This involves pre-assessing a patient in advance of surgery and taking steps to reduce the requirements for transfusion. 'Preparing Patients for Surgery' clinics can also identify medical or social reasons that may have led to an operation being cancelled and therefore increase a hospital's efficiency.

If a patient is anaemic, it is important to address the underlying cause. For example, iron deficiency may be due to a gastrointestinal malignancy. If a patient with iron deficiency anaemia is started on iron, the Hb can be expected to rise by about 1 g/dL per week. It is therefore important to check the blood count sufficiently far in advance of surgery to allow time for treatment to be given if required. Patients presenting for surgery with a normal Hb will require transfusion at a later stage or may even avoid blood transfusion altogether. A personal 'goal' is useful for the patient and their general practitioner; for example, Hb > 12 g/dL prior to elective hip replacement.

Newer formulations of intravenous iron have fewer adverse reactions than were associated with these preparations in the past. Intravenous iron is almost immediately available for red cell production. Research is being undertaken to determine whether administration of intravenous iron as late as the preoperative day can improve red cell production in response to surgical anaemia and thus decrease the use of donor blood.

It is important to consider patient factors that might cause excessive blood loss during surgery and which can be corrected in advance. Patients on aspirin or clopidogrel can stop them 5–7 days before surgery (except if the patient is at high risk of suffering a myocardial infarction or has a drug-eluting coronary stent). Patients in atrial fibrillation on warfarin can: discontinue the drug a few days before surgery. If it is imperative to continue anticoagulation, such as in cases of mechanical heart valve replacement, the patient may be given heparin to cover the surgical period. It is important to take a bleeding history when the patient is seen prior to surgery. Screening tests and specific treatment may be required (see Chapter 30). Bleeding diatheses must be considered in patients with renal or liver disease. Agents such as desmopressin (DDAVP) or tranexamic acid may enhance surgical haemostasis (see Chapter 36).

During surgery: reduction in blood loss

Blood loss in many operations has fallen significantly with advancing surgical and anaesthetic techniques. Use of harmonic scalpels, laparoscopy and careful surgical technique has had a huge impact on blood usage. The maintenance of normothermia ensures optimum coagulation and has also been shown to decrease blood loss.

There are several techniques specific to cardiac surgery, which have been the subject of good-quality clinical trials. Protamine sulphate has an anticoagulant effect when used in excess, so reduced doses are now given following bypass. The dose can be titrated using the activated clotting time, or more simply a 50% dose given. In vascular surgery, heparin is no longer reversed. Heparin bonded bypass circuits can be used to reduce the dose of systemic heparin required. Shed mediastinal blood can be reinfused if washed (see below).

During/after surgery: when to transfuse

No blood transfusion is without risks, but equally the administration of blood may be life-saving. In making the decision to transfuse the balance of risks must be considered for each individual. Factors influencing the decision to transfuse include the Hb, the patient's life expectancy, i.e. age/prognosis (many of the adverse effects of transfusion transmitted infection or immune modulation are delayed) and above all, clinical judgement about the patient's ability to tolerate anaemia including the presence of other factors such as cardiac or respiratory disease and sepsis.

Transfusion triggers

Data from patients who refuse blood on religious grounds or who live in parts of the world where blood is scarce or dangerous have helped our understanding of the effects of anaemia. In otherwise healthy patients the following transfusion triggers for stable anaemia might be considered:
- <4 g/dL: transfuse unless fit, asymptomatic and Hb rising;
- 4–7 g/dL: transfusion usually necessary;
- 7–10 g/dL: transfusion not usually necessary; and
- >10 g/dL: transfusion rarely required.

A randomised trial of patients in intensive care showed that less severely ill patients (Acute Physiology and Chronic Health Evaluation II score <20) and patients under 55 years actually had a survival advantage if the Hb was maintained between 7 and 9 g/dL rather than between 10 and 12 g/dL. For

Table 34.2   Guide to number of units required to achieve the 'target' haemoglobin (Hb).

Amount of Hb in 1 unit of red cells
Example: volume bled 450 mL × average Hb 13 g/dL = 58
  g/unit

	Weight (kg)		
	43	57	71
Blood volume (70 mL/kg in adults)	3 L	4 L	5 L
Increase in Hb after one unit transfusion (g/dL)	1.9	1.6	1.2

patients with clinically significant cardiac disease the mortality was similar in both groups.

For otherwise fit patients with a previously normal Hb who are actively bleeding, the following guidelines are appropriate:
• Blood loss <15% blood volume: give fluids; no need to transfuse.
• Blood loss 15–30% blood volume: consider transfusion.
• Blood loss 30–40% blood volume: transfusion usually necessary.
• Blood loss >40% blood volume: transfusion indicated.

Note that blood volume is about 70 mL/kg in adults, so that 20% of blood volume is approximately 1 L. For patients with a short life expectancy or those with chronic anaemia and impaired red cell production, the main trigger for transfusion should be the patient's *symptoms*.

Transfusion targets

In addition to considering when to transfuse, a target Hb should be established for each clinical scenario using the best data available (see above and Chapter 25). It is also important to consider how many units to give. In other words, the *dose* of blood should depend on the estimated blood volume based on the patient's weight.

When a patient is actively bleeding, replacement of red cells should be guided by an estimate of blood loss. A guide to how many units are required to achieve the target is shown in Table 34.2. Single-unit transfusions have previously been discouraged. However, Table 34.2 shows that it might be reasonable to give one unit to a small elderly woman who is symptomatic with an Hb of 7 g/dL

to bring it up to just under 9 g/dL. The transfusion of blood just because it has been made available for the patient should be avoided. If blood is not used, it can be returned to the blood bank and used for another patient. Near patient testing with a device such as the Haemocue is an *essential* component of modern theatre practice.

Techniques for providing autologous blood

ICS now seems to offer the most cost-effective method of autologous transfusion. Future issues in blood supply and demand combined with the discovery of other blood-borne diseases may change this view and result in a re-examination of PAD and ANH. Autologous blood must be clearly labelled and be distinct from donor blood. An example of an autologous blood label is shown in Figure 34.1; autologous units are more easily identified if their labels are printed a different colour to those used for allogeneic blood.

Cell salvage

Principle
During surgical operations when blood loss is expected, blood can be collected, processed and then returned to the patient. This can be done either intraoperatively or postoperatively depending on the type of operation. This process can be cost-effective even when small volumes of blood (i.e. more than 500 mL) are collected. The amount salvaged not only decreases the use of allogeneic blood but in many instances completely removes the need for allogeneic blood transfusion.

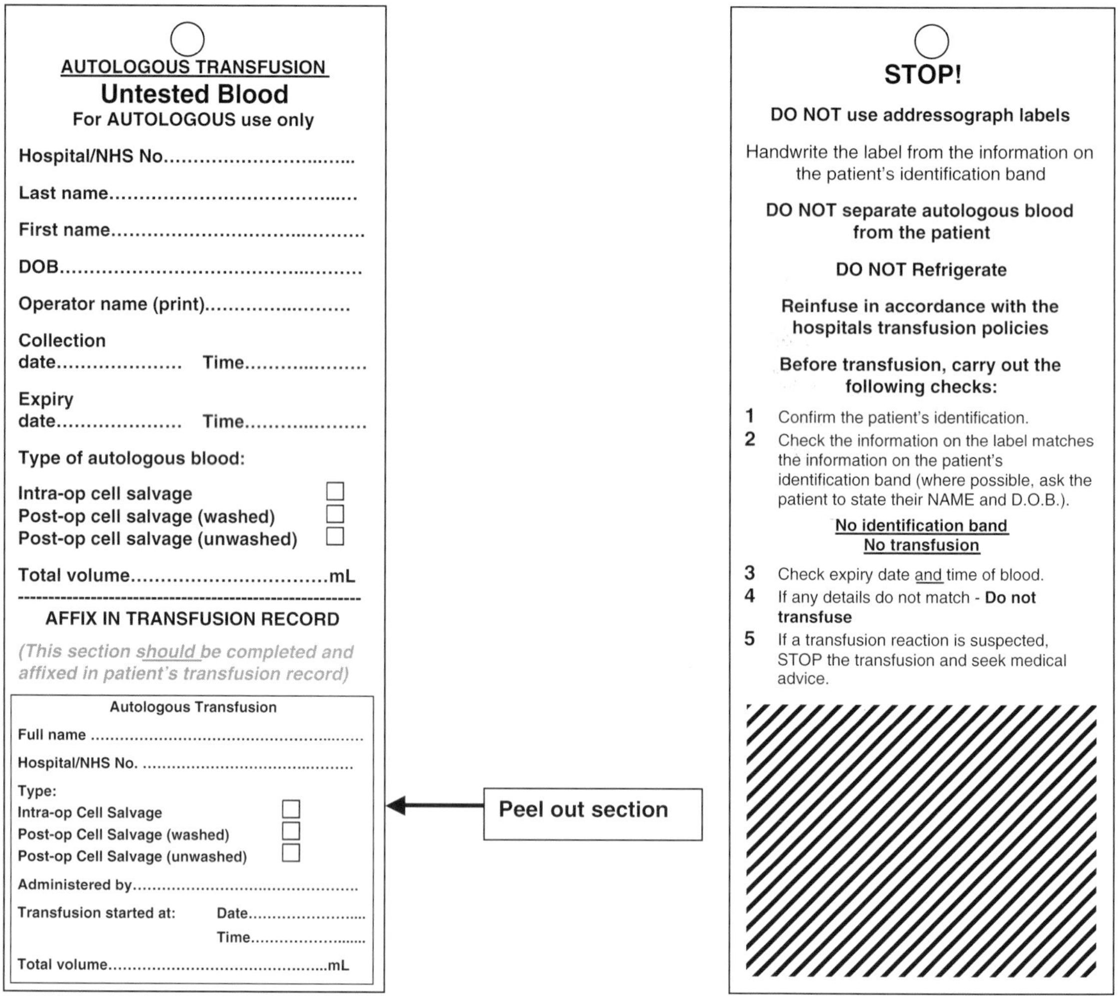
AUTOLOGOUS TRANSFUSION
Untested Blood
For AUTOLOGOUS use only

Hospital/NHS No...............................

Last name..

First name..

DOB...

Operator name (print)..........................

Collection date..................... Time.....................

Expiry date..................... Time.....................

Type of autologous blood:

Intra-op cell salvage ☐
Post-op cell salvage (washed) ☐
Post-op cell salvage (unwashed) ☐

Total volume.................................mL

AFFIX IN TRANSFUSION RECORD

(This section should be completed and affixed in patient's transfusion record)

Autologous Transfusion

Full name ....

Hospital/NHS No. ....

Type:
Intra-op Cell Salvage ☐
Post-op Cell Salvage (washed) ☐
Post-op Cell Salvage (unwashed) ☐

Administered by...

Transfusion started at: Date.........................
Time.........................

Total volume...mL

Peel out section

STOP!

DO NOT use addressograph labels

Handwrite the label from the information on the patient's identification band

DO NOT separate autologous blood from the patient

DO NOT Refrigerate

Reinfuse in accordance with the hospitals transfusion policies

Before transfusion, carry out the following checks:

1 Confirm the patient's identification.
2 Check the information on the label matches the information on the patient's identification band (where possible, ask the patient to state their NAME and D.O.B.).

No identification band
No transfusion

3 Check expiry date and time of blood.
4 If any details do not match - **Do not transfuse**
5 If a transfusion reaction is suspected, STOP the transfusion and seek medical advice.

Figure 34.1 Autologous labels (provided by the UK Cell Salvage Action Group).

Intraoperative cell salvage

Intraoperative cell salvage (ICS) involves the collection and reinfusion of red cells lost during surgery. This may be performed as follows:

• Single-unit reinfusion devices (only used in fully anticoagulated patients). These are simple and cheap for low volume losses.

• Continuous reinfusion of unprocessed blood using dialysis technique. This may be used in conjunction with cardiac bypass but is not of proven benefit and may be associated with risk of haemolysis and high-dose heparin reinfusion leading to coagulopathy.

• Reinfusion of processed blood (discussed below).

There are a number of machines available which wash red cells by centrifugation and resuspend them in saline (examples are shown in Plates 34.1–34.4). Blood is aspirated from the wound site and mixed with heparin or citrate anticoagulant before it enters the reservoir of the machine. The cycle can be either run automatically or controlled manually. In general, about 75% of red cells can be recovered for reinfusion back into the patient. The machines can deliver the equivalent of 10 units of blood per hour. Swabs laden with blood can be wrung out into a bowl of normal saline to further increase yield.

Advantages of ICS

• Considerable reduction in donor blood usage in cases where blood loss is large (>2 L). Suitable operations might include open heart surgery, cystectomy and ruptured ectopic pregnancy.
• Available to *all* patients having appropriate surgery regardless of medical fitness.
• In some situations of uncontrolled blood loss it may be life-saving.
• Unlike other techniques, ICS can be used selectively in cases where the actual, rather than the predicted, blood loss is high.
• Blood can be collected in the reservoir and the decision to use the machine and harness can be deferred until it is clear that the blood loss is sufficient to warrant processing.
• Cell salvage is accepted by Jehovah's Witnesses, provided the collected blood remains in continuity with the patient.

Disadvantages/risks of ICS

• The reinfusion of haemolysed blood is unlikely, providing the wash process is undertaken correctly. Currently, available machines operate an automatic washing process, and a sensor monitors the effluent from the wash cycle, which continues until the liquid being discarded is completely clear, suggesting removal of all free Hb, fragmented red cells and other contaminants.
• There have been no deaths associated with air embolism as a result of improved design and greater awareness of such problems. Air embolism was only reported with very early machines, but collected blood should not be used with pressurised reinfusion devices.
• It does not recover all the blood lost so donor blood may be required in massive haemorrhage. Platelets and coagulation factors are removed by the washing process so supplementation may be required after high volume ICS in the same way as it may be required in high volume bank blood transfusion.
• It requires a capital outlay and trained operators, so ICS can be used only in hospitals with suf-

ficient numbers of suitable operations to become cost-effective. As the cost of donor blood continues to rise with the introduction of safety measures such as universal leucocyte reduction of blood and increasingly sensitive and expensive microbiology testing, cell salvage has become more cost-effective.
• It is important to follow agreed standard operating procedures and to document all stages of the process. Operators should be properly trained according to guidelines (for an example, see http://www.learnbloodtransfusion.org.uk/).

Indications

The primary indication is surgery where expected blood loss is likely to be in excess of 500 mL. Even when blood loss is unpredictable, the collection of operative blood loss may be worthwhile. Providing this blood is anticoagulated, it can be processed and reinfused if sufficient volumes are collected. The processing kits are separately packaged so only the collection reservoir is wasted if small volumes are salvaged with a decision not to wash. ICS is cost-effective providing one unit of packed red cells is reinfused. Even if a small volume of ICS blood is retransfused, raising the patient's Hb level to exceed the agreed transfusion trigger will obviate the need for donor blood.

Relative contraindications

There are a number of situations where the use of cell salvage has been discouraged. However, in the presence of massive haemorrhage, ICS may avoid hypovolaemic shock.
• Malignant cells: Although leucocyte filters may remove the majority of cancer cells, and small numbers may not be clinically significant compared with the numbers that enter the circulation during surgery, some would advocate the use of gamma-irradiation in this setting but this is logistically difficult to arrange. Several studies have reported large numbers of patients receiving cell salvage during cancer surgery, particularly in urology. To date there have been no reports of lung metastasis or decreased survival. The technique should be discussed on an individual basis with patients, with special arrangements for consent. The National Institute for Health and Clinical Excellence (NICE) has now

approved ICS in urological malignancy and all recipients of ICS in cancer surgery should be involved
in audit or clinical trials.

• Infection: Although the balance of risk depends
on the clinical urgency for salvaged blood, antibiotics may be added to the anticoagulant solution
and given parenterally to the patient to treat bacteraemia. Several trials have confirmed the value
of ICS in trauma where the quality of life gain for
younger fitter patients is very high.

• Amniotic fluid in the operative field, which may
cause embolism/disseminated intravascular coagulation. Studies show that circulating amniotic fluid
is common during normal and caesarean delivery.
It is removed during the normal wash cycle and adverse events are rare. ICS can be life-saving in complicated pregnancy such as placenta accreta. Filtering of the salvaged blood removes lamellar bodies
and fetal squames and may enhance patient safety.
NICE now approves ICS in obstetric practice.

• Sickle cell disease: Cells may sickle in the machine due to low oxygen tension and therefore red
cell yield would be low. This is a theoretical reason to avoid using ICS in the presence of sickle cell
disease.

• Where topical clotting agents such as fibrin glue
have been used or iodine has been used to wash out
the abdomen: In practice, these contaminants promote thrombin generation or haemolyse red cells.
Even if these agents are collected they are washed
out during the centrifugal process.

Postoperative cell salvage

Postoperative cell salvage (PCS) involves the collection of blood from surgical drains followed by
reinfusion with or without processing. The blood
recovered is dilute, partially haemolysed and defib-
rinogenated and contains high levels of cytokines
unless washed. There is a clear advantage in terms
of enhanced recovery following knee replacement,
and it may be that cellular activation and enhanced
nitric oxide levels during non-washed PCS are a
positive contributory factor in boosting immunity.
Randomised trials comparing washed and non-
washed PCS with allogeneic blood are awaited. If
the collected wound drainage blood is simply reinfused, some centres limit the quantity reinfused.

Others recommend that all blood is washed and re-
suspended in saline. This can be done either with
the apheresis machines used in the main theatre
suite or with the newer and more compact processing machines that wash collected blood by the patient's bedside.

Key points

1 Autologous transfusion should be considered as
part of a total quality management strategy for
minimising the risk associated with transfusion
for all patients having surgery.
2 Planning and appropriate treatment in advance
of or during surgery can reduce transfusion requirements.
3 Audit of ICS and PCS activity can give useful
local data and inform clinicians about indicated
surgical cases.
4 Before transfusing a patient always consider the
strict clinical indications and how many units are
required.
5 ICS and PCS are the most effective methods of
autologous transfusion.
6 The red cells reinfused are capable of carrying
oxygen immediately.

Further reading

Birkmeyer JD, Goodnough LT, Aubuchon JP, Noordsij PG
& Litenberg B. The cost effectiveness of preoperative
autologous blood donation for total hip and knee replacement. *Transfusion* 1993;33:544–551.

British Committee for Standards in Haematology.
Guidelines for autologous transfusion. 2. Perioperative haemodilution and cell salvage. *Br J Anaesth*
1997;78:768–771.

British Committee for Standards in Haematology. Guidelines for policies on alternatives to allogeneic blood
transfusion 1. Predeposit autologous blood donation
and transfusion. *Transfus Med* 2007;17:354–365.

Calman KC. Cancer: science and society and the communication of risk. *Br Med J* 1996;313:799–802.

Consensus statement. Autologous Transfusion: 3 years
on. What is new? What has happened? *Transfus Med*
1999;9:285–286.

Goodnough LT, Brecher ME, Kanter MH & AuBuchon JP. Transfusion medicine. Part 1. *N Engl J Med* 1999;340:438–447.

Goodnough LT, Brecher ME, Kanter MH & AuBuchon JP. Transfusion medicine. Part 2. *N Engl J Med* 1999;340:525–533.

Goodnough LT, Shander A & Brecher ME. Transfusion medicine: looking to the future. *Lancet* 2003;361:161–169.

Popovsky MA, Whitaker B & Arnold NL. Severe outcomes of allogeneic and autologous blood donation: frequency and characterization. *Transfusion* 1995;35:734–737.

Royal College of Physicians of Edinburgh. Consensus Conference on Autologous Transfusion. *Transfusion* 1996;36:625–667.

Vanderlinde ES, Heal JM & Blumberg N. Clinical review: autologous transfusion. *Br Med J* 2002;321:772–775.

CHAPTER 35

Blood substitutes

Chris V. Prowse[1] & David J. Roberts[2]

[1]National Science Laboratory, Scottish National Blood Transfusion Service, Edinburgh, Scotland
[2]University of Oxford; NHS Blood and Transplant and Department of Haematology, John Radcliffe Hospital, Oxford, UK

Collecting and fractionating human blood for medical use is an expensive and time-consuming process. Large donor panels must be recruited and tested to maintain a constant supply of safe, phenotyped cellular and protein fractions of whole blood. Collection and processing of blood are complex procedures. Moreover, blood transfusion carries risks and has significant, and in some cases unavoidable, adverse effects. There are obvious attractions to the potential replacement of transfusion of cellular components with alternative products that do not have the same dependence on a readily available blood donor population, can be treated to reduce infectious and non-infectious risks, do not require cross-matching, and have a less restrictive shelf life than the current red cell and platelet components provided by transfusion services (Table 35.1). Such products would be of particular interest in battlefield and emergency situations and the armed services have been a major funder of research in this field. Despite research programmes that stretch back to the earlier half of this century, there are only two licenced products in this field: one haemoglobin solution in South Africa and one fluorocarbon product used in Russia and recently licenced in Mexico. An alternative approach of 'virtual blood substitutes' to achieve the desired effect without transfusion is described below.

In broad terms there are three categories of blood substitute under development:
- products that are still based on the use of donor-derived blood cells (human or animal);
- synthetic products that achieve the same endpoint by mirroring the function of the natural product or by novel mechanisms; and
- 'virtual' blood substitutes (Table 35.2), using growth factors to stimulate endogenous haemopoiesis or drugs to secure haemostasis.

The outstanding 'virtual' blood substitutes are the haemopoietic growth factors that can stimulate production of red cells and platelets and mobilise white cells and stem cells. Increasing the effectiveness of circulating platelets using 1-deamino-8-D-arginine vasopressin (DDAVP) or recombinant factor VIIa, inhibiting fibrinolysis by tranexamic acid or ε-aminocaproic acid, or securing haemostasis by the use of fibrin sealant are well-established methods of reducing bleeding and through avoiding red cell and/or platelet transfusion are classic 'virtual' blood substitutes. This chapter discusses the 'real' red cell and platelet substitutes in development. The virtual blood substitutes are covered in Chapters 22, 33, 36 and 43. Understanding the potential role of blood substitutes and the practical and theoretical obstacles to their introduction into clinical practice provides illuminating lessons about the physiology of blood and modern biotechnology.

Practical Transfusion Medicine, 3rd edition. Edited by Michael F. Murphy and Derwood H. Pamphilon. © 2009 Blackwell Publishing, ISBN: 978-1-4051-8196-9.

Table 35.1 Potential 'real' blood substitutes.

Red blood cells
Cross-linked haemoglobin tetramers
Recombinant haemoglobin tetramers
Polymerised haemoglobin
Conjugated haemoglobins
Encapsulated haemoglobin
Perfluorocarbons

Platelets
Freeze-dried platelets
Infusible platelet membranes
Fibrinogen-coated microspheres
Peptide-coated red cells
Glycoprotein receptor-carrying liposomes
Megakaryocytes
In vitro expansion of megakaryocytes

White blood cells
In vitro generation of antiviral and antitumour cytotoxic lymphocytes
In vitro generation of dendritic cells

Stem cells
In vitro expansion of stem cells

Table 35.2 Virtual blood substitutes.

Red blood cells
Erythropoietin
Long acting erythropoietin formulations
Erythropoietin mimetics

Leucocytes
Antibiotics, antiviral and antifungal agents
Active immunisation
G-CSF and GM-CSF
Platelets
Thrombopoietin
Pegylated recombinant human megakaryocyte growth and development factor (MGDF)
Interleukin 11
Thrombopoietin mimetics: microbial peptides

Haemostatic and pharmacological agents
Aprotinin
DDAVP
ε-Aminocaproic acid and tranexamic acid
Recombinant coagulation factor VIIa
Fibrin sealants

DDAVP, 1-deamino-8-D-arginine vasopressin; G-CSF, granulocyte colony-stimulating factor; GM-CSF, granulocyte–macrophage colony-stimulating factor.

Red cell substitutes

Modified haemoglobin-based blood substitutes

Red blood cells have a number of functions beyond oxygen and carbon dioxide transport, including:
• modulation of oxygen delivery under conditions of low pH and/or high p_{CO_2} (the Bohr effect);
• encapsulation of haemoglobin to prolong circulating half-life;
• modulation of vascular tone via effects on nitric oxide (NO) concentration; and
• reduction of methaemoglobin.
These functions depend on a complex and elegant interplay between the haemoglobin molecule, red cell enzymes, the internal milieu and the red cell membrane. Perhaps, not surprisingly, the higher-order functions of the red cell have proved difficult to mimic in artificial components.

Early attempts to transfuse purified unmodified haemoglobin did show that oxygen-carrying ca-

pacity could be restored. However, transfusion of unmodified haemoglobin causes a number of problems as follows.
• Isolated tetramers are unstable and dissociate to globin dimers and monomers. As the tetramers dissociate, the allosteric cooperativity and the modulation of oxygen affinity by bound 2,3-diphosphoglycerate (2,3-DPG) are lost, giving a reduced oxygen-carrying capacity. The P_{50} (partial pressure of oxygen at which haemoglobin is half-saturated with oxygen) is reduced from 26 mm Hg to less than 10 mm Hg (Figure 35.1a). This may be less critical than previously thought as it has recently been shown that molecular size may be more critical than P_{50} for delivery of oxygen to peripheral tissues.
• Globin chains, and to some extent tetramers, are filtered by the kidneys and precipitate in the renal tubules, causing renal dysfunction.
• Isolated tetramers transit the vascular endothelium and by reducing NO availability in the

(a)

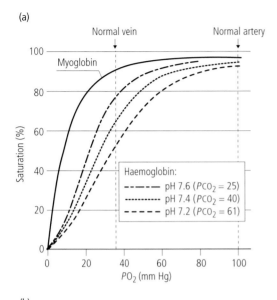

(b)

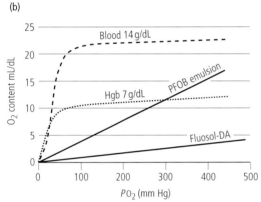

Figure 35.1 (a) Oxygen affinity of haemoglobin tetramers and monomers. Oxygen dissociation curve of myoglobin or dissociated haemoglobin monomers compared with that of haemoglobin at three pH values. Po_2 and Pco_2, partial pressure of oxygen and carbon dioxide. (b) Oxygen affinity of perfluorocarbons. Comparison of oxygen-carrying capacity of whole blood, haemoglobin solution and fluorocarbons. Whole blood with a haemoglobin content of 14 g/dL possesses an arterial oxygen content of 20 mL/dL at a Po_2 of 100 mm Hg. In contrast, fluorocarbon emulsions carry less oxygen at a given partial pressure of oxygen. A 90% perfluoro-octylbromide (PFOB) emulsion can carry 10 mL of oxygen at a Po_2 of 300 mm Hg. Perfluorodecalin (Fluosol-DA 20), which used early emulsification technology to achieve a 20% fluorocarbon emulsion, can only carry 2–3 mL/dL of oxygen at aPo_2 of 300 mm Hg.

extravascular compartment cause vasoconstriction and oesophageal spasm.

Several modifications have been made to free haemoglobin tetramers to overcome these problems. Currently, several second-generation red cell substitutes, including intramolecularly cross-linked haemoglobin, conjugated haemoglobin and polymerised haemoglobin, are in clinical trials and the third generation of substitutes of artificial red blood cells is under development and at the stage of animal trials (for summary, see Table 35.3). In the US, the Food and Drug Administration (FDA) has stated that they will only consider licencing red cell substitutes for three indications:

• regional perfusion, e.g. percutaneous transcoronary angioplasty, enhancing radiation therapy of tumours;
• acute haemorraghic shock; and
• for use in the perioperative period.

As a result, the majority of clinical trials have been in the latter two fields, for which avoidance of allogeneic transfusion is accepted as a surrogate end-point if mortality is not used. In such trials, a haemoglobin 'trigger' level usually determines whom to transfuse and it is worthwhile remembering that a recent systematic review has demonstrated that reducing trigger levels alone can reduce allogeneic transfusion by up to 40%. Since the last edition of this book there have only been two major developments in the field of haemoglobin-based 'blood substitutes' that could be described as having a potential impact in the transfusion world. Firstly, the trauma trial of the cross-linked human haemoglobin (Polyheme) has been completed, although not yet published. Overall this showed no net benefit for its primary end-point of mortality in comparison to crystalloid treatment. Secondly, the ongoing trials of the PEG-modified haemoglobin, Hemospan, have given encouraging results in European trials in surgical patients and further studies in Europe and the US are ongoing. In the case of the bovine cross-linked product, Hemopure, the company with support from the US Navy are still attempting to get the FDA to agree a suitable trial design for a pivotal study in trauma patients.

Table 35.3 Red cell substitutes under trial or development.

	Product/company	Current status[*]
Intramolecularly cross-linked haemoglobin		
Di-aspirin cross-linked haemoglobin	Hemassist, Baxter Healthcare (US)	Failed phase III trials
Recombinant haemoglobin	Optro/rHb2.0, Somatogen Inc. and Baxter (US)	Shelved
Polynitroxylated haemoglobin tetramers	Hemozyme, SynZyme (US)	Preclinical
Sebacoyl-linked haemoglobin tetramers	OxyVita IPBL Pharmaceuticals	Preclinical
Polymerised haemoglobin		
Glutaraldehyde cross-linked haemoglobin	Polyheme, Northfield (US)	Phase III trials show no overall difference from crystalloid in trauma
Glutaraldehyde cross-linked bovine haemoglobin[†]	Hemopure, Biopure (US)	Licenced in South Africa. Completed phase III trials and FDA considering licences in US and UK
O-raffinose cross-linked haemoglobin	Hemolink, Hemosol (Canada)	Failed phase III trials
Conjugated haemoglobin		
Polyoxyethylene – haemoglobin	PHP, Apex Bioscience (US)	In phase III trials
Polyethylene glycol – bovine haemoglobin	Enzon (US)	In phase Ib/II trials
Polyethylene glycol – human haemoglobin	Hemospan, Sangart (US)	In phase II trials
Bovine haemoglobin polymer-containing superoxide dismutase and catalase	PolyHb-SOD-CAT, McGill University	Preclinical
Covalent complex bovine haemoglobin with GSSG, adenosine and ATP	Hemotech, HemoBiotech Inc.	Preclinical
Encapsulated haemoglobin		
Liposome-encapsulated haemoglobin	Terumo (Japan), US Navy	Preclinical
Perfluorocarbons		
Synthetic Perflubron/emulsifer	Pertorfan, Pertorfan Co.	Licenced in Russia and Mexico
	Oxygent, Alliance (US)	In phase III trial; some concerns raised over adverse effects
	Oxycyte, Synthetic Blood/ International Inc.	Phase II orthopaedic surgery trial

GSSG, oxidised glutathione.

[*] Current status is described in clinical trial phase: I is volunteer safety study, II is pilot patient safety and efficacy study, III is pivotal patient efficacy study.

[†] Licenced in South Africa for anaemia therapy.

Intramolecularly cross-linked haemoglobin

Di-aspirin cross-linked haemoglobin

The cross-linking of haemoglobin tetramers with bis-(3,5-dibromosalicyl) fumarate yields di-aspirin cross-linked haemoglobins, with a high P_{50} for good oxygen delivery (e.g. Hemassist). However, haemoglobin tetramers still cause significant smooth muscle spasm, leading to oesophageal spasm and increases in blood pressure. Phase III trials of this product in both trauma and perioperative settings have demonstrated that it can reduce allogeneic transfusion by 19%, but the product has now been withdrawn due to an excess death rate in the trauma trial.

Recombinant haemoglobin

Large-scale production of recombinant haemoglobin in *Escherichia coli* and yeast has been established by Somatogen, who were purchased by Baxter in 1998. Using recombinant DNA technology, the α-globin chains were fused to yield an undissociable 'tetramer'. It was also possible to engineer haemoglobin molecules to reduce NO affinity. Baxter has recently announced withdrawal from this development. Human haemoglobin has also been produced in transgenic pigs, but it proved difficult to separate from the endogenous porcine protein.

Polymerised haemoglobin

Haemoglobin may be cross-linked by bifunctional chemicals to form polymers or haemoglobin molecules can be directly linked to a high-molecular-weight non-protein carrier. In either form renal filtration and smooth muscle dysfunction may be reduced. The oxygen-carrying capacity, reduced by the loss of 2,3-DPG binding, may be restored by other modifications. Three forms of cross-linked polymerised haemoglobin are on trial.

Glutaraldehyde cross-linked haemoglobin

Human haemoglobin has been cross-linked with glutaraldehyde and pyridoxal phosphate added to the 2,3-DPG pocket to increase P_{50} (Polyheme, Northfield, Inc.). The first clinical trials mainly in trauma patients showed that the product was safe and efficacious, reducing transfusion in the first 3 days of hospitalisation. Reduction in mortality has also been demonstrated in patients refusing standard transfusion on religious grounds. These trials used transfusions up to the equivalent of 20 units of red blood cells without serious ill effects. However, the results of a recently completed, pivotal trial of this product in more than 700 at-the-scene trauma patients as announced in press releases indicated an overall mortality of 13%, compared to 9% for the control crystalloid arm. As a result there has been

a dramatic fall in the company share price. There have also been concerns about the ethics of waiving informed consent for the use of a blood substitute in trauma in a hospital where blood itself is readily available. The future design of blood substitutes in these settings will have to be carefully considered.

The second polymerised product is a glutaraldehyde cross-linked bovine haemoglobin (Hemopure). This product is licenced in South Africa and a similar product is already licenced for canine use. Phase III trials have been undertaken in various types of elective surgery using up to 10 units showing, for example, a reduction of allogeneic transfusion of 27% in vascular surgery. An unpublished trial of nearly 700 patients in orthopaedic surgery forms the main basis for a licence application currently under consideration in the US. The FDA has requested further data before considering licensure and the company are in negotiation with them over a suitable design for a clinical trial in trauma patients.

O-raffinose cross-linked haemoglobin

The third form of polymerised haemoglobin is one with oxidised *O*-raffinose cross-linking, which produces a haemoglobin polymer with a high P_{50}. However, the product contains biologically significant amounts of cross-linked haemoglobin tetramers, which can and do cause smooth muscle spasm in the gastrointestinal tract. Trials showing a reduced use of allogeneic blood in orthopaedic and cardiac surgery have been published, but pivotal trials in both indications have recently been curtailed due to an excess rate of myocardial infarction in the patients in the cardiac trial.

Conjugated haemoglobin

Polymeric haemoglobin may also be made by cross-linking haemoglobin not to itself but to high-molecular-weight polyoxyethylene (PHP, Apex Bioscience) or to polyethylene glycol (PEG-Hb, Enzon Inc.; Hemospan, Sangart Inc.). These methods increase the half-life of the preparations and reduce NO-mediated vasoactivity. The Apex Bioscience and Enzon products have been at trial in sepsis and to improve solid tumour radiation therapy. Hemospan is unusual in having a deliberately low P_{50} to prevent the release of oxygen until the haemoglobin reaches the capillaries, and phase I trials have shown that it lacks the vasoactivity of most other preparations that can result in smooth muscle spasm. The product is now entering phase II trials in orthopaedic surgery. These trials have been recently completed without untoward side effects and efficacy studies are now planned in both Europe and the US. Other adaptations under development include cross-linking superoxide dismutase and catalase directly to polymerised haemoglobin to reduce oxygen radical formation and subsequent reperfusion injury.

Artificial red blood cells: encapsulated haemoglobins

The third generation of haemoglobin-based red cell substitutes would be artificial red blood cells. Chang and colleagues pioneered artificial red blood cells using lipid bilayers. The modern formulations have used phospholipid vesicles (0.2 μm in diameter) with sialic acid analogues added to the membranes to reduce clearance by the reticuloendothelial system. Further improvements to microencapsulated haemoglobin under investigation are:
• inclusion of catalase and superoxide dismutase to reduce oxygen radical and methaemoglobin formation; and
• use of biodegradable polylactides and polyglycolides in artificial membranes to increase haemoglobin concentration to 15 g/dL in small nanometer diameter vesicles.

These third-generation haemoglobin substitutes are at the early stage of animal trials. It seems possible that artificial erythrocytes may mimic some of the complex higher-order functions of 'real' red cells in the not too distant future.

Clinical use of haemoglobin-based red cell substitutes

The real dangers of 'natural' red blood cells are low and the safety of substitutes has to be proven in large-scale trials if they are to be accepted for everyday use. In the last 5 years, two major developments, using di-aspirin and *O*-raffinose cross-linked haemoglobin (Hemassist and Hemolink), have failed trials at the last hurdle. A glutaralde-

hyde cross-linked haemoglobin (Polyheme) remains on trial in trauma patients and the equivalent bovine product (Hemopure) awaits a licencing decision for use in elective surgery in the US. Haemoglobin polymerised by cross-linking to polyethylene glycol (Hemospan) uses a promising novel approach and is in preliminary clinical trials. Apart from Hemopure, all these products are still reliant on standard blood donations and their potential advantages will have to outweigh their additional marginal cost.

Perfluorocarbons

Principle

Liquid perfluorocarbons (PFCs) are synthetic hydrocarbons in which most of the hydrogen atoms have been substituted by fluorine atoms. The low intermolecular attractions result in a high capacity to dissolve gases such that the oxygen content of a PFC is up to 20 times that of water.

These chemicals have inherent limitations, including a short intravascular half-life (<12 hours), insolubility in water requiring emulsification with surfactants, and limited oxygen-carrying capacity (the amount of oxygen carried is directly proportional to the inspired oxygen concentration; see Figure 35.1b). This requires that patients breathe oxygen-rich air, limiting their use to operating rooms and intensive care settings.

First-generation fluorocarbons

Fluosol-DA 20, an emulsion of 20% perfluorodecalin, is the only oxygen-carrying volume expander licenced in the US. It was initially hoped that it would gain widespread use but trials showed no efficacy in patients who refused blood transfusions. The only indication for which it has been approved is percutaneous transluminal coronary angioplasty, although some trials showed no benefit in combination with tissue plasminogen activator (tPA) over tPA alone. The inherent limitations of this perfluorocarbon are compounded by the adverse effects, which include:
• marked uptake by the reticuloendothelial system;

- disruption of pulmonary surfactant leading to ventilation–perfusion defects in the lungs; and
- complement activation resulting in anaphylaxis.

The Fluosol product is no longer easily available although a similar product (Pertorfan) has been licenced and used in Russia for some years and has recently been licenced in Mexico.

Oxygent

This second-generation PFC, based on perfluorooctylbromide (PFOB), has been trialled by Alliance Pharmaceutical Company, and contains egg-yolk phospholipids as emulsifier. This composition confers several advantages over previous products, including:

- greater oxygen-carrying capacity (see Figure 35.1b);
- reduced or absent complement activation;
- reduced interference with pulmonary surfactants; and
- improved stability and shelf life.

Trials have been performed in a number of perioperative settings, most notably in cardiac surgery in conjunction with acute normovolaemic haemodilution (ANH). Such trials have shown a delay in the time to reach the trigger levels for allogeneic transfusion, but a large pivotal trial was recently suspended due to concerns about excess rate of stroke. This has now been ascribed to over-enthusiastic ANH rather than the use of the PFC, and the company is now hoping to recommence trials. At present two main studies are planned: the first in Europe aims to use prevention of postoperative ileus as its end-point in patients undergoing major surgery, the other in China is also planned in surgical patients but has an end-point of transfusion avoidance. Adverse effects of flushing and flu-like symptoms and delayed fever, headaches and nausea, as a result of macrophage activation, and a transient thrombocytopenia occur in some patients and may limit clinical applications. The small size of PFCs ($\sim$0.2 μm) has suggested that they may improve oxygenation in ischaemic or infarcted tissues or increase oxygenation in tumours and so enhance sensitisation to radiotherapy or chemotherapy. Other second-generation PFCs, such as Oxycyte, are also at an earlier stage of development.

Platelet substitutes

Platelet concentrates are widely used in the management of thrombocytopenia and abnormal platelet function. These products have allowed the development of chemotherapy regimens that cause prolonged absence of platelet production and have made extracorporeal bypass a safe routine procedure. However, both the supply and use of fresh platelets pose particular problems due to storage being limited to 5–7 days as a result of gradual loss of efficacy and the risk of bacterial contamination. Supply also requires the maintenance of large well-characterised donor panels and specialised centres for apheresis procurement. Repeated platelet transfusions are frequently accompanied by the development of antiplatelet antibodies, usually directed against major histocompatibility complex (MHC) class I antigens or against other platelet surface antigens.

Artificial platelet substitutes hold the promise of avoiding these logistic, technical and medical problems and so achieving cheaper, safer and more readily available therapy for thrombocytopenia. However, as for red cells, replacement of the natural product has not been straightforward. Attempts to replace platelets can again be divided into 'real' and 'virtual' platelet substitutes. Virtual platelet substitutes range from improved clinical guidelines and their implementation (see Chapter 25), through drugs that may reduce blood loss (see Chapters 33 and 36) to compounds that stimulate platelet production (see Chapter 43). Although not strictly speaking a platelet substitute, the development of pathogen reduction technologies for platelets may eliminate bacteria, viruses and leucocytes from this product, so reducing transfusion-transmitted infection, febrile non-haemolytic transfusion reactions and transfusion-associated graft-versus-host disease.

Substitutes for platelets have not yet been licenced but several products are under development (see Table 35.1). The most promising are summarised below, although there has been minimal clinical trial progress in this field over the last 2 or 3 years.

Platelet membrane preparations

In the search for an alternative to fresh platelet concentrates, freeze-dried platelets were initially shown to be superior to frozen and thawed platelets in tests of haemostasis in vitro. Freeze-dried platelets were subsequently shown to be as effective as stored platelets in vitro and to provide haemostasis in thrombocytopenic animals. Clinical evaluation is planned. Compared with platelet concentrates, freeze-dried platelets have the apparent advantage of reduced viral and bacterial load as a result of paraformaldehyde treatment. However, they have some disadvantages such as:

- they must be made from fresh platelets; and
- they may still stimulate an alloimmune response.

Infusible platelet membranes are derived from stored platelets as membrane fragments which seem to promote haemostasis without causing thrombosis in animals. They are the only platelet substitute to have undergone clinical trial and in a small number of patients were effective in individuals refractory to standard platelet transfusions. The advantages of infusible plasma membranes over platelet concentrates include:

- reduced viral and bacterial load;
- reduced expression of human leucocyte antigen (HLA) class I antigens; and
- may be made from outdated platelets.

Synthetic platelets

Beyond the manipulation of platelet membranes, the search for a useful substitute for platelet concentrates has led to a totally synthetic approach. Microspheres of human albumin coated with human fibrinogen (Synthocytes™, Thrombospheres™) reduce bleeding time and acute blood loss in thrombocytopenic animals. They have no immediate toxicity in rodents or primates. Fibrinogen-coated microspheres would have the advantages of:

- sterility;
- production independent of platelet concentrates; and
- absence of HLA class I and platelet surface alloantigens.

Interestingly, these microspheres appear to promote the formation of a platelet plug by interacting with residual normal platelets (Figure 35.2). It seems likely that both lyophilised platelet and infusible plasma membranes may also function in a similar manner. Liposomes with inserted platelet receptors are also under investigation as a platelet alternative.

The efficacy of lyophilised platelets, infusible platelet membranes and fibrinogen-coated microspheres in the prophylaxis of bleeding in severely thrombocytopenic patients will require careful evaluation, and there has been little progress in this field since the first edition of this book. More immediate applications for these platelet substitutes may be in improving haemostasis where the platelet count is moderately reduced and as alternative or adjuvant therapy where patients have become refractory to platelet transfusions through alloimmunisation.

Summary

Real red blood cell and platelet substitutes have yet to reach the clinic. Simple substitutes lack the more complex and important function of whole cells. Nevertheless, modification of haemoglobin by chemical technology has provided products that have been successful or unsuccessful in phase III clinical trials, with one now awaiting a licence decision in the US. The real benefits and safety of these substitutes remain to be shown in clinical practice. One PFC has also reached the stage of pivotal clinical trial.

Progress with platelet substitutes has been much less apparent. Synthetic microspheres that provide platelet-like activity may be free of viral contamination and polymorphic molecules but would seem unlikely to be as effective as fresh platelets with the possible exception of treating haemorrhage, for example in patients with immune platelet refractoriness with no compatible donors.

So, while non-toxic substitutes with reasonable biological activity are likely to be available, it is far from clear whether they will replace cells derived from donors for the majority of clinical uses. At the risk of making speculative assessments, it seems more likely that real blood substitutes will

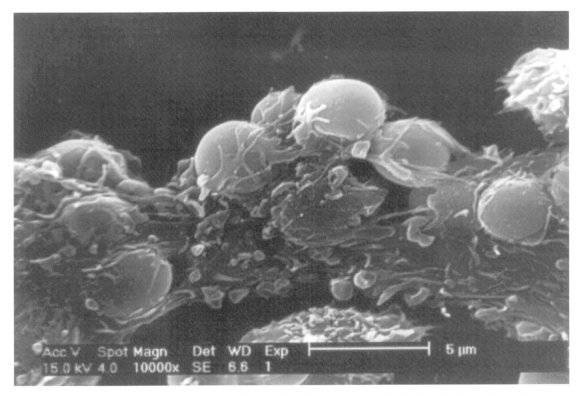

Figure 35.2 Artificial platelet substitutes (Synthocytes™). Electron micrograph showing the interaction of Synthocytes and normal platelets on a collagen surface.

find small niche applications and that virtual blood substitutes and improved prescribing will reduce the use of donor-derived products.

Key points

1 Despite nearly a century of research on blood substitutes there is currently only one licenced haemoglobin solution (in South Africa), and one licenced perfluorocarbon (Pertorfan: in Russia and Mexico) in clinical use.
2 Three haemoglobin-based and one perflurocarbon (Oxygent) product remain in clinical trials for indications that might impact on transfusion practice.
3 Results for one of these (Polyheme) in a recent large trauma trial are not encouraging, whereas another (Hemospan) is just commencing larger efficacy trials.

4 There has only been one small clinical study of a platelet substitute, with little progress being made in recent years on therapeutic products. The products described in this chapter are only to be used in a clinical trial setting except in those countries where they are licenced.

Further reading

Blajchman MA. Novel platelet products, substitutes and alternatives. *Transfus Clin Biol* 2001;8:267–271.

Kipnis K, King NMP & Nelson RM. An open letter to institutional review boards considering Northfield Laboratories PolyHeme® trial. *Am J Bioeth* 2006; 6:18–21.

Kitaguchi T, Murata M, Iijima K, Kamide K, Imagawa T & Ikeda Y. Characterization of liposomes carrying von Willebrand factor-binding domain of platelet glycoprotein Ibalpha: a potential substitute for platelet transfusion. *Biochem Biophys Res Commun* 1999;261:784–789.

Levi M, Friederrich PW, Middleton S *et al.* Fibrinogen-coated albumin microcapsules reduce bleeding in severely thrombocytopenic rabbits. *Nat Med* 1999;5:107–111.

McCarthy MR, Vandegriff KD & Winslow RM. The role of facilitated diffusion in oxygen transport by cell-free hemoglobins: implications for the design of hemoglobin-based oxygen carriers. *Biophys Chem* 2001;92:103–117.

Ness PM & Cushing MM. Oxygen therapeutics: pursuit of an alternative to the donor Blood Cell. *Arch Pathol Lab Med* 2007;131:734–741.

Olofsson C, Ahl T, Johansson T *et al.* A multicenter clinical study of the safety and activity of maleimide-polyethylene glycol-modified Hemoglobin (Hemospan) in patients undergoing major orthopedic surgery. *Anesthesiology* 2006;105:1153–1163.

Prowse CV. Alternatives to human blood and blood resources. *Vox Sang* 1998;74(Suppl 2):21–28.

Reid TJ. Hb-based oxygen carriers: are we there yet? *Transfusion* 2003;43:280–287.

Scigliano E, Enright H, Telen M *et al.* Infusible platelet membrane for the control of bleeding in thrombocytopenic patients. *Blood* 1997;90(Suppl 1):267a (abstract 1170).

Vandegriff KD, Malavalli A, Wooldridge J, Lohman J & Winslow RM. MP4, a new nonvasoactive PEG-Hb conjugate. *Transfusion* 2003;43:509–516.

Winslow RM. Blood substitutes: refocusing an elusive goal. *Br J Haematol* 2000;111:387–396.

CHAPTER 36

Pharmacological agents and recombinant factor VIIa

Beverley J. Hunt

Thrombosis and Haemostasis, Kings College, London; Departments of Haematology, Pathology and Rheumatology, Guy's and St Thomas' NHS Foundation Trust, London, UK

There is rising interest in the use of pharmacological agents to reduce bleeding, in light of the concerns about blood safety. Pharmacological agents have been used in two ways: either to prevent excessive bleeding or to treat established bleeding. The agents used can be broadly classified into three groups, fibrin sealants, antifibrinolytics and desmopressin, which has a unique action.

Antifibrolytics

Aprotinin

The discovery that aprotinin reduced perioperative bleeding in cardiac surgery came from a study at the Hammersmith Hospital, London, where the aim was to assess whether aprotinin's antikallikrein activity would reduce the systemic response of cardiopulmonary bypass (CPB). Kallikrein is formed during the activation of coagulation by CPB and has a central role in the activation of the inflammatory response. However, the investigators noted that the operating fields were 'dry' and there was a dramatic reduction in blood loss, need for transfusion and shorter operating times (due to the reduction in oozing) with aprotinin. Since that time,

Practical Transfusion Medicine, 3rd edition. Edited by Michael F. Murphy and Derwood H. Pamphilon. © 2009 Blackwell Publishing, ISBN: 978-1-4051-8196-9.

aprotinin has been shown to reduce perioperative bleeding in numerous randomised controlled studies, and it obtained a licence to reduce bleeding in high-risk cardiac surgery.

The original and licenced regimen of aprotinin (2M Kallikrein inhibitory units (KIU) to the patient, 2M KIU to the CPB circuit and 50,000 KIU per hour during CPB) reduced postoperative drainage loss by 81%, and total haemoglobin loss by 89%.

Mechanism of action

Aprotinin is a basic serine protease inhibitor extracted from bovine lung. In high doses (150–200 KIU), it inhibits kallikrein; the licenced regimen achieve blood levels of about 200 KIU/mL. However, even in lower concentrations, aprotinin is a powerful inhibitor of plasmin, which appears to be the main mechanism for its effect on bleeding; its molar potency in vitro is 100- and 1000-times that of tranexamic acid (TA) and epsilon aminocaproic acid (EACA). Aprotinin may also have a minor effect in preserving platelet membrane receptors possibly by inhibiting plasmin-mediated degradation.

Monitoring the antikallikrein effect of aprotinin

Aprotinin by inhibiting kallikrein will prolong in vitro tests of the intrinsic system including the activated clotting time (ACT), which is used to monitor heparin during cardiopulmonary bypass. Kallikrein normally operates a positive feedback on the generation of factor XII. In order to allow for adequate levels of heparin, the ACT should be run greater than the normal level of 500 seconds, ideally at 750 seconds to compensate and allow for 'normal' heparin levels. The activator in the ACT has traditionally been celite, but kaolin has been used instead in some ACT tubes, for it is less affected by aprotinin and thus ACTs can be monitored in the normal way.

Administration

Since aprotinin is a bovine protein and thus can provoke an immunological reaction, a test dose should be given. Aprotinin can also be used in established fibrinolytic bleeding; 500,000 KIU intravenous (IV) is a good antiplasmin dose.

Safety

Concerns about aprotinin's safety have led to a voluntary suspension of marketing aprotinin. Several large open studies of the use of antifibrinolytics in cardiac surgery suggested that it was associated with increased risk of death and renal dysfunction compared with other antifibrinolytics. Then a randomised controlled trial comparing aprotinin versus EACA versus TA (the BART study, published in the *New England Journal of Medicine* in 2008) was halted by the data monitoring committee due to concerns about the death rate in patients receiving aprotinin. A total of 74 patients (9.5%) in the aprotinin group had massive bleeding, as compared with 93 (12.1%) in the TA group and 94 (12.1%) in the EACA group (relative risk in the aprotinin group for both comparisons, 0.79; 95% confidence interval (CI), 0.59–1.05). At 30 days the rate of death from any cause was 6.0% in the aprotinin group, as compared to 3.9% in the TA group (relative risk, 1.55; 95% CI, 0.99–2.42) and 4.0 in the EACA group (relative risk, 1.52; 95% CI, 0.98–2.36). The relative risk of death in the aprotinin group as compared with that in both groups receiving lysine analogues was 1.53 (95% CI, 1.06–2.22).

The lysine analogues

The lysine analogues, EACA and TA are competitive inhibitors of plasmin binding to fibrin. A continuous infusion is given perioperatively. The dose of TA that has been used is variable, 2.5–100 mg/kg over 20 minutes preoperatively followed by 0.25–4 mg/kg/h delivered over 1–12 hours and 1 mg/kg for 10 hours. Both drugs can be given to treat established fibrinolysis: the recommended dose for TA is up to 1–2 g by slow IV infusion.

A recent Cochrane review analysed data from over 211 randomised controlled trials of antifibrinolytics in over 20,000 participants. It suggested that TA and EACA were slightly less efficacious in reducing need for transfusion and need for reoperation than aprotinin (as expected from their lower Ki against plasmin). However, the data on TA and EACA were sparse, and the difference failed to reach statistical significance (see Table 36.1). They are cheaper, however, and appear to be safer.

It is not known if antifibrinolytics could be used in trauma. Currently, there is an ongoing randomised controlled study of TA versus placebo in the management of bleeding after trauma aiming to recruit 20,000 patients worldwide. This study is known as CRASH-2 (clinical randomisation of antifibrinolytics in significant haemorrhage). So far,

Table 36.1 The summary statistics from Cochrane review of antifibrinolytic use for minimising perioperative allogeneic blood transfusion.

Agent	Risk reduction in the use of red cell transfusion (85% CI)	Risk reduction in the need for re-operation for bleeding (95% CI)
Aprotinin	34%, i.e. RR = 0.66 (0.61–0.71)	0.48 (0.35–0.68)
Tranexamic acid	0.61 (0.54–0.69)	0.67 (0.41–1.09)
EACA	0.75 (0.58–0.96)	0.35 (0.11–1.17)

CI, confidence interval; EACA, epsilon aminocaproic acid.

over 8000 patients have been recruited and there have been no safety issues. This study will provide the ultimate data on the efficacy and safety of TA.

Fibrin sealants

Fibrin sealants can be used to stop oozing from small, sometimes inaccessible, blood vessels during surgery when conventional surgical techniques are not feasible. The sealants are licenced and used in surgery and trauma including:
- liver and spleen lacerations;
- dental extraction in patients with bleeding disorders;
- gastric ulcers;
- vascular grafts;
- sealing of dural leaks; and
- as an alternative to sutures in plastic surgery.

The sealants mimic the final part of the coagulation cascade in that a source of thrombin is added to fibrinogen concentrates in the presence of calcium and a clot forms. They can be administered by a 'gun' which produces mixing of the reagents. Some sealants have two additional ingredients: factor XIII and aprotinin.

Safety and effectiveness

The initial source of thrombin was of bovine origin, which led to the development of a postoperative bleeding due to the formation of antibodies to bovine thrombin, which cross-react against human factor V leading to acquired factor V deficiency.

Although they are derived from blood products, sealants have a lower risk of transmitting infection than donor blood. A Cochrane review of their efficacy found a total of seven trials, including 388 patients, that showed a reduction of exposure to red cell transfusion by a relative 54%, but the authors felt the trials were of poor methodological quality and that larger more rigorous trials are needed.

Desmopressin

Desmopressin acetate (DDAVP) is a synthetic vasopressin analogue that is relatively devoid of vasoconstrictor activity. It increases the plasma concentrations and activity of von Willebrand Factor (vWF) two- to fivefold by inducing the release of vWF from Weibel Palade bodies in the endothelium. It also stimulates the release of tissue plasminogen activator from the endothelium and promotes platelet activation.

DDAVP shortens the bleeding time in patients with von Willebrand's disease, platelet function defects and uraemia and so is used for these indications.

Despite the success of early trials, a systemic Cochrane review of all 18 randomised controlled trials where DDAVP was given to reduce the use of allogeneic red cells concluded that there was no benefit from DDAVP in minimising perioperative allogeneic red cell transfusion. Side effects include flushing and an antidiuretic effect.

Recombinant-activated factor VIIa

Recombinant-activated factor VII (rFVIIa) was developed as a treatment for bleeding episodes in haemophiliac patients with inhibitors to factor VIII or IX. It is now approved in Europe for this indication and for the management of:
- acquired haemophilia;
- congenital FVII deficiency; and
- Glanzmann's thrombasthenia with antibodies to GPIIb/IIIa or HLA, and with refractoriness to platelet transfusion.

rFVIIa has also been used widely as an 'off label' treatment in patients with platelet dysfunction, thrombocytopenia and massive transfusion after major surgery or trauma in patients without a pre-existing coagulopathy. However, the huge body of evidence for these indications is disappointingly mainly from case reports, case series and only a few randomised trials.

Mechanism of action of pharmacological doses of rFVIIa

About 1% of circulating factor VII is in the activated form and the amount of rFVIIa required to bypass is larger than this. Certainly in haemophilia patients the doses required are much higher than those which generate a plasma concentration adequate for its binding to tissue factor. Disagreement revolves around the issue of whether rFVIIa has an effect independent of tissue factor. It has been demonstrated in vitro that rFVIIa is able to weakly bind activated platelets and cause activation of FX. The explanation of rFVIIa needing to bind to platelets may explain why rFVIIa is located only at the site of bleeding. Others hold the view that VIIA binds to tissue factor in the normal way. Whatever the mechanism, coagulation occurs locally at the site of bleeding without disseminated activation.

Hereditary clotting factor deficiencies

Haemophilia

Like the endogenous protein, rFVIIa has a short half-life, is approximately 2.7 hours in adults, but the half-life in children and in bleeding haemophiliacs is shorter. The dosing interval in treating haemophiliac bleeding episodes is 2 hourly, lengthened up to 4 hourly later in the course of treatment. A loading bolus followed by a continuous infusion of rFVIIa is also used. Even though the recommended dosage is 90 µg/kg, it is clear that the optimal dose and dosing intervals of rFVIIa have not been established with certainty, for higher doses up to 300 µg/kg have proved to be more clinically efficacious.

Whilst the prothrombin time (PT) and activated partial thromboplastin time (APTT) are shortened with pharmacological doses of rFVIIa, these are indirect correlates of its action. The measurement of FVII clotting activity (FVII: C) in the treatment of haemophilia-related bleeding has led to a recommendation of a minimum level of 6–10 IU/mL and peak levels of greater than 30–50 IU/mL when giving IV boluses. These levels appear to be associated with clinical improvement in haemostasis. The use of thromboelastography and thrombin generation has also been explored in trying to find an in vitro measure that correlates with clinical response.

Factor VII deficiency

Bleeding episodes in patients with factor VII deficiency have responded to lower levels than required in haemophiliacs with inhibitors: doses ranging from 15 to 20 µg/kg every 2–3 hours until cessation of bleeding are recommended. Patients with factor VII deficiency are the only known pa-

tients to develop anti-factor VIIa antibodies after treatment.

Other congenital bleeding disorders

There are anecdotal reports of the successful use of rFVIIa in bleeding in von Willebrand's disease. Some consider rFVIIa to be the agent of choice in patients with factor XI deficiency, with similar low doses as used in those with factor VII deficiency.

Platelet dysfunction

Patients with rare, congenital platelet defects have had successful treatment of bleeding episodes and undergone surgery safely with rFVIIa treatment. These include disorders such as Glanzmann thrombasthenia (abnormalities of the platelet fibrinogen receptor glycoprotein IIb/IIIa) and Bernard Soulier syndrome (lack of the glycoprotein Ib platelet receptor).

Platelet dysfunction occurs in uraemia and with aspirin, clopidogrel and glycoprotein (GP) IIb/IIIa inhibitors in acute coronary syndromes. rFVIIa has been reported to control bleeding anecdotally in these situations.

Thrombocytopenia

Anecdotal reports have suggested that those with thrombocytopenia may respond to rFVIIa. One study showed that the bleeding time was reduced by 2 minutes or more in 55 out of 105 thrombocytopenic patients after single doses of 50 or 100 mcg/kg. This effect was significantly more pronounced in patients with a platelet count of greater than $20 \times 10^9/L$, but it was not dose-dependent. Other anecdotal reports have suggested that a dose of 50–100 µg/kg is necessary, and these findings are consistent with a clinical effect due to an accelerated initial rate of thrombin production and thus more rapid activation of residual platelets. However, the vast majority of data are derived from uncontrolled studies and large well-run trials are required to fully assess the benefit of rFVIIa in thrombocytopenia.

Liver dysfunction

Patients with liver dysfunction often have disproportionately low factor VII levels compared to the other vitamin K-dependent factors. rFVIIa normalises the PT in liver disease with a single dose of 5–80 mcg/kg, the dose depending on the patient. In a controlled trial of 245 patients with cirrhosis and variceal bleeding, patients received either 8 doses of 100 μg/kg or placebo. Those who received rFVIIa were most likely to have their bleeding controlled but overall mortality was not affected. A double-blind randomised study of 50–100 μg/kg versus placebo rFVIIa prior to partial hepatectomy made no difference to requirement for red cell transfusion or bleeding.

rFVIIa has also been used in orthotopic liver transplantation. The largest study, a multicentre randomised double-blind study of repeated 60 or 120 μg/kg or placebo intraoperatively in 182 patients showed no effect on intraoperative blood loss or the number of red cell transfused, although there were a significantly higher number of patients who escaped transfusion in the rFVIIa group.

Reversal of over-anticoagulation with warfarin

rFVIIa can reverse over-anticoagulation with warfarin. However, the comparative risk–benefit ratio and health economics of treating patients overdosed with warfarin when compared to standard therapy has not been assessed. There is interesting evidence from an animal model that prothrombinase concentrates are better at restoring in vitro thrombin generation.

Bleeding after trauma

In 1999, there was a report of a soldier with extensive bleeding following a gunshot wound to the abdomen, who despite multiple blood components had a coagulopathy characterised by thrombocytopenia, prolonged APTT and international normalised ratio (INR) and hypofibrinogenaemia, he dramatically responded to two infusions of 60 μg/kg rFVIIa. The same group then presented seven patients with uncontrolled massive bleeding post-trauma in whom rFVIIa 40–120 μg/kg and further doses were used after all surgical, medical and transfusion therapy had failed. All patients displayed evidence of coagulopathy despite multiple transfusions. Diffuse bleeding stopped in all

cases, in some revealing bleeding from larger vessels, which was amenable to further surgery. Three of the seven patients died, one perioperatively and the other two, several weeks after their bleeding episodes. None suffered thromboembolic complications of therapy with rFVIIa. This led to an avalanche of reports of rFVIIa being used in uncontrolled bleeding after surgery and trauma. However, in many reports, it is clear that best practice use of blood components was not used before rFVIIa administration.

A randomised placebo-controlled trial of rFVIIa in blunt and penetrating trauma after patients had been transfused eight units of red cells used doses of 200, 100 and 100 μg/kg of rFVIIa at set time intervals. The patients with blunt trauma treated with rFVIIa needed less red cell transfusion, an estimated 2.6 units of red cells ($p = 0.02$) and there was a non-significant trend to requiring less red cells in those with penetrating injuries. There were no differences in thromboembolic events between rFVIIa and control groups. A further study in progress is looking at rFVIIa usage at an earlier stage in traumatic bleeding. There is increasing data to show that rFVIIa is less effective in those who are acidotic or in severe shock.

Surgical bleeding

The only published randomised controlled trials in the use of rFVIIa to *prevent* perioperative bleeding were carried out in patients undergoing transabdominal retro-pubic prostatectomy. This double-blind study gave 20, 40, 80 g/kg rFVIIa or placebo as a single injection perioperatively. It was found that 40 μg/kg rFVIIa reduced blood loss significantly.

The use of cardiopulmonary bypass to facilitate cardiac surgery may be associated with bleeding complications in 2–8% necessitating re-exploration. Some case reports show control of bleeding after one or two injections of rFVIIa; however, other reports have shown no efficacy. However, many patients undergoing cardiac surgery have risk factors for atherosclerotic disease, which may become unstable in the setting of major cardiac surgery. Such concerns led to a randomised controlled trial, the results of which are awaited.

There are numerous case reports of rFVIIa being used in bleeding patients after all types of surgery and with obstetric haemorrhage where outcomes have been highly variable. Again, more randomised controlled studies are needed. Its use has also been described in surgery in Jehovah's Witnesses where it is an attractive consideration when the use of blood components is denied.

Safety considerations

The mechanism of rFVIIa in initiating haemostasis led to concerns that widespread coagulation could be precipitated, particularly if tissue factor were expressed in atherosclerotic vessels, in which case, administration of rFVIIa could cause acute thrombosis. However, more than 7,000,000 doses of rFVIIa have been given to haemophiliacs with a 1% incidence of serious adverse events including myocardial infarction, stroke and venous thromboembolism. Moreover, a recently published meta-analysis of seven randomised trials using rFVIIa in surgical procedures showed no increased risk of thromboembolism or mortality rates.

Conclusions

Pharmacological agents are now considered part of the management of major bleeding after trauma or surgery, but many key questions pertaining to their safety and efficacy remain unanswered. Practically, TA and EACA seem the safest antifibrinolytics at this current time and have proven efficacy. rFVIIa has also been shown to be much safer than originally thought but the extent of its efficacy, dosage and frequency of use remains unclear. Its use is limited by its cost and lack of licence for many indications. It would seem prudent for each unit to draw guidelines on the use of rFVIIa for 'rescue therapy' whereby it is used only when 'best practice' management of blood component therapy has failed.

Key points

1 Antifibrinolytics have been shown to reduce the use of allogeneic red cells during surgery. At the current time, TA and EACA are recommended over aprotinin in view of concerns about the safety of the latter.

2 Early concerns about the risk of excessive thrombosis with rFVIIa are unsolved.

3 However, the efficacy of rFVIIa in off-licence 'rescue therapy' in bleeding patients is uncertain. It should be used per local protocol after 'best practice' use of blood components therapy has failed.

Further reading

The first paper that discovered aprotinin prevented bleeding

Royston D, Bidstrup BP, Taylor KM & Sapsford RN. Effect of aprotinin on need for blood transfusion after repeat open-heart surgery. *Lancet* 1987;2:1289–1291.

How aprotinin works

Henry DA, Carless PA, Moxley AJ *et al.* Anti-fibrinolytic use for minimising perioperative allogeneic blood transfusion. *Cochrane Database Syst Rev* 2007;CD001886.

Segal H & Hunt BJ. Aprotinin: pharmacological reduction of perioperative bleeding. *Lancet* 2000;355:1289–1290.

How aprotinin upsets the ACT

Hunt BJ, Segal H & Yacoub M. Aprotinin and heparin monitoring during cardiopulmonary bypass. *Circulation* 1992;86:410–412.

Studies of the safety of aprotinin versus other antifibrinolytics

Fergusson DA, Hebert PC, Mazer CD *et al.* A comparison of aprotinin and lysine analogues in high-risk cardiac surgery. *N Engl J Med* 2008;358:2319–2331.

Freemantle N & Irs A. Observational evidence for determining drug safety. *Br Med J* 2008;336:627–628.

Karkouti K, Beattie WS, Dattilo KM *et al.* A propensity score case–control comparison of aprotinin and tranexamic acid in high transfusion – risk cardiac surgery. *Transfusion* 2006;46:327–338.

Mangano DT, Tudor IC & Dietzel C, for Multicentre Study of Perioperative Ischemia Group; Ischemia Research & Education Foundation. The risk associated with aprotinin in cardiac surgery. *N Engl J Med* 2006;354:353–365.

Data on the ongoing CRASH-2 study

CRASH-2 – Clinical randomisation of antifibrinolytics in significant haemorrhage. Available at http://www.crash2. lshtm.ac.uk/.

Reviews of fibrin glue

Banninger H, Hardegger T, Tobler A *et al.* Fibrin glue in surgery: frequent developments of inhibitors of bovine thrombin and human factor V. *Br J Haematol* 1993;85:528–532.

Carless PA, Henry DA & Anthony DM. Fibrin sealant use for minimising peri-operative allogeneic blood transfusion. *Cochrane Database Syst Rev* 2003;CD004171.

Review of desmopressin

Carless PA, Henry DA, Moxet AJ *et al.* Desmopressin for minimising perioperative allogeneic blood transfusion. *Cochrane Database Syst Rev* 2004;CD001884.

Papers on rFVIIa

Boffard KD, Bruno Riou B, Brian Warren B *et al.* Recombinant factor VIIa as adjunctive therapy for bleeding control in severely injured trauma patients: two parallel randomized, placebo-controlled, double-blind clinical trials. *J Trauma* 2005;59:8–15.

Martinowirz U, Kenet G, Lubetski A, Luboshitz J & Segal E. Recombinant activated factor VII for adjunctive hemorrhage control in trauma. *J Trauma* 2001;51:431–438.

Roberts HR, Monroe DM & White GC. The use of recombinant factor VIIa in the treatment of bleeding disorders. *Blood* 2004;104:3858–3864.

Shao YF, Yang JM, Chau GY *et al.* Safety and haemostatic effect of recombinant activated factor VII in cirrhotic patients undergoing partial hepatectomy: a multicentre, randomized, double blind, placebo-controlled trial. *Am J Surg* 2006;191:245–249.

The only study to look at rFVIIa to prevent bleeding

Friederich PW, Henny CP, Messelink EJ *et al.* Effect of recombinant activated factor VII on perioperative blood loss in patients undergoing retropubic prostatectomy: a double-blind placebo-controlled randomised trial. *Lancet* 2003;361:201–205.

An up-to-date review of all the randomised trials of rFVIIa

Ranucci M, Isgro G, Soro G, Conti D & De Toffol B. Efficacy and safety of recombinant activated factor VII in major surgical procedures: systematic review and meta-analysis of randomized clinical trials. *Arch Surg* 2008;143:296–304.

PART 6

Cellular and tissues therapy and organ transplantation

CHAPTER 37

Regulation and accreditation in cellular therapy

Derwood H. Pamphilon[1] *& Zbigniew M. Szczepiorkowski*[2]

[1]NHS Blood and Transplant; Department of Cellular and Molecular Medicine, University of Bristol, Bristol, UK
[2]Dartmouth-Hitchcock Medical Center, Lebanon, New Hampshire, USA

Introduction

In recent years there have been considerable advances in cellular therapies. The most widely used type of cellular therapy has been haemopoietic stem cell transplantation (HSCT) from its inception in 1968. In many cases, patients with haematological and non-haematological diseases are cured after HSCT. There have also been advances in the immunotherapy of cancer and viral infections.

The horizons of cellular therapy are now expanding and stem cell therapies are being applied in the management of patients with solid tumours and degenerative diseases which will affect more than 50% of individuals in Western societies.

A number of different agencies and professional bodies are involved in the regulation and accreditation of cellular therapy in both the US and Europe. The regulations and standards depend on the source of the cell to be transplanted, the way it is used and the nature of any manipulations carried out. As a result of this the last decade has seen a seemingly bewildering growth in regulatory and accreditation requirements and these have put pressure on both clinical and laboratory services. The drivers for these are:

Practical Transfusion Medicine, 3rd edition. Edited by Michael F. Murphy and Derwood H. Pamphilon. © 2009 Blackwell Publishing, ISBN: 978-1-4051-8196-9.

- traceability of products from donor to recipient;
- microbiological safety; and
- enhanced product quality.

There are multiple organisations involved in the process of accreditation and standard setting of haemopoietic stem cell transplant programmes. Figure 37.1 illustrates the timeline of this involvement by different organisations.

Haemopoietic stem cell transplant activity

There has been a marked increase in transplant activity in the last 20 years and estimates are that 45–50,000 HSCT are carried out annually worldwide. In 1990, 4200 HSCTs were reported to the European Blood and Marrow Transplant Group (EBMT); a number that had risen by 2005 to 27,941 (Figure 37.2). Autologous transplants comprised 65% of these, 35% were allografts and the total number of transplants increased by 20%. In Europe, 52% of first-time allografts are now from identical siblings and 41% from unrelated donors. HSCT has increased in all diseases reported to the EBMT and similar bodies with the exception of chronic myeloid leukaemia (CML) where the advent of the tyrosine kinase inhibitor imatinib has reduced the numbers of HSCT (see Chapter 40).

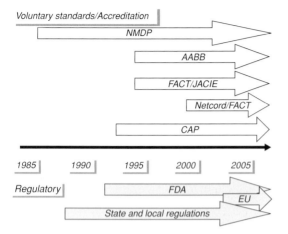

Figure 37.1 Timeline of involvement of different organisations in the field of cellular therapy. AABB, formerly American Association of Blood Banks; CAP, College of American Pathologists; FACT, Foundation for the Accreditation of Cellular Therapy; EU, European Union; FDA, US Food and Drug Administration; JACIE, Joint Accreditation Committee (ISCT and EBMT); NMDP, National Marrow Donor Program.

Other trends in HSCT include the greater use of peripheral blood which is now regarded as the source of choice in 98% of autografts and 74% of allografts in Europe. Umbilical cord blood (CB) now comprises 20% of all HSCT in patients less than 20 years of age and its use is increasing in adults as well.

The structure of SCT programmes

Figure 37.3 shows the journey of an allogeneic stem cell product from a registry or sibling donor or CB unit where a blood sample is typed in the histocompatibility and immunogenetics (H&I) laboratory to determine the HLA type, via the marrow, peripheral blood or CB collection facility and the cell processing laboratory to the clinical transplant unit. The various accreditation and regulatory bodies involved and their areas of involvement are shown.

European Union directives and legislation

In Europe, the need for international standardisation of tissue and cell banking was recognised in a document produced by the Council of Europe (CoE) as long ago as 1978 when it adopted resolution [(78)29]. This suggested the harmonisation of legislation relating to the collection and transplantation of human substances. In 1994, the CoE adopted another recommendation [R(94)1] which identified the variability of quality and safety of tissues and cells in Europe as a key issue and adopted a recommendation which required that there should be functional definitions of tissue banks and that such banks should be:

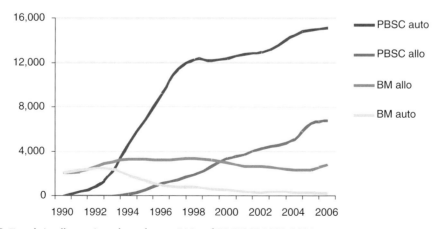

Figure 37.2 Trends in allogeneic and autologous BM and PB HSCT 1990–2006.

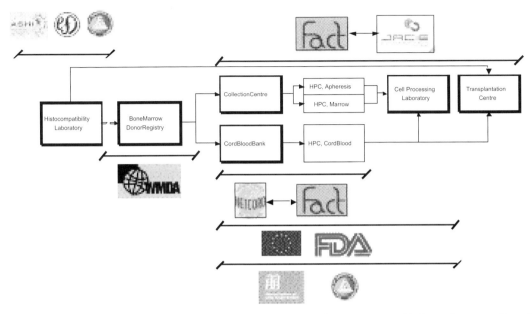

Figure 37.3 Regulatory environment for haemopoietic stem cell transplantation. *Note*: This figure does not reflect all potential regulatory reporting requirements for transplantation centres.

- non-profit making;
- licenced by national health authorities;
- the cells collected should be tested for infectious disease markers (IDMs);
- appropriate records should be kept; and
- there should be consent for removal or collection of cells and tissues.

The CoE's Guide to Safety and Quality Assurance for Organs Tissues and Cells, first published in 2002, is now in its third edition (2007). It is recognised in all CoE member states.

Following this in 2001, the Department of Health in England and Wales published a Code of Practice (CoP) for Tissue Banks, which included cellular therapy laboratories. This was regulated by the Medicines and Healthcare Products Regulatory Agency (MHRA) and it established a voluntary accreditation scheme which promoted the use of good manufacturing practice (GMP). The CoP described standards for cell and tissue bank premises, equipment, personnel, donor selection, quality control, packaging and documentation. Inspection by the MHRA involved examination of the premises, equipment, records, quality management system (QMS) and standard operating proce-

dures (SOP) in the applicant facility. The following year, a European Union (EU) Directive on Tissues and Cells was formally proposed and this was published in 2004 as Directive 2004/23/EC. In 2006, two technical annexes supplying more detailed information were published as Commission Directives 2006/17/EC (donation, procurement and testing) and 2006/86/EC (coding, processing, preservation, storage and distribution). The directives are legally binding with a requirement that they are transposed into European law.

In 2005, Competent Authorities (CAs) were appointed or established in the UK and other European Member States and these subsequently became responsible for the licencing of facilities storing tissues or cells. In the UK, the Human Tissue (Quality and Safety for Human Application) Regulations which translate the EU Directive into UK law were published in 2006 and in 2007; all three directives were fully implemented. The Directive states that it 'lays down standards of quality and safety for human tissues and cells intended for human applications, in order to ensure a high level of protection of human health' and that it was established to 'help to reassure the public that human tissues and cells that are procured in another Member State, nonetheless carry the same guarantees as those in their own country'. The following cells and tissues are included within the scope of the Directive:

• haemopoietic stem cells from peripheral blood, bone marrow and CB;
• donor leucocytes and other cellular therapies;
• adult and embryonic stem cells;
• cardiovascular tissues including heart valves and vessels;
• ocular tissues such as corneas and sclera;
• skin;
• gametes (sperm and eggs) and embryos;
• bone, cartilage, autologous chondrocyte implantation;
• ligaments, tendons, meniscus and other soft tissues; and
• endocrine tissues such as pancreatic islet cells.

The various sections of the Directives describe:

i the requirements for the person in charge of a cellular therapy or tissue facility (the responsible person or designated individual);
ii the arrangements for the facility itself and its staffing;
iii the role of the CA and the need for 2 yearly inspections;
iv consent;
v traceability with retention of key records for a period of 30 years;
vi the reporting of adverse events and reactions to the CA; and
vii conditions to be met when stem cells are imported or exported.

The Human Tissue Act 2004

This key piece of legislation was introduced into the UK in 2006. It repealed and replaced the HT Act of 1961 as well as the Anatomy Act (1989) and Human Organ Transplants Act (1989). It established the Human Tissue Authority (HTA) as the CA for the UK. Its aim is to regulate the collection, storage, use and disposal of human bodies, body parts, organs and tissues.

The Human Tissue Act (HTAct) ensured that consent became the fundamental principle underpinning the lawful storage and use of organs and tissues. In addition, the Act also applies to the removal of transplantable material from the deceased. Consent is required when tissue is removed from the living or deceased for the purposes of:

• anatomical examination;
• determining the cause of death;
• obtaining scientific or medical information about a person relevant to another;
• public display;
• research in connection with disorders or functioning of the human body (unless the material is anonymised and for specific, ethically approved research); and
• transplantation.

The HTAct is supported by two governmental regulations (Statutory Instruments 2006 no. 1659[37] and 2006 no. 1260[38], directions issued by the HTA to help explain and interpret the Act and also a number of Codes of Practice (CoP) of which three are particularly relevant to cell and tissue therapies. These are:

i consent;
ii removal, collection, retention and disposal of organs and tissues; and
iii donation of allogeneic bone marrow and peripheral blood stem cells for transplantation.

Obtaining legally valid consent is extremely important and the HTA states that it is a positive act, that it is voluntary and may be withdrawn at any time. Appropriate information should be provided and the person giving consent must have the capacity to do so. Children may consent if they are competent to do so. Consent prior to death is sufficient for organ and tissue donation and relatives have no legal right to overrule such consent.

The US Food and Drug Administration

The US Food and Drug Administration (FDA) of the Department of Health and Human Services of the US has been involved in area of cellular therapy since early 1990s. Through a series of public meetings and notices in the Federal Register, the FDA recognised the need for regulatory oversight in the area of cell, gene and tissue therapies and products. Initial guidance documents were issued in 1993, 1996, 1997 and 1998 based on the Public Health Service Act, Section 361 (42 USC 264).

FDA Good Tissue Practice (GTP) Regulations for human cells, tissues and tissue-based products (HCT/Ps) require institutions shipping HPC, Cord Blood; HPC, Apheresis; and TC, Apheresis; but not HPC, Marrow; to be registered with FDA as manufacturers. There are specific requirements for donors who may be eligible/ineligible based on a suitability determination and defined in final guidance documents (see below). An annual update is required.

The regulatory approach implemented by the FDA based on the 1997 proposal for regulation included cellular therapy products (named HCT/P – cells, tissues and tissue-based products) with gene therapy and tissues rather than with blood products. This different approach had significant implications for the field by defining minimal requirements for establishments involved in manufacturing of HCT/P. The FDA also introduced a concept of risk assessment which includes (1) the relationship between the donor and the recipient (e.g. autologous, allogeneic related, allogeneic unrelated); (2) the amount of processing and manipulation (non-manipulated, minimally manipulated and more than minimally manipulated); and (3) the purpose for which the tissues are used (homologous and non-homologous use, where homologous use is defined as repair, replacement or supplementation of a recipient's cells or tissues with an HCT/P that performs the same basic functions in the recipients as in the donor.

The last of the aspects of risk assessment has been debated by the cellular therapy community as one which assigns potentially a different level of regulatory scrutiny based on the intended use despite equivalent risk in the first two areas such as donor and the level of manipulation.

For very practical reasons it is common among cellular therapy practitioners in the US to discuss products as '351' and '361' products. This nomenclature relates to two different sections of the Public Health Service Act. The 361 products are covered in 21 CFR 1271 A, B, C, D, E, F (i.e. Good Tissue Practice), while the 351 products are covered in multiple regulations including 21 CFR 1271 C, D; 21 CFR 207.20 (f); 21 CFR 210–211; 21 CFR 807.20 (d); 21 CFR 820.1 (a); 21 CFR 312 [investigational new drug regulations (IND)] and others. The 361 products are defined in 21 CFR 1271.10 as (1) minimally manipulated; (2) intended for homologous use; (3) do not involve combination with a drug or a device, except for a sterilising, preserving, or storage agent, if the agent does not raise new clinical safety concerns; and (4) does not have a systemic effect and is not dependent upon the metabolic activity of living cells for its primary function or has a systemic effect and is for autologous use; or for allogeneic use in a first-degree and second-degree blood relative; or for reproductive use. All products which do not fulfil these requirements are considered 351 products.

Based on the assignment of 351 and 361 products there are different requirements for biological product deviation reporting.

It is important to note that there are tissues excluded from 21 CFR 1271 which include vascularised organs; whole blood and blood components; human milk and minimally manipulated bone marrow. Thus, HPC, Marrow (minimally manipulated) is regulated by different set of regulations which are under the authority of Health Resources and Services Administration (HRSA).

For a thorough discussion of FDA regulatory activities and current guidance documents the reader is referred to the agency website http://www.fda.gov/cber/gene.htm and http://www.fda.gov/cber/tiss.htm.

Non-governmental (voluntary) accreditation

Many programmes elect to be accredited by one of the voluntary accrediting organisations in addition to observing governmental regulations. There are multiple reasons for voluntary accreditation ranging from recognition by health care insurance providers for reimbursement purposes through improved quality of care to fulfilling requirements by some of the local governmental regulations (e.g. Commonwealth of Massachusetts requires FACT accreditation from all Transplantation Centres).

All accrediting organisations require adherence to local and governmental laws and regulations in addition to individual standards established by each of them. Each voluntary organisation has a slightly different approach to accreditation process, but generally an applicant facility needs to meet or exceed standards promulgated by the accrediting organisation. The published standards, which are typically updated in defined time intervals, describe a minimum level of expectations. Table 37.1 summarises major differences (and similarities) between different accrediting organisations.

Standards are prepared by a group of experts within the organisation, typically called 'Standards Committee', which establish minimum expectations for the facilities willing to participate in the accrediting programme. The draft standards are presented for public comments, which then may or may not be incorporated into the final standards. Some organisations, notably CAP, do not present the standards (in this particular case checklist questions) for comments. Once the final version of standards is approved, a tool is created which is used during the inspection process.

The accreditation process generally consists of three phases: phase I – application step, when the applicant facility submits necessary documentation to the accrediting body and certifies that it is compliant with the standards; phase II – confirmation step, when the accrediting body using on-site inspection confirms that the applicant facility truly follows the standards; and phase III – recognition step, when a certificate of accreditation is being issued based on the documentation submitted and the results of on-site inspection and, if necessary, satisfying responses to identified shortcomings in the applicant facility. The accreditation certificate has an expiration date and stipulates that if there are any significant changes in the programme structure and/or performance, these will be promptly reported to the accrediting body. Each

of the accrediting organisations may have additional requirements.

FACT and JACIE

In 1994, the Foundation for Accreditation of Cell Therapy (FACT) in the US initiated a voluntary inspection and accreditation scheme for cell therapy facilities. Five years later, its European counterpart the Joint Accreditation Committee of the ISCT (International Society for Cell Therapy) and EBMT (JACIE) was founded. FACT–JACIE is a voluntary system which accredits clinical transplant programmes as well as the cell collection, processing and banking elements that are covered by current EU legislation. Whilst FACT–JACIE accreditation is not compulsory, there are pressures for the clinical, collection and laboratory parts of HSCT programmes to comply with their requirements in some countries. These include purchasing agreements with health care funders. The primary aim of FACT and JACIE is to improve the quality of HSCT in North America, Europe and elsewhere by providing a means whereby transplant centres, HSC collection facilities and processing facilities can demonstrate high-quality practice. This is achieved through external inspection of facilities to ensure compliance with the FACT–JACIE standards. A further aim is to ensure consistency between the standards and other national and international standards, including the EU Tissues and Cells Directive (Directive 2004/23/EC) and the related Commission Directives 2006/17/EC and 2006/86/EC (see above).

FACT–JACIE accreditation is voluntary but provides a means whereby transplant facilities can demonstrate that they are working within a quality system which covers all aspects of the transplantation process and that they can show compliance with the requirements of insurance companies or national and/or international regulatory authorities. Accreditation of HSC transplant facilities is through on-line submission of documentation and Centres may apply for accreditation as complete programmes comprising a clinical programme, collection facility and processing laboratory or, for example, as a single collection

Table 37.1 Overview of voluntary accreditation/registry organisations.

	FACT	JACIE	Netcord/FACT	aaBB	CAP	NMDP	WMDA
Membership	No	No	No	No	No	Yes	Yes
Accreditation	Yes	Yes	Yes	Yes	Yes	No	Yes
Scope							
Registries	na	na	na	na	na	na	++
Recruitment	na	na	na	na	na	++	+
Donor	+	+	++	+	+	++	++
Collection	++	++	++	++	++	+	+
Processing	++	++	++	++	++	++	na
Transplantation	++	++	na	na	na	++	na
Products							
HPC, Apheresis	Yes	Yes	No	Yes	Yes	Yes	Yes
HPC, Marrow	Yes	Yes	No	Yes	Yes	Yes	Yes
HPC, Cord Blood	No	No	Yes	Yes	Yes	Yes	Yes
TC, Lymphocytes	Yes	Yes	No	Yes	Yes	Yes	No
Other CTCs	No	No	No	Yes	No	No	No
Standards structure	Checklist	Checklist	Checklist	ISO based	Checklist	Checklist	Checklist
Current edition/version*	3rd	3rd	3rd	2nd	2007/10	19th	2007/09
*Accredited facilities (non-US/US)**							
Registries	na	na	na	na	na	na	69
Cord Blood Banks	na	na	5/10†	21/22†	unknown	24	>19
Collection/Processing/Transplant	9/151†	56	na	4/100†	unknown	43/130 tc† 6/84 dc† 17/83 cc† 8/84 ac†	na

FACT, Foundation for the Accreditation of Cellular Therapy; JACIE, Joint Accreditation Committee (ISCT and EBMT); aaBB, formerly American Association for Blood Banks; CAP, College of American Pathologists; NMDP, National Marrow Donor Program; WMDA, World Marrow Donor Association; CTC, Cellular Therapy Products; tc, transplant centre; dc, donor centre; cc, collection centre; ac, apheresis centre; na, not applicable.

*As of 1 June 2008.

†Figures shown as non-US/US.

or processing facility which may serve a number of clinical programmes.

The FACT–JACIE standards

The standards cover all aspects of clinical transplant programmes, bone marrow and peripheral blood stem cell collection facilities and processing laboratories. The standards also apply to the use of therapeutic cells (TCs) derived from the peripheral blood or bone marrow, including donor lymphocytes and mesenchymal stem cells. The standards cover the clinical use of Cord Blood HSC by clinical programmes but not the collection of banking of CB, which are covered by the related Netcord–FACT standards and inspected and accredited by FACT–Netcord (see below). The standards are available on the FACT and JACIE websites, are structured as shown in Table 37.2 and contain essential principles which apply throughout.

• Establishment and maintenance of a quality management programme (QMP).

• Requirement for documentation of policies, procedures, actions and requests which extends to all aspects of transplant activity. For example, the initial diagnosis of a patient must be documented in the clinical notes using source material or reports. A request from the clinical unit to the laboratory for issue of cells must be made in writing. A potential donor must not only be properly evaluated for eligibility, but the programme must have clear written criteria for what constitutes an eligible donor and must clearly document whether the donor meets these criteria.

• Personnel must not only be appropriately qualified, they must be trained in the procedures they regularly perform and their competency to perform the task after training must be assessed and documented.

• Validation of all equipment and procedures. Validation is a term used to describe the activity required to prove that any procedure, process, equipment, material, activity or system actually leads to the expected results. For example, a new apheresis machine must be shown to produce the expected results in terms of cell yields.

Also important is the requirement for close cooperation and interaction between the different parts of the programme, especially important where a clinical programme may use an off-site collection and/or processing facility

Quality management

An active QMP is essential to the FACT–JACIE standards. A QMP is a mechanism to ensure that procedures are being carried out by all staff members in line with agreed standards. In a transplant programme, this ensures that the clinical, collection and laboratory units are all working together to achieve good communication, effective common work practices and increased guarantees for patients. It is a means of rapidly identifying errors or accidents and resolving them so that the possibility of repetition is minimised. It assists in training and clearly identifies the roles and responsibilities of all staff. Once the required level of quality has been achieved, the remaining challenge is to maintain this standard of practice. With a working QMS in place and adequate resources, the fundamental elements necessary to sustain the programme are continued staff commitment and vigilance. The culture and systems for quality management (QM) are well established in laboratories but are relatively new in clinical units and many programmes have experienced difficulty setting up a QMP to cover the clinical programme and collection facility. It is recommended that HSCT programmes have dedicated quality managers.

Experience of centres implementing FACT and JACIE

It was anticipated that implementation of the FACT–JACIE standards would pose some difficulties for applicant centres, particularly in relation to establishing a QMS. It was also anticipated that there would be resource implications in terms of staff time because of the amount of detailed documentation that is required to demonstrate compliance with the standards. To assess this in Europe a survey was designed to assess the difficulties experienced by centres in preparing for JACIE accreditation and the results showed that the most difficult part of preparation was implementing the QMS, adverse event reporting system and other documentation. Lack of a culture of QM was cited as an

Table 37.2 Structure of the FACT–JACIE standards.

Clinical Programme	Collection(MB/PB)	Processing
General	General	General
Facilities	Facilities	Facilities
Personnel	Personnel	Personnel
Quality management	Quality management	Quality management
Policies and procedures	Policies and procedures	Policies and procedures
Donor selection, evaluation and management	Donor selection, evaluation and management	
Therapy administration	Collection procedure (BM/PBPC)	Process controls
	Labelling operations	Labelling operations
Clinical research		Distribution
Data management	Storage	Storage
		Transporation
		Disposal
Records	Records	Records
	Direct distribution	

important problem. The extra resources most frequently required were a quality manager and a data manager. Only 19% of centres needed to improve their physical facilities. There is clearly an important need for training of clinical staff (doctors and nurses) in QM. It is also important for centres to have a designated quality manager who has appropriate experience in QMS.

Improvements clearly depend on the level of existing services, so that failure to demonstrate improvement in, for example, facilities or data management may reflect good pre-existing resources. In other areas, e.g. adverse event reporting, the systems for monitoring performance were only set up as part of implementing JACIE, so that it is difficult to monitor improvements without an established baseline for comparison. Indeed implementation of JACIE may have the paradoxical effect of seeming to increase adverse events because these were not previously adequately reported. All centres felt that accreditation was worth the effort invested. In addition, with the implementation of the EU Directive on Safety of Tissues and Cells (2004/23/EC), it is likely that collection and processing facilities will increasingly view compliance with JACIE standards as important in providing evidence that they are complying with the requirements of the Directive.

Netcord–FACT

In the same way that FACT–JACIE cooperate to produce a globally agreed set of standards and a guidance manual for accreditation of HSCT programmes, FACT collaborates with Netcord which is an international organisation for CB banking. Their combined, international standards, first issued in 2000, are the gold standard for CB banks worldwide. The most recent standards (3rd edition) were published in 2006 and became effective in March 2007. They comprise five sections that cover CB bank QM, operations, donor management and collection, processing, donor selection and release. It should be noted that clinical transplantation is dealt with in the FACT–JACIE standards.

aaBB (formerly American Association of Blood Banks)

Established in 1947, aaBB is an international, not-for-profit association dedicated to the advancement of science and the practice of transfusion medicine and related biological therapies. AABB membership consists of approximately 1800 institutions and 8000 individuals, including physicians, scientists, administrators, medical technologists, nurses, researchers, blood donor recruiters and public relations personnel. Members are located in all 50 states and 80 foreign countries. In 1958, the

Standards for a Blood Transfusion Service was published, and an independent accreditation programme was established. The AABB approach to the field of cellular therapies has aimed to balance flexibility in an outcome-based approach with the need for rigorous evidence-based standards. The standards are written using an ISO-based template. The 10-chapter headings are based on the AABB Quality System Essentials (QSEs), published in 1997 as AABB Association Bulletin # 97-4. The 10 QSEs correlate directly with ISO. The aaBB Standards for Cellular Therapy Services, which are revised and updated every 18 months, cover all cellular therapy product and cell sources including autologous, allogeneic and cadaveric donors.

Under a QMS approach, each chapter progresses from general policies to specific procedures. The chapters are:

• organisation;
• resources;
• equipment;
• agreements;
• process control;
• documents and records;
• deviations and non-conforming products or services;
• internal and external assessments;
• process improvement; and
• safety and facilities.

The chapters open with broad statements (a part of the template for all aaBB standards, which are amended, if necessary, to fit particular field) which are followed by more specific standards and finally, end with reference standards which are most prescriptive. The reference standards are generally presented as tables or lists of activities/requirements.

The aaBB accreditation is valid for 2 years and each accredited institution is assessed every 24 months. Recently, the aaBB following other accrediting organisations introduced unannounced assessments. These occur on any day within 90 days of accreditation expiration date.

College of American Pathologists

The College of American Pathologists (CAP; www.cap.org) is a medical society serving nearly 16,000 physician members and the laboratory community throughout the world. It is the world's largest association composed exclusively of pathologists and is widely considered the leader in laboratory quality assurance. The nearly 16,000 pathologist members of the CAP represent board-certified pathologists and pathologists in training worldwide. More than 6000 laboratories are accredited by the CAP, and approximately 23,000 laboratories are enrolled in the College's proficiency testing programmes. There are two proficiency tests currently offered for the cellular therapy products, SCP (Stem Cell Test) and CBT (Cord Blood Test).

The CAP primarily accredits laboratories in clinical and anotomic pathology; however, the accreditation process also includes other entities such as cellular therapy laboratories, HLA laboratories and reproductive laboratories.

The accreditation process, called Laboratory Accreditation Program, is based on fulfilling the CAP checklist (self-assessment and on-site inspection) which consists of two major parts: general section, which applies to all laboratories and activities; and specific for each laboratory.

The questions on tissue banking were added to the transfusion medicine checklist in 1993. There were five questions covering the following: (1) documentation defining the authority, responsibility and accountability of the program; (2) records documenting the type of processing and infectious disease testing for each tissue stored; (3) procedures defining storage conditions of the different tissues handled and retention of records; (4) records showing proper storage conditions; and (5) records allowing for identification of the donor and recipient for each tissue handled. In 2004, the CAP expanded the Tissues section of the checklist and significantly expanded the Haemopoietic Progenitor Cells section of the checklist. In general, the CAP checklists undergo frequent review by the CAP's scientific resource committees and the Commission on Laboratory Accreditation. New editions are released at least once a year.

The Reproductive Laboratory Accreditation checklist was created in 1993 and contains requirements for gametes and embryos. The September 2007 edition was revised to address or clarify requirements to better prepare CAP-accredited laboratories for their FDA inspections.

The CAP inspections are performed every other year and the inspection team consists of professionals from a CAP accredited facility which is led by a team leader who is appropriately qualified Fellow of the College. The inspections generally last for 2 days.

The World Marrow Donor Association

The World Marrow Donor Association (WMDA) is an international organisation that publishes standards to which HSCT donor registries wishing to achieve accreditation for their activities must adhere. These standards are available on the WMDA website (www.worldmarrow.org). These include benchmark standards with which all registries must comply in order to be accredited for the first time, the rest being optional. For subsequent accreditation, the registry must comply with all of the standards. Important areas described by the standards include general organisation of the donor registry, donor recruitment, assessment, counselling, histocompatibility and immunogenetic characterisation of donors, other testing including infectious disease marker, IT requirements, donor searches, collection and transport of cells. At the present time accreditation is given after detailed review of documentation submitted by the registry by independent reviewers and site visits are not done, although a pilot scheme to introduce them is under way. Accreditation is valid for 5 years.

Histocompatibility accreditation

The American Society for Histocompatibility and Immunogenetics (ASHI) and its European counterpart – the European Federation of Immunogenetics (EFI) accredit H&I laboratories after reviewing documentation and conducting a site visit.

Conclusions: how do HSCT programmes respond to the challenge?

The requirements of regulatory and accreditation bodies place huge demands on transplant programmes. In some cases, they may need to construct new and improved facilities for HSC collection, processing and storage. A key feature is the need to develop robust QMPs as described above which will include detailed policies and procedures to cover all their activities. Initial staff training and ensuring ongoing competency are crucial. HSCT programmes should remember that deficiencies commonly found at inspection involve the QMP, policies and procedures, donor assessment and testing and the labelling of cell therapy products. The interaction between the different component parts of programmes should work seamlessly and where, for example, cell processing or laboratory testing is performed outside the programme by external agencies, then service level agreements will need to be in place. Most units that achieve compliance with regulatory and accreditation standards feel that the exercise has been worthwhile and that the quality of the services that they offer has been improved.

Key points

1 There have been considerable advances in cellular therapy in the last 20 years and newer developments include the use of cell therapy products for regenerative medicine and immunotherapy.
2 The accreditation and regulatory environment has become increasingly complex and its aim is to enhance product quality and safety.
3 The development of robust quality systems is central to achieving compliance with these new requirements.
4 Some regulations are mandatory, e.g. the EU Directive and FDA requirements, whilst others such as FACT–JACIE accreditation are voluntary.
5 Increased resource is required to successfully implement the changes needed to achieve compliance.

Further reading

AABB Standards for Cellular Therapy Services, 3rd edn, 2007. Available at www.aabb.org.

CAP Checklist. Available at www.cap.org under Accreditation and Laboratory Improvement.

Circular of Information for the Use of Cellular Therapy Products, version 2007. Available at www.aabb.org and www.factwebsite.org.

Commission Directive 2006/17/EC implementing Directive 2004/23/EC of the European Parliament and Council as regards certain technical requirements for the donation, procurement and testing of human tissues and cells. Available at www.transfusionguidelines.org.uk.

Commission Directive 2006/86/EC implementing Directive 2004/23/EC of the European Parliament and Council as regards traceability requirements, notification of severe adverse reactions and events and certain technical requirements for the coding, processing, preservation, storage and distribution of human tissues and cells. Available at www.transfusionguidelines.org.uk.

Directive 2004/23/EC of the European Parliament and Council on setting standards of quality and safety for the donation, procurement, testing, processing, preservation, storage and distribution of human tissues and cells. Available at www.transfusionguidelines.org.uk.

FDA documents. Available at www.fda.gov/cber/tiss.htm and www.fda.gov/cber/gene.htm.

Human Tissue Authority (HTA): Codes of Practice for Consent (Code 1), for Donation of Organs, Tissues and Cells (Code 2), for Removal, Storage and Disposal of Human Organs and Tissues (Code 5), for Donation of Allogeneic Bone Marrow and Peripheral Blood Stem Cells for Transplantation (Code 6) and for Import and Export of Human Bodies, Body Parts and Tissue (Code 8). Available at http://www.hta.gov.uk.

Hurley CK. Histocompatibility testing guidelines for haematopoietic stem cell transplantation using volunteer donors: report from the World Marrow Donor Association. Quality Assurance and Donor Registries Working Groups of the World Marrow Donor Association. *Bone Marrow Transplant* 1999;24(2):119–121.

NETCORD-FACT International Standards for Cord Blood Collection, Processing, Testing, Banking, Selection and Release, 3rd edn, 2007. Available at www.factwebsite.org.

Standards for Haematopoietic Progenitor Cell Collection, Processing and Transplantation, 3rd edn, 2007. The Foundation for the Accreditation of Cell Therapy (FACT) and the Joint Accreditation Committee of ISCT-Europe and EBMT (JACIE). Available at www.jacie.org.

Standards for Histocompatibility Testing, 2005. Available at the European Federation for Immunogenetics (EFI) standards. Available at www.efiweb.org.

The Human Tissue Act 2004 (except Scotland), ISBN 0 10 543004 8. Available at www.hta.gov.uk.

The Human Tissue Act 2006 (Scotland), ISBN 0–10-590094-X. Available at www.show.scot.nhs.uk.

World Marrow Donor Association (WMDA) Standards, March 2005. Available at www.worldmarrow.org.

CHAPTER 38

Stem cell collection and therapeutic apheresis

Khaled El-Ghariani

NHS Blood and Transplant and Sheffield Teaching Hospitals NHS Trust; University of Sheffield, Sheffield, UK

The word *apheresis* is derived from the Greek meaning 'a withdrawal'. Therapeutic apheresis is the process of using apheresis technology to manipulate patient's circulatory contents through removal or exchange, to achieve a therapeutic goal. The rationale for this is that it will remove or reduce a substance or substances implicated in the pathology of the disease being treated. Plasma exchange is the process of exchanging part of the patient's plasma with suitable replacement fluid. Different cellular components can be removed with high precision. Red cells can be exchanged, circulating stem cells and lymphocytes can be collected for transplantation and the excess white cells or platelets that are present in myeloproliferative disorders, can be removed. Molecules such as low-density lipoproteins and immunoglobulins can be specifically removed through the use of adsorption columns. A decision to offer these treatments to patients should be based on factors such as temporary benefits of apheresis, potential adverse effects and the availability of other treatment modalities.

Cell separators

Efficient cell separators are currently available. These machines are equipped with sophisticated

Practical Transfusion Medicine, 3rd edition. Edited by Michael F. Murphy and Derwood H. Pamphilon. © 2009 Blackwell Publishing, ISBN: 978-1-4051-8196-9.

software and safety alarm systems to detect air and changes in access or inflow pressure. Apheresis technology is based on either filtration or centrifugal systems. Filtration systems use highly permeable membranes to separate blood into its cellular and non-cellular components by subjecting it to sieving through a membrane with suitably sized pores. An example of a filtration system is the Infomed HF440 (Plate 38.1). Centrifugal systems use G forces to separate blood into different components. Centrifugation of blood within apheresis machines results in sedimentation of its components into distinct layers. Based on increasing density, these layers are plasma, platelets, monocytes, lymphocytes and haemopoietic progenitor cells (HPCs), granulocytes and red cells.

Apheresis machines use either continuous- or intermittent-flow technology. In the continuous-flow machines, blood is continuously pumped into a spinning disposable harness where separation takes place and components are either diverted to a collection bag or returned to the patient as required. These machines often require two points of access to the circulation, one for withdrawal and another for return blood to the subject. Examples of continuous-flow systems are COBE Spectra (Plate 38.2) and Baxter Fenwall CS3000. Intermittent-flow machines collect blood into a bowl during the draw cycle, and then centrifuge it down to separate plasma and cellular components. Different components are diverted to the collection bag or returned to the patient along with replacement fluid during the return cycle. This process requires a single point of access to the circulation. An example of intermittent-flow system is the Haemonetics MCS+. Apheresis systems are primed with normal saline to displace air from the harness and also to ensure isovolumia, an important prerequisite for patients with haemodynamic instability or sickle-cell disease. In children and small adults, the extra-corporeal volume may be relatively high and the system will need to be primed by a mixture of packed red blood cells and normal saline. Cell separators must be validated and maintained according to the manufacture's recommendations and must be operated by trained personal.

Patient assessment and treatment planning

A physician experienced in the use of cell separators should undertake clinical assessment, to weigh the patient's current health status and expected benefit against potential risks and inconveniences. Plasma exchange often provides relief of the patient's symptoms for variable lengths of time and it is usually only part of the patient's treatment plan. Informed consent must be obtained from all competent patients. Minimal laboratory evaluations are required before the first procedure; these include full blood count, coagulation screen and biochemistry. These tests are repeated thereafter as required. Apheresis treatment plans will include the type of vascular access, volume to be exchanged, type of replacement fluid, frequency of procedures and monitoring of response to therapy. Adequate vascular access is crucial. Peripheral veins, usually located in the antecubital fossa, should be evaluated by apheresis staff early in planning and should be used wherever possible, especially for patients requiring a limited number of procedures. Central venous catheterisation is required for patients who have inadequate peripheral veins, or who require frequent procedures. A rigid double-lumen catheter should be used. Trained staff must undertake central vein cannulation and post-insertion catheter care. Maximum effort should be exerted

to avoid failure of vascular access during the procedure; such failure is associated with disappointment to both patients and staff.

Haemopoietic progenitor cell mobilisation

Currently, haemopoietic cell transplantation is more commonly undertaken using mobilised peripheral blood (PB) rather than bone marrow as a source of stem cells. This is because PB-HPC engrafts faster than marrow and without the need for hospital admission or general anaesthesia. In the steady state, HPC circulates in the peripheral blood, albeit in very low numbers, of less than 0.1% of the total white blood cell count. To ensure adequate graft, mobilisation of such cells from the marrow into the peripheral circulation is necessary. Granulocyte colony-stimulating factor (G-CSF) is used to mobilise healthy donors, whereas mobilisation of autologous cells can be achieved by growth factors, mainly G-CSF and/or the administration of chemotherapy such as cyclophosphamide, or disease-specific combination chemotherapy. The mechanism of HPC mobilisation is not completely understood; however, proteolytic enzymes, such as elastase, cathepsin G and matrix metalloproteinase-g, released from neutrophils following administration of chemotherapy and/or G-CSF, are thought to degrade molecules such as CXCR4 and SDF-1, which are important for anchoring stem cells to marrow stroma, and induce mobilisation. Progenitor cells express CXCR4 receptors. The ligand of this receptor is stromal-derived factor 1X (SDF-1), which is present in marrow stromal cells. The association of CXCR4 with its ligand, mediates stem cell homing, trafficking and retention. Also, G-CSF may have an inhibitory effect on expression of CXCR4 mRNA and the reduced expression of CXCR4 receptors enhance mobilisation. Currently, limited data suggest that a single injection of pegylated G-CSF in combination with chemotherapy has the ability to mobilise enough stem cells to allow safe autologous transplantation. Pegylation of G-CSF is a process in which a polyethylene glycol (PEG) moiety is conjugated to G-CSF molecules. This increases its molecular mass, reduces its renal excretion and prolongs its half-life in excess of 30 hours. The role of pegylated G-CSF in stem cell mobilisation needs to be defined. GM-CSF is less effective and more toxic than G-CSF to be used routinely for most donors. It could, however, be used in combination with G-CSF for poor mobilisers. AMD3100 is a reversible inhibitor of the CXCR4 receptor and has been shown to be a powerful mobilising agent. This drug's high efficiency and low-toxicity profile make it a promising future mobilising agent, not only for the old or frail patients but also for healthy volunteers.

Most healthy donors are mobilised by G-CSF at a dose of 10 µg/kg/day. Progenitor cells usually peak after the fourth injection when harvesting starts and the procedure may be repeated until the target number of stem cells is achieved. Donor age, steady-state CD34 levels and both the total dose and schedule of G-CSF, may impact on the CD34+ cell mobilisation. G-CSF used in healthy donors has proven to be both effective and reasonably safe. The most common symptoms are bone pain, headaches, fatigue and nausea. Reduction in arterial oxygenation has also been noted. Rare but serious effects of G-CSF have been reported. Splenic enlargement is common and there are a few case reports of splenic rupture, either spontaneously or precipitated by minor trauma or viral infection. Donors are encouraged to report any pain or discomfort that they may experience over the splenic region. G-CSF has a procoagulant effect and may increase the risk of myocardial infarction, or ischaemic strokes in susceptible individuals. G-CSF should be avoided in donors with a history of autoimmune disorders or sickle-cell disease. The effects of G-CSF on genomic stability and possible long-term leukaemogenesis remain unclear; however, this concern justifies long-term follow-up of G-CSF-stimulated donors.

The response of individuals to mobilisation regimens is variable and some donors fail to mobilise enough HPCs into circulation, to allow collection of an adequate graft. Such poor mobilisation is more common in autologous than allogeneic donors. Stem cell damage due to old age, previous exposure to chemotherapy and radiotherapy, or disease involvement of bone marrow, is associated with poor mobilisation in autologous donors. Stem

cell toxic agents such as melphalan and carmustine (BCNU) and other commonly used chemotherapy agents such as fludarabine are specifically known to impair mobilisation. The percentage of donors who mobilise poorly varies widely between published studies. This is most likely due to inconsistency in the definition of poor mobilisation and the differences in the donor groups studied. Patterns of donors' responses to mobilisation treatment are likely to continue to change in the future, depending on changes in types of diseases treated, the patients' age profiles and co-morbidities. Also, the effects of new cancer treatments need to be defined. A few reports suggested that therapies such as rituximab and bortezomib may not adversely affect mobilisation. The mechanism of poor mobilisation in healthy donors is unclear. However, experiments in mice have suggested a genetic control of the vigour and timing of mobilisation. Individuals who prove to be hard to mobilise may respond favourably to mobilisation at a latter date, or using different mobilisation treatment. If clinically indicated, it is worth undertaking further mobilisation attempts in such individuals. Table 38.1 lists the options available to manage poor mobilisation.

PB HPC collection (leucopheresis)

Leucopheresis, following chemotherapy and G-CSF mobilisation, could commence when WBC counts are rising ($\geq 1 \times 10^9$/L). However, currently, most centres use surface expression of CD34 on PB cells, measured by flow cytometry, to predict the optimal time to start HPC collection, to predict the success of collection and to enumerate HPC in the collected product. CD34 is a heavily glycosylated phosphoglycoprotein expressed on progenitor cells of all lineages within the lymphohaemopoietic system, but not on mature cells. Endothelial progenitors, marrow stromal cells and osteoclasts also express CD34. Approximately, 1.5% of aspirated normal marrow mononuclear cells, less than 0.1% of non-mobilised PB and approximately 0.5% of cord blood cells are CD34+. The function of CD34 molecules remains elusive; however, analysis of its structure indicates that these molecules may have a role in cellular signal transduction and/or cell adhesion. CD34 is a surrogate marker for stem

Table 38.1 Management options for poor mobilisation.

1 Patients should be considered for stem cell mobilisation and harvesting, if required, early in the course of their illness and before stem cell toxic agents is used in their treatment.
2 Leucopheresis is repeated daily for several days and a larger blood volume is processed to maximise yield. Leucopheresis may be started at a lower CD34+ cells level in patients who are likely to be hard to mobilise.
3 Marginally low numbers of stem cells are accepted for transplantation.
4 Bone marrow is harvested instead. However, bone marrow from poor mobilisers may not be of good enough quality and delayed engraftment may follow. At least one study showed that G-CSF-primed marrow is effective in supporting autologous myeloablative transplant.
5 Mobilisation is repeated at a later date to allow marrow recovery using the same mobilisation treatment. Cells obtained from two mobilisation attempts are likely to be adequate.
6 Mobilisation is repeated using a different, usually more intense, mobilisation treatment such as:
  a Chemotherapy and G-CSF
  b Higher dose of G-CSF
  c G-CSF and GM-CSF
7 New agents such as AMD3100 synergises with G-CSF and once licenced, may significantly improve management of poor mobilisation.

cells. Purified autologous CD34+ cells mediate haemopoietic engraftment whereas CD34− cells do not engraft. There is a clear correlation between the number of CD34+ cells infused and the rate of subsequent recovery of both neutrophils and platelets post-transplant. Compared with marrow harvests, G-CSF mobilised grafts contain 3- to 4-fold higher CD34+ cells and about a 10- to 20-fold increase in CD3+ T cells. An optimal number of infused PB HPC required for transplantation is not fully defined. However, to ensure timely engraftment and graft survival, there is a consensus to infuse at least 2.0×10/kg recipient body weight of CD34+ cells for autologous transplant and 2 to 3×10/kg of recipient body weight for allogeneic transplant. A higher allogeneic cell number is required with increased HLA disparity between donor and recipient. In addition, a higher number of cells should be collected if tandem transplant or graft manipulation is contemplated. The maximum number of cells to be infused is not defined. However, in the autologous setting, the inconvenience and cost of harvesting of much higher cell numbers are not justified by improvement of clinical outcome. In some studies, infusion of very high number of allogeneic cells was found to be associated with a higher risk of extensive chronic graft-versus-host disease (GVHD).

Administration of G-CSF just before leucopheresis should be avoided. G-CSF injections are usually followed by temporary reduction of circulating stem cells lasting for about 4 hours. The optimal harvesting time is between 4 and 12 hours after subcutaneous injection of G-CSF. Serial measurement of PB CD34 count in autologous donors is usually obtained as soon as their total WBC approaches 1×10^9/L. Collection, started at a level of 20 CD34+ cells/µL, gives the best yield. However, collection may also start at 10/µL or even 5/µL in donors who may not mobilise so well. Healthy donors usually follow a more predicted course and their peak mobilisation is usually reached at day 5, after four G-CSF injections. Some donors require further injections either because of delayed mobilisation or because not enough cells were collected at the first collection.

Collection of PB HPC is a technically challenging procedure and different machines collect cells with different efficiency and selectivity. Machine efficiency is measured by the percentage of CD34+ cells that can be collected at specific peripheral CD34 count. The collected yield can be enhanced by the machine's ability to process more volumes of donor blood within a reasonable period of time and without inconvenience to the donor. Selective machines manage to target PB HPC with less contamination by other unwanted blood cells. This reduces platelets and red cell contamination of the harvest, which is important in two respects; firstly, such contamination affects stem cell cryopreservation and may increase infusion complications. Secondly, collection of other cells such as platelets may lead to thrombocytopenia in the donor.

Apheresis units should validate new machines against published data, as well as against existing equipment, to ensure that new technologies are safe and convenient to the donors, as well as meeting required product specifications. This is particularly important, in cases where the unit deals with special donor groups such as children, or heavily pre-treated autologous patients, who tend to mobilise poorly.

There are other important operational features of apheresis machines that should be taken into consideration. The volume of the end product should be as small as possible. Smaller volumes are easy to cryopreserve, require smaller storage space and are associated with less dimethylsulfoxide (DMSO) infusion toxicity. Machines that have smaller extracorporeal volumes are less likely to cause transient anaemia and hypovolaemia in small subjects and children and so avert the need to prime with blood. Machines that are using a single point of access to circulation are usually associated with ability to process a smaller volume of blood and so give a lower yield of CD34+ cells.

Several machines, such as Spectra (Gambro BCT), Amicus (Baxter Biotech), Fresenius AS 104 (Fresenius USA) and Haemonetics (Haemonetics Corp), are able to collect stem cells with different efficiencies and selectivity. Spectra machines are available in two versions. Version 4.7 requires visual monitoring of the interface by the operator to ensure optimal PB HPC collection. This version collects cells more efficiently, especially at a low CD34 count. Version 6 is fully automated, has a smaller product volume and smaller extra-corporal volume.

A total of 2–3 patient blood volumes are usually processed by the apheresis machine at each leucopheresis procedure. Large volume leucophoresis, of 3–6 blood volumes or more processed over a period of 6–8 hours, have been tried and shown to collect significantly higher CD34+ yields. This may reduce the number of leucopheresis procedures required and also limit exposure to G-CSF. However, this practice is associated with significant patient inconvenience, citrate toxicity and median platelets loss of 36%.

Plasma exchange

Plasma exchange is an effective treatment for many conditions, mainly immune in nature. Treatment plans include determination of the amount of plasma to be exchanged in relation to the patient's estimated plasma volume and how to space the procedures to ensure efficiency. An exchange of 1.0–1.4 of the patient's plasma volume will exchange 63–75% of their plasma and is therapeutically effective in most situations. Larger volume exchange is associated with inconvenience, use of larger amounts of replacement fluid and brings little extra benefit (Figure 38.1). The frequency and total number of exchanges depend on the disease being treated and on the patient's response. Hyperviscosity, thrombotic thrombocytopenic purpurea (TTP) and Goodpasture's syndrome require daily exchanges; others may respond to a course, for example, five exchanges over 7–10 days. The most commonly used replacement fluid is human albumin solution (HAS) of 4.5%. One-third of the exchange volume can be replaced by normal saline if the patient's starting albumin level is normal, otherwise hypotension and/or peripheral oedema may follow. A therapeutic dose of FFP (10–15 mL/kg) may be included as the last replacement fluid to be infused in cases where repeated exchange with albumin has depleted clotting factors in patients at a high risk of bleeding. Solvent detergent plasma is the recommended replacement fluid for TTP.

Response to treatment varies between patients. Criteria to monitor response to treatment should be agreed early in the treatment plan to avoid under-treatment, over-treatment or the continuation of ineffective treatment. TTP is monitored by measuring the platelet count and other parameters of haemolysis whilst Guillain–Barré syndrome and myasthenia gravis are assessed by clinical neurological improvement. Evidence is accumulating regarding the effectiveness, or otherwise, of different apheresis procedures to treat various disease processes (Table 38.2).

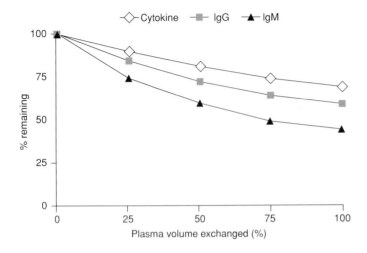

Figure 38.1 Kinetics of plasma exchange. (Reproduced with permission from El-Ghariani & Unsworth 2006.)

Although large randomised trials support the use of plasma exchange in the treatment of Guillain–Barré syndrome, intravenous immunoglobulin (IVIG) is equally effective. Given the ease of administration, IVIG is usually a first-choice therapy. However, either of the two treatment modalities can be used if the other fails. Chronic inflammatory demyelinating polyneuropathy also responds to both plasma exchange and IVIG and the former can be used for maintenance treatment. In myasthenia gravis, plasma exchange has a clear therapeutic effect; however, the disease control is temporary and may be followed by a rebound. Plasmapheresis is used to treat emergencies such as respiratory failure or swallowing difficulties and to prepare patients for thymectomy. Plasmapheresis must be accompanied by an appropriate immunosuppressive regime if it is to be of long-term benefit in myasthenia gravis.

Paraproteinaemia causing clinically evident and progressive hyperviscosity syndrome is a medical emergency requiring urgent plasma exchange to

Table 38.2 Indications of therapeutic apheresis that have been proven by randomised controlled trials.

Plasma exchange
  Thrombotic thrombocytopenic purpura
  Hyperviscosity in monoclonal gammopathies
  Cryoglobulinemia
  Anti-glomerular basement membrane disease (Goodpasture's syndrome)
  Myasthenia gravis
  Paraproteinemic polyneuropathies (IgG/IgA)
  Guillain–Barré syndrome
  Chronic inflammatory demyelinating polyradiculoneuropathy
Red cell exchange
  Life- and organ-threatening sickle crisis
Photopheresis
  Erythrodermic cutaneous T-cell lymphoma
  Heart transplant rejection prophylaxis
Selective lipid removal (usually by adsorption column) for homozygote familial hypercholesterolemia
Leucocytapheresis for hyperleucocytosis causing leucostasis

Other therapeutic apheresis indications, supported by evidence other than randomised controlled trials, are available in the list of further reading.

lower the concentration of the responsible paraprotein. IgM, the largest immunoglobulin and mostly intravascular, is most likely to cause hyperviscosity. IgA and IgG3 tend to aggregate and, after IgM, are more likely than other isotypes or subclasses to be associated with hyperviscosity. One to three treatments will usually alleviate symptoms long enough for chemotherapy to take effect. These patients are often severely anaemic. They should not be transfused until the viscosity has been lowered as a rise in haematocrit can precipitate a serious worsening of their symptoms. Plasma exchange can also be life-saving in cryoglobulinaemia associated with a fulminant clinical picture. Replacement fluids should always be warmed. At the same time, the cause of the cryoglobulinaemia must be determined and definitive chemotherapy instituted if appropriate. Plasma exchange plays a limited role in the treatment of autoimmune cytopenia; however, it is the treatment of choice for TTP and should be started as soon as the diagnosis is made. Daily plasma exchange is needed for at least 2 days after the platelet count has returned to normal. Plasma infusion can also be used to treat TTP if plasma exchange is not available.

Plasma exchange is required as an adjuvant therapy in anti-glomerular basement membrane disease (Goodpasture's syndrome). In the presence of pulmonary haemorrhage, it is important not to overload the patient with replacement fluids as this may provoke further bleeding. Plasma exchange may be used in certain cases of pauci-immune rapidly progressive glomerulonephritis and systemic vasculitis. Such cases need to be discussed with a specialist. Plasma exchange has no proven role in the management of systemic lupus erythematosus (SLE) or uncomplicated rheumatoid arthritis.

Red cell exchange

Red cell exchange involves the removal of a patient's red cells and concomitant infusion of allogeneic donor cells. This procedure, evolved as a manual procedure, can be performed by apheresis machines and is most commonly used to treat sickle-cell disease, polycythaemia and some parasitic infections such as malaria. A major advantage of this automated procedure is the gradual isovolaemic nature of the exchange, which is important in preventing further complications occurring. A single red cell volume exchange removes approximately 60% of the red cells originally present in the patient's circulation. The patient's haematocrit, the fraction of the patient's red cells to be left in circulation after the exchange, the desirable final haematocrit and the haematocrit of the replacement fluid, can be entered into the machine's software, which then calculates the volume of red cells to be removed and estimates the volume of red cells to be used as replacement.

Exchange using normal red cells as a replacement fluid is beneficial in the treatment and prevention of certain sickle-cell crises. Exchange should aim at raising the haemoglobin A to 70–80% to avoid further vasoclusive crises and treat the ongoing one. However, the final haematocrit following exchange should not exceed 30%. Hyperviscosity, associated with a higher haematocrit, is associated with a significant reduction in oxygen delivery. Red cell exchange may not shorten an uncomplicated painful sickle crisis but may be considered in severe and frequent debilitating crises. A patient who survives an acute ischaemic stroke is usually maintained on a regular exchange programme to prevent recurrence. For acute chest syndrome, life- or organ-threatening complications, red cell exchange can provide rapid reduction of sickle haemoglobin and is less likely to cause iron accumulation. Red cell exchange in sickle-cell disease is associated with concerns such as increased requirement of allogeneic blood, which is associated with the risk of viral transmission and red cell alloimmunisation.

Red cell exchange as an adjuvant therapy that should be considered for severely ill patients with malaria if parasitaemia is more than 10% or if the patient has severe malaria manifested by altered mental status, non-volume overload pulmonary oedema or renal complications. Treatment is discontinued after achieving ≤5% residual parasitaemia. Absolute erythrocytosis causing hyperviscosity, thromboembolism or bleeding should be treated by tackling its primary cause and possibly by phlebotomy to maintain a normal haematocrit. However, red cell exchange is also used to treat certain patients with polycythaemia, where removed red cells are replaced with a plasma volume expander to maintain isovolemia. This procedure is particularly useful in patients with polycythaemia vera, complicated by acute thromboembolism, severe microvascular complications or bleeding, especially if the patient is haemodynamically unstable.

Extracorporeal photochemotherapy/photopheresis

Extracorporeal photochemotherapy (ECP) is a process in which the patients' mononuclear cells (MNC) are collected and exposed to ultraviolet A light (UVA) in the presence of photoactivating agents such as 8-methoxypsoralen (8-MOP). This process brings about immunomodulation, which can be therapeutically beneficial to patients with advanced cutaneous T-cell lymphoma (CTCL), GVHD and cardiac transplant rejection. The mechanism of action of ECP is not fully understood; however, the procedure does not lead to an increased incidence of opportunistic infection, a feature that is particularly useful in patients with extensive skin lesions. Collection of MNC can be achieved by an intermittent-flow cell separator such as the Therakos UVAR XTS system. The machine also injects 8-MOP and delivers a calculated UVA radiation dose into the MNC suspension before returning the cells to the patient's circulation. Heparin is usually used as an anticoagulant. This intermittent-flow technology is used for patients weighing more than 40 kg. Standard continuous-flow apheresis machines can be used to collect MNC following oral administration of 8-MOP and the suspension is then exposed to UVA using an irradiation source such as the UV-matic irradiator and then re-infused. This method can be used to treat small patients and children. However, strict adherence to good manufacturing practice (GMP) regulations for re-infused products is required. Oral administration of 8-MOP may cause side effects. However, the US Food and Drug Administration has recently approved the extra-corporeal addition of 8-MOP into the MNC product.

ECP is moderately expensive, time-consuming and approved; indications are restricted. ECP is contraindicated in the presence of psoralen hypersensitivity. There is some evidence for the use of ECP in erythrodermic CTCL and steroid-refractory GVHD, but randomised controlled studies are needed. There is good evidence supporting the use of ECP in preventing cardiac rejection following transplantation. Randomised controlled trials have also shown a therapeutic benefit in type 1 diabetes mellitus but the inconvenience associated with the procedure outweighs the clinical benefit. Patients with advanced CTCL (stage III/IV) typically receive ECP on two consecutive days once per month. For the management of chronic GVHD (cGVHD), an accelerated regimen has been used to gain rapid control of the disease with treatment administered initially weekly with two or three consecutive treatments every 2–3 weeks.

Complications of therapeutic apheresis

Complications occur in up to 10% of procedures, most are mild, but rarely serious complications including deaths have been reported. Given the advances in technology, machine-related problems are unusual. Failure of the machine can result in red cell loss of up to 350 mL of blood. Central catheter-related complications, such as pneumothorax, internal bleeding, thrombosis and infections, are more common and can be serious. Allergic reactions to replacement fluids are uncommon but can be significant. These include anaphylactic reactions, hypotension and urticarial rashes. Reactions to HAS are now rare as the preparations contain lower amounts of significant contaminants than previously, especially of vasoactive kinins. HAS essentially carries no risk of infection and it does not increase the citrate return. Dilution of coagulation factors can occur following repeated plasma exchanges and may require the addition of FFP to the replacement fluid. FFP poses the risk of blood-borne infection (although virally-inactivated products are now available), allergic reactions and also contributes to the citrate load as it contains approximately 14% citrate anticoagulant by volume. Side effects of the citrate anticoagulant, almost universally used, are particularly common. These result from hypocalcaemia and include paraesthesiae (particularly perioral), abdominal cramps and, rarely, cardiac dysrhythmias and seizures. Citrate toxicity usually responds to simple measures such as slowing the rate of return and providing extra calcium orally. Intravenous calcium may be required. Patients with renal failure who are receiving large amounts of citrate during plasma exchange may develop a profound metabolic alkalosis. Patients receiving repeated treatments over a long period of time can lose significant quantities of calcium. Complications during therapeutic apheresis may arise from underlying pathology or co-morbidity. It is important that the clinical status is assessed prior to exchange. Where risks are increased, but benefit is likely, a suitable location for the procedure such as a high dependency unit may be required.

Key points

1 A physician experienced in the use of cell separators should assess the patient's needs to a therapeutic apheresis procedure taking into consideration potential risks and inconvenience.
2 Adequate vascular access is crucial. Central venous catheterisation needs to be undertaken by trained staff to minimise risks to patients.
3 G-CSF with or without chemotherapy is currently the gold standard for HPC mobilisation.
4 Donors who prove to be hard to mobilise may respond favourably to mobilisation at a latter date or by using a different mobilisation treatment.
5 Human albumin solution (4.5%) is the most commonly used replacement fluid for plasma exchange. Occasionally, plasma, usually solvent detergent product, is needed.

6 The mechanism of action of photopheresis is not known; however, this technique induces immunomodulation without immunosuppression.

Further reading

Cashen AF, Lazarus HM & Devine SM. Mobilizing stem cells from normal donors: is it possible to improve upon G-CSF? *Bone Marrow Transplant* 2007;39:577–588.

The American Society for Apheresis. Clinical application of therapeutic apheresis: an evidence based approach. *J. Clin Apheresis (Special Issue)* 2007;22(3).

El-Ghariani K & Unsworth DJ. Therapeutic apheresis – plasmapheresis. *Clin Med* 2006;6(4):P343–P347.

Jantunen E & Kuittinen T. Blood stem cell mobilization and collection in patients with lymphoproliferative diseases: practical issues. *Eur J Haematol* 2008;80:287–295.

Kaplan AA. *A Practical Guide of Therapeutic Plasma Exchange*. Oxford: Blackwell Science, 1999.

Kessinger A & Sharp JG. The whys and hows of hematopoietic progenitor and stem cell mobilization. *Bone Marrow Transplant* 2003;31:319–329.

McKenna KE, Whittaker S, Rhodes LE *et al.* Evidence-based practice of photopheresis 1987–2001: a report of a workshop of the British Photodermatology Group and the UK Skin Lymphoma Group. *Br J Dermatol* 2006;154:7–20.

McLeod BC. (ed) *Apheresis Principles and Practice*, 2nd edn. Bethesda: AABB Press, 2003.

Moog R. Mobilization and harvesting of peripheral blood stem cells. *Curr Stem Cell Res Ther* 2006;1:189–201.

Scarisbrick JJ, Taylor P, Holtick U *et al.* UK consensus statement on the use of extracorporeal photopheresis for treatment of cutaneous T-cell lymphoma and chronic graft-versus-host disease. *Br J Dermatol* 2008;158(4):659–678.

The British Committee for Standards in Haematology. Guidelines on the diagnosis and management of the thrombotic microangiopathic haemolytic anaemia's. *Br J Haematol* 2003;120:556–573.

CHAPTER 39

Haemopoietic stem cell processing and storage

David H. McKenna Jr & Mary E. Clay
Department of Laboratory Medicine and Pathology, University of Minnesota Medical School, Minneapolis, Minnesota, USA

In recent years, haemopoietic stem cell (HSC) transplantation has become an increasingly viable option in the treatment of a growing number of malignant and non-malignant diseases. Reliable methods of HSC processing, cryopreservation and storage are essential to the success of such transplants. The goal of this chapter is to familiarise the reader with these methods while introducing related topics within the field of cell and tissue engineering. This chapter discusses sources of HSCs, processing methods, quality control (QC) testing techniques, cryopreservation and storage, quality assurance (QA) and good manufacturing practices (GMPs).

Sources of HSCs

There are three sources of HSCs for clinical transplant – bone marrow, peripheral blood and umbilical cord blood (see Table 39.1).

Bone marrow

The traditional source of HSCs is bone marrow (BM). Use of BM has decreased over recent years as other sources of HSCs with definite advantages have become available. Despite this decline, however, a role for BM in HSC transplantation does still exist. Target dosage (typically $2-4 \times 10^8$ nucleated cells/kg recipient body weight) is efficiently collected in a single procedure. The harvesting procedure involves aspiration of BM (10–15 mL/kg recipient weight) from the posterior iliac crests under full general, spinal or epidural anaesthesia. Following filtration (typically sequential in-line filters of decreasing filter pore size), the collection is free of bone spicules and other debris and ready for any necessary further processing.

Peripheral blood

Studies performed over 30 years ago showed HSCs to be in the peripheral blood (PB) at very low concentrations. The subsequent discoveries of haemopoietic growth factors (granulocyte-macrophage colony-stimulating factor, or GM-CSF, and granulocyte colony-stimulating factor, or G-CSF) and their role in mobilisation of HSCs from BM led to development of apheresis strategies to collect HSCs from the mononuclear cell fraction of blood. PB has become the major source of HSCs at many transplant centres in both the autologous and allogeneic setting.

PB collection can be less problematic for the donor, as there is no need for anaesthesia or hospitalisation. Venous access (peripheral or central) is utilised in a procedure that lasts roughly 4–5 hours.

Practical Transfusion Medicine, 3rd edition. Edited by Michael F. Murphy and Derwood H. Pamphilon. © 2009 Blackwell Publishing, ISBN: 978-1-4051-8196-9.

Table 39.1 Sources of haemopoietic stem cells.

Source	Characteristics
Bone marrow	Original source of HSCs; decreasing in use
	Used predominantly in allografting (occasional autograft procurement for HSC back-up)
	Requires operating room harvesting procedure to collect 10–15 mL/kg recipient weight (nucleated cell target dose typically $2.0–4.0 \times 10^8$/kg)
	Advantages include need for only one procedure for full collection; a possible advantage is the relatively lower T-cell content
Peripheral blood	Widely used in the autologous setting; surpassing bone marrow as the primary allogeneic HSC source in many/most transplant centres
	Requires mobilisation of stem cells in the patient/donor with chemotherapy, haemopoietic growth factors, or both (CD34+ cell target dose typically 5.0×10^6/kg)
	Advantages include collection without anaesthesia/hospitalisation, more rapid engraftment and, in the autologous transplant setting, possibly lower tumour cell contamination
Umbilical cord blood	Collected from the placenta (in utero or ex utero) following delivery
	Stored either for eventual use by the family or placed into a bank for transplant into unrelated patient
	Minimum CD34+ cell dose: $1.7–2.0 \times 10^5$/kg
	Advantages include decreased incidence of graft-versus-host disease, decreased search time and reduced histocompatibility matching requirements

Modified from Smith BR. Basic biology of hematopoietic progenitor cell transplantation. In: Snyder EL & Haley NR. (eds), *Hematopoietic Progenitor Cells: A Primer for Medical Professionals*. Bethesda, MD: AABB Press, 2000, Table 1-1, p. 8.

Higher numbers of HSCs, relative to typical BM harvests, can be collected, facilitating engraftment. Many centres use rising peripheral white blood cell count and/or peripheral CD34+ cell enumeration (usually 10–20 CD34+ cells/μL) to determine the most efficient collection plan (i.e. date, process volume or length of collection). Using this strategy, most healthy G-CSF-stimulated allogeneic donors need one to two collections to reach the target dose. In the autologous setting, more collections are typically required depending upon the success of mobilisation.

The same apheresis strategies (without growth factor stimulation) may be utilised to harvest PB mononuclear cells for use in the processing/engineering of a variety of other cellular therapies. These therapies (e.g. donor lymphocyte infusion (DLI), natural killer (NK) cells, dendritic cells and antigen-specific T-cell immunotherapies (i.e. cytomegalovirus, Epstein–Barr virus, tumour etc.)) may serve as adjunctive or supportive therapy post-HSC transplant or as therapies altogether independent of HSC transplant. The majority of these ther-

apies are considered investigational at this time. However, as more clinical and manufacturing experience is gained, such therapies will hopefully prove efficacious.

One generally accepted therapy, DLI, is commonly used as post-allogeneic HSC transplant therapy for the prevention of leukaemia relapse or loss of engraftment. DLIs are collected from the original HSC donor. Upon completion of the apheresis procedure, an aliquot from the mononuclear cell product is drawn for lymphocyte quantitation. Dosage is based on lymphocyte content and is calculated using automated or manual differential or flow cytometric analysis (CD3+ cell content), as determined by the institutional protocol. Other than an occasional volume reduction for a small recipient, there is no further processing necessary in the manufacturing of a DLI product.

Umbilical cord blood

Umbilical cord blood (UCB) is the final source of HSCs for transplantation. Since the first clinical transplantation in 1988 into a child with

Fanconi anaemia, use of UCB for haemopoietic re-constitution has steadily increased. Once regarded as biological waste, UCB has been demonstrated to contain HSCs with higher proliferative and self-renewal capacity than those of BM and PB. Due to dose limitations, most patients deemed appropri-ate for UCB transplantation are children or small adults. However, several strategies have been ini-tiated to overcome limitations of dose, including transplantation of two or more units and ex vivo expansion.

UCB is collected by obstetricians or dedicated staff before (in utero) or following delivery (ex utero) of the placenta. A typical UCB collection measures from 50 to 200 mL. Bacterial contam-ination rates, which historically approached 10–20%, have decreased markedly since collection techniques have improved. Most collections now are by 'closed-system' involving umbilical vein can-nulation or venipuncture and direct drainage into a plastic blood bag. The unit then undergoes fur-ther processing and cryopreservation and is stored in liquid nitrogen for eventual use by the family (autologous or related allogeneic) or an unrelated recipient.

In addition to higher potency relative to BM and PB, UCB has several more advantages over these other sources of HSCs. Decreased incidence of graft-versus-host disease and reduced histocompatibil-ity matching requirements are attributable to the naïve immunologic state of the lymphocytes within the UCB. It follows that patients with rare human leucocyte antigen (HLA) types are often success-ful in finding a suitable graft when other sources are not acceptable. Finally, search time is generally decreased, as units are banked and already HLA-typed.

Processing methods

HSC processing involves both routine methods and more specialised, complex methods. The routine methods utilise concepts and equipment well-known to the blood banking profession. Cellular components and plasma are separated based on physical properties (e.g. size and den-sity) using various reagents (e.g. hydroxyethyl starch for red blood cell (RBC) sedimentation), centrifugation-based instruments (e.g. Spectra Apheresis System and COBE 2991 Cell Processor, both from Caridian.BCT, formerly Gambro.BCT) and plasma expressors (see Table 39.2). The more specialised methods involve concepts, reagents and instruments more unique to cell processing/cellular engineering (see Table 39.3).

Routine methods

Volume reduction
Volume reduction (VR), or plasma depletion, is ac-complished with centrifugation and is commonly performed to reduce incompatible plasma (anti-body load) in the case of minor ABO mismatched allografts (BM and PB). Despite plasma compatibil-ity, VR may be necessary in the transplantation of

Table 39.2 Routine HSC processing procedures.

Procedure	Application
Volume reduction (plasma depletion)	Reduction of incompatible plasma (minor ABO mismatch); prevention of volume overload in recipient; concentration of cells for cryopreservation
Red blood cell depletion	Reduction of incompatible red cells (major ABO or other antigen mismatch); maximisa-tion of storage space; limitation of infusion of lysed red cells and free haemoglobin (cryopreserved products)
Buffy coat preparation	Maximisation of storage space; debulking of red cells prior to further manipulation
Thawing, washing and filtration	Preparation of HSC products prior to infusion (see text)

Modified from Law P. Graft processing, storage, and infusion. In: Ball ED, Lister J & Law P. (eds), *Hematopoietic Stem Cell Therapy*. Philadelphia, PA: Churchill Livingstone, 2000, Table 28-1, p. 312.

Table 39.3 Specialised HSC processing procedures.

Procedure	Application
Counterflow centrifugal elutriation	Separation of cell populations by cell size and density; uses include T-cell depletion of HSC grafts and monocyte enrichment for further manipulation
Cell selection systems	Positive and negative cell selection; uses include HSC (CD34+ or CD133+ cells) enrichment with consequent T-cell depletion and a variety of other cell-type enrichments and depletions based on cell surface antigen expression (see the text)
Cell expansion	Expansion of HSCs and progenitors in an effort to enhance engraftment and long-term outcome; utilises culture systems designed to mimic in vivo microenvironment
Other	T-cell depletion and HSC graft purging by monoclonal antibody-based methods and/or physical characteristics; HSC graft purging by pharmacological agents

Modified from Law P. Graft processing, storage, and infusion. In: Ball ED, Lister J & Law P. (eds), *Hematopoietic Stem Cell Therapy*. Philadelphia, PA: Churchill Livingstone, 2000, Table 28-2, p. 313.

patients with current or potential issues of fluid balance/overload (e.g. paediatric and small adult patients, renal/cardiac failure patients). VR may also be employed to reduce product volume or increase cell concentration for purposes of cryopreservation.

Red blood cell depletion

Sedimenting agents (e.g. hydroxyethyl starch or HES) facilitate removal of RBCs. RBC depletion is necessary with major ABO- and other clinically relevant RBC antigen (e.g. Kell, Kidd)- incompatible BM allografts to prevent haemolytic transfusion reactions. Furthermore, in the case of cryopreserved HSCs, RBC depletion prior to freezing limits the amount of lysed RBC fragments and free haemoglobin infused. RBC depletion additionally accomplishes reduction of overall volume, which is useful when storage space is a concern (e.g. UCB banking). RBC depletion typically is not necessary when PB is the source of HSCs; apheresis collections usually result in less than 20 mL of RBCs due to efficiency of instrumentation.

Buffy coat preparation

Buffy coat concentration of BM involves centrifugation and harvesting of the white blood cell fraction. When the RBC volume is large enough, this procedure can be performed with an apheresis or cell washing device using semi-automated processing; HSC loss is minimal with such systems. In instances where RBC volume is too low for machine processing, manual centrifugation suffices. Buffy coat preparation can be used for volume reduction for cryopreservation or as an initial RBC debulking step subsequent to further, more complex procedures (e.g. CD34+ cell enrichment on an immunomagnetic selection device).

Thawing of cryopreserved HSCs

The final processing step prior to infusion of HSCs that have been cryopreserved is the thaw procedure. Depending on institutional policy, this procedure may take place in the laboratory or on the patient care unit. The thaw procedure for all HSCs, regardless of source, is similar. Although quite simple, proper execution is essential, as frozen plastic containers may be prone to breakage for a variety of reasons. The product should be carefully removed from the storage container and inspected to evaluate the integrity of the bag. Following label verification of product identity by two technologists, the unit should be gently placed and tightly sealed within a clean or sterile plastic bag and submerged in a 37°C water bath. The thaw should be performed relatively quickly to prevent recrystallisation and consequent cell damage/death. Gentle kneading of the contents helps to accelerate the process. If a leak is discovered, the site of the break should be determined, and a haemostat should be used to prevent loss of the product. The contents of a broken or leaking bag should be aseptically diverted into a transfer bag, and an aliquot should be sent for culture.

Although it is now common practice to red cell deplete an UCB unit prior to cryopreservation, many institutions continue to perform a post-thaw wash step. Washing serves to remove the minimal lysed red cells, haemoglobin and dimethylsulfoxide (DMSO). Many institutions base their UCB processing methodology, including the wash procedure, on that originally described by Dr Pablo Rubinstein of the New York Placental Blood Program (now National Cord Blood Program). Between institutions there may be slight modifications of this simple procedure, for example, with regard to centrifugation (i.e. rpm, duration of spin etc.) and concentration of solutions used for dilution/resuspension etc. Briefly, the thaw involves slow, sequential addition of a wash solution (e.g. 10% dextran, then 5% albumin), transfer into a bag of appropriate size for centrifugation, and resuspension of cell pellet(s) before delivery to the patient care unit for infusion.

Filtration of HSCs

The issue of filtration of HSCs with a standard blood filter (170 μm) deserves brief mentioning. As noted, BM typically undergoes sequential filtration in the operating room or in the laboratory to remove aggregates/debris. Opinions regarding use of standard blood filters prior to or upon infusion of HSCs from PB or UCB, however, do vary from institution to institution. The decision to use a standard blood filter rests with the individual cell processing laboratory and/or transplant centre. It is recommended, of course, that the laboratories validate their filtration process prior to making filtration a standard policy.

Specialised methods

Specialised cell processing methods generally serve to optimise product purity and potency beyond levels obtained through routine methods and, as mentioned previously, use unique reagents and instrumentation.

Elutriation

Counterflow centrifugal elutriation is a specialised method that separates cell populations based on two physical characteristics – size and density (sedimentation coefficient). A centrifuge is used to separate cell populations of a cell product (e.g. HSC) based on density. Fluid/media is passed through the chamber housing the cells in the direction opposite (counterflow) to the centrifugal force. Adjusting the flow rate of the fluid/media and/or the speed of centrifugation to enable counterflow rate to balance centrifugal force allows for alignment of cells based on sedimentation coefficient. A given cell population can then be diverted as a fraction of the initial product. Beckman Coulter has high-performance centrifuge systems that have elutriation applications, and Caridian.BCT has developed a system called the Elutra.

T-cell depletion has been the traditional application of counterflow centrifugal elutriation, as lymphocytes are readily removed (2–3 log depletion) from an allogeneic HSC collection. Using this method, a specific dose of T cells can be given to a patient as a means to reduce graft-versus-host disease while maintaining engraftment and graft-versus-malignancy effect. There are applications of elutriation aside from T-cell depletion, including monocyte enrichment for dendritic cell generation and subsequent tumour vaccine production.

Cell selection systems

Cell selection systems incorporating monoclonal antibody-based technologies that target cell surface antigens (Isolex 300i Magnetic Cell Selection System, Baxter Healthcare Corp. and CliniMACS system, Miltenyi Biotec) have become the method of cell depletion/enrichment at many institutions. These specialised immunomagnetic methods involve isolation of the cell type of interest by either positive selection (target cells retained) or negative selection (target cells depleted). Cell products manufactured by these methods attain an unequalled level of purity.

The Isolex 300i is limited to positive selection of HSCs (CD34+ cells). Selection is accomplished in four steps. Murine-derived anti-CD34 monoclonal antibody (primary antibody) solution is mixed with cells in suspension. Following washing of un-bound antibody, sheep anti-mouse IgG (secondary antibody)-coated paramagnetic, polystyrene beads (Dynabeads M-450) are added, and CD34+ cell-bead rosette complexes are formed. A magnetic field is then applied to the chamber allowing CD34+ cell-bead complexes to be separated from the rest of the suspension. Finally, a releasing agent, an octapeptide that acts through competitive displacement, is added to separate beads/antibodies from the CD34+ cells. Selection of CD34+ cells with the Isolex 300i accomplishes an ~85% purity of enriched cells and an ~50% CD34+ cell yield with a simultaneous, indirect T-cell depletion (3–4 log).

Miltenyi Biotec technology involves direct capture of target cells. Specific monoclonal antibodies are coupled to 50-nm ferromagnetic particles, comprising the so-called MicroBeads. Magnetically labelled target cells are retained in the process as the cell suspension passes through a column in which a magnetic field is generated. Unlabelled cells pass through the column and are collected in a negative fraction bag. Target cells are then released from the column by removing the magnetic field from the column, allowing passage of the cells into another collection bag. Antibody-coated beads remain on the cell surface with positively selected cell products manufactured on the CliniMACS, as there is no releasing mechanism. In the case of HSCs (CD34+ cells), purity of enriched cells and CD34+ cell yield or recovery are >90% and ~70%, respectively. T-cell depletion consequent to CD34+ cell enrichment is similar to that of the Isolex system (3–4 log).

The Miltenyi CliniMACS system, in contrast to the Isolex 300i, is not limited to CD34+ cell selection. Clinical-grade reagents allow for positive and negative selection of HSCs (CD34+ or CD133+), monocytes (CD14+) and lymphocyte populations (CD3, CD4, CD8, CD19, CD25), for example. With the broadening of this technology, applications to cell therapy/cellular engineering appear limitless.

Cell expansion

Because cell dose (nucleated cell, CD34+ cell and colony forming cell) and patient outcome corre-late positively, much effort has been focused on ex vivo expansion of HSCs and progenitors. It is thought that successful expansion would enhance haemopoietic engraftment while reducing transfusion dependence, risk of infection, and duration of hospitalisation. Further, cell expansion could be exploited to increase the donor pool and to support a variety of clinical applications, such as HSC autograft purging and harvesting of various cell populations for genetic modification and immunotherapy generation.

Most expansion strategies have utilised mobilised PB apheresis collections that have undergone CD34+ cell selection. However, UCB has been the focus more recently due to the higher proliferative and self-renewal capacity of HSCs from this source. Constituents of the cytokine cocktails used to promote expansion have varied, with stem cell factor, flt-3 ligand and thrombopoietin likely being the most integral to true stem cell expansion. Media have differed, as well, with most consisting of human serum or albumin and/or a variety of culture media (e.g. Iscove's modified Dulbecco's medium, Amgen-defined medium). Culture duration has ranged from as few as 4 days to as many as 12 days.

Most of the earlier HSC expansion clinical trials involved patients with breast cancer undergoing autologous HSC transplantation following high-dose chemotherapy. Trial design varied with some involving exclusive use of ex vivo expanded cells (BM and PB) and others involving transplantation of ex vivo expanded cells along with unmanipulated cells of a dose alone usually adequate for engraftment (BM, PB and UCB). Results of more recent trials involving mobilised peripheral blood have been promising. The few trials using ex vivo expanded UCB, as a whole, have shown less promise, though several trials underway are encouraging. Progress to-date has been indicative of successful expansion of short-term repopulating cells with decreases in severity and duration of cytopenias and resultant decreases in neutropenic fever, transfusion dependence and duration of hospital stay. Studies have yet to determine whether long-term repopulating cells (LTRCs), more primitive HSCs that maintain multilineage differentiation capacity and self-renewal, can be successfully expanded to actually improve the overall rate of engraftment and survival. Current efforts are aimed at recreating the in vivo microenvironment (i.e. stroma, extracellular matrix and haemopoietic and non-haemopoietic cytokines etc.) to allow for expansion of true LTRCs.

Additional cell enrichment/depletion techniques

Other techniques for T-cell depletion include monoclonal antibody-based technologies that target surface antigens on T cells (e.g. OKT-3 (anti-CD3), Campath-1H (anti-CD52)) and strategies that exploit T-cell surface characteristics (e.g. soy bean agglutinin/erythrocyte rosette depletion), or both. Complement incubation following antibody binding and coupling of monoclonal antibodies to various molecules (e.g. immunotoxins) have been used to consistently achieve T-cell depletion of 2–3 logs. While effective, most of these T-cell depletion techniques have been replaced by the more efficient and less cumbersome elutriation and cell selection systems.

Approaches in addition to HSC enrichment by cell selection systems, and similar to those mentioned for T-cell depletion, have been attempted in an effort to deplete, or purge, autologous BM and PB HSC grafts of tumour cells. Physical separation (based on size, density etc.), direct exposure of grafts to pharmacological agents (e.g. 4-hydroperoxycyclophosphamide) and monoclonal antibody-based technologies have all been investigated. However, the physical and pharmacological, or chemical, methods lack specificity for malignant cells; as a consequence, HSCs are damaged and lost as evidenced in the laboratory by poor clonogenic assay results and clinically by delayed engraftment.

Monoclonal antibody-based technologies, alternatively, hold great promise as a means of purging autografts, as they offer the advantage of target cell specificity. Malignant cells are depleted while HSCs remain present and functional. Continued recognition of various cell surface antigens and marked improvements in antibody production over the past 5–10 years have propelled antibody-based strate-gies to the forefront of autologous HSC purging. Monoclonal antibodies may be used alone (e.g. Campath 1-H or anti-CD52) or as chemotherapy- or radioisotope-conjugated forms (e.g. HuM195, or anti-CD33, coupled with calicheamicin, anti-CD45 coupled with ^{131}I etc.). While initial approaches have focused on in vitro methods, more recent approaches have included in vivo techniques aimed at eliminating tumour cells prior to HSC collection (e.g. rituximab, or anti-CD20, for B-cell malignancies). Although some clinical trials have been promising, the true benefits of HSC graft purging have yet to be determined. Purging (in vivo or ex vivo) in combination with post-transplant immunotherapy may be the solution in the effort to prevent disease relapse.

Quality control testing techniques

Quality control (QC) testing in the clinical cell therapy laboratory serves two purposes – to determine the suitability and safety of the cellular product for the individual patient and to monitor overall laboratory practices. The level of QC testing performed is dependent on the complexity of the manufacturing process. Testing is aimed at characterising the safety, purity, identity, potency and stability of the cellular product and may include simple tests (e.g. Gram stain and viability) and/or complex tests (e.g. quantitative PCR and functional assays). Here, we present five standard QC tests for HSC products: cell count and differential, CD34+ cell enumeration, viability and clonogenic assays and sterility testing (see Table 39.4 for summary).

Cell count and differential

Nucleated cell (NC) content and the cell differential may be determined with a haematology analyser. Haematology analysers are capable of simultaneously determining several cellular physiochemical characteristics. The majority of these instruments rely on electrical impedance to determine cell size. As cells pass through an aperture located between two electrodes, a change in the electric current occurs, producing a voltage pulse proportional to cell size. Conductivity by

Table 39.4 Quality control testing of HSC products.

Test	Method(s)
Cell counts	Haematology analyser, manual differential
CD34+ cell enumeration	Flow cytometry (single or dual platform)
Viability assay	Dye exclusion (light microscopy), fluorescence microscopy and flow cytometry
Clonogenic assay	CFU (most common in clinical lab) and LTC-IC
Sterility testing	Aerobic/anaerobic culture

high-frequency electromagnetic energy elicits details of chemical composition and nuclear characteristics, and laser scattering characteristics reveals cell shape/surface and cytoplasmic granularity. Because haematology analysers are designed for the purpose of characterising normal (unstimulated) PB, difficulties may arise with analysis of HSCs. For this reason, following determination of NC content with an analyser, a manual differential may be performed to further characterise HSCs and to quantify mononuclear cell content. Flow cytometry-based analysers are becoming more common, and these instruments may be best suited for analysis of cellular therapy products.

CD34+ cell enumeration

It has been known for quite some time that higher CD34+ cell doses lead to greater likelihood of engraftment and successful clinical outcome in HSC transplantation. Although other markers of HSCs (e.g. CD133, aldehyde dehydrogenase) do exist, the CD34 antigen is currently the most commonly used HSC marker in the clinical laboratory. It is a 115-kDa glycoprotein that is present on HSCs, as well as some malignant cells of haemopoietic derivation, vascular endothelium, embryonic fibroblasts and a few unusual tumours. Despite its evident importance as an HSC marker, the function of CD34 has not yet been elucidated.

The International Society for Hematotherapy and Graft Engineering, or ISHAGE (now the International Society for Cellular Therapy, or ISCT), developed *Guidelines for CD34+ Cell Determination by Flow Cytometry* in 1995. The *guidelines* were initially drafted for enumeration of HSCs in peripheral blood by a dual-platform method (i.e. a two-instrument method employing a haema-

tology analyser for determination of total nucleated cell count and a flow cytometer for calculation of % CD34+ cells). They proposed a sequential gating strategy to focus on cells exhibiting low side scatter (low complexity/granularity) and dim CD45 (leucocyte common antigen, or LCA) staining along with CD34-positivity. Many institutions use this strategy or a modification of this strategy for enumeration of HSCs (see Figure 39.1). In more recent years, single-platform methods (i.e. flow cytometry alone), which utilise a known concentration of anti-CD34-coated fluorescent beads, have been introduced. Single-platform methods allow for determination of absolute CD34+ cell counts. These methods appear to be particularly helpful when analysing UCB – the HSC source with characteristically the lowest concentration of CD34+ cells and a preponderance of non-viable cells, cellular debris and nucleated RBCs.

Viability assays

Viability of HSC products may be measured by dye exclusion using vital dyes (e.g. trypan blue, or TB) or with fluorescent stains (e.g. acridine orange/propidium iodide, or AO/PI). Scoring is determined by light and fluorescence microscopy, respectively. Dye exclusion with TB is widely used despite difficulties including variable staining and presence of staining artifact and high background (red cells and debris). The AO/PI method is more reliable with several advantages over dye exclusion using TB. Acridine orange binds to nucleic acids of viable cells and fluoresces green; propidium iodide, alternatively, binds to nucleic acids of non-viable cells and fluoresces orange. Use of fluorescence (dark-field) microscopy precludes

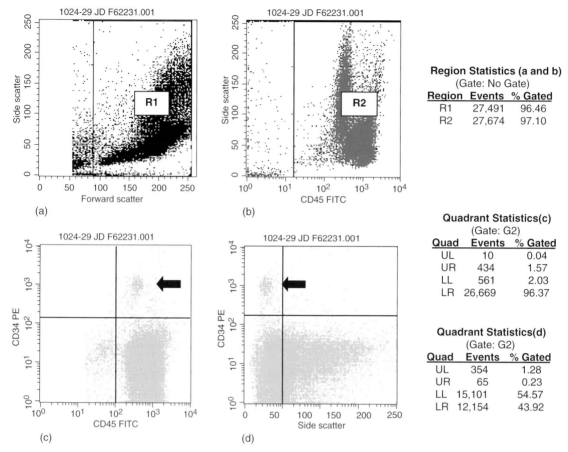

Figure 39.1 HSC (CD34+ cell) enumeration in a mobilised apheresis sample using ISHAGE Guidelines. Fluorochrome-conjugated anti-CD45 antibodies (fluorescein isothiocyanate, or FITC) and anti-CD34 antibodies (phycoerythrin, or PE) are used in this flow cytometric assay. Plot 1 (a) shows the initial gating of all cells with exclusion of visual debris (platelets and cell fragments), or R1. Plot 2 (b) sets CD45-gating (R2) to include only leucocytes for further analysis. Plot 3 (c) shows gating on cells from R2 with addition of anti-CD34-PE. The arrow indicates cells of interest in the upper right (UR) quadrant (CD45+/CD34+ cells = 1.57% of population). This plot serves as quality control in support of the final plot. Plot 4 (d) showing side scatter versus CD34-positivity with gating on R2 is the final plot, and CD34+ cell enumeration is reported as 1.28% (arrow at upper left (UL) quadrant points toward cells exhibiting low side scatter and CD34-positivity). (Courtesy of Dr W. Jaszcz and M. Kraft-Weisjahn, University of Minnesota Medical Center.)

background interference. Less variable staining and simultaneous visualisation of both viable and non-viable cells allows for greater readability and more accurate interpretation.

Although the AO/PI method has proven to be superior to that of TB, both methods measure only nucleated cell viability, and, therefore, are not necessarily informative of the condition of the HSCs. For this reason, the most relevant viability assay utilises flow cytometry with dyes such as 7-amino actinomycin D (7-AAD) or PI. With proper gating, viability of the HSC population (i.e. CD34+ cells) may be determined.

Clonogenic assays

Although CD34+ cell content has become the accepted surrogate marker for graft potency, clonogenic assays remain the only truly functional

QC tests. Therefore, a role for these assays in the evaluation of graft adequacy does still exist. Colony-forming unit (CFU) and long-term culture-initiating cell (LTC-IC) assays are the most commonly performed clonogenic assays, the CFU assay being most practical in the clinical laboratory. Most clinical laboratories limit analysis to CFU-granulocyte, macrophage (GM), as multiple studies have shown correlation between engraftment and dose of CFU-GM. CFU assays require expertise and unique equipment (e.g. CO_2 incubator and dissecting microscope), materials and reagents (e.g. culture media). A 14- to 16-day incubation ($37°C/5\%$ CO_2) limits its usefulness, though with proper planning, timely analysis of cryopreserved products may be accomplished. Many laboratories limit performance of CFU assays to monthly QC testing. However, routine testing of cryopreserved HSC products, particularly UCB, may prove useful.

Sterility testing

A small volume of the HSC product is removed for sterility testing. Aerobic and anaerobic cultures are set up; fungal/yeast cultures may be initiated as well. Microbial contamination may occur at any point from collection (e.g. donor bacteremia, lack of aseptic technique at collection etc.) through processing. Therefore, to assure efficient detection of contamination, the aliquot is removed from the final product shortly before infusion. For products undergoing cryopreservation, a sample is taken for microbial culture just prior to freezing. Most laboratories employ automated microbial detection systems, which offer many advantages over older methods, including more rapid identification of contaminants. If an HSC product is contaminated, immediate notification should be given to the patient's physician. Factors to be weighed by the physician and the medical director of the clinical cell therapy laboratory include condition of the patient and identity, virulence and antibiotic sensitivities of the organism(s). Medical necessity may occasionally dictate that a contaminated cryopreserved HSC product be infused into the patient.

Cryopreservation and storage

Although HSCs may be processed and infused within a few hours of collection, components collected for autologous or allogeneic HSC transplantation may need to be transported to processing centres for short-term (a few hours to a few days) or long-term (weeks to years) storage. Cryopreservation is not required for short-term storage of HSCs, but it is the most appropriate process for the long-term storage of HSCs regardless of their source. Fundamental to preserving HSC integrity and viability during the freezing process is the utilisation of proper cryoprotective solutions, procedures and freezing rates that prevent intracellular ice crystal formation and cellular dehydration. Cryopreservation techniques that are optimal for HSCs will not preserve mature blood cells such as granulocytes, platelets and red cells that are often present in HSC components. Since damaged cells may cause infusion-related toxicities, HSC cryopreservation can be enhanced by the pre-freeze removal of the mature blood elements or setting concentration limits. Although HSC cell concentrations used by different programmes and protocols vary widely, they tend to focus on practical issues such as the need to freeze more than one bag or minimise the total volume of components stored.

HSC cryopreservation has generally required: (1) DMSO as an intracellular cryoprotectant, with or without extracellular cryoprotectants such as hydroxyethyl starch (HES) or human serum albumin (HSA); (2) cooling at $1–3°C/min$; and (3) storage at $−80°C$ or colder. Although DMSO is a reasonably well-tolerated agent, it does have the potential for HSC and clinical toxicity, thus supporting conservative usage procedures. Traditional cryopreservation techniques have used 10% DMSO, but there have been multiple reports showing that it is possible to cryopreserve HSCs using a combination of 6% HES and 5% DMSO.

The cryopreservation process requires the use of special bags constructed with material capable of withstanding the temperature range of freezing and thawing and either controlled-rate or non-controlled-rate freezing methods. Computer-assisted controlled-rate freezing chambers allow a progressive temperature reduction of 1°C/min through the liquid/solid phase change (which occurs at approximately −8°C) to −60°C and then a 3°C/min reduction to −80°C or −100°C followed by storage in a mechanical freezer at −80°C or −135°C or colder conditions in either a liquid or vapour phase of nitrogen. It is advisable to store cells at colder temperatures, and, in fact, some standards require storage at less than −135°C or −150°C. Liquid nitrogen freezers have the advantage of maintaining a very consistent storage temperature (−196°C), but they may serve as reservoirs of infectious agents. Therefore, centres storing HSC components in liquid nitrogen must have procedures to prevent cross-contamination between stored products. Vapour phase storage reduces the risk of cross-contamination but specific procedures, materials and systems must be employed to minimise the temperature gradient that may form within these freezers (i.e. −100 to −190°C).

Controlled-rate freezing and storage at temperatures attainable with liquid nitrogen (liquid or vapour phase) are highly recommended. However, several investigators have established that HSC products can be cryopreserved with the use of a single-step non-controlled-rate freezing procedure and stored at −80°C for extended periods of time without compromising engraftment potential. This technique is less costly and does not require investment in programmable freezers and liquid nitrogen filler tanks or freezers. Although −80°C freezers are easier to maintain, they are prone to mechanical malfunction and significant temperature fluctuations, especially when the door is opened. Most HSC components stored at −80°C are cryopreserved with a mixture of DMSO and HES. Storage of cells in mechanical freezers may be most appropriate for non-clinical, research samples.

All storage freezers should have: (1) continuous temperature monitoring and recording, (2) an alarm system for detection of temperature range deviations or equipment failure, (3) a racking and inventory system and (4) restricted access. Although cryopreservation results in an immediate loss of some portion of the HSCs, the loss is not progressive over time if the storage conditions are appropriate. Several studies have now shown that the duration of HSC storage may be indefinite if adequate storage temperatures are maintained and appropriate cryopreservation techniques used.

Quality assurance and good manufacturing practices

Quality assurance (QA) is the sum of activities planned and performed to provide confidence that all systems that influence product quality are reliable and functioning as expected. The QA, or quality, programme defines the policies and environment necessary to attain minimum quality and safety standards. The basic components of a programme include standard operating procedures (SOPs), documentation/recordkeeping and traceability requirements, personnel qualifications and training including a continuing education programme, building and facilities/equipment QC, process control, auditing and investigation, and error and accident system/management (see Table 39.5 for summary of elements of a quality system). Regulatory authorities worldwide, realising the importance of QA, have placed major emphasis on the establishment of an effective quality programme. It is expected that the HSC collection/processing centre's quality programme will ensure a laboratory's compliance with regulations.

Table 39.5 Elements of a quality system.

Quality plan
Quality assessments/audits
Documentation/recordkeeping
Facility design/maintenance
Process control
Validation
Personnel training
Equipment
Materials management
Receipt/storage/distribution
Labelling
Safety/safety training
Deviations
Adverse events

At a cellular therapy/processing laboratory, the quality programme is the means by which regulatory requirements, such as good manufacturing practices (GMPs), are instituted. GMPs are scientifically sound methods or procedures that are followed and documented throughout product manufacturing. Initially developed for enforcement in the pharmaceutical industry, GMPs have been applied to cellular therapies to minimise lot-to-lot variation, allowing for guarantee of safety, purity and potency. The GMP programme is a QA programme and, as such, includes requirements and specifications for production facilities, staff, supplies and reagents, equipment, laboratory controls, finished product controls, and records and reports. GMPs are not dissimilar from the ISO 9000 approach, and facilities that achieve ISO 9000 certification should also comply with GMP requirements.

Conclusions

The cell processing laboratory is a highly specialised Transfusion Medicine manufacturing centre that employs both standard, blood bank-based and unique methods of manufacturing in support of a rapidly evolving field. As novel cell therapies move into the Transfusion Medicine environment, cell processing facilities move beyond routine HSC processing and storage and increasingly function as translational research/development centres supporting more than blood and marrow transplantation programmes. The challenges exceed the technical realm and include extensive evaluations of the scientific/medical merit as well as the quality and regulatory pathways necessary for success.

Key points

1 There are three sources of HSCs – bone marrow, peripheral blood and UCB; UCB is gaining favour as a source of HSCs for treatment of a variety of haematological and non-haematological diseases.

2 Cell processing is based upon both basic, blood bank-type methods and newer, specialised techniques; the field is expanding rapidly with these cell therapy-specific technologies.

3 QC testing of cell therapy products is critical; it determines the safety, purity, identity, potency and stability of the products. Standard QC tests for HSCs include cell count and differential, CD34+ cell enumeration, viability and clonogenic assays, and sterility testing.

4 Sound methods for cryopreservation are essential to assure integrity of the cell therapy product; most laboratories use 10% DMSO, controlled-rate freezing and liquid nitrogen storage tanks.

5 A QA programme serves as the foundation for a clinical cell therapy laboratory's activities.

Further reading

Austin EB, Guttridge M, Pamphilon D & Watt SM. The role of blood services and regulatory bodies in stem cell transplantation. *Vox Sang* 2008;94(1):6–17.

Bock TA. Assay systems for hematopoietic stem and progenitor cells. *Stem Cells* 1997;15(Suppl 1):185–195.

Brunstein CG, Setubal DC & Wagner JE. Expanding the role of umbilical cord blood transplantation. *Br J Haematol* 2007;137(1):20–35.

Fleming KK & Hubel A. Cryopreservation of hematopoietic and non-hematopoietic stem cells. *Transfus Apheresis Sci* 2006;34(3):309–315.

Keeney M & Sutherland DR. Stem cell enumeration by flow cytometry: current concepts and recent developments in CD34+ cell enumeration. *Cytotherapy* 2000;2(5):395–402.

Khuu HM, Patel N, Carter CS, Murray PR & Read EJ. Sterility testing of cell therapy products: parallel comparison of automated methods with a CFR-compliant method. *Transfusion* 2006;46(12):2071–2082.

Loren AW & Porter DL. Donor leukocyte infusions after unrelated donor hematopoietic stem cell transplantation. *Curr Opin Oncol* 2006;18(2):107–114.

McKenna DH, Sumstad D, Bostrom N *et al.* Good manufacturing practices production of natural killer cells for immunotherapy: a six-year single-institution experience. *Transfusion* 2007;47(3):520–528.

Mohle R & Kanz L. Hematopoietic growth factors for hematopoietic stem cell mobilization and expansion. *Semin Hematol* 2007;44(3):193–202.

Smith L & Lowdell MW. Quality issues in stem cell and immunotherapy laboratories. *Transfus Med* 2003;13(6):417–423.

Sutherland DR, Anderson L, Keeney M, Nayar R & Chin-Yee I. The ISHAGE guidelines for CD34+ cell determination by flow cytometry. *J Hematother* 1996;5(3):213–226.

Verfaillie CM. Hematopoietic stem cells for transplantation. *Nat Immunol* 2002;3(4):314–317.

Suggested textbook

Thomas ED, Blume KG & Forman SJ. (eds) *Hematopoietic Cell Transplantation*, 3rd edn. Malden, MA: Blackwell Science, 2004.

CHAPTER 40

Haemopoietic stem cell transplantation

I. Grant McQuaker[1] & Ian M. Franklin[2]
[1]Bone Marrow Transplant Unit, Beatson West of Scotland Cancer Centre, Glasgow, Scotland
[2]University of Glasgow; Scottish National Blood Transfusion Service, Glasgow, Scotland

Introduction

Although the treatment of haematological malignancies has improved significantly in the past 30 years, many patients have diseases that are incurable with conventional therapeutic approaches. Bone marrow cells are exquisitely sensitive to chemotherapy and radiotherapy, and the recognition that radiation could kill bone marrow function permanently while other organs recovered or were largely unaffected suggested that bone marrow transplantation (BMT) might be feasible. Initially, the pre-transplant chemo-radiotherapy *conditioning* of the patient was thought to provide 'space' for the incoming cells to engraft, as well as killing any residual cancer cells. The transplant itself was perceived only as haemopoietic 'rescue'. Subsequently, it was recognised that the person's own (autologous) bone marrow cells could be used for the same purpose. However, it became apparent that allogeneic transplants (between different individuals) produce an immune-mediated graft-versus-leukaemia (GvL) effect, because patients with chronic graft-versus-host disease (GvHD) had improved disease-free survival. Allogeneic BMT is therefore a combination of the chemotherapy and/or radiotherapy with an immune-mediated effect against the leukaemia or other malignancy.

Practical Transfusion Medicine, 3rd edition. Edited by Michael F. Murphy and Derwood H. Pamphilon. © 2009 Blackwell Publishing, ISBN: 978-1-4051-8196-9.

Later, it was shown that some patients with chronic myeloid leukaemia, who had relapsed after an allogeneic haemopoietic stem cell transplant (HSCT), could return to full molecular remission after infusions of immune competent lymphocytes from the original donor. This provided more direct proof of a GvL effect. Allogeneic BMT is now seen as more of an immunotherapy, in which the transplant itself is a major component in keeping the disease under control. This is why allogeneic BMT has a much lower recurrence rate, but also a higher incidence of post-transplant infections and immune-associated complications, than an autologous transplant. Reduced intensity conditioning (RIC) transplants have been developed to harness the immunological benefits of allogeneic transplants, while avoiding much of the toxicity. The RIC is insufficient to eradicate bone marrow cells, but immune tolerance is induced to ensure engraftment of the incoming donor transplant. Although these RIC transplants are sometimes known as 'mini-transplants', they are still arduous procedures requiring great commitment from the patient.

Principles of HSCTs

The original bone marrow-derived transplants are now more likely to be performed using peripheral blood stem cells (PBSCs) or even cord blood. The term *haemopoietic stem cell* is now more appropriate. HSCT is used:

Table 40.1 Comparison of sources of stem cells.

	Sibling	Unrelated adult volunteer	Umbilical cord blood
Availability	~1:3 have a sibling donor match	>11 million donors world-wide. About 70% chance of finding a matched donor for those of Western European origin	~400,000 banked worldwide; 99% chance of finding a 4/6 HLA A,B,DR match
Matching requirements	Increasingly molecular matching with 9/10 allele match acceptable	Molecular matching with 9/10 allele match acceptable	Most data describe 4/6 matching by serology for class 1 and molecular for class 2(DR)
Speed of availability	3–4 weeks, can be quicker	3–4 mo, can be quicker but difficult	Potentially available in days from identifying the preferred cord blood(s)
Engraftment	PBSC ~14 days; BM ~21 days	As for sibling	~20–30 days. Platelets may be slower in adult size recipients
Acute GvHD (grade II–IV)	25–50% (highest with multiparous female donors)	30–70%	30–70%
Chronic GvHD	30–40% for BM; 40–70% for PBSC (highest with multiparous female donors)	40–50% for BM; 50–70% for PBSC	20–50%
Second donations/DLI availability	Availability dependent on donor	Availability dependent on donor	Unavailable
Risk to the donor	Small	Small	None
Pre-transplant testing complete (HLA and virology)	Once donor identified; it takes a week or so	Once donor identified and requested; it may take several weeks	At time of cryopreservation and unit available for issue

HLA, human leucocyte antigen; PBSC, peripheral blood stem cells; BM, bone marrow; GvHD, graft-versus-host disease; DLI, donor lymphocyte infusion.

• to enable intensification of chemotherapy and radiotherapy so that toxicity to the bone marrow is no longer an important factor in determining outcome; and/or
• to ensure complete engraftment of the donor marrow through immunosuppression of the host (patient), thus permitting tolerance to develop; and
• to promote a GvL (or other tumour) effect.

Sources of stem cells
• *Allogeneic stem cells*: These come from another individual, traditionally a sibling. There is an increasing use of alternative donors, mainly unrelated adults from donor registries but also cord blood-derived cells (see Table 40.1). Unrelated transplants use volunteer donors from national and international registries. The toxicity and results of these procedures are improving steadily. Human leucocyte antigen (HLA) compatibility testing using molecular typing and sequencing of patient and recipient genes has resulted in much improved transplant outcomes. The use of umbilical cord blood, from unrelated donor cord blood banks, is increasing worldwide. It is still, in the main, for individuals with low body weight (<50 kg) because of the small number of stem cells in a cord sample.

Using two-cord donations may lead to more rapid engraftment and much reduced failed engraftment (10%) and means that cord blood transplants for adults are now a realistic option. The advantage of cord blood is that it is obtained from an immune naïve source so that HLA and other mismatches are tolerated with less GvHD than would be expected if an adult donor were used.

• *Syngeneic cells*: These come from an identical twin. Similar attributes to autologous stem cells.

• *Autologous*: These come from the patient.

The donor

Donors must always be treated with respect and not as a means to an end. In particular, the patient must not be used as a conduit to transmit information to a potential sibling donor. Ideally, a physician separate from the transplant team should take responsibility for donor care. Both the Human Tissues Authority (HTA) and the Joint Accreditation Committee of EBMT and the International Society for Cytotherapy (ISC)–Europe (JACIE) have recommendations regarding donor care, and where the donor is a child and an independent assessor is essential. Doctors involved in advising donors, whether family or unrelated, must be aware of current guidance and legislation in this area.

Often, especially if the donor is a sibling, there is only one available. But if there is a choice of donor, a range of factors must be considered before selecting the best donor including the degree of HLA matching between donor and recipient, the gender and age of the donor, CMV status and blood group. Young male donors are preferred. Multiparous female donors can increase the risk of GvHD, and usually have a lower body weight.

Collecting haemopoietic stem cells

Bone marrow cells may be obtained either directly by aspiration or from the peripheral blood (PBSCs). Bone marrow harvesting involves bone marrow aspiration from both posterior iliac crests (under general anaesthesia). A minimum of 2×10^8/kg nucleated cells provides reliable engraftment post-transplant. PBSC mobilisation is increasingly used instead of marrow harvesting, although some donors may be unfit for one method or the other, or express a preference, which should be respected. In healthy donors, this is achieved using the growth factor G-CSF, in patients undergoing autologous procedures, following chemotherapy and growth factor. It is likely that PBSC allografts produce more chronic, but not acute, GvHD, than bone marrow transplants in siblings. This may be associated with less relapse in patients at high risk of recurrent disease – advanced phase chronic myeloid leukaemia (CML), for example – and so will still be favoured. Comparative data in unrelated donor transplants also suggest that the use of PBSC is associated with more chronic GvHD but no difference in long-term survival.

Indications for HSCTs

Stem cell therapy is generally used when conventional dose treatment has failed or is expected to have a high likelihood of failure. The failure of primary therapy when a disease recurs is a clear end point. A perception that failure is likely is more subjective, although some objective evidence may be present. Examples would be chromosome abnormalities known to be associated with poor outcomes, such as the Philadelphia chromosome or 4;11 translocations in acute lymphoblastic leukaemia (ALL), and chromosome 7 deletions in acute myeloid leukaemia (AML). A slow initial response to treatment may suggest that relapse will be likely, as might a high tumour load (bulky disease or a high leucocyte count).

The indications for HSCT have changed over time, and will continue to do so. Current indications for HSCT in 2008 are shown in Table 40.2.

Complications of transplantation

Patients who are being considered for any form of HSCT must be given full information about the procedure prior to giving consent. Although results are improving, all HSCT procedures carry major risks of mortality, morbidity and long-term complications. Some of these risks will be lifelong. The chronology

Table 40.2 Classification of indications for blood and marrow transplants.

Degree of consensus	Allogeneic HSCT	Autologous HSCT
Very high level of agreement	Poor risk AML CR1	Multiple myeloma first response
	AML other than CR1	Relapsed Hodgkin disease
	Adults <35 years with ALL CR1	Relapsed aggressive NHL
	ALL other than CR1	
	CML CP1 if poorly responsive to TKI	
	CML other than CP1	
	Poor risk myelodysplasia	
	Very severe aplastic anaemia in children and young adults	
Some variation in practice between BMT units/nations	Multiple myeloma	AML CR1
	Chronic lymphocytic leukaemia	AML other than CR1
	Low-grade NHL	
Little consensus as to evidence in support of indication. Clinical trials highly appropriate in these conditions	Hodgkin's disease	CML CP1
		CML other than CP1
		Myelodysplasia
		Chronic lymphocytic eukaemia

All transplant procedures are arduous, even though mortality has fallen over the past years. In addition, the use of allogeneic donors causes major problems with immune reconstitution such that few patients over 60 years would be considered for such transplants. With improved tissue matching, the difference between sibling and unrelated transplants is less apparent. Reduced intensity conditioned transplants have increased these age thresholds. For autografting, some groups have extended the limit to 75 years and the authors have experience up to 69 years. Fitness of the patient and the likelihood of benefit are the most important considerations.
HSCT, haemopoietic stem cell transplant; AML, acute myeloid leukaemia; NHL, non-Hodgkin lymphoma; ALL, acute lymphoblastic leukaemia; CR, complete remission; CR1, first complete remission; CP, chronic phase of CML; BMT, bone marrow transplantation.

of the major complications of allogeneic HSCT is shown in Figure 40.1.

Regimen-related toxicity

This refers to the immediate toxic effects of the radiotherapy or chemotherapy used for the transplant. Even the RIC protocols are sufficient to cause toxicity. Organs at risk of damage include the gut, with severe mucositis a major problem. Less commonly, liver, heart, lungs and kidneys may suffer transient or even permanent damage. Careful pre-transplant assessment of each patient is essential. Damage to these tissues by the conditioning may

be more likely to elicit an immune response from the donor cells, adding to the toxicity of the procedure. The use of RIC transplants does reduce this toxicity and enables some patients to receive transplants who might be unfit for full chemotherapy and radiotherapy conditioning.

Rejection

Rejection is an immune-mediated event in which the pre-transplant conditioning and immuno-suppression are insufficient to prevent residual recipient immune cells eliminating donor cells. It only occurs in allogeneic transplants, although

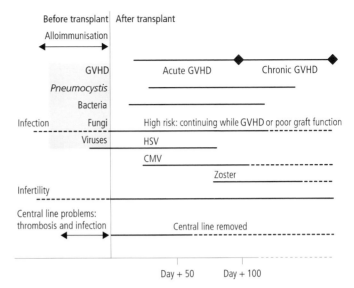

Figure 40.1 Relationship of the major complications of BMT to the time before and/or after transplant. Such a diagram can give only a broad view of the most common periods of relatively uncomplicated transplants. Those using an unrelated or other alternative donor will have greater risks of graft failure, graft-versus-host disease (GvHD) and thus continuing likelihood of infections. CMV, cytomegalovirus; HSV, herpes simplex virus; Zoster, varicella-zoster virus.

graft failure due to inadequate numbers of stem cells in the transplant and/or pre-existing damage to the marrow microenvironment can occur in autografts. HLA incompatibility between patient and donor, and prior sensitisation of the patient to HLA or other marrow cell antigens are risk factors for rejection. HLA sensitisation should be prevented, by using leucocyte-reduced blood components from presentation onwards. The kinetics of HSCT engraftment are shown in Figure 40.2.

Graft-versus-host disease

GvHD is caused by immune-competent T lymphocytes in the donor recognising antigens in the patient as foreign, a process that begins with tissue damage caused by the conditioning therapy. This is followed by antigen recognition, clonal T-cell expansion and then cytokine release, which increases and perpetuates the response. Despite immunosuppression of the patient to prevent it, more than half of patients receiving allogeneic transplants will develop acute GvHD in the first 100 days post-transplant. Acute GvHD is characterised by involvement of skin, liver and gut.

- Skin: From an erythematous sunburn-like rash to a blistering, exfoliative erythroderma.

- Liver: Typically the bile ducts are attacked and an obstructive jaundice-type picture develops. Milder forms may lead to elevated transaminases and cause considerable difficulties with diagnosis.
- Gastrointestinal tract: Classically profuse watery diarrhoea develops, bloody in the most severe cases. Upper gastrointestinal upset is not uncommon, with nausea and sickness.

Relapse

Despite the intensive preparation for transplant, a significant proportion of patients will suffer recurrent disease post-transplant. Patients at special risk are those not in remission at the time of transplant, or patients with more advanced disease, i.e. has already relapsed once after chemotherapy. An absence of a GvL effect, as in autologous HSCT or when no GvHD is seen, is also at higher risk.

Infectious complications

The immune system of the transplant recipient must be suppressed to allow the graft to be accepted, and anti-tumour therapy such as total body irradiation (TBI) ensures that the patient has minimal immune function at the time of the transplant.

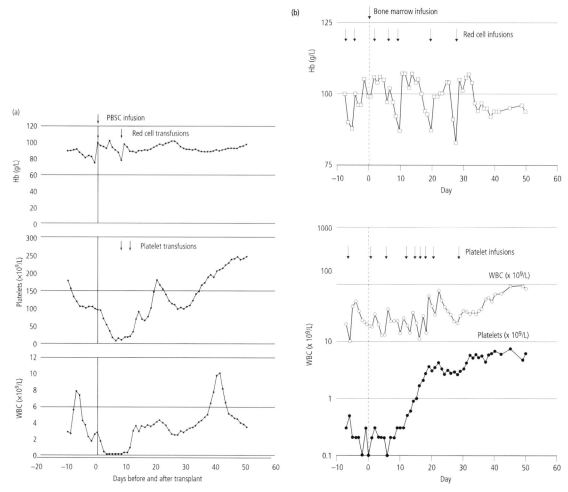

Figure 40.2 (a) A patient with chronic myeloid leukaemia who received a peripheral blood stem cell (PBSC) allogeneic transplant from a sibling using reduced-intensity conditioning. The blood count falls following the chemotherapy (fludarabine and melphalan) and recovers quickly once engraftment begins. The patient had minimal acute graft-versus-host disease and the marrow graft has remained robust. Molecular evidence of chronic myeloid leukaemia was detected some 9 months after the transplant and was treated with low-dose donor lymphocyte infusion. The patient is alive and disease-free 6 months later. Hb, haemoglobin; WBC, white blood cells. (b) A patient with severe aplastic anaemia secondary to hepatitis. Blood counts are low before the transplant, reflecting the aplasia and are relatively slow to recover. Severe acute graft-versus-host disease occurred but was controlled eventually with corticosteroids and antilymphocyte globulin. The patient is alive and well 4 years later. Hb, haemoglobin; WBC, white blood cells.

Even the RIC transplants have this risk, because they utilise intensive immunosuppression in order to ensure that the transplant is not rejected. The agents used (fludarabine and anti-T cell or pan lymphoid monoclonal antibodies) induce prolonged and profound immune deficiency. Haemopoietic recovery takes at least 2–3 weeks (see Figure 40.2), but recovery of neutrophils is only part of the reconstitution of the immune system that must occur for full recovery. BMT-related immune problems may be divided conveniently into three phases as follows. Immune deficiency is compounded at any point after BMT by the presence of active GvHD.

Immediate post-BMT phase

This phase is characterised by neutropenia as well as lymphopenia and hypogammaglobulinaemia. During this period, the patient is managed with:

- protective isolation; filtered air to reduce fungal contamination is especially important;
- prophylactic antifungal, antiviral and antibacterial therapy is routine;
- pre-emptive use of therapeutic antimicrobials; broad-spectrum antibacterial agents at the first sign of fever, followed by antifungal treatment empirically in the absence of prompt resolution;
- intravenous immunoglobulin may be used in some patient groups; and
- prophylactic neutrophil infusions are not used routinely. Trials are needed urgently but are very difficult to design and deliver.

Early post-engraftment period

The patient will now have some marrow function and, if GvHD is absent or controlled, may be able to leave hospital. Although patients having autologous transplants rarely have major problems after this time, vigilance is necessary. Allogeneic HSCT recipients remain at risk of:

- bacterial infections related to central lines;
- fungal infection;
- cytomegalovirus (CMV): most units will monitor for emerging CMV using a polymerase chain reaction (PCR)-based test, and treat positive results before there is evidence of disease. Such pre-emptive strategies are very effective and CMV is becoming a much less important cause of mortality after allogeneic SCT. Such monitoring is also applied to other viruses such as adenovirus and Epstein–Barr virus (EBV), which are becoming more important considerations as current SCT techniques produce more profound pre- and post-transplant immunosuppression;
- other viruses, especially respiratory syncytial virus (RSV) and other herpes viruses such as herpes zoster (HZV); and
- *toxoplasmosis* and *pneumocystis*.

Later problems

Patients who have active GvHD requiring immunosuppressive therapy will continue to have im-

paired immunity to pathogens, and most patients who have received unrelated donor transplants will have detectable abnormalities of the immune system. However, by 3 years' post-transplant almost all patients not taking immunosuppressive drugs will have virtually normal immunity.

- (Re-)vaccination has a role to play but those patients still on immunosuppression will not respond optimally.
- Continued prophylaxis and vigilance are required.
- Hyposplenic cover: Patients who have had allogeneic transplants are hyposplenic and must receive vaccine against organisms such as *Pneumococcus*, *Meningococcus* and *Haemophilus influenzae B* (HIB), as well as receiving lifelong chemoprophylaxis, e.g. with amoxicillin.

Late effects

It might be thought that having endured a life-threatening primary disease followed by the immediate risks of HSCT outlined above, that survivors might be entitled to a respite from further problems. Unfortunately, a litany of potential problems can and do occur, including the following:

- cataracts (total body irradiation only);
- endocrine problems such as
  - ○ hypothyroidism
  - ○ growth retardation in children (especially TBI ± steroids)
  - ○ infertility
- sexual dysfunction;
- second malignancies; this remains a risk even 20 years after the transplant;
- transfusion-transmitted viruses, e.g. hepatitis C; and
- iron overload and liver dysfunction from red cell transfusions.

These problems mean that HSCT recipients require lifelong follow-up at a centre familiar with the range of late complications and with a sufficiently large practice to ensure that emerging problems are identified promptly.

BMT outcome

A discussion of the results of BMT for the wide range of indications now accepted is beyond the scope of this chapter. Current results from the International Bone Marrow Transplant Registry (IBMTR) are available on their website, and should be referred to so that only the most up-to-date information is used.

CML

Historically, CML has been one of the major and widely accepted indications for allogeneic HSCT, and excellent results were achieved, especially in young patients transplanted early after diagnosis. Since the advent of tyrosine kinase inhibitors (TKIs), such as imatinib, disease control is excellent in the majority of patients and so HSCT is no longer considered to be standard first-line treatment if a good response to TKI is achieved. Patients with more advanced stage CML or those who fail to respond or lose a response to TKI are considered for allogeneic SCT (see Figure 40.3).

Acute leukaemia

For acute leukaemia, the precise details of each case are needed before a recommendation can be made. These include chromosome analysis and phenotype. For example, very few patients with Philadelphia chromosome-positive ALL will be cured without an allogeneic transplant.

Results for all patient groups at 3 years for leukaemia-free survival (LFS) in acute leukaemia in adults are of the order of:

• 50–60% in first complete remission (CR1): relapse risk 25%;
• 35–40% for second or subsequent complete remission: relapse risk 46%; and
• 20–25% for patients transplanted not in remission: relapse risk 68%.

Registry data are of great importance but cannot replace the careful assessment of individual patients in the light of their specific prognostic factors. These may serve to improve or worsen the risks for a particular case, e.g. coexistent disease, toxic effects of prior chemotherapy and previous invasive fungal infection. Also, registries report only mature data, usually with a minimum of 3 years' follow-up. The value of more recent developments requires the scrutiny of primary research publications and reports to specialist meetings.

Post-BMT chimerism and molecular monitoring

It has been possible to monitor leukaemic clones using sensitive molecular techniques for over 10 years now. More recently, molecular techniques have been applied to routine monitoring of donor and recipient chimerism post-transplant. RIC transplants often exhibit a period of mixed chimerism early post-transplant, when the presence of both residual host and donor haemopoiesis is detectable. Capillary electrophoresis detection systems allow accurate quantitation of the relative contributions of host and donor to haemopoiesis, by detecting

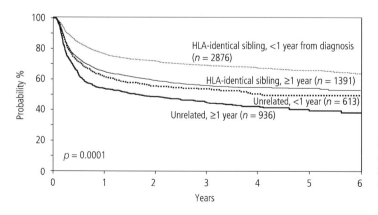

Figure 40.3 Probability of survival after allogeneic transplants for chronic myeloid leukaemia in chronic phase by donor type and disease duration, 1994–1999.

short tandem repeats (STRs). Mixed chimerism is believed to be associated with a higher risk of graft rejection or relapse and optimal GvL responses are dependent upon full donor chimerism. Donor lymphocyte infusions (DLIs) of graded numbers of T lymphocytes can be used to switch patients from mixed to full donor chimerism.

By using DLI early in relapse of CML after allogeneic HSCT, and giving a specific dose of cells, it is possible to separate GvL from a GvH response, although the particular subset of T cells that will generate GvL without the risk of GvHD has not been identified. DLI has been tried in numerous diseases with varying success. In multiple myeloma, there is good evidence of re-induction of remission although the number of cases remains small. Also, it appears to be necessary to use rather more lymphocytes, e.g. 1×10^8/kg. In other diseases, such as acute leukaemia and myelodysplasia, the impact of DLI has not been great.

Cytotoxic T-cell therapy

It has been known for some time that DLI targeted against EBV can be used to treat lymphoproliferative disorder (LPD) in children who have received an unrelated donor HSCT. In these cases, intensive immunosuppression is given to ensure that the graft was not rejected and this led to increased reactivation of EBV, which triggered the LPD. By isolating T cells and exposing them to EBV in vitro, it is possible to generate clonal cytotoxic T cells that recognise EBV antigens and kill the LPD cells. In the main, this treatment has been highly effective in both the prophylactic and therapeutic management of EBV LPD.

Although it is possible to generate sufficient antitumour effect to induce remissions in LPD, the one disease that has been treated effectively with immunotherapy is a virus-associated malignancy. In the past few years, more progress has been made in developing strategies for using cytotoxic T cells against viruses in the HSCT setting, particularly CMV, than for anti-tumour indications. Viruses possess foreign antigens not possessed by the human patient, and the relative lack of progress in anti-tumour immunotherapy, beyond basic DLI ap-

proaches, suggests that identifying and exploiting tumour antigens remain elusive.

Regulatory aspects of haemopoietic stem cell transplantation

An awareness of current regulations regarding HSCT is essential for medical, nursing and scientific staff responsible for the various parts of the service.

In the UK, the HTA regulates tissue banks, which includes processing and storage of HSC. The HTA is the competent authority to ensure the European Union Directive on Tissues and Cells is implemented, and has legal powers. A professional organisation, JACIE, inspects and sets standards for the clinical and laboratory HSCT process. Although not having legal force, JACIE compliance is seen as essential to an active HSCT programme.

Conclusion

At present, there are still no clearly developed indications or proven strategies for cellular immunotherapy other than for generating GvL against CML (and possibly myeloma) using DLI and for the prevention and treatment of EBV LPD. The exploitation of increasing knowledge of the immune system has not been easy. The most likely application appears to be in a more refined approach to the use of DLI post-transplant, and the application of RIC transplants to more non-malignant diseases where immune modulation may have a role.

Meanwhile, what is the long-term future for HSCT generally? These transplants can save life in many patients with incurable leukaemia and lymphomas. Patients who survive the first 3 years are likely to enjoy long-term survival, although life expectancy does not return to normal. RIC transplants extend the benefits to more patients who might have been unfit to undergo the rigours of a myelo-ablative procedure. Whether the use of RIC transplants in a wider range of malignant diseases is effective will become apparent in the next few years. Autologous transplants seem set to decline further in importance as improved chemotherapy, immunotherapy (Rituximab) and improved allogeneic HSCT reduce the number of patients for which they are applicable. Additional approaches are still needed to deal with those patients whose primary disease is poorly responsive to current chemo-radiotherapy.

Key Points

1 The increasing use of cord blood transplants generally, and particularly, for adult/larger patients >50 kg.
2 The declining role for autologous transplants due to improvements in conventional treatment (myeloma and lymphoma) or a greater emphasis on allogeneic stem cell transplantation (adult acute leukaemia).
3 The importance of treating donors of stem cells as individuals and not as a means to an end.
4 The stem cell transplantation field is becoming increasingly regulated in Europe by both professional and statutary bodies.
5 Although reduced intensity/non-myeloablative transplants have less immediate toxicity than conventional radiation therapy-based transplants, they remain arduous procedures with many short- and medium-term complications.
6 The randomised controlled clinical trials remain the best way to produce definitive data as to the relative merits of treatments in blood and lymphoid malignancies.

Further reading

Barker JN, Weisdorf DJ, Defor TE, Blazar BR, Miller JS, Wagner JE. Rapid and complete donor chimerism in adult recipients of unrelated donor umbilical cord blood transplantation after reduced-intensity conditioning. *Blood* 2003;102;1915–1919.

Barrett AJ & van Rhee F. Graft-vs.-leukaemia. *Baill Clin Haematol* 1997;10:337–355.

Dazzi F & Goldman JM. Adoptive immunotherapy following allogeneic bone marrow transplantation. *Ann Rev Med* 1998;49:329–340.

Goldman JM, Schmitz N, Niethammer D & Gratwohl A., for Accreditation Sub-Committee of the European Group for Blood and Marrow Transplantation. Allogeneic and autologous transplantation for haematological diseases, solid tumours and immune disorders: current practice in Europe in 1998. *Bone Marrow Transplant* 1998;21:1–7.

Gratwohl A, Baldomero H, Schmid O, Horisberger B, Bargetze M, Urbano-Ispizua A. Hematopoietic stem cell transplantation for hematological malignancies in Europe. *Leukaemia* 2003;17:941–959.

Greten TF & Jaffee EM. Cancer vaccines. *J Clin Oncol* 1999;17:1047–1060.

Kolb HJ & Holler E. Hematopoietic transplantation: state of the art. *Stem Cells* 1997;15(Suppl 1):151–157; discussion 158.

Laupacis A & Fergusson D., for The International Study of Peri-operative Transfusion (ISPOT) Investigators. Erythropoietin to minimize perioperative blood transfusion: a systematic review of randomized trials. *Transfus Med* 1998;8:309–317.

Slavin S. Immunotherapy of cancer with alloreactive lymphocytes. *Lancet Oncol* 2001;2;491–498.

Socie G, Stone JV, Wingard JR *et al.* Long-term survival and late deaths after allogeneic bone marrow transplantation. *N Engl J Med* 1999;341:14–21.

Storek, Joseph A, Espino I *et al.* Immunity of patients surviving 20 to 30 years after allogeneic or syngeneic bone marrow transplantation. *Blood* 2001;98:3505–3512.

Thomas ED. Does BMT confer a normal life span? *N Engl J Med* 1999;341:50–51.

Web resources

European Group for Blood and Marrow Transplantation (EBMT). Available at http://www.ebmt.org/.

International Bone Marrow Transplant Registry (IBMTR) and the Autologous Blood and Marrow Transplant Registry (ABMTR). Available at http://www.ibmtr.org. Web site of the International Allogeneic database and the Autologous database for North and South America.

CHAPTER 41

Cord blood transplantation

Leandro de Padua Silva, Marcos de Lima, Elizabeth J. Shpall & Susan Armitage
Department of Stem Cell Transplantation and Cell Therapy, The University of Texas MD Anderson Cancer Center, Houston, Texas, USA

Rationale for cord blood transplantation

A variety of malignant or severe genetic diseases of the bone marrow (BM) or immune system can be treated by allogeneic haemopoietic stem cell (HSC) transplantation. This, however, is only an option if there is a suitable human leucocyte antigen (HLA)-matched donor. Approximately, 30% of patients requiring an allogeneic HSC transplant have a suitable family donor, the rest rely on unrelated BM registries. Unfortunately, many patients, particularly those from racial and ethnic minority groups that are underrepresented on donor registries, are unable to find a suitable donor. The reason for this is that a donor is more likely to be found within the same ethnic group as that of the patient. Moreover, the donor search process requires a significant amount of time (median 4 months) and a substantial proportion of donors are not available at the time of the request. Over the last decade, cord blood (CB) has increasingly been used an alternate source of HSC for such patients who otherwise would not find an HLA-matched donor.

Types of CB banking

CB can be collected and stored in a bank for a number of reasons:

Practical Transfusion Medicine, 3rd edition. Edited by Michael F. Murphy and Derwood H. Pamphilon. © 2009 Blackwell Publishing, ISBN: 978-1-4051-8196-9.

- Public banks collect altruistic donations for a potential match to any patient who has a disease treatable with allogeneic HSC therapy. This is a proven and increasingly common practice of social value.
- Sibling programmes store donations for a biological sibling who has a disease treatable by allogeneic HSC transplantation. This is also a proven medical practice.
- Commercial banks store CB for the following purposes:
  - Donor or the family may need them in the future for a disease treatable by HSC therapy. It should be noted that the likelihood of the stored blood being used is low, estimates range from 1 in 1400 to 1 in 20,000. Autologous CB may not be the best option – pre-leukaemic mutations or leukaemic cells may be present.
  - Possible future use in regenerative medicine: at present, although unique cell populations have been isolated in CB that have potential for tissue regeneration, there is no evidence that these cells can be used therapeutically for this purpose.

Advantages of CB as a source of haemopoietic stem cells

- Generally considered a waste product, CB is abundantly and readily available and can be harvested with no risk to either the donor mother or infant.

- Ethnic minority groups that are markedly underrepresented in BM donor registries can be targeted for CB collection. For example, the MD Anderson Cord Blood Bank stores approximately 50% of donations derived from minorities compared to only 22% in the National Marrow Donor Program.
- Ability to store fully tested and HLA-typed CB units (CBU) in the frozen state for immediate use, reducing the morbidity and mortality in patients associated with the long procurement times for BM.
- Absence of donor attrition.
- Low risk of viral transmission.
- Higher degree of HLA mismatch appears to be acceptable with a comparatively reduced risk of acute and chronic graft-versus-host disease (GVHD), possibly due to the naivety of the cells. This relative tolerance reduces the tissue-matching requirement and enables larger numbers of recipients to find a donor, resulting in the need for fewer CBU to be banked than the number of donors required for an effective BM registry.
- Strong graft-versus-leukaemia (GVL) effect.

Disadvantages of CB as a source of haemopoietic stem cells

- Only one donation can be obtained; the donor cannot be contacted again; impossibility of using donor lymphocytes for immunotherapy.
- The number of haemopoietic progenitor cells in a CBU is limited and is reflected by longer engraftment times compared to bone marrow transplant (BMT). Eurocord group recommend a minimum nucleated cell (NC) dose of 3×10^7/kg for malignant diseases and 4.9×10^7/kg for non-malignant disorders.
- The donor may have a genetic disease of the marrow or immune system, which is not apparent at the time of donation, but could be transmissible by transplantation.

Ethics and consent issues of CB banking

The ethical issues associated with CB banking are complex and include the following.

- 'Ownership' of CB and issues of consent, with varying views on who 'owns' the cord: the neonate, the mother, the CB bank or the community.
- Controversy exists regarding the most appropriate method of collection. With in utero collection, there is less delay, increase in the collection volume and reduced incidence of clotted collections. Issues of privacy and intrusion complicate collection at this time for the mother in the delivery suite and a potential conflict of interest on the part of the professionals caring for the mother/infant pair as they undertake the collection.
- Intrusion into the confidentiality and convenience of the donor, especially with regard to infectious and genetic testing, must be balanced against safety of the recipient.
- In the context of directed collections, antenatal tissue typing and screening for genetic diseases could be undertaken on potential donors, and result in the elective abortion of fetuses with genetic disease or those which are not a tissue-type match for the intended recipient.
- The content of the informed consent process should include all the aspects detailed in Table 41.1.

Operation of CB banking

The process of CB banking is conducted in different ways at different centres. Figure 41.1 details the operational processes common to banks. Close collaboration and clear definition of roles and responsibilities between the bank and the participating obstetric units is essential, whether the obstetric unit staff participate in the collection and donor interview process or these steps are carried out independently by CB bank staff.

On release from quarantine, following review of all donor and donation data, CB units are made available for search through national and international registries.

A number of sources provide guidance regarding quality standards that should be applied to CB banking, developed to establish good practice, facilitate donor search and improve the quality of the graft. A large majority of banks follow either the international FACT (Foundation for the Accreditation

Table 41.1 Consent for unrelated cord blood banking.

- Collection and storage of CB for transplantation into unrelated individuals worldwide
- Possible risks and benefits to mother and/or infant, including medical and ethical concerns
- Maintenance of linkage for the purpose of notifying infant family of communicable or genetic diseases
- Examination of the mother's and infant's relevant medical notes and dialogue with relevant clinical professionals
- Permission for microbiological testing, including for HIV, and for the donor to be counselled in the event of results relevant to their health
- Storage of samples for future testing
- Storage of personal information
- Right of the mother to refuse without prejudice
- Research and development use if the donation is unsuitable for clinical use

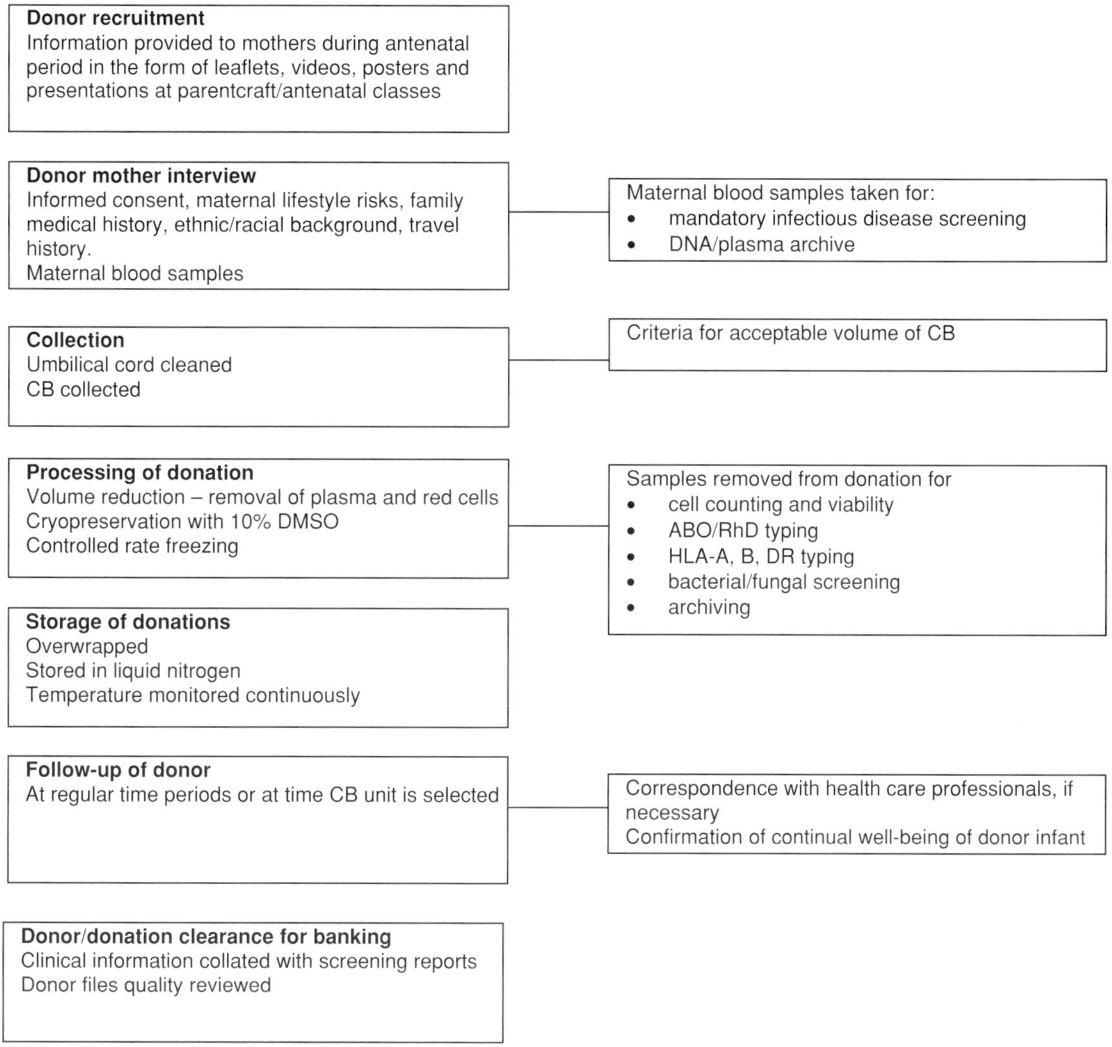

Donor recruitment
Information provided to mothers during antenatal period in the form of leaflets, videos, posters and presentations at parentcraft/antenatal classes

Donor mother interview
Informed consent, maternal lifestyle risks, family medical history, ethnic/racial background, travel history.
Maternal blood samples

Maternal blood samples taken for:
- mandatory infectious disease screening
- DNA/plasma archive

Collection
Umbilical cord cleaned
CB collected

Criteria for acceptable volume of CB

Processing of donation
Volume reduction – removal of plasma and red cells
Cryopreservation with 10% DMSO
Controlled rate freezing

Samples removed from donation for
- cell counting and viability
- ABO/RhD typing
- HLA-A, B, DR typing
- bacterial/fungal screening
- archiving

Storage of donations
Overwrapped
Stored in liquid nitrogen
Temperature monitored continuously

Follow-up of donor
At regular time periods or at time CB unit is selected

Correspondence with health care professionals, if necessary
Confirmation of continual well-being of donor infant

Donor/donation clearance for banking
Clinical information collated with screening reports
Donor files quality reviewed

Figure 41.1 Cord blood banking operations.

of Cellular Therapy)–Netcord or American Association of Blood Banks (AABB) standards for CB Banking. The EU Directive on Tissues and Cells requires Member States to have inspection and accreditation systems in place to ensure that all facilities providing these services comply with an agreed set of standards. The Food and Drug Administration (FDA) in the US has also proposed new regulations for human cellular and tissue-based products and is developing licensure for CB banking.

Reducing the risk of transplant-transmitted disease and infection

Strategies are required to minimise the risk of infections and genetic disease transmission through cord blood transplantation (CBT). Volunteer BM donors would probably manifest any genetic disease at the time they volunteer. This may not be the case for the infant donor of CB; hence, the need arises for specific screening for haematological abnormalities including thalassaemia and sickle-cell disease, particularly in donors from ethnic/racial groups known to be at higher risk for these conditions.

Donor testing

Mandatory infectious disease screening of the CB donation is performed by testing the donor mothers at the time of donation for human immunodeficiency virus (HIV) type 1 and 2, hepatitis C virus (HCV), human T-cell leukaemia virus (HTLV) I and II, hepatitis B virus (HBV), cytomegalovirus (CMV) and syphilis. Additional testing may be required at the time of selection of a unit for transplantation to include the requirements of the transplant centre, e.g. toxoplasmosis and Epstein–Barr virus (EBV). It is common practice to screen samples of the CB unit for these mandatory markers at the time of selection.

Extra mandatory tests or improved testing technologies may have been introduced in the period between donation and selection, or the country of import may have additional testing requirements. For such purposes, aliquots of both maternal and CB samples are archived.

Clinical results of CB transplantation

The first successful sibling CB transplant, for Fanconi's anaemia, in 1988, paved the way for other sibling transplants, followed by unrelated transplants. It has been estimated that over 10,000 patients have undergone CBT worldwide. The majority of studies reported over the last few years were retrospective multi-centre analyses; the vast majority of the transplants report 1–2 HLA antigen mismatches between donor and recipient, with significant number of patients in advanced stage of disease and with relatively short follow-up. Neutrophil and platelet recovery after CBT are significantly delayed compared with BM; the median time to neutrophil recovery ranges between 20 and 30 days, and cumulative rates of engraftment between 80 and 90%. Multiple studies demonstrate the devastating impact of low NC dose on engraftment, transplant-related mortality (TRM) and survival. This limiting cell dose particularly contributes to the inferior haemopoietic recovery and increased TRM in adults receiving a single unit CBT.

Increasing data demonstrates the critical importance of HLA match on CBT outcome. Increasing the cell dose overcomes the effect of HLA mismatches, conversely improved HLA match can compensate for lower cell dose. In non-malignant diseases, survival is affected by HLA mismatches. However, in malignant diseases, HLA mismatches were found not to influence survival because of the need for a GVL effect.

CBT in children

Clinical studies demonstrate slower but complete haemopoietic reconstitution in the majority of patients (see Table 41.2). Factors associated with speed of neutrophil recovery vary between studies, but most include NC dose. The incidence of severe acute GVHD is lower, despite HLA mismatches. TRM, relapse rate and overall survival are at least comparable with BM. Reports from the Institute of Medicine in the US indicate that CB is now the primary source of HSC for transplantation in children.

Table 41.2 Summary of studies comparing CBT with HSC sources in paediatric patients.

Author	HSC source	n	Median age (range)	Cell dose (range) ($\times 10^7$/kg)	Time to ANC >500 × 10^3/mL (days)	aGVHD II–IV (%)	Severe cGVHD (%)	Relapse (%)	Survival (%)	TRM (%)
Rocha *et al.*	CB related	113	5 (<1–15)	4.7 (<10–36)	26	14	6		14	64*
	BM related	2052	8 (<1–15)	35 (<10–410)	18	26	16		12	66*
Rocha *et al.*	CB unrelated	99	6 (2.5–10)	3.8 (2.4–36)	32	26	25	38		35†
	BM unrelated	262	8 (5–12)	42 (14–56)	18	39	46	39		49†
	T-cell depleted BM unrelated	180	36 (6–12)	38 (11–53)	16	30	12	47		41†

* 3 years' survival
† 2 years' survival

HSC, haemopoietic stem cell; aGVHD, acute graft-versus-host disease; cGVHD, chronic graft-versus-host disease; TRM, transplant-related mortality; BM, bone marrow; ANC, absolute neutrophil count.

Related CB transplantation

• Primarily of interest in the unrelated setting, CB has been successfully used in related transplants for malignant and non-malignant diseases. An early study of 102 children receiving CBT for acute leukaemia reported 42 children received a related donor transplant; 12 received a mismatched graft; neutrophil engraftment was 84% and a 2-year event-free survival was 41%. An NC dose of 3.7×10^7/kg correlated with engraftment.

• Eurocord analysed results of 44 children receiving related CBT for thalassaemia ($n = 33$) and sickle-cell disease ($n = 11$). Engraftment was obtained in 86.4% of transplants, no patient died and one patient with sickle-cell disease did not have sustained donor engraftment as compared with seven of the thalassaemic patients. The 2-year probability of event-free survival is 79% for thalassaemia and 90% for sickle-cell disease. Thalassaemia and sickle-cell disease are among the most common genetic disorders, affecting several million children and young adults worldwide and may be well suited to treatment with related CBT, where the need for a GVL effect is not required.

• Although there have been no randomised studies between CB and BM transplantation, retrospective matched-pair analyses have been performed. Rocha and colleagues compared 113 related CB recipients with 2052 related BM recipients treated for both malignant and non-malignant diseases. The incidence of acute and chronic GVHD was significantly reduced after CBT compared with BM – 15% and 6% compared to 24% and 16%, respectively. The mortality was similar between the two groups.

Unrelated CB transplantation

• A series of 562 recipients in multiple centres, transplanted with CB provided by the New York CBB was published in 1998. In this analysis, 20% of patients were under 2 years of age, 47% between the ages of 2 and 11 and 18% were over 18. In all 67% of recipients had leukaemia or lymphoma and 24% had genetic diseases. The most common leukaemias were acute lymphoid leukaemia (ALL) and acute myeloid leukaemia (AML). Genetic diseases included Fanconi's anaemia, severe combined immune deficiency and a variety of rarer disorders such as Hurler's syndrome and

Wiskott–Aldrich syndrome. Engraftment was 81% and risk of grade III–IV acute GVHD was 23%. The study indicated that younger age and a higher infused NC dose correlated with improved engraftment and survival.

- A study reported results of CBT in children with acute leukaemia. Analysis of 95 children with AML demonstrated a 2-year leukaemia-free survival (LFS) of 42% in patients transplanted in first remission, 50% in second remission and 21% in children not in remission. Analysis of 195 children with ALL produced a 2-year LFS rate of 36% in patients transplanted in remission and 15% in patients transplanted in relapse. A comparative study of children transplanted for acute leukaemia with either unrelated 1 or 2 antigen mismatched CB, unrelated matched or 1 antigen mismatched BM or unrelated T-cell depleted BM, showed delayed engraftment and an increased number of early deaths in the first 100 days in the CB group and decreased GVHD in the CB and T-cell depleted groups. The 2-year disease-free survival was comparable.

- A retrospective study compared the outcome of 503 children transplanted with CB (35 matched and 468 mismatched) for acute leukaemia to 282 BM recipients (116 matched and 166 mismatched) treated between 1995 and 2003. Typing of CB was at antigen level for HLA-A and -B and allele level for HLA-DR; BM was matched at allele level for HLA-A, -B, -C and -DR. The objective was to compare LFS. The median follow-up of survivors of BM and CB was 59 and 45 months, respectively. Rates of acute and chronic GVHD were similar in both groups. TRM rates were higher following transplant of the two antigen mismatched CB and one antigen mismatched CB with a cell dose of $<3 \times 10^7$/kg. Relapse rates were lower following the two antigen mismatched CBT which could be consistent with a more potent GVL effect. The 5-year LFS rate was 60% for matched CB, 45% one-antigen mismatched, CB with a cell dose $> 3 \times 10^7$/kg, 38% for matched BM, 37% for mismatched BM, 36% for one-antigen mismatched CB with a cell dose $< 3 \times 10^7$/kg and 33% for two-antigen mismatched CB.

- CBT has also been shown to be effective in a number of congenital and metabolic storage disorders, including Hurler syndrome, Krabbe disease and immunodeficiency. One of the advantages of using CB in these situations is that rapidly progressive disorders can be treated quickly. Martin *et al.* described outcomes of the 69 paediatrics patients transplanted for lysosomal and peroxisomal storage diseases (LSDs), without prior treatment. The median age of the patients was 1.8 years median cell counts were total nucleated cell (TNC) 8.7×10^7/kg and CD34+ 2.4×10^5/kg and matched at a minimum of three out of six HLA loci with high resolution typing. Overall survival was 72% in 1 year, with median neutrophil engraftment of 25 days. Acute GVHD was the primary cause of death, with infections as a contributing cause. CBT offers a good option to young patients with LSD without previous therapy.

CBT in adults

Progress of CBT in adults has been slower. Initial reports were poor, largely due to a combination of advanced disease status, low cell dose and high degree of HLA mismatch, which manifested in slow engraftment, high TRM and poor survival. Recent studies have established CBT as a safe and feasible alternative to BMT in adults when no sibling donor is available.

- A retrospective analysis of data provided to the Eurocord–Netcord group by 63 centres in 13 countries, on 171 uprelated cord blood transplants (UCBT) in adults with haematological malignancies was reported. In this analysis, 110 (64%) patients received an irradiation-based conditioning regimen and 61 (36%) busulfan-based conditioning. HLA disparities were a minimum of three out of six by high resolution, the medium CD34+ and TNC cells infused were 1.0×10^5/kg and 2.1×10^7/kg, respectively. The medium neutrophil recovery was 28 days. The cumulative incidence (CI) was 32% for acute GVHD grade II–IV at 100 days post-transplant and for chronic GVHD 36% at 2 years. CI for relapse, overall survival and disease-free survival was 22%, 33% and 27%, respectively, at 2 years. The chance of being alive with no disease at 2 years was 41%, 34% and 18% for patients transplanted in early, intermediate and advanced phase of disease, respectively.

• Three retrospective studies reported in 2004, one single centre and two registry based, compared CBT with unrelated BMT in adults (Table 41.3). The age range between the groups was similar but the NC dose was one log less in the CB grafts. Neutrophil and platelet recovery was significantly delayed and graft failure was higher following CBT. Despite a higher degree of mismatch of the CBU incidence of grade II–IV, acute GVHD was similar or lower to that seen with BM. Relapse rates were similar. However, TRM and survival results are less conclusive (see Table 41.3). It should be noted that only two key studies evaluated patients receiving transplants after 1998, following published data indicting improved criteria for the selection of CBU. The superior results in the Japanese study may reflect the smaller cohort size and the genetic homogeneity of the population.

• The Eurocord group analysed 682 adults with acute leukaemia reported to the Eurocord and the European Blood and Marrow Transplant group from 1998 through 2002. Ninety-eight patients received CB and 584 patients received BM. The recipients of CB were younger than BM recipients (median 24.5 versus 32 years of age) and had more advanced disease at transplant (52% versus 33%). The BM group was HLA-matched and 94% of CB grafts were HLA-mismatched. The incidence of acute GVHD, TRM, relapsed rate and leukaemia-free survival was not significantly different between either groups (see Table 41.2).

Multiple CBT

To address the problem of low cell dose, particularly in adult patients, the use of multiple CBT was proposed. Double transplant, using partially matched CBU, in both the myeloablative and non-myeloablative setting has been shown to be both safe and efficacious. Data indicate that rapid neutrophil engraftment, with the ultimate predominance of a single CB is achieved. There are still a number of questions to be answered relating to the degree of acceptable mismatch between the two CBU and the patient, the effects of acute GVHD and risk of relapse.

• A study comparing outcomes from single or double CBT for patients with acute leukaemia reported

sustained neutrophil engraftment and TRM were virtually the same. However, there was a three-fold higher incidence of grades III–IV acute GVHD among recipients of the double CBT, but no difference in incidence of grades III–IV or chronic GVHD. Results of multivariate analysis indicated that double CBT was associated with a 10-fold lower risk of relapse than single transplants.

• The same group reported the use of double CBT in the non-myeloablative setting, extending the availability of transplantation to those patients who are unable to find a suitable BM donor and are at increased risk of regimen-related toxicity and TRM, such as the older or heavily treated patients.

CB expansion

Expansion of CB progenitor cells ex vivo could potentially ameliorate inadequate haemopoietic recovery by generating higher numbers of cells responsible for short-term reconstitution. Preliminary clinical results have demonstrated safety of infusing ex vivo expanded cells into patients. Ongoing preclinical and clinical studies will hopefully define the optimal culture conditions to enable this technology to be used in CBT.

Future directions

Novel strategies currently under investigation are focused on developing strategies to further improve engraftment, immune reconstitution, transplant-related mortality, risk of relapse and survival following CBT:

• ex vivo cell expansion to augment HSC and progenitor cell number;
• use of haploidentical HSC to ameliorate the prolonged period of neutropenia following CBT;
• methods to minimise non-specific loss of circulating HSC and enhance homing to the marrow; and
• adoptive immunotherapy.

A potential future use for CB may be in the regenerative medicine field. A number of workers have revealed the possibility of differentiating CB stem cells into diverse tissue-specific stem cell progenitors with bone, fat and neural markers, under specific culture conditions.

Table 41.3 Summary of studies comparing CBT with other unrelated HSC sources in adult patients.

Author	Study period	HSC source	n	Median age (range)	Cell dose (range) ($\times 10^7$/kg)	aGVHD II–IV (%)	Severe cGVHD (%)	Relapse (%)	TRM (%)	LFS (%)	Time to ANC > 500 × 10^3/mL (days)
Takahashi et al.	1998–2001	CB	68	36 (16–53)	2.5 (1.1–5.3)	22	30	13	16	9	74
		BM matched	45	26 (16–50)	33 (6.6–50)	18	30	14	25	29	44
Rocha et al.	1998–2002	CB	98	25 (15–55)	2.3 (0.9–6.0)	26	26	30	23	44	33
		BM matched	584	32 (15–59)	29 (<10–90)	19	39	46	23	38	38
Laughlin et al.	1996–2001	CB	150	(16–60)	2.2 (1.0–6.5)	27	41	33	17	63	23
		BM matched	367	(16–60)	24 (0.2–170)	18	48	52	23	46	33
		BM mismatched	83	(16–60)	22 (0.1–58)	20	52	71	14	65	19

HSC, haemopoietic stem cell; aGVHD, acute graft-versus-host disease; cGVHD, chronic graft-versus-host disease; TRM, transplant-related mortality; BM, bone marrow; LFS, leukaemia-free survival.

Summary

Early reports of CBT left a number of unanswered questions and obstacles regarding the reliability of CB stem cells to provide long-term haemopoietic and immune reconstitution. It has become clear over the last decade that CB is an effective and safe alternative source of HSC for transplantation to patients lacking a suitable related or unrelated BM donor, in both the paediatric and adult settings. Literature shows that following CBT with a well-selected unit, the relapse rate, disease-free survival and overall survival of patients with myeloid malignancies are similar to other HSC sources. Initial concerns regarding the potency of the GVL effect of CB have been dismissed by several publications showing relapse rates similar to those with other HSC sources. Improving the engraftment rate by increasing cell dose and optimising HLA match is the key to expanding the use of CB. Increasing cell dose improves survival and decreases the effect of HLA mismatches.

With development of new strategies and a better understanding of selection of a CBU, it is anticipated that in the next few years the use of CB will expand as a useful source of HSC and as a source of immune effectors cells or non-HSC populations.

Key Points

1 CB is an effective and safe alternative source of HSC for transplantation in patients lacking a suitable related and unrelated bonor marrow donor, this is of particular importance for racial and ethnic minorities.

2 CB has the potential to resolve the limitations of search time, donor availability and the lack of suitable matched donors for many patients.

3 The incidence of severe acute GVHD, following a CB transplant, is lower, despite HLA mismatches. TRM, relapse rate and overall survival are at least comparable with BM.

4 Increasing data demonstrates the critical importance of HLA match on CBT outcome. Increasing the cell dose appears to overcome the effect of HLA mismatches, conversely improved HLA match can compensate for lower cell dose.

5 New preparative regimens combined with double CB transplants have demonstrated improved engraftment and survival in larger children and adult patients.

Further reading

Barker JN, Weisdorf DJ, DeFor TE *et al.* Transplantation of 2 partially HLA-matched umbilical cord blood units to enhance engraftment in adults with hematologic malignancy. *Blood* 2005;105:1343–1347.

Boelens JJ. Trends in haematopoietic cell transplantation for inborn errors of metabolism. *J Inherit Metab Dis* 2006;29:413–420.

Brunstein CG, Barker KS & Wagner JE. Umbilical cord blood transplantation for myeloid malignancies. *Curr Opin Hematol* 2007;14:162–169.

Brunstein CG, Setubal DC & Wagner JE. Expanding the role of umbilical cord blood transplantation. *Br J Haematol* 2007;137:20–35.

Eapen M, Rubinstein P, Zhang MJ *et al.* Outcomes of transplantation of unrelated donor umbilical cord blood and bone marrow in children with acute leukemia: a comparison study. *Lancet* 2007;369:1947–1954.

Gluckman E & Rocha V. Donor selection for unrelated cord blood transplants. *Curr Opin Immunol* 2006;18:565–570.

Laughlin MJ, Eapen M, Rubinstein P *et al.* Outcomes after transplantation of cord blood or bone marrow from unrelated donors in adults with leukemia. *N Engl J Med* 2004;351:2265–2275.

Locatelli F, Rocha V, Reed W *et al.* Related umbilical cord blood transplantation in patients with thalassemia and sickle cell disease. *Blood* 2003;101:2137–2143.

Martin PL, Carter SL, Kernan NA *et al.* Results of the Cord Blood Transplantation Study (COBLT): outcomes of unrelated donor umbilical cord blood transplantation in pediatric patients with lysosomal and peroxisomal storage diseases. *Biol Blood Marrow Transplant* 2006;12:184–194.

Rocha V, Cornish J, Sievers E *et al.* Comparison of outcomes of unrelated bone marrow and umbilical cord blood transplants in children with acute leukemia. *Blood* 2001;97:2962–2971.

Rocha V, Labopin M, Sanz G *et al.* Transplants of umbilical cord blood or bone marrow from unrelated donors in adults with acute leukemia. *N Engl J Med* 2004;351:2276–2285.

Takahashi S, Iseki T, Ooi J *et al.* Single-institute comparative analysis of unrelated bone marrow transplantation and cord blood transplantation for adult patients with hematologic malignancies. *Blood* 2004;104:3873–3820.

CHAPTER 42

Recent advances in clinical cellular immunotherapy

Mark W. Lowdell[1] & Emma Morris[2]

[1]University College London Medical School; Royal Free Hospital, London, UK
[2]Department of Immunology and Molecular Pathology, University College London Medical School, University College London Hospitals NHS Trust, London, UK

Introduction

Immunotherapy in the form of vaccination has been part of medical practice since Jenner in the eighteenth century. This, so-called, 'Active' immunisation requires that the recipient has the capacity to mount an immune response against the antigens within the vaccine. In contrast, the infusion of antibodies or immune cells raised in other animals or individuals, in response to deliberate vaccination or prior antigen exposure, into patients at risk of infection; 'Passive' immunisation allows treatment of immunodeficient or immunocompromised patients.

Until recently, infusion of pathogen-specific anti-sera was the only routine form of passive immunotherapy; equine anti-tetanus anti-sera is a well-known example. Successful passive cellular immunotherapy requires precise matching of donor–recipient histocompatibility antigens and thus advances in human leucocyte antigen (HLA)-typing over the past 40 years has allowed this form of immunotherapy to move closer to routine treatment.

Practical Transfusion Medicine, 3rd edition. Edited by Michael F. Murphy and Derwood H. Pamphilon. © 2009 Blackwell Publishing, ISBN: 978-1-4051-8196-9.

Cellular immunotherapy in haemopoietic progenitor cell transplantation

The anti-leukaemic activity of allogeneic bone marrow transplantation was first described, in murine experiments, more than 40 years ago but was appreciated in the clinic only in the late 1970s when attempts at preventing graft-versus-host disease (GvHD) by T-cell depletion were sometimes frustrated by an increase in the risk of leukaemia recurrence. The clinical anti-leukaemic effect of GvHD was first reported in 1979 and confirmed later by registry data from the International Bone Marrow Transplant Registry (IBMTR). The observed benefit of GvHD was particularly evident in patients transplanted for chronic myeloid leukaemia and led to the trial of post-transplant infusions of donor leucocytes (DLIs). The first peer-reviewed report of DLI therapy included a single patient who achieved molecular remission with no evidence of clinical GvHD, supporting the hypothesis that graft-versus-leukaemia (GvL) could be directed at leukaemia-specific or leukaemia-restricted target antigens. GvHD after DLI remained a significant clinical problem which has been somewhat ameliorated by the use of incremental doses of DLI but the search for the 'holy grail' of leukaemia-specific GvL in the complete absence of GvHD continues to be an active research theme.

Non-specific T-cell immunotherapy

A pragmatic approach to the dissection of GvHD from GvL was the concept of removal of alloreactive T cells from donor grafts whilst retaining non-alloreactive cells which could mediate GvL and anti-viral responses. These approaches were all based upon ex vivo stimulation of allogeneic donor T cells with normal haemopoietic cells from the recipient to provoke a clinical-scale mixed lymphocyte response. Reacting T cells were then identified by the expression of one or more activation antigens (e.g. CD25 and CD69) and depleted by immunotoxin or immunomagnetic selection. Whilst possibly successful in the reduction of GvHD, the clinical trials of this approach showed no evidence of a GvL effect although anti-viral immune responses have been enhanced in some cases. The principal criticism of these studies was that too few allodepleted T cells were infused to definitively test the hypothesis that GvHD was prevented. Subsequently, an extremely thorough study of the nature of alloreactive T-cell activation in vitro in a mixed lymphocyte reaction concluded that the oligoclonal T-cell response is random and hence unpredictable from day to day. These data demonstrated that not all alloreactive T-cell clones will activate in a single mixed cell reaction and thus clinically relevant minor alloreactive T cells are likely to remain and induce GvHD upon infusion.

Another non-specific approach has been the selective depletion of CD8 T cells from DLI. Based upon the fact that the target cells of GvHD mostly lack expression of HLA class II, it has been considered that infusions of allogeneic CD4 T cells induce less GvHD. Many haemopoietic malignancies express HLA class II antigens and are potential targets for CD4 T cells. Evidence of GvL, resolution of mixed T-cell chimerism and improved anti-viral immunity in the absence of GvHD have all been reported in the clinical trials of CD8-depleted DLI. Trials of this form of immunotherapy are continuing and are reporting encouraging results with respect to reversal of mixed chimerism and GvL.

Tumour-specific or tumour-restricted T-cell immunotherapy

Unselected DLI currently remains the mainstay of anti-tumour cellular immunotherapy following haemopoietic progenitor cell (HPC) transplantation; however, tumour antigen-specific T-cell responses can be generated by vaccination or by the generation of tumour antigen-specific T cells for adoptive transfer. T-cell-recognised tumour antigens can be divided into two main categories:

• The first is known as tumour-specific antigens (TSAs), and the genes encoding TSA are present only in tumour cells and not in normal tissues.
• The second group, called tumour-associated antigens (TAAs), is expressed at elevated levels in tumour cells but are also present in normal cells.

The majority of T-cell-recognised tumour antigens in humans are TAAs. The significance of this is that a low level of gene expression in normal cells can lead to the inactivation of high avidity T cells by immunological tolerance mechanisms. As a consequence, low avidity T-cell responses in patients are often inadequate in providing tumour protection. Therefore, TSAs are theoretically the most desirable target antigens for cellular immunotherapy (vaccination or adoptive transfer), as there is no pre-existing immunological self-tolerance, and TSA-specific immune responses are unlikely to damage normal tissues. Unfortunately, TSAs with specific mutations are often invisible to cytotoxic T lymphocyte (CTL) as a result of impaired antigen presentation due to competition with normal cellular antigens for proteasomal degradation, transportation by TAP molecules and binding to major histocompatibility complex (MHC). To date, most tumour antigens identified as CTL targets are TAAs.

The majority of anti-tumour vaccination trials in humans have been against melanoma antigens and not in the context of stem cell transplantation. In these situations, vaccination can lead to TAA or TSA reactive CTL responses, but this has rarely corresponded to a clinical benefit.

Recently, vaccination against Wilms' tumour antigen 1 (WT1, a leukaemia-associated antigen) has been shown to induce WT1-specific T-cell responses in patients with myeloid malignancies. In the next 5 years, it is anticipated that phase I/II clinical trials will test whether vaccination against WT1 epitopes early post-transplant can augment the reconstitution of WT1-specific CTL and act as maintenance immunotherapy.

T-cell receptor gene transfer

The inability to generate antigen-specific T cells is a serious limitation of adoptive cellular therapy for cancer. As discussed above, tumour antigens are often poorly immunogenic and patients are frequently immunocompromised as a consequence of tumour burden or as a result of previous therapies. T-cell receptor (TCR) gene transfer offers a strategy to produce antigen-specific T cells independent of precursor frequency. Over the last 5 years, TCR gene transfer has been demonstrated to reliably redirect the antigen-specificity of a given population of T cells via the introduction of a cloned TCR using retroviral transduction. This allows for the rapid generation and expansion of tumour antigen-specific T cells. Both the specificity and avidity

of the TCR-transduced T cells are similar to the parental CTL clone from which the TCR has been isolated. Tumour antigen-specific TCR-transduced T cells have been shown to provide tumour protection in murine models and result in re-call responses up to 3 months post-adoptive transfer. Recently, the first clinical trial using TCR-transduced T cells has been published which demonstrated that TCR-transduced autologous T cells can have an anti-tumour effect in melanoma patients. Patient T cells were transduced with a retroviral construct encoding the alpha- and beta-chains of the MART-1-specific TCR. This milestone study demonstrated the feasibility and potential of TCR gene therapy. However, further modifications are required to the approach in order to maximise the clinical benefit. These include modifications of the TCR construct to enhance cell surface expression of the introduced TCR and reduce the incidence of mis-pairing with endogenous alpha- and beta-chains (Figure 42.1), optimisation of the conditioning regimen used prior to adoptive transfer and the generation of functional TCR-transduced helper T cells.

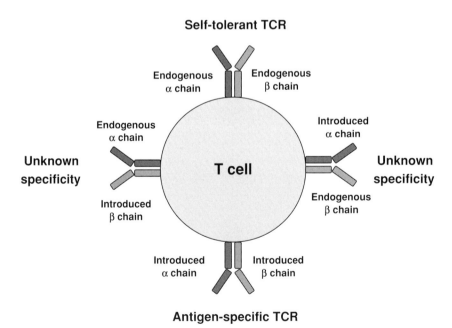

Figure 42.1 Schematic illustrating mis-pairing with endogenous TCR chains by the introduced TCR chains following retroviral TCR gene transfer.

Tumour-restricted natural killer cell immunotherapy

Some of the earliest trials of anti-tumour cellular immunotherapy were based upon infusion of NK cell-activating cytokines or of ex vivo activated NK cells. Most of the early trials were in the autologous setting and, with the notable exception of a single report of acute myeloid leukaemia (AML) patients after autologous HPC transplant, were uniformly disappointing. However, these early trials were conducted before the complex mechanisms underlying NK cell function were understood.

Human NK cells are controlled by a variety of inhibitory and stimulatory signals through cell surface receptors which allow them to distinguish between normal and malignant or infected cells. These receptors fall into one of four families:

• killer immunoglobulin-like receptor (KIR);
• C-type lectins;
• immunoglobulin-like transcript (ILT); and
• natural cytotoxicity receptors (NCRs).

The first two families include both inhibitory and activating receptors whilst the ILT and NCR families contain only activating receptors. All human NK cells express multiple receptors from each family and it is now apparent that functional subsets of NK cells exist.

In the 1980s, Klaus Karre first demonstrated that murine NK cells preferentially lysed MHC class I-negative tumours. This led him to construct his 'missing self' hypothesis in which he proposed that NK cells are inhibited from lysis of normal cells which express MHC class I, but are capable of lysing MHC class I-negative tumour cells. Murine NK cells express surface receptors for MHC class I molecules and their ligation transduces inhibitory signals which prevent NK-mediated lysis. As implied above, the human NK regulatory system is more complex. KIRs bind to HLA class I molecules and the majority transduce inhibitory signals upon ligation by their specific HLA class I ligand. KIR molecules are classified on the basis of the number of extracellular domains and the length of the intracellular domain. For example:

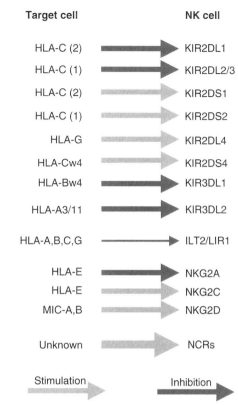

Figure 42.2 Ligands controlling NK cell activation and triggering.

• KIR2DL1 is a molecule with 2 extracellular domains and 1 long intracellular domain. This KIR binds to the family of HLA-C molecules with asparginine in position 77, the so-called 'type 2' HLA-C. The inhibitory signal is via an immunoreceptor tyrosine-based inhibitory motif (ITIM) in the long intracellular domain;
• KIR2DL2, in contrast, binds to the remaining 'type 1' HLA-C molecules, those with a serine in position 77;
• KIR3DL1 binds to HLA-Bw4 alleles;
• KIR3DL2 binds HLA-A3 or A11 alleles; and
• other KIRs have been shown to bind HLA-G (Figure 42.2).

In a co-culture of NK cells, autologous normal cells and HLA class I-deficient tumour cells, one can demonstrate the co-localisation of the KIR:HLA interaction between the NK and normal cell whilst the tumour cells show no such signalling

Given the concept that NK cells are 'kept in check' by inhibitory signals initiated through binding HLA molecules on normal somatic cells one might imagine that the KIR repertoire of any given individual is determined by their HLA type. This is not, however, the case and many healthy individuals will maintain NK cell clones which lack the appropriate inhibitory KIR molecules. However, the C-type lectin, NKG2A, which forms a heterodimer with CD94, appears to be universally expressed on human NK cells and presumably can provide the requisite inhibitory signals through its ligation to HLA-E.

The clinical relevance of the understanding of NK cell inhibition is evident in haploidentical HPC transplantation where certain HLA class I mismatches generate a situation of HLA:KIR incompatibility. Highly significant reductions in relapse have been reported among AML patients receiving HLA:KIR incompatible haploidentical HPC grafts compared to patients receiving grafts in which the donor NK repertoire is matched to the HLA type of the patient.

Whilst these data stand on their own merit, much remains to be done to understand the mechanisms behind their results since the KIR effect seems to be limited to excessively T-cell-depleted haploidentical grafts and there is little or no role for CD94/NKG2A or for the activating receptors which appear so important in autologous NK cell function.

The implication from the haploidentical transplant data is that the lack of KIR-mediated NK cell inhibition is sufficient to initiate NK activation and lysis. However, since the patients with known KIR:HLA incompatibility did not experience NK-mediated GvHD, one must assume that normal cells failing to inhibit NK cells were spared. NK-activating signals may be provided via numerous receptors although their ligands remain largely unknown. Recent published work has shown that, like T cells, NK cells generally require more than one signal to initiate cytokine secretion or lysis and that these signals may need to be provided sequentially to the cell.

Despite the lack of a complete understanding of human NK biology, the clinical trials of allogeneic NK immunotherapy are already underway and some have been reported.

A remarkable study in which minimally conditioned patients with AML received bolus infusions of partially enriched IL2-activated NK cells from HLA-mismatched donors without concomitant HPC transplant showed engraftment of donor NK cells in the presence of recipient T, B and myeloid cells. At the highest NK dose and the greatest level of pre-infusion conditioning with cyclophosphamide and fludarabine 5 of 19 patients achieved complete remission. Donor NK cells were detected in their peripheral blood and bone marrow. Despite the engraftment of haplo-mismatched NK cells, the patients maintained normal bone marrow function and normal levels of autologous T cells, B cells and granulocytes.

The anti-leukaemic effect was relatively short-lived in this trial, but the data support the safety of such an approach and it is possible that such patients could receive multiple courses of NK cell infusions to maintain control of residual disease. The concept of repetitive passive cellular immunotherapy is novel and contrary to the design of most current approaches which have been conceived within a mindset of 'cure by vaccination'. However, most tumour antigens elicit relatively weak immune responses and the physiological immune response to tumours may be one of control rather than eradication.

Passive cellular immunotherapy of infectious disease

Possibly the most remarkable clinical results from cellular immunotherapies have been seen in the treatment of opportunistic viral infections in immunocompromised patients. Most of these trials have been in the post-transplant setting, particularly in recipients of allogeneic HPC grafts:
• the earliest studies involving infusion of enormous numbers of cloned cytomegalovirus (CMV)-reactive CD8 T cells which caused resolution of refractory CMV disease in patients post-allogeneic

haematopoietic progenitor cell transplant (HPCT); and

• subsequently, others elegantly demonstrated the specific resolution of post-transplant EBV-driven lymphoma following infusion of donor-derived anti-Epstein Barr Virus (EBV) CTLs.

Ex vivo generation of very large numbers of anti-viral T cells is complex and expensive. However, in 2003, a phase I trial of allogeneic donor-derived CMV-reactive T cells grown for 21–28 days ex vivo on monocyte-derived dendritic cells which were pulsed with fixed whole CMV was reported. These expanded cells were infused into patients with molecular evidence of CMV reactivation post-allogeneic HPCT and 8 out of 16 patients resolved the reactivation without recourse to anti-viral chemotherapy. No patient received a dose greater than 10^5 T cells per kilogram body weight and the average dose of CMV-specific T cells in each dose was no greater than 200–300 per kilogram. Despite this incredibly low dose of cells, virus-specific T cells were detectable in the peripheral blood of responding recipients at levels equivalent to a 35,000-fold expansion. The small numbers of cells infused in this demonstrated that the production of donor-specific cell therapies could be cost-effective.

Despite the acknowledged clinical success of these trials, neither led to the wide-scale adoption of cellular therapy due to the extreme technical complexity of cell therapy production. However, with recent advances in the availability of clinical-grade reagents and disposables, the translation of laboratory-grade procedures to clinical application has advanced rapidly. For several years, immunologists have been able to immunomagnetically select specifically activated T cells on the basis of the secretion of gamma-interferon and its capture on the cell surface with a bi-specific antibody. This patented technology is now produced to clinical grade and is already central to a number of trials including a phase III trial of allogeneic immunotherapy of CMV reactivation post-HPCT; the first multicentre randomised the clinical trial of directed donation cellular immunotherapy.

There is undoubted promise in the clinical application of cellular immunity and the field has advanced very substantially in the last 5 years. How-ever, the true potential of adoptive cellular immunotherapy remains constrained by the perceived need for directed donations (autologous or HLA-matched allogeneic) and by confusion over the regulatory framework in which the therapies fall. The first issue is the greatest barrier although some recent studies do support the feasibility of the ultimate goal of 'off the shelf' products. Haploidentical NK study discussed above used NK cells from HLA-mismatched donors and demonstrated transient engraftment. A group in Edinburgh recently used 'off the shelf' HLA-mismatched T-cell lines to treat post-transplant EBV lymphoma in recipients of renal transplants.

Technical advances facilitating translational research in cellular immunotherapy

In Europe, since the ratification of the EU Clinical Trials Directive in Member States in 2004, cellular immunotherapies have becomes susceptible to regulation as investigational medicinal products (IMPs). Whether a specific cell therapy product constitutes an IMP is determined by the relevant authority in each member state; but once a product is regulated as an IMP then production must meet good manufacturing practice (GMP) and this has been difficult in the field of cellular immunotherapy. However, a number of European companies now manufacture CE-marked reagents, consumables and devices for clinical-grade cell production. Closed and semi-closed systems are available for handling large volume cell suspensions. Gas-permeable cell culture and expansion bags allowing closed-system culture are now widely available and the availability of clinical-grade cytokines is improving.

One of the most significant advances in the field has been the development of CE-marked clinical-grade immunomagnetic cell sorters. These are now widely used for the specific selection of subsets of HPCs and other leucocytes and can even select antigen-reactive cells on the basis of cytokine secretion, multimeric HLA-peptide reagents or expression of activation markers.

As the regulatory position becomes clearer, more trials will be conducted to good clinical practice and the regulatory authorities will gather more evidence and experience of the field. In the not too distant future hospital blood banks may become more of a 'cell pharmacy' than ever before.

Key points

1 Allogeneic GvL by DLI is proof of principle of cellular immunotherapy.
2 Cellular immunotherapy of viral infections is becoming an alternative to anti-viral chemotherapy.
3 Need for HLA-matching may not be necessary.
4 Technical and regulatory difficulties in production of cell therapies are being overcome.

Further reading

Cobbold M, Khan N, Pourgheysari B *et al.* Adoptive transfer of CMV-specific CTL to stem cell transplant patients after selection by HLA-peptide tetramers. *J Exp Med* 2005;202:379–386.

Haque T, Wilkie GM, Jones MM *et al.* Allogeneic cytotoxic T cell therapy for EBV-positive PTLD: results of a phase II multicentre clinical trial. *Blood* 2007;110:1123–1131.

Horowitz MM, Gale RP, Sondel PM *et al.* Graft-versus-leukemia reactions after bone marrow transplantation. *Blood* 1990;75:555–562.

Kolb HJ, Mittermueller J, Clemm C *et al.* Donor leukocyte transfusion for treatment of recurrent chronic myelogenous leukemia in marrow transplant patients. *Blood* 1990;76:2462–2465.

Leen AM, Myers GD, Sili U *et al.* Monoculture-derived T lymphocytes specific for multiple viruses expand and produce clinically relevant effects in immunocompromised individuals. *Nat Med* 2006;12:1160–1166.

Mackinnon S, Thomson K, Verfuerth S, Peggs K & Lowdell MW. Adoptive cellular therapy for cytomegalovirus infection following allogeneic stem cell transplantation using virus-specific T-cells. *Blood Cells Mol Dis* 2008;40:63–67.

Miller JS, Soignier Y, Panoskaltis-Mortari A *et al.* Successful adoptive transfer and in vivo expansion of human haploidentical NK cells in patients with cancer. *Blood* 2005;105:3051–3057.

Shimoni A, Gajewski JA, Donato M *et al.* Long-term follow up of recipients of CD8-depleted DLI for the treatment of CML relapsing after allogeneic progenitor cell transplantation. *Biol Blood Marrow Transplant* 2001;7:568–575.

Xue SA & Stauss HJ. Enhancing immune responses for cancer therapy. *Cell Mol Immunol* 2007;4:173–184.

CHAPTER 43

Cytokines in transfusion practice

Derwood H. Pamphilon[1] *& Michael F. Murphy*[2]

[1]NHS Blood and Transplant; Department of Cellular and Molecular Medicine, University of Bristol, Bristol, UK
[2]University of Oxford; NHS Blood and Transplant and Department of Haematology, John Radcliffe Hospital, Oxford, UK

Introduction

Cytokines are soluble or membrane-bound factors that stimulate the growth of cells and tissues, including cells of the haemopoietic and lymphoid systems. They belong to a number of cytokine superfamilies and act as lineage-specific, multilineage, stem cell or accessory factors (Table 43.1). Many cytokines are produced using recombinant DNA technology (see Chapter 31).

The two principal ways in which cytokines are relevant to transfusion medicine are as stimulants of either haemopoietic or lymphopoietic activity.

1 *Haemopoietic activity*: Cytokines may be used to prevent or reduce cytopenia, e.g. the anaemia of chronic renal failure, and the neutropenia following chemotherapy for cancer. In these and other settings, cytokines are used to avoid the need for the transfusion of red cells, platelets and perhaps also granulocytes. This may help to minimise the risks associated with transfusion of blood components, e.g. microbiological contamination, acute lung injury and others discussed in previous chapters. The use of cytokines to mobilise peripheral blood stem cells (PBSCs) into the bloodstream also reduces the requirement for transfusion since PBSCs are associated with a shorter engraftment time than bone marrow stem cells (see Chapter 40).

Practical Transfusion Medicine, 3rd edition. Edited by Michael F. Murphy and Derwood H. Pamphilon. © 2009 Blackwell Publishing, ISBN: 978-1-4051-8196-9.

2 *Lymphopoietic activity*: Cytokines are used in the generation of dendritic cells and cytotoxic T lymphocytes for the immunotherapy of cancer and viral infections. The use of cytokine-generated immunotherapeutic cells such as dendritic cells does not impact directly on routine aspects of transfusion practice. However, it has become clear that blood centres have an important role to play in utilising their expertise in good manufacturing practice for the production of such cells.

This chapter is devoted mainly to the use of cytokines to reduce transfusions of donated blood components. It focuses on the use of erythropoietin (Epo) for the treatment of anaemia, thrombopoietic agents for the treatment of thrombocytopenia, and granulocyte colony-stimulating factor (G-CSF) for granulocyte collection and for the mobilisation of PBSC.

Erythropoiesis

Red cell development occurs during a 2-week period. The earliest erythroid precursor is the burst-forming unit, erythroid (BFU-E). These cells are small without specific cytological features and express the CD34 antigen found on most haemopoietic stem cells. Maturation occurs into the colony-forming unit, erythroid (CFU-E), which has deeply basophilic cytoplasm and represents about day 7 of development, immediately prior to the time of haemoglobinisation. Following this, cell size

Table 43.1 Cytokine superfamilies.

	Factor	Name(s)	Chromosome	Action	Application/clinical use
Lineage-specific factors	G-CSF*	Granulocyte colony-stimulating factor	17q11.2–21	Produces *granulocyte* colony-forming units in in vitro cultures	Mobilisation of peripheral blood stem cells Increases neutrophil counts after chemotherapy and BMT Granulocyte collection
	M-CSF (also known as CSF-1)	Monocyte colony-stimulating factor	1p13–21	Monocyte stimulation	No clinical applications
	EPO*	Erythropoietin	7q11–22	Stimulates erythropoiesis	Anaemia of renal failure Some effect in anaemia of malignancy As adjunct to autologous transfusion regimens
	TPO	Thrombopoietin	3q27–28	Stimulates platelet production	Platelet collection May speed platelet recovery after chemotherapy/BMT Immunogenicity of one TPO analogue has slowed clinical development
Multilineage factors	IL-5	Interleukin 5	5q31	Eosinophil stimulator	Research applications only
	IL-3	Multi-CSF	5q23–31	Acts on all lineages at colony-forming cell (CFC) stage	Actions on mast cells and basophils produce problematic adverse effects Likely value in in vitro culture applications in future
	GM-CSF*	Granulocyte – macrophage colony-stimulating factor	5q23–31	Acts on all CFCs in vitro	Mobilisation of PBSC Similar applications to G-CSF but more adverse events Possible role in management of fungal infections and wound healing

Stem cell factors	SCF	Steel factor, stem cell factor, *kit* ligand	12q2–24	Has synergistic effects on primitive precursor cells with IL-3, IL-6, IL-11	Clinical trials bedevilled with adverse events due to mast cell activation in vivo (asthma etc.) Likely use will be in vitro in haemopoietic stem cell expansion protocols
	FL	Flk2/Flt3 ligand	13q12–13	Synergistic with a range of cytokines on primitive and committed haemopoietic progenitors	Likely to be confined to in vitro cell expansion
Accessory or synergistic factors	IL-1D IL-1E	Interleukin 1	2q13	Synergistic with SCF, IL-3 on primitive progenitors	None as yet
	IL-6	Interleukin 6	7p15	Synergistic with IL-3, SCF Myeloma cell growth factor	Trialled as megakaryocyte stimulator, but not clinically effective
	IL-11	Interleukin 11	19q13.3–13.4	Also synergistic with SCF and IL-3	Megakaryocyte stimulator Licensed in USA for post-chemotherapy thrombocytopenia

* Growth factors licenced for clinical use in the UK.
BMT, bone marrow transplantation; PBSC, peripheral blood stem cells.

reduces and the nucleus is extruded. The cytokines interleukin (IL)-3 and stem cell factor (SCF) are intimately associated with the first 7–9 days of erythroid differentiation. The predominant erythropoietic cytokine is Epo, which acts on erythroid progenitors from day 2 onwards and is the only cytokine capable of differentiating BFU-E. Epo is a glycoprotein growth hormone encoded on chromosome 7q21 and largely produced by the peritubular capillary endothelium of the kidney in response to reduced oxygen content in the renal arterial circulation. Some Epo is also produced by hepatocytes. Endogenous Epo levels are increased in patients with primary polycythaemia and reduced in patients with renal failure (see below). It binds to receptors on the surface of erythroid progenitors. Epo is available in Europe and the US as the short-acting epoetin alfa (Eprex, Janssen-Cilag; Epogen and Procrit, Amgen) and beta (NeoRecormon, Roche) and the long-acting darbepoetin alfa (Aranesp, Amgen); the latter is achieved by modifying the glycosylation of the molecule.

Clinical indications for Epo therapy

Epo is used as treatment to prevent or reduce the requirements for red cell transfusion in patients with:

- chronic renal failure;
- anaemia in HIV-infected patients treated with zidovudine;
- cancer chemotherapy-related anaemia; and
- pre-surgery to increase the procurement of autologous blood and so reduce exposure to allogeneic transfusions.

In chronic renal failure, anaemia results in part from chronic inflammation leading to cytokine dysregulation. Epo has been used in this setting for nearly 20 years. The rate of rise of the haematocrit is dependent on time, the dose of Epo given and individual patient variation. A recent meta-analysis has shown that Epo administration resulted in a rise in haemoglobin from <8.0 g/dL to >11.0 g/dL, an improvement in quality-of-life measures of between 10 and 70% and reduced hospitalisations and transfusions.

Epo preparations are indicated and licenced for the treatment of anaemia related to therapy with zidovudine in HIV-infected patients. Studies show that it is effective in reducing the transfusion requirement and increasing the haematocrit in patients with low endogenous serum Epo levels compared with patients who receive placebo. An additional benefit is that patients may maintain a satisfactory haemoglobin without the need for a significant reduction in their zidovudine dose.

Epo has been used to treat patients with anaemia secondary to malignant diseases. The aetiology is multifactorial and due to blood loss, nutritional deficiency, bone marrow infiltration or suppression from chemotherapy and cytokine dysregulation leading to functional iron deficiency. Epo therapy reduces transfusion requirements and improves quality-of-life parameters in patients with cancer, but meta-analyses show no benefit in survival or outcome. Epo therapy often depletes iron stores, but oral iron preparations are ineffective and parenteral iron therapy may be required. The need for this can be guided by measurement of serum ferritin, transferrin saturation and zinc protoporphyrin. Weekly epoietin alpha/beta or 2-weekly darbepoietin therapy is effective.

Recent studies have shown a poorer outcome with increased mortality and tumour progression in some Epo-treated cancer patients. However, they all had high target haemoglobin levels and in two studies those patients who received Epo tended to have more aggressive disease. As a result of this, the American Food and Drug Administration (FDA) issued a 'black box' warning in 2006, requiring Epo to be withheld from patients with a haemoglobin >12 g/dL. Guidance published in 2007 by the American Societies of Haematology and Clinical Oncology recommends that an erythropoiesis-stimulating agent (ESA) is used in patients with chemotherapy-associated anaemia when the haemoglobin approaches or falls below 10 g/dL. An ESA is also recommended in low-risk myelodysplasia patients. The guidance states that there is no evidence to show that treating at haemoglobin levels >10 g/dL reduces the requirement for transfusion or improves quality of life. Use of an ESA in patients who are not receiving chemotherapy is not advised since trials show that the risks of thromboembolism and cancer recurrence are increased in some recent studies. The mechanism of tumour recurrence or progression is not clearly understood although it may be due to the expression of Epo receptors on the tumour cells. Caution is advised in the use of Epo in this setting and further studies are needed.

Patients scheduled for major elective surgery, such as hip replacement, may be treated with Epo to increase the haematocrit and allow collection of more autologous blood. This is discussed in greater detail in Chapters 33 and 34. This approach reduces the number of units of allogeneic blood required and may totally avoid the requirement for allogeneic blood transfusion.

Risks of Epo therapy
• Iron deficiency due to rapid expansion in the number of erythroid cells.
• Increased blood pressure.
• Thrombosis: meta-analysis has shown that the risk is doubled, but this does not impact on overall morbidity or mortality.
• Cancer recurrence: this is described above.
• Pure red cell aplasia: this is important although uncommon adverse effect occurred largely with the Eprex preparation. It appears that the administration caused the formation of anti-Epo antibodies, which cross-reacted with the recipient's own Epo leading to destruction of erythropoietic cells.

Thrombopoiesis

The major haemopoietic growth factor responsible for maintaining normal platelet levels in the blood is thrombopoietin (Tpo) isolated in 1994. A number of other cytokines are important in platelet development. These include IL-3, G-CSF, granulocyte-macrophage (GM)-CSF and SCF which act at the progenitor cell stage. IL-6 acts late in megakaryocyte maturation and Tpo together with IL-11 stimulate all stages of megakaryocyte development. Tpo is also known as c-Mp1 ligand and megakaryocyte growth and development factor (MGDF). The clinical use of recombinant(r) Tpo was extensively studied in the 1990s, but the development of neutralising antibodies against endogenous Tpo and

severe thrombocytopenia in healthy subjects who received rMGDF eventually led to the development of novel second-generation thrombopoietic agents.

Thrombopoietin
Tpo is a glycoprotein of molecular mass of 30 kDa. The gene encoding it is located on chromosome 3q27. The amino-terminal residues have 21% sequence identity and 46% overall sequence similarity with human Epo and it is this domain that binds to c-Mpl (the Tpo receptor). Recombinant human Tpo (rTpo) is a full-length polypeptide while rMGDF, also used in clinical studies, is a truncated protein containing the receptor-binding region modified by addition of polyethylene glycol (PEG). Tpo is primarily synthesised in the liver, while lesser amounts are seen in the kidneys, brain and testes. Circulating Tpo levels are inversely related to platelet mass. Platelets contain an avid Tpo receptor that removes it from the circulation; therefore, normal or high platelet levels prevent the action of Tpo on the bone marrow by binding to circulating receptors. In bone marrow failure states, e.g. aplastic anaemia, Tpo levels are high whereas in immune thrombocytopenic purpura (ITP) they are low or normal, since Tpo is rapidly removed from the circulation by platelets with a short circulation span. The principal action of Tpo is to increase the megakaryocyte mass and circulating platelet count.

Clinical trials of first-generation thrombopoietic agents
Both rTpo and rMGDF were administered to patients with solid tumours with few immediate adverse effects. If given prior to chemotherapy, there was marked stimulation of platelet production. Studies showed that the duration of thrombocytopenia was shorter and the nadir of platelet count higher in patients given Tpo compared with control during a first cycle of chemotherapy. However, in patients with more intense myelosuppression, e.g. acute myeloid leukaemia undergoing chemotherapy, rTpo and rMGDF failed to reduce the duration of thrombocytopenia or the number of days of platelet transfusions. Tpo given in conjunction with other cytokines such as G-CSF could increase

the mobilisation of stem cells into the peripheral blood. Administration of rTpo to apheresis donors elevated their platelet counts and increased the number of platelets that could be harvested in a single apheresis procedure. However, this approach was abandoned following the development of severe immune-mediated thrombocytopenia in volunteer donors.

Second-generation thrombopoietic agents

These molecules have been developed in the last 5 years. They all bind to and activate the Tpo receptor in different ways but with subsequent signalling via the JAK2/STAT pathway to produce a dose-dependent rise in the platelet count (Figure 43.1). Two types have been studied in man:

• Tpo peptide mimetics: This group includes the compounds AMG 531, Fab59 and Peg-TPOmp. They were developed by screening peptide libraries for sequences that stimulated Tpo-dependent cell

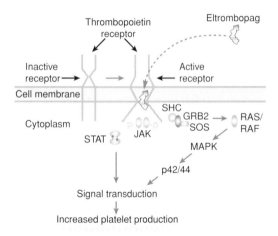

Figure 43.1 Mechanism of activation of Tpo receptor by some Tpo non-peptide mimetics. Tpo non-peptide mimetics such as eltrombopag activate the Tpo receptor by a mechanism different from Tpo (see 'Tpo non-peptide mimetics'). Although drawn here to suggest direct binding of eltrombopag to the TM region of the Tpo receptor, eltrombopag may bind elsewhere on the Tpo receptor but may have its effect mediated by unique structures in the TM region. Most Tpo non-peptide mimetics do not compete for binding with rhTpo and have a biologic effect additive to that of rhTpo. (Illustration by Paulette Dennis.)

lines and lacked sequence homology with Tpo itself. These linear peptides are short-lived in the circulation and an effective half-life has been obtained by their insertion into human Fab or Fc constructs or by pegylation. All stimulate thrombopoiesis and elevate the platelet count although Fab 59 has not yet been studied in humans (Figure 43.2).

• Tpo non-peptide mimetics: This group includes eltrombopag and AKR-501. They were developed after screening of libraries of small non-peptide molecules for their ability to stimulate genes such as STAT in Tpo-dependent cell lines. They are highly species-specific, activate the Tpo receptor in a different way to Tpo and have an additive effect to it. Both are active after oral, once daily administration and are currently being studied in patients with ITP, liver disease and chemotherapy-induced myelosuppression (see Figure 43.1).

Clinical trials with second-generation Tpos

AMG 531 and eltrombopag have been studied in patients with ITP looking at safety and their ability to elevate the platelet count. A recent, large, multicentred, randomised and open-label study of AMG 531 in splenectomised ITP patients has shown efficacy with weekly dosing compared to placebo and an overall response rate of 79% versus 0%. The requirement for rescue therapy was reduced and more patients were able to reduce or discontinue other medications. Patients in the placebo arm had more bleeding episodes. A 1-year follow-up study of more than 100 subjects is ongoing. The main side effect is mild headache; platelet counts return to baseline after stopping. In a randomised, double-blind, placebo-controlled phase 2 study in ITP patients eltrombopag, at the highest dose given, raised the platelet count to a median of 183×10^9/L. A similar effect was seen in patients with chronic hepatitis C liver disease. Again the counts return to baseline on stopping.

Potential adverse effects of second-generation Tpos

(modified from Kuter, 2007)

• Thrombocytosis;
• Thrombosis;

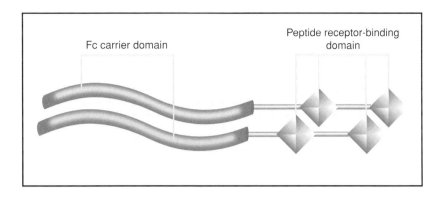

Figure 43.2 Structure of AMG 531. The left hand of the diagram shows the IgG Fc carrier portion of the module. The right hand shows the peptide that binds to the Tpo receptor (not shown in figure). There are four binding sites in the peptide portion. (From Bussel JB *et al. N Engl J Med* 2006;355:1672–1681.)

- Stimulation of leukaemic cell growth – there is no evidence for this at present; and
- Autoantibody formation.

Granulopoiesis

The production of mature granulocytes from stem cells is controlled by G-CSF, SCF, IL-3 and GM-CSF. G-CSF is a glycoprotein encoded for by a gene on chromosome 17. Recombinant G-CSF is indicated for the treatment of neutropenia after chemotherapy and stem cell transplantation, mobilisation of PBSC, severe congenital neutropenia, cyclic and idiopathic neutropenia when there is a history of severe infection, and persistent neutropenia in advanced HIV infection. It may be given by subcutaneous injection or intravenous infusion, stimulating:

- granulocytic precursors to produce mature granulocytes and
- more primitive precursors, so that CD34 cells are released into the bloodstream.

Granulocyte collection

Patients receiving chemotherapy and stem cell transplantation for cancer often have prolonged periods of neutropenia and are susceptible to life-threatening bacterial and fungal infections. Granulocytes collected by steady-state apheresis of healthy donors or made from buffy coat preparations have been used to prevent or treat such infections. However, the dose administered is usually only about $5–10 \times 10^9/L$. Increments in the patient's granulocyte count are uncommon although recently-developed, optimised buffy coat granulocyte preparations are in clinical trial (see Chapter 21).

Corticosteroids elevate the peripheral granulocyte count and increase by two to four times the dose of granulocytes that can be collected. Priming donors with a single dose of G-CSF increases the average dose collected to $50–100 \times 10^9/L$ and often good count increments are seen. There is now considerable interest in this approach, but further prospective randomised studies of both prophylactic and therapeutic therapy are required before definite recommendations can be made. In the meantime, it is reasonable to give granulocytes collected by apheresis from mobilised donors to patients with severe neutropenia and bacterial or fungal infections unresponsive to 2 days or more of appropriate antimicrobial therapy. G-CSF is given to donors as a single dose, either alone or plus a single dose of dexamethasone 12–24 hours prior to apheresis.

Stem cell collection from healthy volunteer donors

Roughly, 70% of all allogeneic stem cell transplants from family and unrelated donors use mobilised PBSC. There are in excess of 12 million donors on the Bone Marrow Donors Worldwide (BMDW) database at the present time and nearly all registries now sanction the use of G-CSF for stem cell collection by apheresis. Ordinarily, the cytokine is given for 4 or 5 days with careful donor monitoring and then one or two apheresis procedures are carried out (see Chapter 40 for further details).

Risks of G-CSF

G-CSF is a non-toxic agent which, as a naturally occurring hormone, is present in health at low levels. Common short-term effects include:

- bone pain;
- headache;
- myalgia;
- fatigue;
- nausea and vomiting;
- minor alterations in blood chemistry; and
- leucocytosis.

The first three of these occur in up to 80% of healthy people given G-CSF and can be treated with regular paracetamol. Leucocytosis may be marked and can increase blood viscosity, causing leucostasis. When it is given to healthy people, the dose should be omitted if the neutrophil count exceeds 80×10^9/L.

Rare events include:

- spontaneous rupture of the spleen reported in five healthy donors and due to rapid expansion of myelopoiesis;
- flare-ups of autoimmune disease; and
- precipitation of sickle-cell crisis.

There is also a theoretical risk of stimulating the growth of leukaemic cells in patients predisposed to develop myeloid malignancy, e.g. severe congenital neutropenia (SCN). Mutations in the G-CSF receptor gene have been described in some SCN patients, and are believed to define the subgroup of patients with an increased susceptibility to myelodysplastic syndrome (MDS)/acute myeloid leukaemia (AML). The risk of this in SCN appears to increase with the duration of G-CSF therapy and the cumulative incidence is 36% after 12 years of treatment. However, the exact role of G-CSF administration in this process remains controversial and malignancy occurs also in patients who do not receive cytokines. In vitro cytogenetic studies in samples from PBSC donors suggested that they had changes similar to those seen in patients with cancer, possibly resulting from genomic instability. Three cases of AML have been reported in healthy sibling donors who received G-CSF for stem cell mobilisation. However, review of stem cell registry and other data indicates that the occurrence of haematological malignancy in donors is not increased compared to bone marrow donors (who do not receive G-CSF) or normal non-donor populations. No case of MDS/AML is known to have occurred in a healthy, unrelated, volunteer donor.

Cytokine in lymphpoiesis and immunotherapy

This increasingly important category of cellular therapy products includes dendritic cells, cytotoxic T lymphocytes (CTLs), natural killer cells and T-regulatory cells. Immunotherapy is used in the treatment of cancer, viral infections and possibly also in autoimmune disease. In malignant disease, the paradigm for an anti-tumour effect was the observation that in chronic myeloid leukaemia relapsing post-stem cell transplant, a further remission could be induced after infusions of lymphocytes from the donor. More sophisticated therapy requires the production in culture systems or in vivo of 'educated' CTL and other cells that specifically recognise and kill either tumour or virus-infected cells. This can be done, for example by culturing the mononuclear cell fraction from patients to generate dendritic cells that are effective in presenting antigen to T cells. These are then cultured ('pulsed') in the laboratory with some form of tumour antigen and incubated with T cells from the patient or an allogeneic donor. This causes proliferation of cells in response to antigen recognition, with production of tumour-specific cells which can then be reinfused to the patient. Alternatively, dendritic cells may be primed with antigen and injected, causing the proliferation of CTL and other cells in vivo. Growth factors for dendritic cells include SCF, IL-4, GM-CSF, anti-CD40 ligand and transforming growth factor-β. The principal cytokine that drives T-cell growth ex vivo is IL-2 (see Chapter 42 for more details of immunotherapeutic approaches).

Key points

1 Epo is the main regulator of erythroid development and has been used for the treatment of anaemia in patients with cancer, renal failure and HIV infection as well as patients scheduled for elective surgery to reduce red cell transfusion requirements.

2 Caution is advised when prescribing Epo in cancer patients, particularly those who have not had chemotherapy. Recent guidelines are available to help guide decision-making.

3 Established side-effects of Epo use include iron deficiency, hypertension and thrombosis.

4 Tpo has been withdrawn from use, but newer second-generation thrombopoietic agents such as AMG 531 and eltrombopag show promise in the management of ITP and deserve further study.

5 Potential side-effects of these newer thrombopoietic agents include thrombocytosis and thrombosis.

6 G-CSF is used to mobilise granulocytes for transfusion and further studies are needed to establish the role of such transfusions in patients with neutropenic sepsis.

7 PBSC can be mobilised efficiently using G-CSF. Healthy donors who receive it should be carefully monitored for common and rarer adverse effects.

8 Cytokines have a key role in the generation of cells for immunotherapy.

Further reading

Bennett CL, Evens AM, Andritsos LA *et al.* Haermatological malignancies developing in previously healthy individuals who received haematopoietic growth factors: report from the Research on Adverse Drug Events and Reports (RADAR) project. *Br J Haematol* 2006;135:642–650.

Blau CA. Erythropoietin in cancer: presumption of innocence. *Stem Cells* 2007;25:2094–2097.

Greaves P & Agrawal S. Safe and efficacious use of recombinant human erythropoietin in malignancy. *Clin Med.* 2007;7:617–620.

Jones M, Ibels L, Schenkel B *et al.* Impact of epoetin alfa on clinical end points in patients with chronic renal failure: a meta-analysis. *Kidney Int* 2004;65:757–767.

Kaushansky K. Use of thrombopoietic growth factors in acute leukemia. *Leukaemia* 2000;14:505–508.

Kolb HJ, Schmidt C, Barrett AJ & Schendel DJ. Graft-versus-leukaemia reactions in allogeneic chimeras. *Blood* 2004;103:767–776.

Kuter DJ. New thrombopoietic growth factors. *Blood* 2007;109:4607–4616.

Kuter DJ & Begley CG. Recombinant human thrombopoietin: basic biology and evaluation of clinical studies. *Blood* 2002;100:3457–3469.

Lyman G, Castro LG & Djulbegovic B. *Cochrane Database Syst Rev* 2003;3:CD003039.

Macdougall IC. Erythropoietin and renal failure. *Curr Hematol Rep* 2003;2:459–464.

Rizzo JD, Somerfield MR, Hagerty KL *et al.* Use of epoetin and darbepoetin in patients with cancer: 2007 American Society of Hematology/American Society of Clinical Oncology clinical practice guidelines update. *Blood* 2008;111(1):25–41.

CHAPTER 44

Tissue banking

Ruth M. Warwick[1] & Deirdre Fehily[2]
[1]NHS Blood and Transplant, Edgware, Middlesex, UK
[2]National Transplant Centre, Rome, Italy

The provision of tissue banking services has been a natural development for many blood services, where so much of the expertise and infrastructure required already exists for the banking of blood. The safe banking of human tissues such as bone, skin, corneas, tendons and meniscus, heart valves and amnion requires expertise in donor recruitment, consent, donor selection and testing as well as comprehensive quality management. The National Blood Services in the UK have greatly increased their involvement in tissue banking over the last 15 years. Blood centres in many other European countries also contribute significantly to the provision of tissue banking services.

There are some important features of tissue banking, however, that make it distinctly different from blood or cord blood banking. A large proportion of tissue donors are deceased, which presents different challenges particularly in relation to donor history, collection and donor testing. Tissue processing is by necessity very open, and therefore the requirements for processing facilities are much more stringent than for blood. Tissues can be sterilised when cell viability is not required.

Tissue banking services are also provided by many hospital departments and, in the US particularly, by independent organisations, some of which operate for profit. Where deceased donor tissues

Practical Transfusion Medicine, 3rd edition. Edited by Michael F. Murphy and Derwood H. Pamphilon. © 2009 Blackwell Publishing, ISBN: 978-1-4051-8196-9.

are banked, there is usually some degree of collaboration with organ transplantation programmes and in some cases organ and tissue donation is coordinated in a fully integrated way, though this is unusual in the UK. Recent organisational changes in the UK have greatly enhanced the potential for closer working between UK organ and tissue procurement with the merger of UK Transplant and the National Blood Service to form National Health Service Blood and Transplant (NHSBT).

This chapter aims to identify the key considerations for a blood centre embarking on the banking of human tissues.

Regulation of tissue banking

In the European Union, legally binding tissue and cell directives (known as the TCDs) have been adopted and are in the process of being transposed into the national legislation of all 27 Member States. The original, or 'mother', Directive (Directive 2004/23/EC) is largely aimed at the Health Authorities of Member States. It requires all Member States to have inspection and accreditation systems in place which ensure that all banks providing these services comply with certain technical requirements. These technical requirements are detailed in two further Directives: Directive 2006/17/EC, which defines the requirements for donor selection, donor testing and tissue procurement, and Directive 2006/86/EC, which defines the requirements for the accreditation/

designation/authorisation/licencing of tissue establishments, the reporting of serious adverse events and reactions, coding and for import and export. Together these are often referred to as the 'daughter' directives. The adoption of these directives by the European Union has resulted in a high level of organisational activity both at individual Member State level and through EU-wide initiatives aimed at common interpretation and implementation.

In England, the Human Tissue Act 2004 established the Human Tissue Authority (HTA) as the English competent authority for tissues and cells (excluding reproductive cells), which operates a system of inspection and licencing. The HTA has responsibility for ensuring compliance with the TCDs as well as the Human Tissue Act; the latter predominantly relates to issues of consent. During 2006 and 2007, the HTA published Codes of Practice, which provide guidance in a number of areas pertinent to tissue banking including on consent, donation of organs, tissues and cells for transplantation, import and export of human bodies, body parts and tissue, removal, storage and disposal of tissues and organs (http://www.hta.gov.uk/guidance/codes_of_practice.cfm). The Human Tissue (Scotland) Act 2006 has provisions on living donation almost identical to those in the English Act. The HTA has UK-wide (including Scotland by agreement with Scottish ministers) responsibility for approving donations from the living of whole organs, bone marrow and peripheral blood stem cells. The HTA is also the Competent Authority for Scotland under the Human Tissue (Quality and Safety for Human Application) Regulations 2007 (the Regulations 2007). The Regulations 2007 transposed the European Union Tissues and Cells Directives into UK law on 5 July 2007.

Legally binding regulation is also in place in the US, where the Food and Drug Administration (FDA) has published a number of relevant rules (listed in Table 44.1), most recently their good tissue practices (GTPs) which enlarge on the pre-existing requirements for the assessment of donor suitability by adding detailed requirements for quality management at all stages of the process.

Guidance and standards are available from a number of professional sources (see Table 44.1). International perspectives on the ethics and regulation of human cell and tissue transplantation have been reviewed at a WHO expert meeting and a summary published in the WHO Bulletin.

Consent

Patients undergoing surgery for joint replacement or heart transplantation can donate tissues, femoral heads and heart valves, respectively. Amniotic membrane can be donated at the time of caesarean section. Written consent for all the relevant aspects of tissue donation, testing and/or for research use should be obtained, separately from the consent for surgery, in advance of tissue retrieval.

The legal requirements for obtaining permission for the retrieval of tissues after death vary from country to country. However, even where 'opting out' or 'presumed consent' systems are operated, it is considered best professional practice to confirm that no relatives object to the donation proceeding. In the UK, the Human Tissue Act 2004 gives precedence to the wishes of the donor as registered prior to their death, over the wishes of their bereaved relatives. It also defines a hierarchy of individuals who may give consent on behalf of the deceased for a donation after death if the potential donors did not register their wishes when alive. There are special provisions to protect those who are not competent to give consent. The NHS Organ Donor Register provides an opportunity for individuals to record their wish to donate after death and a significant proportion of the UK population, over 14 million, had registered by March 2007.

Consent should be taken only by those trained to do so and the discussion before consent should provide information on the following areas:
- the intended clinical use of the donation, in general terms;
- the need for virological testing and the implications of any positive results;
- the possible need for a review of medical records held elsewhere; and
- if applicable, the potential use of the tissue for research and development, if it proves unsuitable

Table 44.1 Regulations and guidance in the field of tissue banking.

Committee on Microbiological Safety of Blood and Tissues for Transplantation (MSBT), Department of Health. August 2000. Guidance on the microbiological safety of human tissues and organs used in transplantation. NHS Executive. The MSBT Committee itself has been re-formulated as the **Advisory Committee on the Safety of Blood, Tissues and Organs (SaBTO) and it is likely that the MSBTO guidance 2000 will be reviewed by the new body.**

American Association of Tissue Banks (AATB). 2006. Standards for Tissue Banking, 11th edition, McLean, VA.

Directive 2004/23/EC of the European Parliament and of the Council of 31 March 2004 on setting standards for quality and safety in the donation, procurement, processing, preservation, storage and distribution of human tissues and cells. *Official Journal of the European Union* L 102/48 07/04/2004.

Commission Directive 2006/17/EC of 8 February 2006 implementing Directive 2004/23/EC of the European Parliament and of the Council as regards certain technical requirements for the donation, procurement and testing of human tissues and cells. *Official Journal of the European Union* L 38/40 09/02/2006.

Commission Directive 2006/86/EC of 24 October 2006 implementing Directive 2004/23/EC of the European Parliament and of the Council as regards traceability requirements, notification of serious adverse reactions and events, and certain technical requirements for the coding, processing, preservation, storage and distribution of human tissues and cells. *Official Journal of the European Union* L 294/32 25/10/2006.

United States DHHS Federal Register 21 CFR Parts 16, 1270, and 1271 Current Good Tissue Practice for Human Cell, Tissue, and Cellular and Tissue-Based Product Establishments; Inspection and Enforcement; Final Rule FDA. 2004.

FDA guidance for Industry, US. http://www.fda.gov/bbs/topics/news/2004/NEW01070.html.

UK Blood Transfusion Services. 2005. Guidelines for the UK Blood Transfusion Services, 7th edition. http://www.transfusionguidelines.org.uk.

The Human Tissue Act, 2004 (UK).

The Human Tissue Act (Scotland) 2006.

Human Tissue Ethical and Legal Issues published by the Nuffield Council on Bioethics 1995.

Ethical Aspects of Human Tissue Banking. Opinion of the European Group on Ethics in Science and New Technologies to the European Commission (21 July 1998).

Council of Europe. 2007. Guide to Safety and Quality Assurance for the Transplantation of Organs, Tissues and Cells. 3rd edition (available at www.coe.int).

American Association of Tissue Banks (AATB). 2006. Standards for Tissue Banking, 11th edition, McLean, VA

for clinical use. The information provided about research should describe the various types of research including whether the donation may be used in a commercial research setting.

Donor selection

Living donors

Where patients can be interviewed face to face, the selection process can be very similar to blood donation but should also include a review of the patient's hospital notes.

Deceased donors

The primary source of donor selection information for deceased donors is the interview with someone who knew the donor well; usually, but not always, a relative. Additional information should be sought from the family doctor as an added security

measure required in the absence of a face-to-face interview with the donor. Where a postmortem examination has been performed or is scheduled, the results should be reviewed as part of the donor selection process.

Interviews with donors or their families should include enquiries as detailed in Table 44.2.

Detailed donor selection guidance for living and deceased donors is available for the tissue banks operating within the UK Blood services and this guidance is reviewed and updated regularly. It is available at http://www.transfusionguidelines.org.uk.

Donor testing

Living donors

In many countries, including the UK, there is a requirement to quarantine living tissue donations and to obtain a further blood sample from the

Table 44.2 Enquiries to be made of tissue donors or their families.

Enquiry category	Information sought and outcome	Notes, examples and special circumstances
General past medical history	Malignancy specifically excludes	Exceptions are cured in situ cancer of the cervix and basal cell carcinoma. Primary brain tumours should be excluded unless benign nature is confirmed histologically due to the risk that a solitary metastasis might be mistaken for a primary. Brain tumour diagnostic procedures during life may increase the chance of extracranial metastases by breaching the blood–brain barrier
	Diseases of unknown aetiology are reason to exclude	For example, sarcoidosis, Crohn's disease and ulcerative colitis have some features in common with some infectious disorders
	Diseases of neurodegenerative aetiology specifically exclude	Pakinson's disease and multiple sclerosis are common diseases in this category
	Diseases of known infectious origin usually exclude	Examples include systemic bacterial infections such as fulminant pneumonia (although small foci of infection associated with ventilation, even if currently being treated, may not exclude the donor), septicaemia, acute myocarditis and active tuberculosis
	Multisystem autoimmune diseases exclude donation	Examples include rheumatoid arthritis, systemic lupus erythematosus and polyrteritis nodosa. These may affect the quality of the tissues. May be treated with drugs that may affect the quality of the tissues. May be treated with immunosoppressants that may affect validity of test results. Are of unknown aetiology possibly with an infectious trigger
Medication	Enquiries primarily aimed at identifying underlying disease that may make the donor ineligible	Long-term steroid therapy can affect the quality of skin and bone and immunosuppression may render antibody-based tests invalid
Hepatitis and HIV transmission risk	Exposure to behavioural risks such as acupuncture, tatooing, ear or body piercing, sex for money or between males or intravenous drug abuse. Reciept of an organ, cornea, sclera or dura mater transplant excludes donation	In the case of acupuncture, tatooing or piercing, living donors with these risks can be accepted although retesting should be conducted at least 6 months after the risk event (assuming that anti-HBc was performed on the donation sample as required in the EU, otherwise retesting should be performed at least 1 year after the risk event).
CJD	Enquiries should elicit any family history of CJD and any brain or spinal surgery before 1992. Hormone treatment for infertility or growth before 1985	Details and dates of brain or spinal surgery should be recorded and further investigations made with the hospital concerned
		In the UK, potential tissue donors, except those donating skin, corneas and heart valves, who have been transfused since 1980 are excluded to reduce the risk of vCJD transmission

(Continued)

Table 44.2 *(Continued)*

Enquiry category	Information sought and outcome	Notes, examples and special circumstances
Travel (malaria and chagas' disease)	The rules for history-taking, acceptance and malarial antibody testing of blood donors should be applied equally to tissue donors	It is nor clear whether any risk of malaria transmission remains in non-viable tissues. Cornea banks do not exclude donations on the basis of malarial risk
Tissue-specific medical history	Depending on the tissues to be donated, enquiries should be made to exclude donors on the basis of a medical history which may imply that the quality of the specific tissue is compromised	For example, previous eye surgery in eye donors, or previous hip surgery in femoral head donors
Recent history	Enquiries should establish circumstances surrounding the death, including whether a hospital or coroner's postmortem is to be performed	

CJD, Creutzfeldt-Jakob disease.

donors at least 180 days following their initial donation. Virology testing at donation and after quarantine should be as for blood donors, though Directive 2006/17/EC also requires anti-hepatitis B core testing of all donors and allows for repeat testing to be replaced by NAT for HIV, HBV and HCV at donation.

Deceased tissue donors

The quality and nature of blood samples from deceased donors vary considerably due to autolysis and haemolysis and there is documented observation of a high rate of false positivity in serological microbiological assays and a significant rate of inhibition in NAT assays. Standardising the site and method of sample collection and minimising the time period between cessation of the circulation and blood sampling can reduce problems in testing deceased donor samples; most standards require sampling within 24 hours after death. Samples taken close to an intravenous administration or central line may be diluted even if the donor has not received a significant amount of fluids. Wherever possible, antemortem blood samples should be taken, as long as they can be reliably identified. Where there is a concern regarding the identity of a premortem sample, the use of molecular finger printing such as short tandem repeat (STR) analysis may be used to confirm the origin of the sample

by comparing with a bone marrow sample from a donated bone.

DNA extraction techniques can be adapted to remove the inhibitors present in deceased donor blood samples which can interfere in NAT assays. Where test kits are available that have been licenced for use with deceased donor samples then they should be used. Test kits for both mandatory and discretionary testing should be validated for use with deceased donors.

Fluids administered in the 48 hours prior to death must be recorded to allow an estimation of any plasma dilution effect. It is generally accepted that a blood sample which is more than 50% dilute should not be considered valid for microbiological testing. An algorithm can be applied in the calculation of plasma dilution for deceased donors (Table 44.3).

Both the FDA 'Guidance for the Industry 2005' and Directive 2006/17/EC permit the acceptance of donors where a screening test for syphilis is reactive but confirmatory testing indicates an absence of infection.

Testing of the donor for variant Creutzfeldt–Jakob disease (vCJD) or classical CJD has not yet been validated, but a pilot is under way in NHSBT using deceased donor tonsil as an analyte for vCJD using a Western blot assay. For deceased tissue donors, the testing of tonsil or other

Table 44.3 Calculation of plasma dilution.

Interval prior to sampling	Volume infused (mL)	Per cent retained	Volume retained (mL)
Crystalloid infused			
>24 h	—	0	None
2–24 h	—	25	—
1–2 h	—	50	—
<1 h	—	75	—
Total crystalloid retained = Blood/colloid infused			
24–48 h	—	100 (blood)	—
	—	50 (colloid)	—
0–24 h	—	100	—
Total blood/colloid retained =			
Estimated total blood volume	70 mL/kg body weight		

$$\%Haemodilution = \frac{\text{Crystalloid} + \text{blood/colloid retained} \times 100}{\text{blood volume}}$$

reticulo-endothelial tissue for vCJD may carry significant potential benefits over blood testing. Animal model studies have shown that it is likely that reticulo-endothelial tissue will contain abnormal prion before infected individuals demonstrate clinical disease and before it is detectable in blood. Tonsil procurement can be difficult when rigor mortis is established, but the procedure is quick and not technically challenging. There are a number of ethical issues that limit which donors can be tested. In the UK pilot, vCJD testing is limited to donors of tissue who are not also organ donors because the time taken to obtain test results may be longer than the time to implantation of the organs and reactive results would pose difficult management problems for recipients of organs from tested donors.

Tissue procurement

Living donors

By necessity, living donations are retrieved during surgery by the operating team. Clear written instructions, staff training and standard sterile kits should be provided by the tissue bank for tissue collection, with regular auditing to ensure compliance with agreed procedures, detailed in a written agreement between the tissue bank and the hospital. A critical aspect of the retrieval is the iden-

tification of the donor, the donation and the associated blood samples for donor testing and tissue samples for bacteriology and fungal testing. The use of bar-coded donation number labels for donations, samples and associated documentation greatly increases the security of this step.

Deceased donors

The donor must be positively identified by means of a wristband, toe-tag or by the mortuary staff. The appearance of the donor's body must match with the description of the donor and the circumstances of death, e.g. age, gender, ethnicity etc. Where tissues are to be processed in the tissue bank, with a decontamination or terminal sterilisation step, it is common practice for the tissue recovery to be conducted in a mortuary. However, sterile instruments should be used and a local sterile field created.

Before the tissue recovery commences, a thorough external examination of the donor body appearance should be conducted and recorded and the findings included as part of the donor selection assessment. The examination should include detection and recording of:

- tattoos;
- jaundice;
- evidence of intravenous drug use;
- skin or mucosal abnormalities;
- body piercing;

- open wounds or signs of infection;
- scars and trauma;
- intravenous cannula sites; and
- operation incision sites.

In general, tissues should be recovered within the shortest possible period of time from death. Standards vary around the world from 12 to 48 hours depending on the tissue and the processing method to which it will be subjected. If the donor body was not refrigerated within a certain period after death, the recovery should be started earlier. The limits applied for time from death to refrigeration are stipulated in guidelines and should be validated for the circumstances pertaining to the individual tissue bank. Delayed tissue recovery increases the risk that bacterial contamination from the deceased donor's internal organs will spread via the large blood vessels to donated tissues. It is preferable for the tissue recovery to be undertaken prior to any autopsy, as long as circumstances allow, avoiding contamination of tissues by gut contents. Bacterial contamination may pose significant clinical risk as clearly shown in the reports of transmission of Clostridia by soft tissue allografting.

Minimising bacterial cross-contamination is further ensured by staff gowning, draping the donor body (see photograph of retrieval, Plate 44.1) and by applying normal aseptic technique during the tissue recovery process.

An important aspect of tissue recovery is the careful reconstruction of the donor body. Extendible plastic prostheses can be used to replace large bones. Tissue recovery may be undertaken in a postmortem room, a dedicated recovery suite resembling an operating theatre, or a hospital operating suite. In all cases, precautions must be taken to create a clean immediate environment by the use of sterile drapes and equipment. Where feasible, disposable sterile equipment should be used.

NHSBT Tissue Services has recently developed a dedicated tissue recovery suite at one of its tissue processing facilities (see Plate 44.2). Staff can be supervised more closely in this environment and senior expertise is available on-site. The environment is controlled to a defined specification and is easier to maintain and monitor. Staff travelling time is reduced and staff can rotate between tissue recovery and other duties more effectively. Next of kin are asked if they object to the movement of their relative to a specified site for tissue recovery and the donor is returned to the hospital or other location according to the family's wishes within a designated time period. The NHSBT facility in Liverpool is shown in the picture.

Tissue processing

If tissues have been recovered in an operating theatre, and validated bacteriological testing reveals absence of bacterial or fungal contamination, they may be frozen and transplanted without further processing (e.g. femoral heads). If, however, there is evidence of bacterial contamination, or the tissues have been retrieved in a mortuary, they should be further processed. In a case of a multi-organ, multi-tissue donor in the US, from whom HIV was transmitted by organs and frozen bone grafts, there was no transmission by bone which had been processed by cleaning, shaping or grinding and freeze-drying, even though it had not been subjected to terminal sterilisation.

Processing reduces the risk of disease transmission by the removal of blood and marrow and by reducing or eliminating contamination by chemical and physical means (Plate 44.3).

Pooling of donations during processing is not permitted by standards in Europe or the US. Each tissue facility should have a policy for acceptance of rejection of tissues where contamination by certain organisms is found at particular stages in processing. The policy should be based on the pathogenicity of the organism and the validated effectiveness of any subsequent decontamination or sterilisation step.

Processing facilities

The required standard of EU tissue processing facilities is defined in Directive 2006/86/EC and is recognised as a key factor for the safety of tissues at risk of contamination. In general, the directive defines the minimum air quality in which tissues are exposed as Grade A (as defined in the European

Guide to Good Manufacturing Practice, annex 1) with a minimum background air quality of Grade D (Plate 44.4). The directive defines a number of circumstances where a lower standard can be applied though the chosen standard must be justified and shown to give adequate protection to the tissue. Individual Member States may apply more stringent criteria and many require a background of Grade B for some or all tissues exposed to the environment without terminal sterilisation.

Supply and traceability of tissues

Directive 2006/86/EC requires the development of a European Coding system which will facilitate tracking of tissue from the donor all the way to the recipient. A variety of different coding systems are currently in use, some using manually recorded codes and others using computerised systems with bar coding. The use of the ISBT 128 coding standard for blood is widespread in blood services in Europe and in the US and has been further developed to include a tissue product nomenclature (see www.iccbba.org).

Currently, most tissue banks supply tissues direct to operating theatre departments and it is the responsibility of the receiving hospital to track from receipt of the tissue to the graft's ultimate fate. Many tissue banks supply the hospital with a recipient record to be completed for each graft and returned to the bank. The users should always be advised:
- to keep a log of tissue received and used;
- to record any allograft unit numbers in the patient's notes; and
- to inform the tissue bank immediately of any adverse reaction that might be attributable to the tissue graft.

In most cases, tissues are supplied for specific cases and stocks are not held in theatres, the notable exception to this being freeze-dried bone which can be kept at ambient temperature. In the UK, surgical facilities requiring urgent stocks on site, such as acute burns units, are required to obtain HTA licences for storage of grafts if they keep tissue for more than 48 hours.

Relevant experience in the storage and recording of human tissue for clinical use is available in the hospital blood bank. If hospital haematology departments are also willing to receive, store and distribute tissues in the future, then existing blood computer systems can be used to increase the security of tissue tracking within the hospital. The American Association of Tissue Banks has provided guidance for the handling of tissues once they arrive in hospitals.

Serious adverse events and reactions

Directive 2006/86/EC requires Member States to have systems for reporting adverse reactions and events related to the procurement, processing, storage, testing or distribution of the tissue, which might seriously affect the recipient. The TCD definitions are as follows.

Adverse event:

Any untoward occurrence associated with the procurement, testing, processing, storage and distribution of tissues and cells that might lead to the transmission of a communicable disease, to death or life-threatening, disabling or incapacitating conditions for patients or which might result in, or prolong, hospitalisation or morbidity.

Adverse reaction:

An unintended response, including a communicable disease, in the donor or in the recipient associated with the procurement or human application of tissues and cells that is fatal, life-threatening, disabling, incapacitating or which results in, or prolongs, hospitalisation or morbidity.

In England, the HTA has developed an electronic reporting system for tissue and cell facilities, in line with the requirements of Directive 2006/86/EC. Each tissue bank receiving information about such a reaction or an event must report it to the HTA when it comes to their attention, and then again when the investigation of the event is completed. Such reactions and events can also be reported by the organisation applying the graft, direct to the HTA.

Summary

The banking of non-blood tissues is increasing within blood services where expertise in donor selection, donor testing and quality management is being applied to the banking of many tissues including bone, tendons, heart valves and skin. Living donors can donate bone, amnion and heart valves during joint replacement, delivery of an infant or heart transplant surgery, respectively. All other types of tissue donation are made after death. For deceased donors, a thorough medical and behavioural history from a number of alternative sources is recorded to compensate for the lack of a face-to-face donor interview. This additional information should be sought from the donor's family doctor and the postmortem examination report (where applicable). Great care should be taken in blood sample collection and the acceptance of test results where tests were performed on blood samples taken from deceased donors.

Tissue processing is necessarily open and usually involves decontamination or terminal sterilisation. As a minimum, facilities for tissue processing in the EU should be designed to achieve class C for tissues destined for terminal sterilisation and class A, with class D background, for the manipulation of tissues in the absence of a terminal sterilisation step but following chemical or antibiotic decontamination. Many EU Member States apply more stringent requirements.

Traceability is an essential aspect of the quality chain and should be supported by machine-readable identification codes. If these are compatible with blood coding systems, traceability within the transplanting hospital can be greatly enhanced. Requirements are now in place for the reporting of serious adverse events and reactions to regulatory authorities to support the further enhancement of safety and quality in tissue banking.

Key points

1 Many donors of tissue are deceased resulting in many important features of tissue banking that make it different from blood banking notably in relation to donor history, collection and testing and processing.

2 EC Directives have been or are being transposed into the national legislation of the EC's 27 Member States requiring EC Member States to have inspection and accreditation systems to ensure that all tissue banks comply with mandated technical requirements.

3 Consent should be taken only by those trained to do so and the associated discussion should include information on intended clinical use of the tissue including research use, virological testing and the implications of positive results.

4 The primary source of donor selection information for deceased donors is the interview with someone who knew the donor well and this may not necessarily be the person who gives consent for the donation. Where a postmortem examination has been performed or is scheduled, the results should be reviewed as part of the donor selection process.

5 To avoid unnecessary loss of tissue due to poor labelling of hospital samples of donor blood, the identity of a premortem sample can be confirmed by use of molecular finger printing such as STR analysis to compare the sample and DNA from the donor's tissues such as bone marrow from a bone cavity.

6 An external examination of the donor body should be conducted, recorded and form part of the donor selection assessment prior to the tissue recovery. After tissue recovery, it is important to carefully reconstruct the donor body.

7 Processing tissue reduces the risk of disease transmission by removing blood and marrow and by reducing or eliminating contamination by chemical and physical means. Pooling of donations during processing is not permitted by standards in Europe or the US.

Further reading

Eastlund DT & Eisenbrey AB. (eds) *Guidelines for Managing Tissue Allografts in Hospitals*. Bethesda, MD: American Association of Blood Banks, 2006.

Eastlund T. Viral infections transmitted by tissue transplantation. In: Kennedy JF, Phillips GO & Williams PA.

(eds), *Sterilization of Tissue Using Ionizing Radiations*. Cambridge, UK: Woodhead Publisher, 2005.

Eastlund T & Strong DM. Infectious disease transmission through tissue transplantation. In: Phillips GO, Kearney JN, Strong DM, von Versen R & Nather A. (eds), *Advances in Tissue Banking*, Vol. 7. Singapore: World Scientific Publishing, 2003.

Fehily D, Delvecchio C, Di Ciaccio P *et al*. The EUSTITE project: working towards harmonised implementation of European regulation of tissues and cells. *Organs Tissues Cells* 2007;10(1)31–36.

Fehily D, Ashford P & Poniatowski S. Traceability of human tissues for transplantation – the development and implementation of a coding system using ISBT 128. *Organs Tissues* 2004;7(2):83–88.

MMWR Update: Allograft-Associated Bacterial Infections – United States, 2002. Available at http://www.cdc.gov/mmwr/preview/mmwrhtml/mm5110a2.htm.

Padley DJ, Lucas SB & Saldanha J. Elimination of false negative HCV RNA results by removal of inhibitors in cadaver donor blood specimens. *Transplantation* 2003;76(2):432–434.

Schulz-Baldes A, Biller-Andorno N & Capron AM. International perspectives on the ethics and regulation of human cell and tissue transplantation. *Bull World Health Org* 2007;85:941–948.

Simonds RJ, Holmberg SD, Hurwitz RL *et al*. Transmission of human immunodeficiency virus type 1 from a seronegative organ and tissue donor. *N Engl J Med* 1992;326:726–732.

Warwick RM, Eastlund T & Fehily D. Role of the blood transfusion service in tissue banking. *Vox Sang* 1996;71:71–77.

Warwick RM & Eglin R. Should deceased donors be tested for vCJD? *Cell Tissue Banking* 2005;6(4):263–270.

CHAPTER 45

Transfusion strategies in organ transplant patients

Anneke Brand[1] *& Derwood H. Pamphilon*[2]

[1]Department of Immunohaematology and Blood Transfusion, Leiden University Medical Center and Sanquin Blood Supply, Leiden, The Netherlands
[2]NHS Blood and Transplant; Department of Cellular and Molecular Medicine, University of Bristol, Bristol, UK

Immunomodulatory effects of pre-transplantant blood transfusions on solid organ transplantation

Before the 1980s, recombinant human erythropoietin (RhEpo) was not available. Consequently, patients with renal disease were often anaemic and received transfusions whilst dialysis dependent. Moreover, these transfusions were not leucocyte-reduced.

In 1973, Opelz and Terasaki showed in a multivariate analysis of observational studies that cadaver kidney graft survival in multiply transfused patients was significantly better when compared to non-transfused patients. This effect was irrespective of matching at human leucocyte antigen (HLA)-A, -B or -DR antigens, although the benefit of transfusion was greatest when there were more mismatches between recipient and kidney graft. Even today, there are different views on the mechanism of this 'transfusion effect', e.g. whether it is due to immunomodulation or, because transfusions elicit HLA antibodies, the benefits are due to better selection of kidneys from cross-match-negative donors. The possibility that allogeneic leucocytes play a

causal role was supported by a study showing that a single blood unit containing leucocytes improved graft survival, in particular when the blood donor and recipient shared an HLA haplotype.

The transfusion effect has been found in living-related donor kidney transplantation where it is called donor-specific transfusion (DST), as well as in heart, combined pancreas–kidney and liver transplantation, irrespective of the development of highly effective immunosuppressive drugs and anti-T-cell monoclonal antibodies to prevent and treat rejection episodes.

There have been many studies on the effects of pre-transplant transfusions in the last 30 years. Of 19 retrospective studies published between 1973 and 2005, 14 reported that pre-transplant transfusion reduced acute graft rejection and/or improved graft survival. In seven prospective studies, of which, only two were randomised, five showed a modest positive effect of transfusion. Because of the differences between the studies, a meta-analysis was impossible and definite recommendations cannot be made. Deliberate, pre-transplant third-party non-leucocyte-reduced transfusions have been virtually abandoned, mainly because of lack of solid evidence, concerns about transmissible diseases and HLA antibody formation. When DSTs are given, 8–13% of patients become sensitised, and fewer if concurrent treatment with

Practical Transfusion Medicine, 3rd edition. Edited by Michael F. Murphy and Derwood H. Pamphilon. © 2009 Blackwell Publishing, ISBN: 978-1-4051-8196-9.

immunosuppressive drugs is given. Graft and patient survival of 90% at 5 years following DST has been reported where combinations of immunosuppressive drugs were given after transplantation.

It has also been shown that transfusion of donor bone marrow cells to patients who receive kidney, liver or heart transplants reduces the incidence of acute cellular graft rejection and lowers reactivity against donor cells in the mixed lymphocyte reaction. This suggests that specific tolerance may be maintained due to the persistence of donor cells, which can be detected by sensitive molecular analysis of chimeric status.

Although the clinical effect of third-party pre-transplant blood transfusions still awaits convincing randomised controlled studies, many animal studies to determine the mechanisms have been performed. The main reason to utilise blood transfusion to achieve tolerance to the organ donor, is to avoid or reduce the use of intensive immunosuppression, which may enhance the development of post-transplant malignancies such as non-Hodgkin's lymphoma, which occurs in patients after transplantation 35–40 times more frequently than in the general population.

Proposed mechanisms for induction of tolerance by blood transfusion are:
• induction of suppressor cells;
• reduction by apoptosis or deletion in the number of cytotoxic T-effector lymphocytes reactive with donor-type HLA;
• induction of anergy; and
• formation of anti-idiotype antibodies, counteracting the formation of HLA antibodies.

These putative mechanisms do not explain the role of HLA sharing between donor and recipient and why a single blood transfusion may downregulate the response against a third-party organ donor. A hypothetical model is that the patient's T cells recognise foreign allogeneic peptide presented by the HLA-DR (which the donor and patients share) on donor antigen presenting cells (APCs). These APCs which may be slightly modified by blood processing and storage initiate induction of memory regulatory T cells (Tregs). Such Tregs may downregulate an effective immune response towards a subsequently transplanted organ sharing a peptide

with the transfusion donor, which is quite likely given the large number of shared peptides among random individuals (Figure 45.1).

Sensitisation of potential transplant recipients

Transplant rejection may occur as:
(i) (hyper)acute rejection mediated by pre-existing antibodies; and
(ii) acute and chronic cellular and/or humoral rejection which require immunosuppressive drugs for their prevention.

The effect of HLA matching and the harm caused by HLA antibodies differs depending on the type of organ graft:
• HLA matching is most important in kidney transplantation.
• DR-shared heart transplants have a better outcome than DR-mismatched grafts.
• In liver transplantation, HLA matching hardly plays a role.

For all prospective transplant recipients, HLA alloimmunisation should be avoided because a positive lymphocytotoxic cross-match between donor lymphocytes and the patient's serum compromises the outcome. Options for antibody depletion in sensitised patients include:
• plasma exchange with or without antibody absorption columns;
• intravenous immunoglobulin (IVIG);
• monoclonal antibodies, e.g. rituximab; and
• other immunosuppressive drugs.

Major ABO compatibility is required for all solid organ grafts, although in group O or B recipients, with low titre anti-A antibodies, blood group A2 grafts have acceptable survival. Where other risk factors for HLA immunisation and red cell alloimmunisation by pregnancies and previous graft rejection cannot be circumvented, immunisation by transfusion should be prevented as much as possible.

Potential renal transplant recipients
All end-stage renal patients currently receive recombinant human RhEpo and therapeutic

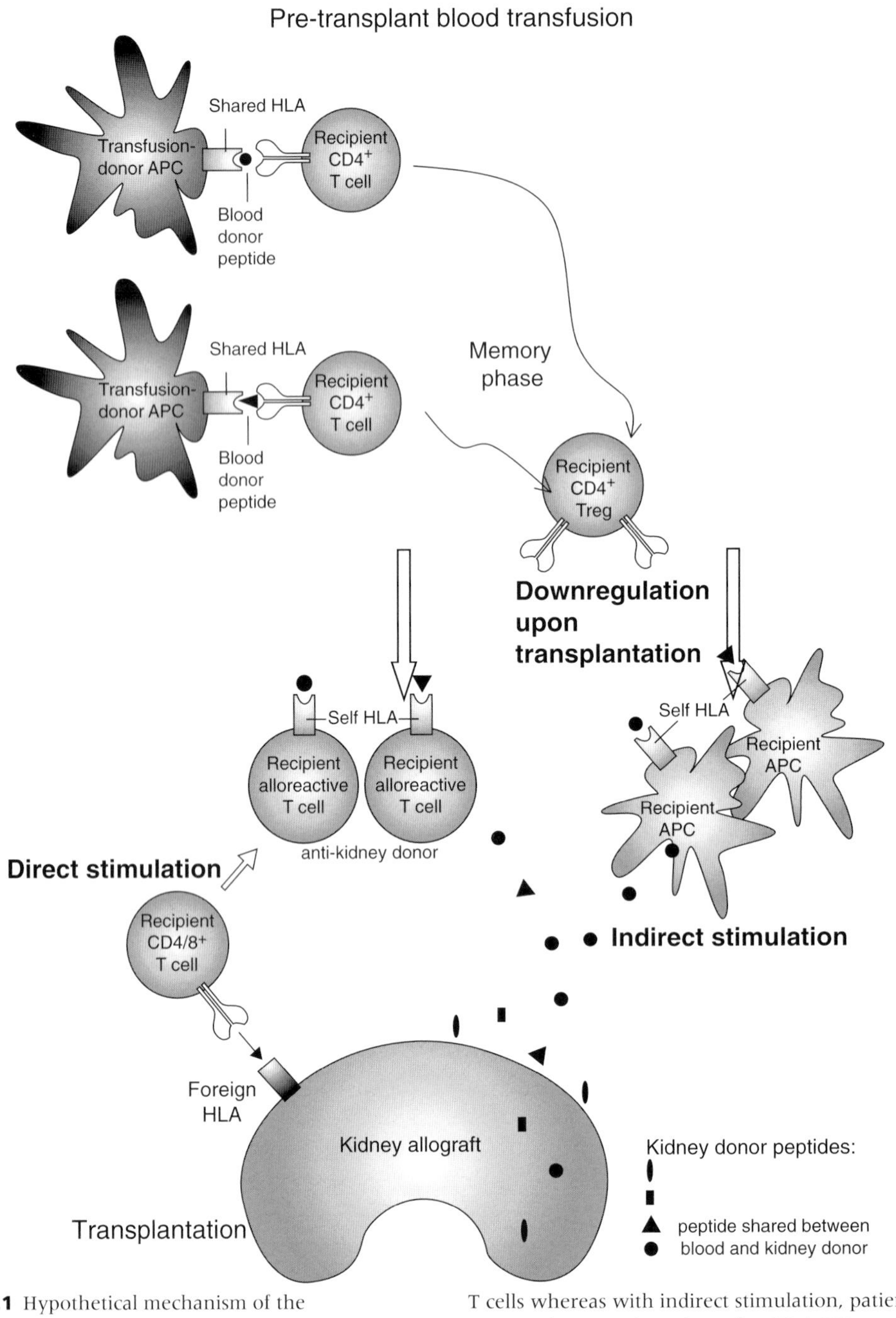

Figure 45.1 Hypothetical mechanism of the pre-transplantation transfusion effect dampening allograft rejection. Antigen presenting cells (APCs) from a 1 HLA-DR shared blood donor induce a recipient immune response against one or more transfusion donor peptides which leads to specific CD4+ regulatory T cells in the recipient. After organ transplantation, the patient's T cells can be stimulated by direct or indirect pathways. After direct stimulation, HLA-DR is induced on recipient T cells whereas with indirect stimulation, patient APCs present donor antigens bound to HLA-DR to self-T cells. If the organ donor shares peptides with the transfusion donor, the regulatory T cells that have memory for specific peptides from the donor are activated and downregulate an effective immune response against the shared peptide(s). (Drawing provided by Marloes Waanders, Leiden University Medical Center.)

transfusions are required only for patients do not respond to it. These therapeutic transfusions are now routinely leucocyte-reduced by filtration in Western Europe. Although leucocyte reduction significantly reduces HLA alloimmunisation induced by platelet transfusions by more than 70%, this has not been demonstrated for leucocyte-reduced red cell transfusions. Before transplantation, transfusion should be restricted as much as possible, because HLA alloimmunisation is a major threat for kidney graft recipients. Recently, concern has been raised because of thrombotic complications resulting from the use of RhEpo, in particular when the haemoglobin (Hb) concentration is corrected to normal. However, reaching Hb levels that avoid transfusions is an important achievement which:

• improves the quality of life; and
• minimises the risk of broad HLA alloimmunisation which can lead to prolonged waiting times for a suitable kidney and impaired graft survival.

Moreover, some red cell antigens such as Duffy, Kidd and Lewis are expressed outside the haemopoietic lineage and can act as minor transplantation antigens which are of particular relevance for chronic rejection.

Potential orthotopic liver transplant recipients

Liver transplantation accounts for more than 10,000 transplants each year in Europe and the US. It has a long-term survival of about 70% and is performed for:

• end-stage chronic liver failure;
• acute liver failure;
• unresectable primary liver tumours; and
• metabolic diseases.

Depending on the underlying disease, patients may receive multiple transfusions preoperatively for correction of anaemia, thrombocytopenia and coagulation factor deficiency; although there is lack of evidence for the benefit of prophylactic correction of abnormal bleeding times or coagulation tests. The key points regarding HLA matching are:

• HLA matching between donor and recipient does not influence the outcome.

• The presence of HLA antibodies and a positive lymphocytotoxic cross-match with the organ donor is not a contraindication for transplantation.
• Combined liver and kidney transplantation can be performed where there is a positive cross-match since the liver can absorb harmful antibodies.
• Although a positive cross-match with the liver donor is associated with poorer graft survival, in general, acute graft rejection episodes with orthotopic liver transplant (OLT) have been described in only up to 15% of patients, while graft loss from rejection is a rare event.

Alloimmunisation to red blood cell antigens (reported in 6–14%) of prospective OLT patients may pose a problem and results from published studies have identified worse patient survival where there is a history of red cell antibodies. In Caucasians, antibodies to Rh and K1 dominate and while not currently included in guidelines, prospective matching with compatible Rh/K units for patients with liver diseases may be considered in the future.

Potential cardiac transplant recipients

HLA antibodies must be avoided as a strongly positive lymphocytotoxic cross-match with the heart donor is associated with rejection. Primary cardiac transplantation without prior cardiac surgery poses hardly any problems of alloimmunisation towards HLA or red cell antigens. After prior coronary artery bypass surgery, leucocyte antibodies have been found in 10–15% and red cell antibodies in 3–5% of the patients. In particular, patients who have left ventricular assist devices (LVADs) implanted as a bridge to transplantation need multiple blood components and approximately 30% develop HLA antibodies, reducing the chance of a cross-match-negative graft. Several approaches to reduce the titre of allo-HLA antibodies, in the same way as for kidney transplant patients, are currently being studied. For patients with LVAD, it is important to check the presence and specificity of irregular red cell antibodies because these patients will need further transfusions during the transplant procedure.

Blood component transfusion during transplantation surgery

Renal transplantation

The risk of transfusions in kidney transplantation is low and apart from the group and screen procedure, blood is generally not requested unless the preoperative haemoglobin is below 9 g/dL, e.g. in RhEpo refractory patients. As transfusions are infrequently required during surgery, the use of cell salvage or pharmacological agents to reduce blood loss is not appropriate.

Orthotopic liver transplant

The liver produces and regulates many proteins of the coagulation and fibrinolytic cascades. Normally these two cascades are in balance, but they are disturbed in chronic liver disease. Patients with terminal liver failure usually have disordered coagulation and thrombocytopenia due to portal hypertension before transplantation. There are three phases of liver transplantation surgery:

• In the *pre-anhepatic phase* of surgery, bleeding is largely determined by preoperative haemostatic disorders. Frequent findings are prolonged prothrombin and activated partial thromboplastin times and thrombocytopenia. However, most clotting tests estimate procoagulant activity only and because anticoagulant activity is also impaired many centres do not correct an abnormal PT or a low platelet count prior to transplantation and decide on the use of blood component therapy if there is excessive bleeding.

• During the *anhepatic phase*, coagulation factors are not produced or cleared. Bleeding in this phase is mainly the result of primary hyperfibrinolysis because of reduced clearance of tissue-plasminogen activator (t-PA). Increased t-PA stimulates plasminogen conversion to plasmin, which in turn, converts fibrinogen to split products leading to enhanced destruction of formed clots.

• In the *reperfusion phase*, t-PA normalises, but ischaemia-reperfusion injury decreases the platelet count and causes bleeding associated with thrombocytopathy.

Knowledge of these coagulation disturbances and the use of anti-fibrinolytic drugs, such as aprotinin and tranexamic acid and intraoperative blood salvage, have all contributed to a reduction of blood loss and transfusion requirements. Currently, approximately one-third of patients do not need red cell transfusions during OLT and the average need has been reduced from 12 to 3–4 units of red cells, and to an average of 6–12 units of fresh frozen plasma (FFP) and 1–2 platelet transfusions. FFP treated with solvent–detergent processes to inactivate viruses is as effective as standard FFP in OLT (see Table 45.1).

A reduction in transfusions is important, as red cell transfusions are associated with worse graft function in the immediate postoperative period, an increased incidence of infection, gastrointestinal and intra-abdominal complications, respiratory syndromes, rejection and a lower overall survival. However, up to 15% of patients still require more than 20 red cell units and a minority even more than 40 units. If because of preceding blood transfusions, multiple red cell antibodies are present this adds to the difficulty of providing large inventories of compatible red cells. Timely identification of red cell antibodies is needed so as not to delay the procedure and to collect a stock of compatible units. Cooperation between the surgical team and transfusion service is needed as after 5–10 compatible units, in case of massive bleeding, incompatible units (if the patient has antibodies) or RhD-positive units to RhD-negative recipients may be used to allow 5–10 compatible units to be reserved for transfusions that are expected to remain in the circulation.

Cardiac transplantation

The key points are:

• Red cell antibodies are reported in 1–1.5% of patients.

• Heart transplantation requires similar transfusion support as coronary artery bypass surgery.

• In primary transplants, 0–2 units of red cells are required.

• Twice this amount is generally needed when there has been prior surgery.

	Red cells	FFP	Platelets*
Renal	0–1	—	—
Liver (85%)	3	6–12	2
Liver (15%)†	>20	>30	>6
Heart	2–4	1–6	1
Heart after LVAD/heart–lung	8	12	2
Pancreas	1–2	—	—

Table 45.1 Blood component usage in organ transplantation.

*As therapeutic dose 4–6 donor unit equivalents.
†10–15% of patient need >20 units.
FFP, fresh frozen plasma; LVAD, left ventricular assist device.

• Patients with prior LVAD support will often need multiple transfusions of red cells (more than 6 units) plus FFP and platelet transfusions. Because these patients may have already received 50 units of red cells or more (depending on the length of LVAD support), regular screening will reveal red cell antibodies prior to transplantation.

• Although in general, red cell antibodies do not pose major problems in cardiac transplant patients, these patients have the highest risk for passenger lymphocyte syndrome (PLS) and post-transplantation haemolysis occurs in 2–5%.

Autologous blood

Autologous blood salvage is routinely used in liver and heart transplantation. It has been shown that the haemodynamic status in patients, with cardiac or pulmonary disease, who were candidates for cardiac transplants was comparable with controls following autologous blood donation. This may, therefore, be an appropriate strategy to reduce the requirement for allogeneic blood products during surgery. Blood collection could be augmented by the use of RhEpo, although this is expensive. For a more detailed discussion of autologous transfusion strategies, see Chapters 33 and 34.

Platelet concentrates may be collected immediately preoperatively in the anaesthetic room, using an apheresis machine, and infused during surgery. There is evidence that this will reduce the requirement for allogeneic platelets and may also impact on transfusion requirements since the platelets are fresh.

Viral infections

Because of immunosuppressive therapy, viral infections, in particular those that need life-long T-cell immunity, are of clinical importance after transplantation. Most important from a clinical point of view as well as by virtue of their transmission by transfusions or the organ graft are the herpes viruses CMV (cytomegalovirus) and EBV (Epstein–Barr virus). Hepatitis viruses will be discussed in the context of liver transplant patients.

Cytomegalovirus
Renal transplantation

CMV is of importance after organ transplantation and can be acquired from:

• the donor kidney if seropositive;
• CMV-positive blood transfusions; and
• reactivation of the patients' CMV.

CMV infection can be prevented in CMV-seronegative donor–recipients by:

• provision of CMV-seronegative blood components; and
• leucocyte reduction to less than 5×10^6 leucocytes/transfused component.

A review of 1145 renal transplant patients showed active CMV infection in 85% of those with, and 53% of those without, CMV antibodies at the time of transplant, suggesting that latent virus is reactivated during the transplant process. Reactivation itself does not appear to be detrimental to graft survival. If CMV-seronegative blood is given to CMV-seronegative donor–recipient pairs, then no CMV infection results. Primary infection transferred with the donor kidney is of greater severity than infection associated with reactivation. In one report, 26 of 74 patients who received CMV-seronegative blood and a kidney from a donor of unknown CMV-serostatus developed primary infection, 20 of the 26 were symptomatic, and three died.

In 'at-risk' transplants, i.e. where either the patient or donor is CMV-seropositive, administration of ganciclovir or valaciclovir for 3 months is effective in preventing CMV disease. Intravenous immunoglobulin from CMV hyperimmune globulin (CMVIg) may reduce the chance of CMV infection, but its role is controversial.

Orthotopic liver transplant

Liver transplant recipients who are CMV-seronegative may acquire infection via a seropositive graft or via blood transfusions. The former route seems to be of greater importance. Recipients of CMV-seropositive grafts are more likely to have:
- CMV pneumonia;
- CMV hepatitis;
- invasive fungal infections; and
- reduced survival.

The incidence of CMV pneumonia has been shown to correlate with both the total number of units of blood and the number of CMV-positive units transfused perioperatively. CMV infection is also associated with an increased chance of graft rejection. CMV infection may also occur because of reactivation in CMV-positive recipients. It appears that seroconversion to human herpes virus (HHV)-6 is a marker for CMV disease.

In patients at risk of CMV infection, use of CMVIg has been shown to reduce severe CMV-associated disease and improve long-term survival. In addition, the use of prophylactic ganciclovir in at-risk patients significantly reduces the incidence of CMV disease.

Cardiac transplantation

CMV infection adversely affects the outcome of cardiac allografting. In 91 of 301 patients who developed CMV infection at one centre over an 8-year period there was an increase in:

- graft rejection; and
- development of atherosclerosis resulting in decreased survival.

Epstein–Barr virus

EBV is the major cause of post-transplant lymphoma (post-transplant lymphoproliferative disease or PTLD) complicating all kinds of allogeneic solid organ and haemopoietic stem cell transplantations after an average interval of 3 years (range 1 month to 15 years). It does not originate from transfused blood components as most adult patients and organ donors are EBV-seropositive and leucocyte reduction of blood products removes latently infected leucocytes. It is due to immunosuppression, in particular with ATG, anti-T-cell response modifiers and drugs, and maybe enhanced by an allogeneic effect. EBV-associated non-Hodgkin's lymphoma has a strikingly increased incidence in the transplant population. Currently, some centres apply novel treatment with donor-specific anti-EBV cytotoxic T lymphocytes (CTLs) after stem cell transplantation. Research is ongoing into the use of unrelated HLA compatible random donor anti-EBV CTLs in solid organ transplant recipients. This approach may in the future also be useful to treat severe disease manifestations caused by other herpes viruses, such as CMV and varicella zoster virus. This would be particularly useful for children who may be seronegative for herpes viruses and transplanted with grafts from seropositive donors.

Hepatitis viruses

HCV and hepatitis B (HBV) can be acquired from blood transfusion. An increased incidence of post-transplant liver disease has been reported in HCV-seropositive patients, but this does not appear to influence either the graft or patient survival.

A number of patients with HCV infection develop severe liver disease and undergo OLT. The overall outcome in this group of patients is excellent, with survival as high as 75% at 5 years after transplantation. Surprisingly, grafts from HCV-seropositive donors do not result in decreased survival when compared with grafts from HCV-seronegative donors and there is no difference in the rate of graft rejection. HBV-positive recipients are also eligible for OLT after antiviral treatment to reduce the viral load. Provided after transplantation, the viral load is kept low with antiviral treatment often including hepatitis B immunoglobulin, graft and patient survival is excellent.

Postoperative complications associated with perioperative blood transfusions

• Red cell transfusions in liver transplantation and after open-heart surgery are dose-dependent and associated with poorer graft function in the immediate postoperative period, an increased incidence of infection, gastrointestinal and intra-abdominal complications, respiratory syndromes, rejection and lower overall survival.
• Although a causal role is unknown, it has been shown that leuco-reduction of red cell products are associated with less complications as compared to leucocyte-containing transfusions.
• Cellular blood components used in the pre-, per- and postoperative setting thus must be leucocyte-reduced to reduce HLA immunisation and CMV transmission and impair post-perfusion complications after liver and cardiac surgery.
• It is not necessary to irradiate cellular blood components to prevent transfusion-associated graft-versus-host disease.

Passenger lymphocyte syndrome
(also see Chapter 7)

After organ grafting, graft-derived memory B cells, which encounter incompatible antigens in the recipient, can rapidly produce very high titres of allo-antibodies mainly against red cell antigens, but platelet or even solid tissue antigens can be the target of donor-derived antibodies. Even primary donor B-cell responses have been reported. Haemolysis most often occurs in minor ABO-incompatible grafts, but severe haemolysis due to RhD antibodies has also been described. IgG antibodies typically appear after 7 days to 3 weeks af-

ter transplantation and dependent on the size of the graft disappear after 1 month, but may last longer than 6 months. Passive haemolysis most frequently occurs after heart transplantation, followed by liver transplantation, kidney transplants and is rare after visceral transplants. Patients typically receive ciclosporin and/or tacrolimus. Antithymocyte immunoglobulin and mycophenolate mofetil do not protect against PLS. Often there is only mild haemolysis associated with a positive direct antiglobulin (DAT) test, although severe haemolysis causing renal failure or even death has been observed. It is important to consider this phenomenon in any unexpected haemoglobin decrease after transplantation. Treatment consists of recipient and donor compatible transfusions, although corticosteroids, plasma exchange and rituximab may be needed.

Key points

1 All cellular blood products for transplant patients must be leucocyte-reduced.
2 Leucocyte-containing transfusions for immunomodulation should be given only in clinical studies.
3 Leucocyte-reduced red cell transfusions can still induce HLA antibodies and their use must be restricted for prospective renal and heart transplant patients.
4 Liver transplant patients may possess multiple red cell antibodies, this should be identified prior to transplantation.
5 Consideration should be given to transfusing prospective liver transplant recipients with Rh- and K-matched red cells.
6 Abnormal coagulation tests in patients with liver failure do not predict bleeding and FFP correction of a prolonged PT prior to transplantation is not indicated.
7 In case of haemoglobin decrease after transplantation, haemolysis due to passive lymphocyte syndrome should be considered.
8 Blood transfusions, provided leucocyte reduction is used, play a minor role in post-transplantation viral diseases.

Further reading

Blajchman MA & Singal DP. The role of red blood cell antigens, histocompatibility antigens, and blood transfusions on renal allograft survival. *Transfus Med Rev* 1998;3:171–179.

Chavers B, Sullivan EK, Tejani A & Harmon WE. Pre-transplant blood transfusion and renal allograft outcome: a report of the North American Paediatric Renal Transplant Cooperative Study. *Pediatr Transplant* 1997;1:22–28.

Deeg HJ & Sayers MH. Transfusion support in transplant patients. In: Pamphilon DH. (ed), *Modern Transfusion Medicine*. Boca Raton, FL: CRC Press, 1995, pp. 177–192.

Gratton MR, Moreno-Cabral CE, Starnes VA, Oyer PF, Stinson EB & Shumway ME. Cytomegalovirus and its association with cardiac allograft rejection and atherosclerosis. *JAMA* 1998;261:3561–3566.

Kanj SA, Sharara AI, Clavien P-A & Hamilton JD. Cytomegalovirus infection following liver transplantation: review of the literature. *Clin Infect Dis* 1996;22:537–549.

Lisman T, Caldwell SH, Porte LJ & Leebeek FW. Consequences of abnormal hemostasis tests for clinical practice. *J Thromb Haemost* 2006;4:2062–2063.

McCarthy JF, Cook DJ, Massad MG *et al.* Vascular rejection post heart transplantation is associated with positive flow cytometric cross-matching. *Eur J Cardiothorac Surg* 1998;14:197–200.

Molenaar IQ, Warnaar N, Groen H, Tenvergent EM, Slooff MJ & Porte RJ. Efficacy and safety of antifibrinolytic drugs in liver transplantation: a systemic review and meta-analysis. *Am J Transplant* 2007;7:185–194.

Palomo Sanchez JC, Jimenez C, Moreno Gonzalez E *et al.* Effects of intraoperative blood transfusion on postoperative complications and survival after orthotopic liver transplantation. *Hepatogastroenterology* 1998;45:1026–1033.

Salgar SK, Shapiro R, Dodson F *et al.* Infusion of donor leucocytes to induce tolerance in organ allograft recipients. *J Leuk Biol* 1999;66:310–314.

PART 7

Development of the evidence base for transfusion

CHAPTER 46

The design of interventional trials in transfusion medicine

Paul C. Hébert, Alan T. Tinmouth & Dean Fergusson
[1] University of Ottawa; University of Ottawa Center for Transfusion Research, Clinical Epidemiology Program, The Ottawa Health Research Institute, Ottawa, Ontario, Canada

Introduction

Randomised controlled clinical trials (RCTs) have evolved to become the 'gold standard' clinical research design used to distinguish the risks and benefits of therapeutic interventions. In 1948, for the first time a controlled clinical trial made use of random allocation, a control group and blinding. Additional principles guiding the design of RCTs were first elaborated by Sir Austin Bradford-Hill in the 1960s.

Many important questions regarding the use of blood products and alternatives such as blood conservation therapies have not been the subject of well-designed and executed RCTs. Consequently, clinicians frequently base their therapeutic decisions on suboptimal levels of clinical evidence, including observational studies, poorly controlled clinical trials or laboratory studies, and personal experience or observations, which are not evidence based. There are a number of plausible reasons why there are so few large clinical trials in transfusion medicine:

• transfusion medicine has historically been a laboratory-based specialty with research focused on the product;

Practical Transfusion Medicine, 3rd edition. Edited by Michael F. Murphy and Derwood H. Pamphilon. © 2009 Blackwell Publishing, ISBN: 978-1-4051-8196-9.

• a dearth of clinical epidemiologists and clinical trialists interested in transfusion medicine;

• difficulty in obtaining funding for research of a supportive as opposed to a curative therapy;

• many of the products have been in standard use for years; and

• there are few industry partners willing to invest in large clinical trials given that products are already in wide use.

It could also be postulated that unique difficulties in the field may have impeded the development of important clinical studies. In this chapter, we outline some of the methodological issues central to the development and conduct of interventional trials and RCTs in transfusion medicine.

What is unique about transfusion medicine?

There are a number of unique difficulties in transfusion medicine that require consideration in the development of clinical research. First and foremost, transfusion medicine as a discipline is largely based upon the provision of supportive interventions in the treatment of a wide variety of acute illnesses as opposed to disciplines such as cardiology or oncology where interventions are evaluated in well-defined diseases. Furthermore, studies are conducted by trialists trained within a specific discipline (e.g. oncologists, cardiac surgeons). In comparison, blood products are indicated in response to conditions such as anaemia or coagulopathy induced by medications or disease entities. The supportive nature of transfusions leads to consideration of outcomes that may not be directly clinically relevant to the underlying disease process. In addition, most benefits and risks of care would not be attributed to supportive interventions.

Conditions that require blood products, such as anaemia and coagulopathies, occur in a broad range of diseases. This raises significant difficulties in designing studies and setting a research agenda. If one tries to evaluate a transfusion intervention in many diseases, then larger sample sizes and more robust outcomes are required to account for the variation within the patient population. Alternatively, many smaller trials in targeted populations may also be considered. However, this strategy will limit the generalisability of the study as the conclusions may not be applicable to patient groups outside the studied target population.

A further concern is the complex biological nature of blood products. For instance, red cell concentrates are prepared using a variety of techniques and storage media, and intravenous immunoglobulins are manufactured by different companies using different processes. This leads investigators to consider whether studies evaluating a transfusion intervention should only be done with one product or preparation, or with many different preparations. Indeed, there may be unforeseen or unexpected clinical consequences due to different approaches to the preparation of blood products. In the planning of studies, one must carefully consider whether products are sufficiently similar to consider including in the same study. Regulatory concerns within or between jurisdictions may also impact on the choice of products included in the study.

As discussed in subsequent sections, regulations may not permit the conduct of randomised trials for studies assessing the clinical consequences of different products or testing procedures. Under such constraints, quasi-experimental designs such as before-

and-after studies or time-series analyses should be considered.

One of the remaining unique aspects of conducting clinical research in transfusion medicine is that transfusions are often incorporated into complex care paths or within therapeutic algorithms of care. The evaluation of transfusions with many other interventions and diagnostic tests increases the complexity of any clinical evaluation.

Types of studies

To ascertain the effectiveness of an intervention, the RCT remains the preferred study design as it minimises the most important biases if properly conceived and executed. Despite being the gold standard, there are often practical, legal, financial and ethical limitations to the use of clinical trials. For instance, exposing subjects to undesirable and dangerous interventions such as cigarettes and toxins would not be permitted in an RCT. While many of these limitations have been well described, one unique obstacle encountered in transfusion medicine is the conduct of an RCT when an intervention is universally implemented, such as a new processing method or testing procedure for the entire blood supply. By implementing an intervention such as universal prestorage leucocyte reduction or universal polymerase chain reaction (PCR) testing for hepatitis C, an RCT becomes impossible within that population. If an RCT is not possible, other study designs including quasi-experimental and observational designs should be considered.

Observational studies

Two types of observational designs are often considered in clinical research, case–control studies and cohort or prognostic studies (Figure 46.1). A case–control study refers to a study where one identifies a group of individuals with an outcome and another group of individuals who would be considered at risk of developing the outcome. Once both groups have been identified, investigators usually seek to identify potential risk factors in

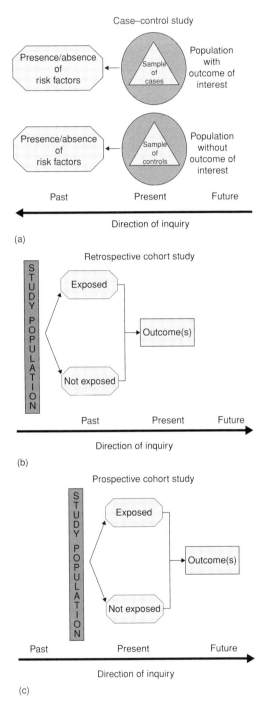

Case–control study

Presence/absence of risk factors ← Sample of cases — Population with outcome of interest

Presence/absence of risk factors ← Sample of controls — Population without outcome of interest

Past   Present   Future

Direction of inquiry

(a)

Retrospective cohort study

STUDY POPULATION

Exposed

Not exposed

→ Outcome(s)

Past   Present   Future

Direction of inquiry

(b)

Prospective cohort study

STUDY POPULATION

Exposed

Not exposed

→ Outcome(s)

Past   Present   Future

Direction of inquiry

(c)

Figure 46.1 Observational study designs: case–control and cohort studies. (Adapted from Tay and Tinmouth *Transfusion* 2007;47(7):1115–1117.)

both the group with the outcome and the controls. This classic epidemiological design is ideally suited to the investigation of rare diseases and the identification of potential aetiological or risk factors particulary if there is a long latency period. In transfusion medicine, case–control studies would be ideally suited for the initial study of rare conditions such as transfusion-related acute lung injury (TRALI) and the association between blood transfusion and variant Creutzfeldt–Jakob disease (vCJD). By definition, this study design is always retrospective in nature. Cases, controls and potential risk factors are identified from historical records or past events. By comparing 46 cases of patients with TRALI (cases) and 225 randomly selected transfusion recipients without TRALI (controls), Siliman *et al.* were able to identify that certain diagnoses (haematological malignancies and cardiac disease) and the age of the platelets were associated with TRALI. In a smaller subset of cases and controls, the implicated units also had greater neutrophil priming activity as compared with controls. While these results demonstrate an association between neutrophil priming activity, which increases in older platelets, and TRALI reactions, the case–control design does not allow causation to be determined.

Despite some of the potential advantages of this study design, it is also difficult to do well and is fraught with potential biases. A systematic review of case–control studies attempting to establish the association between blood transfusion and vCJD demonstrated that blood transfusion had a protective effect. Such a protective effect makes little sense and is probably the result of some biased approach to the sampling of controls.

The second observational design choice is a cohort study. In this type of study, individuals are identified well in advance of developing a disease and followed forward in time. Ideally, information on potential risk factors would be gathered from patients throughout the period of observation until the occurrence of an outcome or the end of the study. If subjects are identified well in advance of the development of a disease, then comparing individuals who have a given risk factor with individuals who do not may provide important clues to the aetiology of a disease or health state. It may also lead to a better understanding of the course of the disease and its incidence. If patients are identified and followed once a disease has developed, then this design may also provide invaluable prognostic information.

Cohort studies follow patients forward in time and evaluate outcomes based on a known exposure, risk factor or treatment. This design is most powerful when all eligible individuals are identified early, followed prospectively and without any losses to follow-up. A number of cohort studies have examined the relationship between anaemia, red cell transfusion and outcomes such as hospital mortality. These studies illustrate both positive and negative attributes of cohort studies. A retrospective study conducted by Carson and colleagues evaluated the relationship between increasing degrees of anaemia, the presence of ischaemic heart disease and mortality rates. In 1958, Jehovah's Witness patients, the adjusted odds of death increased from 2.3 (95% confidence interval (CI) 1.4–4.0) to 12.3 (95% CI 2.5–62.1) as preoperative haemoglobin concentrations declined from 10.0–10.9 g/dL to 6.0–6.9 g/dL in patients with cardiac disease as compared with patients without cardiac disease. This study shows a clear relationship between increasing anaemia and death.

In comparison, the risks of anaemia and benefits of transfusions may be quite complex. This interdependence is often referred to as confounding by indication. Observational studies in transfusion medicine have attempted to compare clinical outcomes at varying haemoglobin concentrations in transfused and non-transfused patients in various clinical settings. Previous studies have major limitations including confounding by indication. Wu *et al.* retrospectively studied Medicare records of 78,974 patients older than 65 who were hospitalised with a primary diagnosis of acute myocardial infarction. The authors then categorised patients according to their admission haematocrit. Although anaemia defined in the study as a haematocrit of less than 39% was present in nearly half the patients, only 4.7% (3680 of 78,974) patients received a red cell transfusion. Lower admission haematocrit values were associated with increased 30-day mortality, with a mortality rate approaching 50% among patients with a haematocrit of 27% or lower who did not receive a red cell transfusion. Even though the study was published in a prestigious journal, there were several major limitations making it difficult to draw useful conclusions:

• confounding by indication may have been a major concern;
• admission haematocrits rather than haematocrits prior to transfusion were used in the analysis;
• the timing and number of transfusions were unknown;
• few adjustments for other sources of confounding were undertaken because of the retrospective nature of the study; and
• inability to adjust for important but unmeasured variables.

One of the positive aspects of the study by Wu and colleagues was their approach to analysis. They did not presume that the risks of anaemia and transfusion would be similar at all degrees of anaemia. This was one of the most important limitations of a recent study by Vincent and colleagues. These authors completed a prospective observational cross-sectional study involving 3534 patients admitted to 146 western European intensive care units (ICUs) during a 2-week period in November 1999; 37% of patients received a red cell transfusion during their ICU admission, with the overall transfusion rate increasing to 41.6% over a 28-day period. For those patients who were transfused, the mean pre-transfusion haemoglobin concentration was 8.4 ± 1.3 g/dL. In an effort to control for confounding created by illness severity and the need for transfusion, these investigators employed a strategy of matching transfused and non-transfused patients based on their propensity to receive a transfusion, thereby defining two well-balanced groups (516 patients in each group) to determine the influence of red cell transfusions on mortality. Using this approach, the associated risk of death was increased instead of decreased by 33% for patients who received a transfusion compared with similar patients who did not receive blood. However, as pointed out in the accompanying editorial, the results may have differed if the propensity scores were derived separately for categories of pre-transfusion haemoglobin concentrations (e.g. <8, 8–10 and >10 g/dL) instead of haemoglobin concentrations at ICU admission. For example, if one were to consider groups of patients with a pre-transfusion haemoglobin concentration below 6.0 g/dL, it is unlikely that the observed 33% increase in mortality would similarly hold true or blood transfusion would never have been recommended.

The use of cohort studies in the evaluation of a universally implemented intervention such as pre-storage leucocyte reduction requires either that subjects be sampled over a period of time prior to and after the implementation of the programme (a 'before-and-after' or interrupted time-series study) or that sampling occur among subjects who received leucocyte-reduced blood products and another population that did not receive such products (standardised incidence study). In this type of study, a standardised incidence ratio is calculated by comparing (standardising) the incidence of an outcome in a defined exposed population with that of another population. In the standardisation procedure, care is taken to adjust for important confounders. Using universal leucocyte reduction as an example, the incidence of nosocomial infection in Canadian patients receiving a transfusion could be compared to a Japanese population of transfused patients receiving non-leucocyte-reduced blood products. In comparison, a before-and-after study design measures the frequency of an outcome in a specified population during a period of time when the exposure is absent followed by a measurement in the same population during a period of time where exposure is present. Consecutive periods before and after the implementation of a treatment are often compared. One type of before-and-after study is the interrupted time-series design that proposes to make determinations of an outcome at multiple time points, rather than only one, before and after the implementation of an intervention.

Well-executed case–control studies may provide clues about the aetiology or risk factors associated with the development of a disease or a complication. A cohort study may provide the best estimate of incidence, prognosis and risks associated with the development of a disease or its complications. Both designs provide weak inferences regarding specific therapeutic interventions because many forms of bias and confounding remain even after complex multivariable analysis. Before-and-after studies and time-series analysis, both quasi-experimental designs, may provide some inferences regarding clinical consequences attributed to the implementation of a universal programme when a randomised trial is not possible. Inherent in both case–control and cohort studies is the inability to determine causality between a risk factor or treatment and a specific outcome.

Randomised controlled trials

Overall design approaches for RCTs

Clinicians, hospital administrators and policy-makers should always seek to identify the best evidence for decision-making. Researchers should aspire to conduct the highest-quality studies. For therapeutic interventions, there is little debate that this should be an RCT. However, there should be an awareness that randomised trials may be complex. The question being addressed, the many choices and compromises made by the investigators pertaining to different study manoeuvres, such as the selection of patients and centres, may affect inferences made from the results of the trial. In this section, a conceptual framework is provided for randomised trials that should assist providers and consumers of clinical research.

The ideal RCT establishes whether therapeutic interventions work and determines the overall benefits and risks of each alternative in predefined patient populations. This is accomplished by minimising the influence of chance, bias and confounding through appropriate methodology. In addition, the ideal RCT should attempt to fulfil its objectives with the fewest patients possible (often termed 'statistical efficiency'). Unfortunately, these objectives are often in direct conflict rather than complementary. More importantly, economic considerations often limit our ability to fulfil all these objectives. For instance, by maximising the efficiency of a study,

Table 46.1 Comparison of study characteristics using either an efficacy or an effectiveness approach when designing a study.

Study characteristics	Efficacy trial	Effectiveness trial
Research question	Will the intervention work under ideal conditions?	Will the intervention result in more good than harm under usual practice conditions?
Setting	Restricted to specialised centres	Open to all institutions
Patient selection	Selected, well-defined patients	A wider range of patients identified using broad eligibility criteria
Study design	Smaller RCT using stringent rules	Larger multicentre RCT using simpler rules
Baseline assessment	Elaborate and detailed	Simple and clinician friendly
Intervention	Tightly controlled	Less controlled
	Optimal therapy under optimal study conditions	Therapy administered by investigators using accepted approaches
Treatment protocols	Rigorous and detailed	Very general
	Compliance	Non-compliance tolerated
Endpoints	Disease-related	Patient-related such as all-cause mortality or quality of life
	Related to biologic effect	
	Surrogate endpoints	
Analysis	By treatment received	Intention to treat
	Non-compliers removed	All patients included
Data collection	Elaborate	Minimal and simple
Data monitoring*	Detailed and rigorous	Minimal

*Data monitoring refers to the review of source documents and adjudication/verification of outcomes.
RCT, randomised controlled clinical trial.

investigators might sacrifice their ability to draw conclusions in clinically important subgroups because of inadequate sample size.

The most important consequence of these conflicting objectives is that choices made in the design of RCTs must focus on whether an intervention works or whether it results in more good than harm for patients. Trials that attempt to determine therapeutic *efficacy* address the question 'Will the therapy work under ideal conditions?' Trials attempting to determine therapeutic *effectiveness* address the question 'Will the therapy do more good than harm under usual practice conditions in all patients who are offered the intervention?' Clearly, both questions will yield useful information for health practitioners. Efficacy is often established first, and then the intervention is evaluated for its effectiveness. In pivotal RCTs used in the final phase of obtaining regulatory approval (phase III trials), pharmaceutical companies primarily wish to demonstrate that their product has proven

efficacy; rarely are attempts made to demonstrate therapeutic effectiveness.

The design characteristics of efficacy and effectiveness trials tend to differ considerably (Table 46.1). As a consequence of design choices, inferences and threats to the validity of effectiveness and efficacy trials are different. Therefore, one of the first steps in planning an RCT is to determine which of these two design approaches will best reflect the primary study question. Efficacy trials often opt for restricted eligibility, rigorous treatment protocols, and disease-specific outcomes responsive to the potential benefits of the experimental intervention. By using this approach efficacy studies attempt to maximise internal validity, defined as the extent to which the experimental findings represent the true effect in study participants. As a consequence, this design approach will often lack the ability to maximise external validity, defined as the extent to which the experimental findings in the study represent the true effect in the target.

Hence, there is often a trade-off between the two forms of validity in any one study.

As an example of an efficacy trial, Rivers and colleagues undertook an RCT in which they randomly allocated 263 patients with early sepsis and septic shock to receive either goal-directed therapy using a monitor of continuous central venous saturation in one group or standard care in the other arm of the trial. Both groups received fluids, vasopressors such as noradrenaline (norepinephrine), inotropic agents such as dobutamine, and red cell transfusions according to a strict clinical algorithm. In addition to the clinical algorithm, the goal-directed therapy arm was required to maintain mixed venous saturation greater than 70%. Saturations below 70% suggest an ongoing oxygen debt and shock. In the first 6 hours of care in the emergency department, the experimental group received more fluids (4981 mL versus 3499 mL, $p < 0.001$), more inotropic agents (13.7% versus 0.8% of patients, $p < 0.001$) and more red cell transfusions (64.1% versus 18.5% of patients, $p < 0.001$). As a result of the multiple interventions including red cells, in-hospital mortality was decreased from 46.5 to 30.5% ($p < 0.009$). In this efficacy study, many of the study manoeuvres were tightly controlled. Specifically, the trial was conducted in a single tertiary centre, by a small number of experts, in a well-defined patient population using elaborate treatment algorithms in both the experimental and standard of care groups. This efficacy approach may be contrasted with large cardiovascular trials such as the International Study of Infarct Survival trials in acute myocardial infarction which enrolled thousands of patients. One of the major shortcomings of effectiveness trials is the limited data collection and the limited control imposed on most aspects of the study design, thereby increasing biological variability, minimising information on biological mechanisms and curtailing the possibility of understanding negative results or the influence of cointerventions and confounding on study outcomes. At this juncture, there are no published RCTs in transfusion medicine that have opted for a large simple trial design approach. There is, however, a recently published large randomised trial of 7000 critically ill patients that compares 4% albu-

min to saline in a wide variety of patients. This trial found that mortality did not differ between the two groups. There was no evidence of harm by albumin, but the lack of benefit of albumin makes the use of albumin, which is expensive and hard to justify in this group of patients.

Many trials opted for a hybrid approach between large simple trials and tightly controlled clinical studies. The Transfusion Requirements in Critical Care trial provides such an example. This was an 838-patient trial that randomly allocated patients to either a restrictive or a liberal transfusion strategy. The study was conducted in 25 clinical centres, enrolled patients using broad eligibility criteria, followed simple treatment strategies for the administration of red cells and ascertained mortality rates and rates of organ failure.

RCT design alternatives

Once investigators have chosen whether an efficacy, effectiveness or a hybrid approach will best answer the research question, there are several design options that may be considered (Table 46.2). A two-group parallel design is the most common of RCT design choices (Figure 46.2a). In this design, patients are randomly allocated to one of two therapeutic interventions and followed forward in time. It is the simplest to plan, implement, analyse and, most importantly, interpret. Therefore, a parallel group design is the most frequently adopted choice of RCT design. Parallel group designs may also be used to independently compare three or more treatments.

The use of factorial designs may also be considered when a number of therapies are being evaluated in combinations. For instance, in a two-by-two (2×2) factorial design, two interventions are tested both alone and in combination, and compared with a control group (usually a placebo) (Figure 46.2b). This means that investigators can efficiently test two interventions with only marginal increases in sample size. In addition, the benefits of treatment combinations can be evaluated in a controlled manner. This design is most useful when interactions are either very strong or nonexistent. Thus, before embarking on a large, more

Table 46.2 Types of randomised controlled clinical trial (RCT) designs.

Type of RCT	Description	Advantage	Disadvantage
Two group parallel	Patients randomised to one of two groups	Simplest approach widely used and accepted	Limited to simple comparisons
Factorial (2 × 2)	Patients randomised to one of four groups; therapy a, therapy b, therapy a + b or control	Combinations of therapy may be compared	Larger sample size required. More complex design
Sequential study	Pairs of outcomes continuously compared in patients randomised to one of two therapies	Ongoing evaluations of therapy	Limited uses (efficacy only)
			Not a well-accepted approach
			Sample size unpredictable
Two period crossover	Patients allocated to one of two therapies then receive other therapy in second treatment period	Smaller sample required	Limited to reversible outcomes
			Major concern with carry-over effect
N-of-study	Single patient sequentially and repeatedly receives a therapy and a placebo	Optimal method of determining if a therapy is beneficial to a given patient	Results not generalisable
		Difficult in unstable patients	
		Very labour intensive	
Cluster design	Groups of patients are randomised	Ideal for programme or guideline evaluation	Less well accepted in clinical practice
			Difficult to implement when large variability between clusters

complex factorial study, investigators should expect either strong additive or synergistic effects from combined therapy or none at all. Prospective investigators should realise that detecting interactions is also more difficult and requires much larger sample size as compared with comparison of either therapy with a placebo. Factorial designs have been used very successfully to evaluate thrombolytic therapy in combination with an antiplatelet agent in acute myocardial infarction and unstable angina.

Factorial designs imply concurrent comparisons between at least two therapies. It is also possible to implement a design that compares interventions sequentially. For example, two therapies in the early treatment of a disease could be compared, followed by the evaluation of a second intervention in the late phase of care several days later. The authors are not aware of a study in transfusion medicine that has made use of a factorial design. An example of a factorial trial would be to randomise patients to an algorithm of care versus standard care in addition to either a conservative or liberal transfusion threshold. Traditionally, the factorial design is used to answer two unrelated study questions.

Both the simple parallel group design and a factorial design are designed using classical or frequentist statistical approaches, where the sample size is fixed according to pre-established assumptions (anticipated outcomes in treatment and control group, power and significance levels) prior to

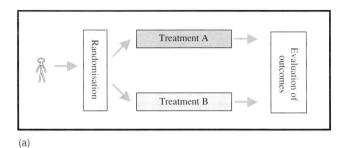

(a)

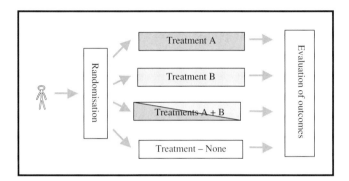

(b)

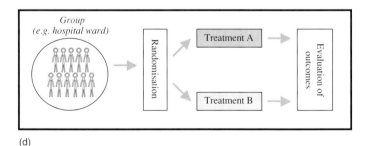

(c)

(d)

Figure 46.2 Design approaches for randomised controlled trials. (Adapted from Tinmouth and Hebert, *Transfusion* 2007;47(4):565–567). (a) Randomised two-group parallel design: subjects randomly assigned to treatment A or B. (b) Factorial design: all subjects randomly assigned to treatment A, treatment B, treatment A + B or no treatment. (c) Randomised crossover design: subjects randomly assigned to treatment A followed by treatment B (after washout period) or treatment B followed by treatment A. (d) Randomised cluster design: all subjects in one group/area (e.g. by physician, by hospital, by ward) are assigned to treatment A or B.

the commencement of enrolment. There are other experimental designs that are more responsive to patient outcomes as the study progresses. Sequential designs use frequentist statistical methods to set boundaries for significance levels which consider the increasing number of comparisons and sample size throughout the study. True sequential studies randomly allocate patients to receive one of two therapies. Pairs of patients are then sequentially compared. The study is terminated as soon as one of the significance boundaries is crossed. One of the major concerns with this design may be its inability to conceal the randomisation process and the uncertainty of not knowing the exact sample size in advance. From this methodology, several biostatisticians have developed methods of performing interim analyses in large clinical trials, referred to as group sequential methods. A Bayesian statistical approach offers an alternative methodology. In a Bayesian analysis, previous beliefs about the effectiveness of a therapy are combined with the observed data from the trial to provide a new revised set of likely values for the effectiveness of the therapy. This approach allows for repeated or continuous monitoring of study results as patients accrue. As a result, predetermined sample sizes are not required and enrolment continues until the results meet predetermined significance levels. This can allow for increased trial efficiency as studies will not enrol additional patients unnecessarily or terminate the study prematurely. A Bayesian approach has also been advocated for interim analyses of large clinical trials.

Another RCT design option particularly amenable to an efficacy evaluation is a two-period crossover study in which patients are used as their own controls. In a two-period crossover trial, patients are randomised to one of two therapies for a fixed period of time and then proceed to receive the other therapy in a second comparable interval (Figure 46.2c). Minimising 'between-subject' variability in this manner makes significant gains in efficiency. Crossover studies are therefore best suited to relatively stable conditions (stability is required during the study), interventions with rapid onset of action and a very short half-life (the biological effect must disappear

prior to the second treatment period), and rapidly modifiable end points such as haemodynamic and respiratory measures. An example of a crossover trial in transfusion medicine would be the evaluation of a modified red cell product (e.g. bacterially inactivated or pegylated red cells) in patients with transfusion-dependent congenital anaemias. The time to next transfusion or red cell survival could be measured in patients who receive, in a random order, standard red cell transfusions and modified red cell transfusions for fixed periods of time. An appropriate washout time between the two interventions is required to ensure there is no contamination of the modified red cells during the period of standard transfusions.

All designs discussed so far have described the evaluation of interventions for individual patients. However, it is sometimes necessary to evaluate therapies, protocols, guidelines or treatment programmes for groups of individuals. Using this design, groups or 'clusters' such as ICUs, wards, hospitals and physician practice are randomised to receive an intervention or control (Figure 46.2d). Cluster design may be the most appropriate design for evaluating complex or multi-dimensional interventions such as the implementation of educational interventions, care paths and approaches to auditing transfusion practices. For these evaluations, the cluster is a more natural method of allocation than the individual. Cluster trials are advantageous when there is a real risk of the intervention will be implemented in all patients rather than only the patients assigned to receive the therapy. When individuals in the control group receive the intervention or elements of the intervention, this contamination biases the results of the study. This may easily occur when one is evaluating guidelines, educational interventions, interventions designed to modify health provider behaviour and administrative changes to systems. However, the allocation of interventions to groups rather than individuals comes at a cost. The sample size is usually larger as a result of the non-independence within the group and it is often difficult to infer what happened at an individual level. As a result, this design has many detractors. In addition, one of the major concerns in cluster trials is the possibility of large variations

Table 46.3 Considerations in determining which design approach to implement in transfusion trials.

Criteria to consider	Choice of design	
	Favouring efficacy	Favouring effectiveness
Evidence	Limited evidence	Efficacy well documented
Importance of the question	Rare and less serious	Common and serious problem
Feasibility	Not demonstrated	Adequate accrual and confirmed feasibility
Risks	Unknown or significant consequences	Minimal or acceptable risks given benefits
Benefits	Limited or unknown benefits	Significant benefits anticipated

between clusters that may make it difficult to detect actual differences between therapies.

In a 2007 study, Murphy *et al.* randomised wards at different hospitals to receive units of red cells with labels reminding nurses to check the patient and component identification. The randomisation by wards was important to ensure that transfusions given without the reminder were not given by nurses who had been previously exposed to the intervention (reminders tags). In this study, the reminders tags did not result in an improvement in the bedside check for transfusion.

Selecting a study population

In transfusion medicine, most blood products are currently used in a wide variety of diseases and conditions. The choice of study population will invariably depend on the study question, the underlying hypothesis and on a number of other factors. The choice of a hypothesis that will address either therapeutic efficacy or effectiveness will have a substantial impact on the selection of the study population. Specifically, in choosing an efficacy approach, investigators usually perform the study in a well-defined patient population where the intervention has the highest probability of demonstrating an effect. This may be done by narrowly defining the patient population through the use of restrictive eligibility criteria and disease definitions, as well as selecting specialised centres with clinical expertise in the field. Choosing a narrowly defined study population will decrease overall variability attributed to patient selection but may have adverse consequences such as hampering patient recruitment and jeopardising the generalisability of

study results. When defining the eligibility criteria for an effectiveness trial, investigators should consider utilising more liberal criteria in a wide range of clinical settings. Thus, as the study is being designed, medical or surgical critically ill patients with a broad range of primary diagnoses (or underlying conditions) from a range of tertiary care centres might be considered for enrolment in the study.

On the spectrum between highly selected patients (efficacy) and large patient population (effectiveness), investigators should consider a number of factors in making the decision (Table 46.3). The spectrum of biological activity of the intervention is an important consideration. For instance, a narrow spectrum of biological activity should translate into restricted eligibility while a broad spectrum of biological activity should yield more liberal eligibility criteria. Eligibility may also be restricted through the selection of study centres. In efficacy trials, highly specialised units should be sought while studies evaluating the effectiveness of an intervention would require the inclusion of a large number of non-specialised centres. In practice, investigators should first focus on therapeutic efficacy and seek to first study the intervention in high-risk and/or well-defined patient populations initially.

Selecting outcomes (Table 46.4)

In most clinical trials, the clinical investigative team should consider a number of potential outcomes, both fatal and non-fatal. An outcome is defined as a measurement (e.g. haematocrit) or an event (e.g. death) potentially modified following the implementation of an intervention. If all are given equal

Table 46.4 Guides to the choice of outcome measure in a randomised controlled clinical trial.

1   Is the outcome causally related to the consequences of the disease?
2   Is the outcome clinically relevant to the health care providers and/or patients?
3   Has the validity of the outcome (for complex outcomes such as scoring systems or composite outcomes) been established?
4   Is the outcome easily and accurately determined?
5   Is the outcome responsive to changes in a patient's condition?
6   Is the outcome measure potentially able to discriminate between patients who benefit from a therapy from patients in the control group?

consideration, concerns arise about multiple comparisons and interpretation of a study with heterogeneous findings. Thus, it is important to choose a primary outcome that will determine an intervention's therapeutic success or failure, as well as secondary outcomes that will provide supportive evidence in secondary analyses. As a corollary, a predefined hierarchy implies that the investigators believe that clinically or statistically important differences in secondary outcomes, in the absence of important changes in the primary outcome, will not be interpreted as strong evidence of therapeutic benefit. The primary outcome is also essential in determining the sample size requirements in a clinical trial. Thus, once a decision has been made to determine either therapeutic efficacy or effectiveness (or possibly a combined approach), the second task facing investigators is ranking outcomes as primary and secondary.

The choice of study outcome is one of the most important design considerations to be made by investigators. However, there are a number of factors that should be considered prior to selection of an outcome. The primary outcomes should be considered clinically important and easily ascertained. By fulfilling these two criteria, the investigator will have a much greater chance of influencing clinical practice once a study has been completed and published.

Outcomes should also measure what they are supposed to measure (validity) and be precise and reproducible. An outcome must be able to detect a clinically important true positive or negative change in the patient's condition following a therapy. In a study evaluating erythropoeitin-α in 1302 critically ill patients from 65 American centres, Corwin and colleagues, after consultation with the Food and Drug Administration (FDA) and the pharmaceutical sponsor, opted to compare the proportion of patients who received at least one red cell unit once randomised. The study documented a 10% decrease in the proportion of patients avoiding a transfusion (60–50%, $p < 0.05$). They were unable to detect differences in any clinically important outcomes beyond transfusions. As a consequence, erythropoeitin has not received approval for general use in ICU patients by the FDA and has not been widely adopted into clinical practice in critical care.

Using mortality as an outcome, the sample size in a clinical trial comparing two therapies is based on the baseline event rate, the expected incremental benefit or difference, the level of significance (α) and the power to detect differences ($1 - \beta$). Establishing the incremental benefit of a new therapy is vitally important because of the enormous sample size repercussions. A sample size calculation for an RCT requires that the investigators establish the minimum therapeutic effect detectable within the trial. This difference in outcomes between interventions is referred to as the minimally important difference (MID) or minimal clinically important difference (MCID). The MID is essentially establishing the level of discrimination in the study population who are exposed to the interventions given acceptable levels of type I (finding a difference when one does not truly exist) and type II (not finding a difference when one truly exists) errors and the baseline event rate. Too often, investigators calculate a sample size based on very large and unrealistic expected differences in outcomes. To determine a plausible effect size,

Table 46.5 Suggestions when planning a randomised controlled clinical trial (RCT) in transfusion medicine.

1	Explicitly determine whether you are primarily interested in establishing therapeutic efficacy or effectiveness.
2	Whenever possible, undertake an RCT as part of a broader research programme.
3	If the study intervention is complex (or risky) or if other aspects of study feasibility are questionable, a pilot study should be considered.
4	Whenever possible, investigators should use simple rather than complex designs (two groups parallel design vs. factorial design).
5	The study population should be tailored to the intervention.
6	Ideally, the study intervention and treatment protocols should not aim to substantially modify or affect usual clinical practice.
7	Given the complexity of RCTs, data collection should aim to clearly describe the study population, describe co-interventions and all major study outcomes.
8	In choosing primary study end points investigators should focus on patient-oriented outcomes rather than surrogate or biological markers.
9	If you are planning a seminal RCT, you may only have one chance to get it right. When making compromises, always opt to answer questions that most clinicians consider most important.
10	In establishing the minimally important difference, select a potentially achievable benefit.

investigators should ask themselves the following questions.

• What difference or incremental benefit can be realistically expected of the experimental therapy? (Anticipated biological effect of therapy)

• Are the required number of patients available to participate in the clinical trial? (Feasibility)

• How much of a survival benefit, given the added costs and expected adverse effects of therapy, would be required for clinicians, patients and administrators to adopt a new therapy? (Overall benefit of therapy)

As a concrete example, assuming that a given study population has an expected mortality rate of 25% in the standard therapy group while the experimental therapy is expected to decrease mortality by an absolute difference of 12.5% (a 50% relative risk reduction), the total number of patients required would be approximately 250. Most therapies used in the ICU would not be expected to decrease mortality so dramatically. More realistic expectations may be in the range of a 5% absolute decrease (a 20% relative risk reduction) which would require a total sample size of 2200 patients respectively if the baseline mortality was 25%. Investigators need to consider whether an absolute incremental benefit in the range of 5–10% is attainable using the experimental therapy. If not, another more discriminating outcome should be sought.

Conclusion

In this chapter on interventional studies in transfusion medicine, several major RCT design characteristics have been discussed. Study design issues of special interest to health professionals interested in transfusion medicine have been outlined. Suggestions when planning an RCT in transfusion medicine are provided in Table 46.5. Observational and quasi-experimental studies may provide invaluable information in transfusion medicine. Although RCTs provide the most unbiased and accurate assessment of the efficacy and effectiveness of therapeutic and preventive interventions, they remain challenging and expensive to conduct. As more research groups form to address unanswered therapeutic questions in transfusion medicine, investigators will invariably better understand the strengths and limitations of different RCT design characteristics.

Key points

1 Properly conducted RCTs are the best means to evaluate the risk and benefits of therapeutic interventions.

2 Observational studies can be useful when RCTs are not feasible: case–control studies are

particularly useful to evaluate rare outcomes and cohort studies can examine outcomes following known exposures, risk factors or therapies; however, all observational studies are prone to biases and cannot show causation.

3 The design of an RCT depends on whether the investigators wish to evaluate the *efficacy* or the *effectiveness* of an intervention.

4 A two-group parallel group design is the simplest RCT to design, execute and evaluate, but alternative designs can be useful in specific circumstances.

5 Selecting the appropriate study population and the outcomes are critical to ensure both the feasibility of completing the RCT and the generalisability and clinical relevance of the study results.

Acknowledgements

Dr Hébert is a Career Scientist of the Ontario Ministry of Health. Dr Fergusson is supported by a Canadian Institutes of Health Research New Investigator Award. Alan T. Tinmouth is supported by a Canadian Blood Services/Canadian Institutes of Health Research New Investigator Award. We wish to thank our students, teachers and colleagues who contributed many of the ideas outlined in this manuscript.

Further reading

Campbell DT & Stanley JC. *Experimental and Quasi-experimental Designs for Research*. Chicago: Rand McNally College Publishing Company, 1966.

Carson JL, Duff A, Poses RM *et al.* Effects of anaemia and cardiovascular disease on surgical mortality and morbidity. *Lancet* 1996;348:1055–1060.

Corwin HL, Gettinger A, Pearl RG *et al.* Efficacy of recombinant human erythropoietin in critically ill patients: a randomized controlled trial. *JAMA* 2002;288:2827–2835.

Friedman LM, Furberg CD & Demets DL. *Fundamentals of Clinical Trials*, 3rd edn. St Louis: Mosby-Year Book, 1996.

Guyatt GH, Sackett DL & Cook DJ. Users' guides to the medical literature II. How to use an article about therapy or prevention. A. Are the results of the study valid? *JAMA* 1993;270:2598–2601.

Haynes RB, Sackett DL, Guyatt GH & Tugwell P. *Clinical Epidemiology: A Basic Science for Clinical Medicine*, 3rd edn. Philadelphia: Lippincott Williams & Wilkins, 2006.

Hébert PC & Fergusson DA. Red blood cell transfusions in critically ill patients. *JAMA* 2002;288:1525–1526.

Hébert PC, Wells G, Blajchman MA *et al.* for the Transfusion Requirements in Critical Care investigators for the Canadian Critical Care Trials Group. Transfusion Requirements in critical care: a multicentre randomized controlled clinical trial. *N Engl J Med* 1999;340:409–417.

Murphy MF, Casbard AC, Ballard S *et al.* Prevention of bedside errors in transfusion medicine (PROBE-TM) study: a cluster randomized, matched-paired clinical areas trial of a simple intervention to reduce errors in the pretransfusion bedside check. *Transfusion* 2007;47:771–780.

Sackett DL. Bias in analytic research. *J Chronic Dis* 1979;32:51–63.

Sackett DL. The competing objectives of randomized trials. *N Engl J Med* 1980;303:1059–1060.

Sackett DL & Gent M. Controversy in counting and attributing events in clinical trials. *N Engl J Med* 1979;301:1410–1412.

Sackett DL, Haynes RB, Guyatt GH & Tugwell P. *Clinical Epidemiology: A Basic Science for Clinical Medicine*, 2nd edn. Boston/Toronto/London: Little, Brown and Company, 1991.

Silliman CC, Boshkov LK, Mehdizadehkashi Z *et al.* Transfusion-related acute lung injury: epidemiology and a prospective analysis of etiologic factors. *Blood* 2003;101:454–462.

The SAFE Study Invetigators. A comparison of albumin and saline for fluid resuscitation. *N Engl J Med* 2004;350:2247–2256.

Vincent JL, Baron J-F, Reinhart K *et al.* Anemia and blood transfusion in critically ill patients. *JAMA* 2002;288:1499–1507.

Wu WC, Rathore SS, Wang Y, Radford MJ & Krumholz HM. Blood transfusion in elderly patient's with acute myocardial infarction. *N Engl J Med* 2001;345:1230–1236.

CHAPTER 47

Getting the most out of the evidence for transfusion medicine

Simon J. Stanworth, Susan J. Brunskill, Carolyn Doree & Chris J. Hyde
NHS Blood and Transplant, John Radcliffe Hospital, Oxford, UK

What is meant by evidence-based medicine?

Evidence-based medicine (EBM) is a relatively recent phrase which Sackett describes as 'the integration of best research evidence with clinical expertise and patient values' (see Further Reading). Proponents of EBM have particularly highlighted the nature of the evidence that is used to make clinical decisions, i.e. where is it from, how believable is it, how relevant is it to my patient and can it be supported by other data? However, evidence is only one of the factors driving clinical decision-making, and each clinician will also need to consider the available resources and opportunities, the values and needs (physical, psychological and social) of the patient, the local clinical expertise and the costs of the intervention. In some clinical situations, the judgement of the clinician will determine that the available evidence for a specific clinical problem is not relevant.

EBM should not be thought of as just about obtaining and evaluating clinical research evidence; it is also a means by which effective strategies for self-learning can be applied, aimed at continuously improving clinical performance. The focus of this chapter will be a discussion of some of the core

elements of the practice of EBM. Particular reference will be made to the appraisal of all identified clinical research evidence in a systematic and transparent way. Although these points are initially described in a general way, they apply to transfusion medicine as much as to any other branch of medicine.

What is meant by optimal clinical evidence?

Optimal evidence is the best evidence available to answer a question. Since the first randomised controlled trial (RCT) was published comparing two different treatment plans for pulmonary tuberculosis in 1948, this form of experimental study has been generally regarded as the 'gold standard' design for providing evidence of the effectiveness of an intervention; in other words, to establish a cause-and-effect relationship for this intervention. This is because if the process of randomisation (including allocation concealment) is undertaken correctly, the differences observed between the groups of patients randomised in the trial should be attributable to the intervention being studied and not to other confounding factors related to the patients, study setting or quality of care. Other forms of experimental study design, of which the RCT is one, do exist, e.g. crossover, cluster, factorial, N-of-1 study or before and after studies, but a fuller

Practical Transfusion Medicine, 3rd edition. Edited by Michael F. Murphy and Derwood H. Pamphilon. © 2009 Blackwell Publishing, ISBN: 978-1-4051-8196-9.

description of these types of studies is beyond the scope of this chapter (see Chapter 46).

The most common (and simple) design for an RCT is a parallel design, in which participants are randomly allocated to one of two groups. But, even these RCTs are not without their difficulties:

• Randomised trials are costly to undertake, and a number of logistic problems can arise if these studies are conducted at multiple centres (which is often necessary if large numbers of participants need to be enrolled).

• Small studies, although easier to develop, may overestimate any observed intervention effect, and may place too much emphasis on those outcomes with more striking results.

• Small studies may be designed to look for unreasonably large differences in the effects of an intervention (which they will never be able to show because of the size of the study).

• Randomised trials with negative results may never be fully reported, or only found in abstract form (publication bias).

• Intervention effects can be overgeneralised and misapplied to different and unstudied patient populations.

• RCTs are not suited to investigating (lower frequency) adverse effects of an intervention, or to studies of prognostic factors, prevalence or diagnostic criteria.

• These points illustrate the need for an important phase in the reading of a trial, that is appraisal of the study, including the methodological quality, and this will be discussed below.

Observational studies

Observational studies, such as cohort or case–control, and whether prospective or retrospective in nature, may demonstrate an association between intervention and outcome, but it is often difficult to be sure that this association does not reflect the effects of unknown confounding factors. It is recognised that the influence of confounding factors and biased participant selection can dramatically distort the accuracy of the study findings in observational studies. However, this does not mean that findings from well-designed observational studies should be disregarded. Such study designs can be very effective in establishing or confirming effects of large size. However, interpretation is more difficult when the observed effects are smaller. As mentioned, clinical questions addressing possible aetiology or monitoring adverse effects may be more suited to observational studies.

Appraisal of primary research evidence for its validity and usefulness

One component of EBM is the critical appraisal of evidence generated from a study. Published RCTs should provide sufficient detail to allow the reader to make an independent assessment of the trial's strength and weaknesses. Guidelines and checklists have been designed to help a reader to complete an assessment of the findings in RCTs. As shown in Table 47.1, the key components of this appraisal process for clinical trials relate to the methodology of the study (the participants, interventions and comparators, the outcomes and the methods used in the randomisation process, the sample size, blinding) and the presentation of the results (numbers analysed/evaluated, the role of chance, i.e. confidence intervals). Poor study methodology and presentation of results will lead to bias at selection, bias at detection and bias due to unacceptable attrition losses and result in a risk of inaccurate conclusions being drawn by readers. Appraisal guidelines could also be useful to authors of primary research because they define the relevant information from studies which should be included in publication.

One aspect of trial appraisal that requires emphasis concerns the understanding of chance variation and the sample size calculation. One needs to distinguish between 'no evidence of effect' and 'evidence of no effect' and this relates to the issue of whether the trial was adequately powered to evaluate the intervention in the first place. Information about sample size calculations should be provided in the published report for each clinical trial.

Table 47.1 Key components of the critical appraisal process for clinical trials.

Did the study ask a focused question?

Was the allocation of participants to the study arms appropriate?

Were the study staff and participants unaware (blind) to the treatment allocation?

Were all the participants who entered the study accounted for within the results?

Were all the participants followed up and data collected in the same way?

Was the study sample size big enough to minimise any play of chance that may occur?

How are the results presented and what is the main result?

How precise are the results?

Were all the important outcomes for this patient population considered?

Can the results be applied to practice/different populations?

From the Critical Appraisal Skills Programme worksheets, Milton Keynes Primary Care Trust, 2002.

Reviews: literature and systematic

Reviews have long been used to provide evidence for clinical practice. For many readers, they are looked upon as summary statements of the whole evidence, including the quality of the evidence for a particular topic. Often written by experts in the field, literature or narrative reviews can provide a good overview of the relevant findings, as well as being educational and informative. However, in the 1980s, researchers began to question the completeness of the literature in these reviews and the level of bias and selectiveness of the data included, and systematic reviews evolved in response.

Systematic reviews aim to be more explicit and less biased in their approach to reviewing a subject than traditional literature reviews. Systematic reviews can enable the results of primary trials to be made more accessible to clinicians, and provide clearer and more transparent evidence for clinical decisions and policy. Systematic reviews also feed back into the next important stage of clinical trial design, as a means of hypothesis testing and as a valuable guide for optimising the development of a trial protocol based on lessons that can be learned from previous studies. Systematic reviews are not substitutes for good clinical trials, but should be considered as complementary methods of clinical research.

There are generally accepted 'rules' about how to undertake a systematic review, which include:
- developing a focused review question;
- comprehensively searching for all (published and unpublished) material relevant to this question;
- using explicit criteria to assess the eligibility and methodological quality of identified studies;
- citing, with reasons why some studies have been excluded from the review;
- acknowledging any methodological weaknesses and differences in the included studies; and
- using explicit methods for combining data from studies including, where appropriate, a meta-analysis of the study data.

Meta-analysis in this chapter, strictly speaking, refers only to quantitative analysis within a review. It should be noted that for many readers in the US, meta-analysis refers to the whole systematic review process, including quantitative analysis. As such, many systematic reviews may not (and indeed should not) require this form of analysis. For example, if there are insufficient trials or if the review has pointed out major concerns about the quality of the trials, then meta-analysis is clearly inappropriate.

Results from each trial within a systematic review are typically presented in the form of a graphical display, termed a 'forest plot'. A hypothetical example is shown in Figure 47.1. The result for the outcome point estimate in each trial is represented

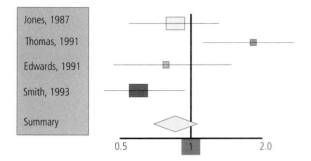

- The figure shows a forest plot display for four hypothetical studies.
- The point estimates for each trial have been presented as a relative risk for an outcome with discrete data. The blocks for the point estimates are different sizes, in proportion to the weight that each study takes in the analysis. Weighting is used in order to draw the reader's eye to the more precise studies.
- The relative risk (RR) is the ratio of risk in the intervention group to the risk in the control group. A RR of one (RR = 1.0) indicates no difference between comparison groups. For undesirable outcomes an RR that is less than 1 indicates that the intervention was effective in reducing the risk of that outcome.
- The diamond shape represents a summary point estimate for all trials. The vertical line corresponds to no effect of treatment. Thus if the 95% confidence interval crosses the vertical line, this indicates that the difference in effect of intervention therapy compared t o control is not statistically significant at the level of $p > 0.05$ (please note there will be a 1 in 20 chance that the confidence interval do es not include the true value). Such is the case in this example.
- Perhaps, the most important aspect of displaying the results graphically in this way is that it helps the reader look at the overall effects for each trial. Therefore, in this example, it should prompt the reader to ask why the results for one trial seem to be so different from the others (Thomas, 1991)?

Figure 47.1 A hypothetical forest plot.

by a square, together with a horizontal line that corresponds to the 95% confidence intervals (CIs). For summary statistics of binary or discrete data, effect measures are typically summarised as either a relative risk or an odds ratio (for definitions, see Figure 47.1). The 95% CI provides a very useful measure of effect, in that it represents the range of values that will contain the true size of treatment effect in 95% of the occasions, should the study be repeated again and again. The solid vertical line corresponds to no effect of treatment (or a relative risk of 1.0 for the analysis of discrete data, see Figure 47.1). Forest plots, therefore, readily allow a reader the opportunity to make visual comparisons of the size of treatment effects between different trials, and to allow the reader to see whether:

- the lower limits of the confidence interval for trials exceed or overlap the minimal clinically important benefit;

- the treatment effects in multiple trials are consistent in the same direction, or disparate (opposite in effect), with some trials suggesting no benefit, others significant benefit; and
- the results from some trials appear unexpectedly different compared with other trials.

Figure 47.2 provides an overall guide for assessing the validity of evidence for treatment decisions for the different types of studies, trials and reviews mentioned in this section. Although sometimes criticised for their overemphasis on methodology at the expense of clinical relevance, and the inappropriate use of meta-analysis, systematic reviews do have a place in clinical practice as a means of transparently evaluating evidence from multiple trials. Again, as for RCTs, key components of a critical appraisal process for systematic reviews have been developed based on the QUOROM statement and CASP (Critical Appraisal Skills Programme) worksheets (Table 47.2).

A hierarchy of evidence for effectiveness

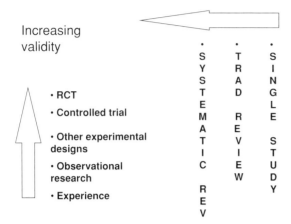

Figure 47.2 A guide for judging the validity of evidence for treatment decisions from different types of studies and reviews.

Evidence base for transfusion medicine

So, how good is the evidence base for transfusion medicine? As a first step, identification of all relevant RCTs in transfusion medicine would be essential. Such an approach has been made much easier by the Cochrane Collaboration, as a database of RCTs exists and is constantly being updated. This database uses sensitive literature search filters that aim to identify all RCTs that have been catalogued on MEDLINE from 1966 and on the European medical bibliographic database, Embase, from 1980. High-level evidence can be derived not only from methodologically sound RCTs but also from systematic reviews of RCTs. In addition, other databases of reviews for clinical evidence exist for clinicians, e.g. Bandolier (a print and Internet journal about health care using EBM techniques). Table 47.3 presents a list of sources that can be searched to identify relevant reports of clinical trials and reviews.

The total number of published systematic reviews relevant to the broad theme of transfusion medicine was approximately 300 at the time of searching in 2008. These identified reviews cover topics ranging from the effective use of blood components and fractionated blood products to alternatives to blood products used to minimise the need for blood in a surgical setting and to blood safety. It should be noted that the searching filters for this exercise excluded some potentially relevant areas (e.g. stem cells) and that the boundaries between transfusion medicine and other branches of medicine do overlap, e.g. a systematic review of resuscitation fluids is relevant to both the fields of transfusion medicine and anaesthesia. The search strategy also identified a number of areas of transfusion practice where few published systematic reviews exist, e.g. areas of donation screening and donor selection. In paediatric transfusion practice, there is a general lack of evidence on which to base decisions derived from randomised trials

Table 47.2 Key components of the critical appraisal process for systematic reviews.

Did the review ask a clearly focused question?
Did the reviewers try to identify all relevant studies?
Were the eligibility criteria of the included studies detailed in the review?
Did the reviewers assess the quality of the included studies?
Have the results of the studies been combined and was it reasonable to do so?
How many studies were included in the review?
What is the main result for each outcome?
How precise are the results?
Were all the important outcomes for the review question considered?
How applicable are these results to clinical practice?

From the Critical Appraisal Skills Programme worksheets, Milton Keynes Primary Care Trust, 2002; Systematic Review Initiative NBS in-house worksheets.

Table 47.3 List of selected sources that can be searched to identify reports of trials and clinical evidence.

Source	How to access?
Electronic Databases	
Cochrane Central Register of Controlled Trials (CENTRAL) (four issues published per year)	Within the Cochrane Library, available through medical libraries or at: www.library.nhs.uk, or from Wiley Interscience at: www3.interscience.wiley.com/
Cochrane Database of Systematic Reviews (four issues published per year)	Within the Cochrane Library, available through medical libraries or at: www.library.nhs.uk, or from Wiley Interscience at: www3.interscience.wiley.com/
Database of Abstracts of Reviews of Effects	Within the Cochrane Library, available through medical libraries or at: www.library.nhs.uk. Most up-to-date version at: www.crd.york.ac.uk/crdweb/
MEDLINE (US database produced by the National Library of Medicine; references dating from 1950)	Available through medical libraries or at: http://www.ncbi.nlm.nih.gov/pubmed/
EMBASE (European equivalent of Medline, approximately 40% overlap) references dating from 1974)	Available through medical libraries or at: www.embase.com (subscription required)
BMJ Clinical Evidence	clinicalevidence.bmj.com (subscription required)
Evidence-Based Medicine	ebm.bmj.com (subscription required)
Websites of Guidelines and Ongoing Trials	
UK Transfusion Guidelines	www.transfusionguidelines.org
National Library of Guidelines	www.library.nhs.uk/guidelinesfinder/
National Guidelines Clearinghouse	www.guidelines.gov
International Network of Agencies of Health Technology Assessment (INAHTA)	www.inahta.org
metaRegister of Controlled Trials (CCTR)	www.controlled-trials.com/mrct
ClinicalTrials.gov	www.clinicaltrials.gov/ct2/search
UK Clinical Research Network Portfolio Database	public.ukcrn.org.uk/search
UK Clinical Trials Gateway	www.controlled-trials.com/ukctg
IFPMA Clinical Trials Portal	clinicaltrials.ifpma.org
WHO International Clinical Trials Register Platform	www.who.int/trialsearch/Default.aspx
Trials Central	www.trialscentral.org/index.html
Other	
Abstracts from subject-relevant conferences	Websites or paper copies; often published alongside leading subject journals
Follow-up from the reference lists of identified studies	Relevant papers: trials, narrative or systematic reviews
Relevant pharmaceutical companies	Personal communication
Selected experts in the particular fields	Personal communication
Bandolier	www.jr2.ox.ac.uk/Bandolier

or systematic reviews. Even when systematic reviews were identified, many were only able to draw upon information from a very limited number of relevant randomised trials. Therefore, overall, the RCT and systematic review evidence base for much of transfusion practice appears weaker than one might wish to admit.

Evidence base for transfusion medicine: individual examples

Frozen plasma

Two recent relevant systematic reviews have attempted to address evidence relevant to the clinical use of FFP. The first asked the question about the evidence for whether abnormalities in coagulation tests predict an increased risk of clinical bleeding, as such abnormalities are important drivers for decisions to transfuse FFP. All relevant publications describing bleeding outcomes in patients with abnormalities in coagulation tests prior to invasive procedures were assessed. Overall, the published studies did not support evidence for a predictive value of PT/INR for bleeding.

The second systematic review was undertaken to identify and analyse all RCTs examining the clinical effectiveness of FFP. Comprehensive searching of the databases MEDLINE (1966–2002), Embase (1980–2002) and the Cochrane Library (2002, issue 4) and detailed eligibility criteria identified 57 RCTs as relevant for inclusion and analysis.

The analysis focused on:
• Studies of interventions comparing FFP with no FFP/plasma. These studies would be expected to provide the clearest evidence for a direct effect of FFP.
• Studies of interventions comparing FFP with a non-blood product (e.g. solutions of colloids and/or crystalloids).
• Studies of interventions comparing FFP with a different blood product or different formulations of FFP, e.g. solvent–detergent and methylene-blue treated.

Few of the identified studies included details of the study methodology (method of randomisation, blinding of patients and study personnel). The sample size of many included studies was small (mean range 8–78 patients per arm). Few studies took adequate account of the extent to which adverse events might negate the clinical benefits of treatment with FFP. Taken together, many of the identified trials in groups such as cardiac, neonatal and other clinical conditions evaluated a prophylactic transfusion strategy. When these trials evaluating prophylactic usage were more closely assessed as a group in the systematic review, irrespective of clinical setting, it appeared that there was evidence (including from larger trials) for a *lack of effect* of prophylactic FFP. The overall finding of the review was that for most clinical situations of the RCT base for the clinical use of FFP is very limited.

Platelets

A number of different systematic reviews have more critically evaluated the evidence underpinning the following questions:

1 What is the appropriate threshold platelet count to trigger prophylactic platelet transfusions?

2 What is the optimal dose for platelet transfusions?

3 What is the evidence that a strategy of prophylactic platelet transfusions is superior to the use of platelet transfusions only in the event of bleeding? The results from the three identified trials in one systematic review evaluating different thresholds do not provide assurance that a 10×10^9/L threshold is as safe and effective as 20×10^9/L for all clinical outcomes, and indeed raise the critical question as to whether the combined studies have sufficient power to demonstrate equivalence in terms of the safety of the lower prophylactic threshold. This is because the combined results of the quantitative meta-analysis have confidence intervals which include both detrimental and beneficial effects. The analysis of identified dose studies also raises uncertainty about the optimal dose of platelets for transfusion, although ongoing larger studies should help answer this question and would be added into updated systematic reviews.

The more fundamental question about whether a prophylactic platelet transfusion policy is any better than a therapeutic policy based on the aggressive use of platelet transfusions to treat the onset of clinical bleeding is unproven. The older age of the published identified randomised studies addressing this question raises questions of their applicability to current clinical practice, since the trials were conducted at a time when product specifications and quality control were very different, when supportive care for chemotherapy patients was less advanced and when antipyretics with antiplatelet activity, such as aspirin, were in common use. In addition to the small number of patients randomised in the trials, there was also considerable heterogeneity in the study population in relation to the indications for platelet transfusion, the definition of clinically significant bleeding, the threshold in the prophylaxis arm and in the dose of platelets given. Taken together, these analyses cast doubt on the validity of the data from published trials aimed at evaluating evidence for the effectiveness of prophylaxis.

Common practices of transfusion and interventions to improve transfusion practice

Systematic reviews may also be applied to important questions about the evidence base for common or well-established practices in transfusion. For example, some recent reviews have addressed:

• What is the maximum time that one unit of RBCs can be out of the fridge before it becomes unsafe?
• How often should blood administration sets be changed while a patient is being transfused?
• Blood transfusion administration: 1- or 2-person checks – which is the safest method?

It is surprising and salutary to realise that some of these common recommendations appear to have little firm basis, yet are commonly reproduced in guidelines and protocols.

Are there limitations to evidence-based practice?

It is important to acknowledge some of the limitations of EBM that have been discussed by critics and supporters alike. Evidence-based practice alone cannot provide a clinical decision. The findings generated from EBM are one strand of input driving decision-making in clinical practice. Each clinician will also need to consider the available resources and opportunities, the values and needs (physical, psychological and social) of the patient, the local clinical expertise and the costs of the intervention. Patients enrolled in clinical trials are not always the same as the individual patients requiring treatment, and generalising to different clinical settings may not be appropriate. It has also been said that within EBM there is an overemphasis on methodology at the expense of clinical relevance, with the risks of generating conclusions that are either overly pessimistic or inappropriate for the clinical question. Perhaps we need to get away from the 'there is no good RCT evidence available to answer this clinical question' to thinking more about why this should be so, what can be learned from those studies that have already been completed, and what design of trial would answer the main area of uncertainty in this transfusion setting.

This chapter has attempted to explain why it is essential to assess the quality of primary clinical research and consider the risks of evidence being misleading, e.g. in the case of few trials or a failure to identify appropriate clinical research questions. Systematic reviews can be a useful tool to achieve this but, like trials themselves, can be outdated, and based on clinical protocols developed many years prior to publication. Transfusion medicine is no different to many other branches of medicine, and the evidence base for much of the practice has not developed to the point at which it can be universally applied with confidence. There is a need to recognise these uncertainties, and to consider the responses and in particular those transfusion issues that really require high priority for clinical research.

Finally, appraising the evidence base for transfusion medicine is one part of improving practice, another is the effective dissemination of the evidence to clinicians. For example, clinicians may not have the time to search and evaluate the evidence themselves given the increasing numbers of publications and journals. As many of the sources are web-based, access at any one moment may be easier but the skills of appraisal need to be regularly maintained. Chapter 48 discusses aspects of changing practice in more detail.

Summary

There has been growing recognition that research, especially empirical research (that based on observing what has happened), has been underutilised in making health care decisions at all levels. This appears to be as true for transfusion medicine as much as other clinical areas. EBM is an approach to developing and improving skills to identify and apply research evidence to clinical decisions. Even the most ardent proponents of EBM have never claimed it is a panacea, and there is recognition that it should amplify rather than replace clinical skills and knowledge, and be a driver for keeping health care workers up to date.

Systematic reviews can help bring together all relevant literature on a particular problem and assess its strengths, weaknesses and overall meaning. Such reviews can be used in different ways including improving the precision of estimates of effect, generating hypotheses and providing background to new primary research. Progress is being made in ensuring most areas in transfusion medicine are being systematically reviewed and some of these have encouraged plans for new RCTs.

Key points

1 The process of EBM consists of question formulation, searching for literature, critically appraising studies (identifying strengths and weaknesses) and application to the patient.
2 It is essential to assess the quality of primary clinical research and consider the risks of evidence being misleading, e.g. in the case of few trials or a failure to identify appropriate clinical research questions.
3 Systematic reviews of RCTs combine evidence most likely to provide valid (truthful) answers on particular questions of effectiveness, and form an important component to the evaluation of evidence-based practice in transfusion medicine.
4 There is a common perception that much of transfusion medicine practice is based on limited evidence, but this is changing, and systematic reviews are an important tool to collate, analyse and update the evidence base.

Further reading

Carson JL, Hill S, Carless P, Hébert P & Henry D. Transfusion triggers: a systematic review of the literature. *Transfus Med Rev* 2002;16(3):187–199.

Cid J & Lozano M. Lower or higher doses for prophylactic platelet transfusions: results of a meta-analysis of randomized controlled trials. *Transfusion* 2007;47(3):464–470.

Egger M, Davey Smith G & Altman DG. *Systematic Reviews in Health Care. Meta-analysis in Context*, 2nd edn. London: BMJ Publishing Group, 2001.

Guyatt GH & Rennie D. *Users' Guide to the Medical Literature: Essentials of Evidence-based Clinical Practice*. Chicago, IL: American Medical Association, 2002.

Heddle NM. Evidence-based clinical reporting: a need for improvement. *Transfusion* 2002;42:1106–1110.

Hyde CJ, Stanworth SJ & Murphy MF. Can you see the wood for the trees! Making sense of the forest plot. 1. Presentation of the data from the included studies. *Transfusion* 2008;48(2):218–220.

Hyde CJ, Stanworth SJ & Murphy MF. Can you see the wood for the trees! Making sense of the forest plot. 2. Analysis of the combined results from the included studies. *Transfusion* 2008;48(4):580–583.

Moher DF, Schulz KF & Altman DG. The CONSORT statement: revised recommendations for improving the quality of reports of parallel-group randomised trials. *Clin Oral Investig* 2003;7(1):2–7.

Sackett DL, Strauss SE, Richardson WS, Rosenberg W & Haynes RB. *Evidence Based Medicine: How to Practice and Teach EBM*, 2nd edn. Edinburgh: Churchill Livingstone, 2000.

Stanworth SJ, Brunskill SJ, Hyde CJ, Mcllelland DBL & Murphy MF. Is fresh frozen plasma clinically effective? A systematic review of randomized controlled trials. *Br J Haematol* 2004;126:139–152.

Stanworth SJ, Hyde C, Heddle N, Rebulla P, Brunskill S & Murphy MF. Prophylactic platelet transfusion for haemorrhage after chemotherapy and stem cell transplantation. *Cochrane Database Syst Rev* 2004, Issue 4. DOI: 10.1002/14651858.CD004269.pub2.

Segal JB & Dzik WH. Paucity of studies to support that abnormal coagulation test results predict bleeding in the setting of invasive procedures: an evidence-based review. *Transfusion* 2005;45:1413–1425.

Tinmouth AT & Freedman J. Prophylactic platelet transfusions: which dose is the best dose? A review of the literature. *Transfus Med Rev* 2003;17(3):181–193.

von Elm E, Altman DG, Egger M, Pocock SJ, Gøtzsche PC & Vandenbroucke JP, for STROBE Initiative. The Strengthening the Reporting of Observational Studies in Epidemiology (STROBE) statement: guidelines for reporting observational studies. *Ann Intern Med* 2007;147(8):573–577.

Watson D, Murdock J, Doree C *et al.* Blood transfusion administration – 1 or 2 person checks, which is the safest method? *Transfusion* 2008;48(4):783–789.

CHAPTER 48

How to influence clinicians' use of blood – improving transfusion practice in hospitals

Simon J. Stanworth[1], *J.J. Francis*[4], *M.P. Eccles*[5], *Chris J. Hyde*[1], *Michael F. Murphy*[2] *&*
Alan T. Tinmouth[3]

[1]NHS Blood and Transplant, John Radcliffe Hospital, Oxford, UK
[2]University of Oxford; NHS Blood and Transplant and Department of Haematology, John Radcliffe Hospital, Oxford, UK
[3]Department of Medicine and Pathology and Laboratory Medicine, University of Ottawa; University of Ottawa Centre for Transfusion Research, Clinical Epidemiology Program, Ottawa Health Research Institute, Ottawa, Ontario, Canada
[4]Health Services Research Unit, University of Aberdeen, Aberdeen, Scotland
[5]Institute of Health and Society, Newcastle University, Newcastle, UK

Background

Changing established patterns of transfusion practice is not easy. However, as the evidence base for transfusion medicine advances, there is an increasing need to ensure that important new research is rapidly implemented and that practice which is shown to be less effective (or cost-inefficient) is discontinued. Many of the methods used to deliver change in clinical behaviour are familiar to hospital health care workers in the field of transfusion medicine. They include:

- guideline adoption and dissemination;
- educational materials or teaching sessions;
- the use of audits with feedback; and
- reminders.

But which is best – or put another way, which intervention delivers effective and sustained change in transfusion prescribing behaviour in a cost-effective manner? Answers are needed to address common questions at meetings, such as 'Is it worthwhile writing up yet another set of local transfusion guidelines', or 'What is the point of doing yet another audit of this area of transfusion practice?'

Perhaps surprisingly, the general literature surrounding changing professional medical practice is vast. Moreover, the wider volume of literature relevant to promoting clinical effectiveness and the uptake of effective practice is now increasing substantially. This chapter will attempt to summarise some of these issues with regard to reducing inappropriate practice. All hospital health care workers in the field of transfusion medicine spend considerable time developing or undertaking different interventions or 'treatments' aimed at improving transfusion practice, but there remain questions about which are most effective. Unfortunately, the volume of literature directly relevant to changing transfusion practice is limited.

Interventions to change practice

The different means of achieving changes in practice have been reviewed by many groups, and

Practical Transfusion Medicine, 3rd edition. Edited by Michael F. Murphy and Derwood H. Pamphilon. © 2009 Blackwell Publishing. ISBN: 978-1-4051-8196-9.

cover a wide range of candidate 'strategies'. One (empirically-based) general taxonomy of interventions developed and used by the Cochrane Collaboration Effective Practice and Organisation of Care (EPOC) Group is reproduced below, to illustrate the breadth of different interventions.

(a) Professional
  - audit and feedback;
  - reminders;
  - educational – groups, meetings, outreach visits;
  - patient-mediated interventions; and
  - local opinion leaders.

(b) Financial
  - fee-for-service and
  - provider incentives.

(c) Organisational
  - clinical multidisciplinary teams and
  - changes to the setting/site of service delivery.

(d) Regulatory
  - changes in medical liability and
  - peer review.

Professional interventions represent the main group of 'strategies' with which health care workers in transfusion are familiar. Audit and feedback is defined by EPOC as 'any summary of clinical performance of health care over a specified period of time. The summary may also have included recommendations for clinical action'. Audit and feedback is a very well-established tool for evaluation and improvement of the quality of clinical care and quality assurance in hospitals, which can be applied at local or regional or national level. There are many different examples of audits reported (both prospective and retrospective) in transfusion. These have looked at changes in number of appropriate transfusions and total number of transfusions. If the methods used for undertaking audit to evaluate care or compliance are deficient or not appropriate, there is a risk of bias, and a lack of credibility and hence the whole cycle of modifying practice becomes flawed. The method of feedback (for example, at individual or team level) is acknowledged as critical to delivering change.

Educational outreach involves the 'use of a trained person who met with providers in their practice settings to give information with the intent of changing the provider's practice'. Educational meetings are defined by EPOC as 'participation of healthcare providers in conferences, lectures, workshops or traineeships'. Other examples of interventions include the use of local opinion leaders who are 'providers nominated by their colleagues as educationally influential'. Reminders are 'patient- or encounter-specific information, provided verbally, on paper or on a computer screen, which is designed or intended to prompt a health professional to recall information. Computer-aided decision supports are included'. In transfusion, reminders have been incorporated into transfusion request forms or computer order entry.

Practice change may also be instigated by combinations of these interventions, and multifaceted interventions include 'any intervention including two or more components'. Multifaceted interventions are inevitably likely to be more costly than single-component interventions.

A recent example by Rothschild et al. of a combined approach to changing and improving transfusion decisions was a report of a study examining transfusion practices before and after a conventional educational intervention followed by a randomised controlled trial of a decision support intervention based on computerised physician order entry. Education and computerised decision support both decreased the percentage of inappropriate transfusions, although, of note, the residual amount of inappropriate transfusions remained high.

Organisational interventions are also widely used to deliver change in some areas of transfusion practice. In contrast to professional interventions looking at usage of blood, organisational interventions have been designed to deliver safer transfusion practice. Examples might include the introduction of two-person pre-transfusion bedside checking, or patient identification using bar coding. Aspects of wider quality assurance systems for delivering safer transfusion practice might also be considered as organisational interventions for change, but these categories will not be considered further in this chapter.

Comparing interventions to change practice

Different forms of behavioural interventions are undertaken by hospitals and blood transfusion services worldwide with the aim of changing transfusion practice, but there are few data on their relative or absolute effectiveness. The broad principles of clinical research should be applied to evaluate these interventions as for any pharmaceutical intervention in medical care. The literature for practice change can then be appraised in the context of formal clinical studies and systematic reviews.

For example, a controlled trial by Soumerai et al. of an intensive educational outreach programme (based around printed materials, presentations and face-to-face visits by transfusion medicine specialists) indicated good evidence for improved appropriateness of blood-product use, although in this study there were perhaps unanswered questions regarding the sustainability of changes and overall cost-effectiveness.

Systematic reviews (see Chapter 47) to identify and appraise all relevant publications evaluating different interventions in transfusion have been undertaken and published. Not surprisingly, the identification of the eligible literature in the field of practice improvement is challenging because of the wider numbers of potentially relevant journals and the lack of specific indexing to trials trying to change transfusion practice. In addition, as studies may report multiple and different endpoints, or define appropriateness of transfusion in different ways, data synthesis can be complex, and narrative summaries may be preferred, but this complicates any more detailed evaluations of, for example, cost-effectiveness implications.

The systematic reviews of all studies determining the relative effectiveness of different interventions to change transfusion practice reported mixed findings. The clinical studies evaluated guidelines, audit and feedback, audit with approval, a new transfusion request form and education (at different levels). Most of the identified studies assessed multifaceted, not single interventions. All interventions for the reduction of transfusion studied in clinical trials seemed to be effective; with a reported reduc-tion in inappropriate transfusions of 12–83% and 9–77% for the total number of units transfused. No specific types of intervention appeared to be more effective than others and there was no clear benefit of multifaceted interventions (see Table 48.1).

However, there were significant limitations to the quality of this evidence. Most of the studies were not controlled trials, but 'before-and-after' studies with no controls which do not account for changes that may occur over time for other reasons, and are more prone to bias in favour of the intervention. Most were single-centre studies and many were performed more than 10 years ago. The common success in the published studies also raises the possibility of a 'Hawthorne effect' which describes an initial improvement in performance due to the simple act of observing the performance. These concerns about the true effectiveness and the durability of the effect of these interventions were raised in one study, which reported a return to the baseline rate of transfusions 3 months after the completion of the intervention, and a follow-up report from another study that reported a return to previous transfusion practice. None of the studies formally reported cost-effectiveness comparisons, which is an increasingly important assessment in any health care system. Finally, it is likely that this topic area may be liable to 'publication bias' in that studies with negative results may not have been submitted for publication.

The results of the systematic reviews described above support the concept that interventions can be successful in changing physicians' transfusion practice. These findings are similar to other studies that have examined the effects of interventions to change physician practice in other settings. However, given the limitations in the design of the studies, there is uncertainty as to the nature of the 'active ingredients' of interventions (or combinations of ingredients) that have the maximum effectiveness in delivering sustained (and cost-effective) changes in transfusion practice.

Variation in practice

That there is variation in transfusion practice should not be a surprise to any health care

Table 48.1 Relative reductions (%) in blood product utilisation (red blood cells, frozen plasma or platelets) following introduction of behavioural interventions to change transfusion practice.

Intervention	Solitary intervention				As part of multifaceted intervention			
	Inappropriate transfusions (n)	pts (n)	Units/pt (n)	Units (n)	Inappropriate transfusions (n)	Pts (n)	Units/pt (n)	Units (n)
Guidelines	—	—	—	—	−13% to −49% (3)	−43% to −79% (2)	−12% to −65% (4)	+64% to −77% (7)
Education	—	−17% (1)	−20% (1)	−14% (1)	−13% to −49% (3)	−17% to −43% (2)	−12% to −65% (4)	+64% to −77% (8)
Retrospective audit/feedback	−73% (1)	—	—	—	—	−21% to −29% (3)	−12% to −29% (3)	−9% to −77% (5)
Prospective audit/approval	—	—	0 to −55% (1)	—	−48% to −82% (2)	−27% (1)	−22% to −55% (1)	−9% to −52% (4)
Reminders	+40% to −50% (1)	—	—	+5% to 0% (1)	−48% to −82% (2)	−27% (1)	−12% to −35% (3)	−9% to −52% (5)

n, number of trials; pts, patients.

professional involved in this area of hospital medicine. Indeed in a wider context all health care systems experience inappropriate variation in treatments and treatment rates which suggest there is considerable inappropriate practice. Alongside the public and political anxiety surrounding blood transfusion, this variation in practice has arguably been more comprehensively documented over a longer period of time for transfusion medicine than other areas of health care, and is frequently reported as a key rationale for the need for and use of interventions to change practice.

Historically, one of the more commonly quoted studies on this topic was reported by The Sanguis Study Group. They evaluated the use of blood components for elective surgery at multiple European hospitals, and reported large differences between hospitals and clinical teams in the use of red cell transfusion for the same surgical procedures, with no clear explanation based on patient and clinical factors such as age, preoperative haemoglobin or perioperative blood loss.

Variation in usage also has been reported for other blood components. In a comparison of plasma use in a number of countries, the ratio of frozen plasma (FP) units to red blood cell units transfused varied from 1:3.6 in the US to 1:8.5 in France. Other studies have reported wide variation in the use of plasma and platelets among centres within the same country, including patients undergoing cardiac surgery and critical care patients. Moreover, in one study, lower use of FP in critical care patients did not correlate with lower use in cardiac surgery patients suggesting that important variation also exists within hospitals. Other studies have suggested that FFP may be associated with the highest rate of inappropriate transfusion, with some studies indicating a rate of inappropriate transfusions as high as 50%.

However, the reasons for variation in transfusion practice are complex. Arguably some of this variation may be expected given the complicated nature of health care and wide differences between patients and their responses to intensive medical or surgical treatments, which are frequently the setting for transfusion. Although a degree of variation is therefore to be expected in any health care setting, it is variation against an explicit set of criteria or guidelines based on good evidence that is the key issue. In other words, it is variation against an underlying body of clinical evidence defining appropriate use that would be a significant concern. Questions about understanding variations in transfusion practice need to be addressed alongside a better appreciation of appropriate use.

Appropriate use of blood

Defining appropriate use of blood and what is clearly inappropriate use is frequently a challenge for transfusion practice. The transfusion medicine community has perhaps focused historically on documenting the risks of transfusion, with relatively fewer resources devoted to evaluating the effectiveness of transfusion. However, one of the most effective ways to deliver safe transfusion is to define which patients really need transfusion in the first place, thereby minimising the risk of exposure to unnecessary transfusions.

Both underuse and overuse of transfusions expose patients to unnecessary risks. Regarding overuse, this is a widely recognised problem with finite risks for adverse events associated with unnecessary transfusion, as well as considerations of cost and wastage. Concerns about wastage may become increasingly important given that blood is a scarce resource and that there are real concerns about a diminishing donor base in the future, reflecting in the UK, additional worries about introducing screening tests for vCJD. In contrast, the extent of under-transfusion and risks associated with under-transfusion have been less clearly defined as a whole.

For example, one simple recent regional audit of different centres in the UK (see Murphy & Stanworth) evaluated patients undergoing primary hip replacement surgery and found that the proportion of patients receiving transfusions varied from 23% to 58%. The majority of transfusion patients received only one or two units of blood and a number were discharged with haemoglobin concentrations of above 10 g/dL, raising concern about over-transfusion.

Many of the risks of transfusion are delayed adverse events and therefore unlikely to be observed by the physicians who prescribed the blood. Physicians are more likely to be involved in managing acute reactions to blood, but more severe acute reactions are generally uncommon and most are readily treated at the bedside, e.g. febrile reactions, fluid overload. Even the greater awareness of low-frequency errors in the process and administration of blood transfusion as a major problem is unlikely to have high salience in many individual prescribers' minds. Attempting to change transfusion practice solely on the basis of increasing individual physician understanding of the risk of harm related to transfusion is unlikely to be effective by itself.

Physicians may tend to focus on laboratory measures such as haemoglobin, platelet count or standard coagulation tests as the main drivers for the decision to transfuse. It seems such an intuitively desirable outcome to improve or optimise these figures in sick patients by transfusion. Although the evidence base for transfusion practice based on clinical outcomes is still poorly developed in many fields, an increasing number of trials are now being undertaken and reported. Interestingly, these trials are beginning to challenge some of the preconceived notions of benefit for transfusion. For example, the transfusion in critical care (TRICC) trial compared two transfusion thresholds for adult patients admitted to Canadian intensive care units; the results showed a trend towards lower 30-day mortality in the restrictive transfusion group. In the paediatric intensive care unit setting, a similar restrictive transfusion strategy was also found to be at least equivalent to a more liberal strategy in terms of outcomes and multiple organ dysfunction. Comparable trials evaluating red cell transfusion strategies in neonates have also been published. As a broad generalisation, the combined weight of evidence from these trials of red cell transfusion does not support unrestricted use of red cell transfusions in many patient groups and therefore appears to argue against the intuitive desire to raise haemoglobin levels.

Models of behaviour and change

It is important to systematically study the wider influences on decisions to transfuse in the context of

the considerable variation in practice. At one level, inappropriate variation in blood usage may reflect poor knowledge by physicians. However, there are likely to be many other different influences on clinical practice and a number of ways to improve and optimise transfusion practice that may not focus solely around knowledge (or the lack of it).

It has been suggested that the clinical actions of health care professionals are influenced by the same factors that influence human behaviour in general. Models of change can then be used to better understand the behaviour of health professionals and to inform the development of interventions to change behaviour. Some current models propose that the ways in which people think about a particular action, and not just their knowledge, will influence their behaviour. For example, applying one such psychological model (the Theory of Planned Behaviour) to clinical practice suggests that three factors influence the clinician's intention to take action, based on the following questions:

1 *Is it good practice?* What is my understanding of the evidence about effectiveness versus risk? How do I weigh up the pros and cons? What might be the consequences of the action? (Consequences for the patient, for other patients in the unit, for me or for the clinical team.)

2 *What are the views of other important or relevant people?* Would my senior colleagues make the same judgement? What will be the views of staff coming on to the ward on the next shift? Do the patients' relatives have strong views?

3 *Do I have the capacity and resources to take the action?* Am I confident about my judgement and skills? Do I have the staff I need to take action? Do I have access to the products, equipment and time to carry out the procedure?

The influence of specific beliefs on clinical practice has been explored in few studies with reference to transfusion. One interview-based survey of over 100 surgeons and anaesthetists attempted to identify gaps in transfusion knowledge as well as the different non-clinical factors that affected decisions to transfuse e.g. organisational, attitudes and staff relationships.

A behavioural perspective on enhancing the uptake of evidence-based transfusion practice may not only help unravel the complexities of decisions to transfuse, but lead to new strategies for influencing clinicians' use of blood. For example, different domains influencing behaviour change can be elaborated further in ways that could identify the major drivers of decisions about whether or not to transfuse in a specific situation. These drivers focus on how individual clinicians might weigh up the relative importance of various factors to do with transfusion. Attitudes arise not only from the perceived advantages and disadvantages of transfusing, but also on how individuals balance them up against one another. It might be understandable if immediate adverse events were weighed more heavily than delayed adverse events, even though the likelihood of the delayed event may be greater. Similarly, the influences of other people with different views (say, the patient's family) is likely to be greater when those people are present in the ward than when they are distant. Further, factors influencing the clinician's control over the behaviour may exert different amounts of influence. For example, time constraints will have a more powerful influence when other critically ill patients are in greater need of attention.

Implementation research

There is increasing recognition that the findings from clinical research will not change population health outcomes unless health care systems and professionals adopt them in practice. But a consistent finding from many groups and organisations is that this transfer of research findings into practice is unpredictable and in many cases slow and haphazard. There is no reason to believe that this is any different for transfusion medicine, and the problem of slow uptake will become more important as new primary research is published. Recognition of this quality gap in practice has led to much more interest in active quality improvement strategies over the last 10 years, and a body of implementation research has developed in many different health care areas. As a generalisation, this again demonstrates that interventions can be effective, although providing less information to guide the choice or to optimise the interventions in actual practice.

The starting position for implementation research is the recognition that identifying factors predictive of clinicians' behaviour that are amenable to change may guide the design and choice of interventions with the highest chance of success. However, our understanding of potential barriers and enablers to quality improvement is largely limited in transfusion, and hindered by a lack of a 'basic science' relating to determinants of professional and organisational behaviour and potential targets for intervention. A systematic investigation of the beliefs associated with inappropriate transfusion practice and barriers to change could therefore point to potentially effective ways to optimise practice.

Conclusions

Many health care professionals are becoming more aware of the need to practise evidence-based transfusion medicine. But there remains considerable variation in transfusion practice against explicit criteria and guidelines. Some teams carry out even major procedures without blood transfusion by attention to patient care throughout the perioperative period. For example, a combination of educational support for algorithms for blood management and restrictive transfusion thresholds may offer a more effective approach to blood conservation than the implementation of more complex (or costly) single interventions, but better evidence on the relative effectiveness of these (or other) different strategies is required. While interventions to change transfusion practice can be aimed at a number of levels (individual health care professionals; health care groups or teams; organisations providing health care; the larger health care system; or environment), the majority of interventions have been aimed at individual practitioners, as ultimately it is the individual clinician who dictates much of the patient-facing decision-making. More resources need to be devoted towards a better understanding of the promotion of clinical effectiveness and the uptake of clinically effective transfusion practice (*evidence-based implementation*). Evidence of 'what to do' is one thing, but learning 'how to implement' this is another.

Key points

1 The evidence base for transfusion practice is poorly developed but is improving. As it increases, changes in transfusion behaviour will need to be enacted more frequently.
2 Transfusion practice is also characterised by variation against explicit criteria and guidelines.
3 The decision to transfuse is a complex process, and knowledge is unlikely to be the only influence; research into these factors is generally sparse.
4 A better understanding of the determinants of transfusion behaviour should better guide the design and choice of interventions to deliver changes and improvements in transfusion practice. These need to be evaluated in rigorous clinical studies.

Further reading

Ajzen I. The theory of planned behaviour. *Organ Behav Hum Decis Process* 1991;50:179–211.

Canadian Agency for Drugs and Technologies in Health. The *Rx for Change* database summarizes current research evidence about the effects of strategies to improve drug prescribing practice and drug use. Available at www.rxforchange.ca.

Eisenstaedt RS. Modifying physicians' transfusion practice. *Transfus Med Rev* 1997;11:27–37.

Effective Health Care. Bulletin on the effectiveness of health service interventions for decision makers. Centre for Reviews and Dissemination. The Royal Society of Medicine. Available at www.york.ac.uk.

Grimshaw JM, Thomas RE, MacLennan G *et al.* Effectiveness and efficiency of guideline dissemination and implementation strategies. *Health Technol Assess* 2004;8(6):1–84.

Grol R. Implementation of changes in practice. In: Grol R, Wensing M & Eccles M. (eds), *Improving Patient Care: Implementing Change in Clinical Practice*. Oxford: Elsevier, 2004.

Kirplani H, Whyte RK, Anderson C. The Premature infants in need of transfusion (PINT) study: a randomised controlled trial of a restrictive (low) versus liberal (high) transfusion threshold for extremely low birthweight infants. *J Pediatr* 2006;149:301–307.

Michie S, Johnston M, Abraham C *et al.* Making psychological theory useful for implementing evidence based practice: a consensus approach. *Qual Saf Health Care* 2005;14:26–33.

Murphy MF & Stanworth SJ. Global perspectives in transfusion medicine. In: Lozano M, Contreras M & Blajchman M. (eds), *Transfusion Practice*. Bethesda: AABB Press.

Rothschild JM, McGurk S, Honour M *et al.* Assessment of education and computerised decision support interventions for improving transfusion practice. *Transfusion* 2007;47:228–239.

Sanguis Study Group. Use of blood products for elective surgery in 43 European hospitals. *Transfus Med* 1994;4:251–268.

Salem-Schatz SR, Avorn J & Soumerai SB. Influence of clinical knowledge, organisational context and practice style on transfusion decision making: implications for practice change strategies. *JAMA* 1990;264:476–483.

Soumerai SB, Salem-Schatz SR, Avorn J *et al.* A controlled trial of education outreach to improve blood transfusion practice. *JAMA* 1993;270:961–966.

Stanworth S & Tinmouth A. Plasma transfusion and use of albumin. In: Simon TL, Snyder EL, Stowell CP, Strauss RG, Solheim BG, Petrides M. (eds), *Rossi's Textbook of Transfusion Medicine*, 4th edn. Wiley-Blackwell, *AABB* Press (in press).

Tinmouth A, MacDougall L, Fergusson D *et al.* Reducing the amount of blood transfused. *Arch Intern Med* 2005;165:845–852.

Wilson K, MacDougall L, Fergusson D, Graham L, Tinmouth A & Hebert, PC. The effectiveness of interventions to reduce physician's levels of inappropriate transfusion: what can be learned from a systematic review of the literature. *Transfusion* 2002;42(9):1224–1229.

CHAPTER 49

Scanning the future of transfusion medicine

Walter H. Dzik

Blood Transfusion Service, Massachusetts General Hospital; Harvard Medical School, Boston, Massachusetts, USA

Doctors must learn to translate between disease, which is what's in a textbook, and illness, which is the experience of a human being in trouble.

– Daniel Federman, Harvard Medical School

Introduction

The pace of change in biological sciences and health care has never been greater. This acceleration of innovation and discovery applies equally to transfusion medicine. New technology is being introduced that is changing the way blood is collected, processed and used for therapeutic benefit. This chapter briefly summarises some of the ongoing and anticipated changes coming to our profession. In considering what may lie ahead, it is often of value to assess what has just occurred. Some changes which seem at first to be inconsequential or of limited impact can, with time, take on much greater importance. Other innovations, which at first seem to be on the near horizon, encounter obstacles to implementation that keep them forever just beyond the reach of application. Numerous obstacles lie in the path of those who seek to implement new technology in health care. New technology is rarely

Practical Transfusion Medicine, 3rd edition. Edited by Michael F. Murphy and Derwood H. Pamphilon. © 2009 Blackwell Publishing, ISBN: 978-1-4051-8196-9.

seen as cost-effective. Regulatory requirements for safety are stringent, as they should be, and safety is often difficult to prove especially for low-frequency adverse events. For these reasons and others, the pace of change is slower than the pace of innovation and prediction of the future is no better now than it ever has been. The author apologises to the reader for errors of omission and comission or for over-optimism. If both author and reader are fortunate, we shall be able to learn in 2015 just what really happened. Table 49.1 lists recent developments in transfusion medicine during the last few years, those anticipated to arrive in the next 7 years, and those considered to be still further in the offing.

Changes in transfusion medicine since 2000

Donor collections

The increasing application of apheresis technology for routine donor collections has characterised the last decade. In the US, for example, platelets collected by apheresis have overtaken whole blood-derived platelets. In most regions, blood suppliers have completely stopped supplying whole blood-derived platelets as part of the implementation of universal leucocyte reduction. Perhaps as a result, platelet shortages have become commonplace in many hospitals. The loss of whole blood-derived platelets may be seen as a serious

Table 49.1 Changes in transfusion medicine in nations with advanced technology.

	Since 2000	Before 2015	After 2015
• Donor collections • Infectious risk	• Increased apheresis collections • Bacterial screening • West Nile virus screening • *T. cruzi* screening	• Changing donor demographics • Limited introduction of pathogen reduction for components • Early research of DNA chips for pathogen testing	• National blood donors • Chemical pathogen reduction for increased numbers of zoonoses due to encroachment on non-human habitats • DNA chips for pathogen screening
• Non-infectious risk	• General measures for TRALI risk reduction	• Specific measures for TRALI risk reduction • Shared databases of patient transfusion requirements	• ABO antigen removal • Conversion from FFP to recombinant factors • Attempts at artificial platelets
• Process risk	• Increased sophistication of haemovigilance data • Emergence of machine-readable patient ID • Increased laboratory automation	• Policy decisions based on haemovigilance data • Deployment of machine-readable patient ID • Laboratory automation • Computer-based decision support	• Machine-readable patient ID becomes standard • Computer-based decision-making • Computer simulation • Robotic surgery
• Diagnostics	• DNA diagnostics • Emerging proteomics • Imaging technologies • Microarray technology	• Limited use of chip-based blood genotyping • Increased use of HLA testing • Advances in diagnostic radiology and minimally invasive surgery	• Nanotechnology sensors • Personalised genomic medicine • Proteomics
• Therapeutics	• Off-label use of rituximab • Off-label use of rVIIa • Increased use of stem cells	• Early use of eculizimab • Early use of thrombopoietin • New anticoagulants • Increased organ and stem cell transplantation • Continued development of gene therapy research • Early use of haemoglobin-based oxygen carriers	• Liposome encapsulated haemoglobin • Specific immunotherapy • Tissue regeneration • Antigen-specific tolerance • Biomechanical organs • Limited gene therapy
• Clinical practice	————	• Clinical trials medicine and clinical specialists	————

This table is composed with contributions from Nancy Heddle, McMaster University; George Garratty, American Red Cross, Los Angeles; Jay Menitove, Community Blood Center of Greater Kansas City; Paul Ness, John Hopkins University; Gerald Sandler, George Washington University; and Ronald Strauss, University of Iowa.
TRALI, transfusion-related acute lung injury; HLA, human leucocyte antigen.

disadvantage to providing an adequate blood supply. For example, in the US, approximately 12 million whole blood donor units are collected each year because of demand for red cells. In contrast, only approximately 6 million platelets are required. Therefore, if blood suppliers were to prepare whole blood-derived platelets from even a *portion* of whole blood donations and these platelets were used to supplement collections made with apheresis, then there would be a substantial platelet supply to meet patient needs at very little incremental cost. While chronic shortages of group O red blood cells (RBCs) have fostered the development of double-unit RBC collections, double-unit RBC collections remain only a very small fraction of the RBC supply.

Product changes – infectious risk

Attention since the year 2000 was focused largely on three forms of transfusion-transmitted infection:
- bacteria;
- West Nile virus (WNV); and
- *Typanosoma cruzi*, the agent responsible for Chagas disease.

Bacterial contamination of blood components was recognised as an unusual but important hazard resulting uncommonly in serious patient morbidity or mortality. Bacterial risk was reduced by strategies that included diversion of the donor's initial blood from the final collection product and the pre-release screening of platelets by culture. Bacterial screening represents an example of an infectious disease screening test targeted to specific blood components (platelets) rather than to the donor sample.

WNV emerged after 2000 as a transfusion-transmitted infection affecting a very low number of transfusion recipients, including those with impaired immunity. WNV was the first example in which the initial screening test for the blood supply was based on nucleic acid technology. Originally tested in minipool format, individual donor testing by nucleic acid testing (NAT) was subsequently introduced.

In the US, *T. cruzi* testing was begun as a serologic test for high-risk individuals. While clinical Chagas disease resulting from *T. cruzi* infection acquired by transfusion would be an extraordinarily remote event in North America, the increased migration of people who are *T. cruzi* carriers prompted screening to reduce the risk of transfusion-transmitted infection.

Chemical pathogen reduction saw gradual implementation in the past few years. In addition to widespread use of methylene blue-treated plasma, there was limited introduction of a psoralen-based system for apheresis platelets. Readers are referred to a Canadian Consensus Conference on Pathogen Inactivation, which summarised the state of the art in 2007 (see Further Reading; Hebert *et al.*). The conference panel recommended against widespread implementation of pathogen inactivation but signalled the importance of additional research in this area.

The spectacular reduction in the risk of transfusion-transmitted diseases has been limited to the affluent nations, and transfusion-transmitted hepatitis and HIV remain major worldwide threats in nations with emerging economies. For example, in Africa, where HIV donor screening may be incomplete, the prevalence of HIV among blood donors ranges from 0.09% in South Africa to 8% in Zambia. In some regions, no screening for HCV exists. For more information, see: http://www.pepfar.gov/.

Product changes – non-infectious risks

Transfusion-related acute lung injury (TRALI) has come into better focus since 2000. Criteria for the diagnosis were improved as a result of NIH and Canadian Consensus Conferences on the topic. Haemovigilance programmes such as the SHOT programme in England have better documented its incidence. In response to these data, blood centres in the US, UK and European nations have taken general measures designed to reduce the frequency of TRALI. In some cases, this has included diversion of plasma donated by females away from the stock of fresh frozen plasma (FFP). The benefit of this approach will need to be assessed in relation to the loss of blood donors and to any unintended consequences resulting from the shift towards more male-donated plasma. While the infusion of anti-leucocyte or anti-HLA (human leucocyte antigen) antibodies reactive with antigens found in the recipient is, without doubt, a major mechanism for the induction of TRALI, research continues on alternative pathways to lung injury as well as a better understanding of the factors that influence the severity of the reaction.

Other non-infectious risks of transfusion continue to merit attention. Data on the frequency and morbidity of both acute and delayed haemolytic reactions resulting from antibodies to non-ABO antigens have emerged from both the SHOT programme and the Quebec haemovigilance programme. These haemovigilance systems document substantial numbers of haemolytic events due to antigens other than ABO. In contrast, recent data suggest a decrease in the incidence of transfusion-associated graft-versus-host disease. Whether this latter finding results from more widespread use of gamma irradiation or from an effect of leucocyte reduction is uncertain.

Process changes

Since the year 2000, data from haemovigilance programmes throughout the world continue to document that process weaknesses and human error are significant causes of for mis-transfusion events that lead to serious patient morbidity and mortality. In recent years, haemovigilance data has become more sophisticated and programmes such as those in Canada, England and France have used the results to guide data-driven policy decisions for regional blood services.

To address the problem of mis-transfusion, a number of companies developed and are marketing devices for bedside reading of bar codes from patient wristbands and blood containers. These devices are expected to decrease the frequency of clerical error at the time of transfusion (see Further Reading; CAP Today). Nevertheless, the deployment of machine-readable technology for the bedside transfusion check has been limited to a relatively small number of 'early adopters'.

Within the laboratory, the last several years has witnessed increased automation. The hospital transfusion service, long relegated to manual tube testing, has begun a transformation based on increased use of robotic sample handling and machine-readable assay reactions. These technologies are expected not only to reduce clerical errors in the laboratory, but also to increase throughput in a profession where the number of qualified medical technologists continues to diminish.

New diagnostics: genomics and microarrays

Sequencing the human genome represented the landmark medical milestone of the last decade. The sequencing project promoted the development of high-throughput technology for nucleic acid sequencing that is the basis for genomics. The beginning of the new century saw the emergence of proteomics and microarray technology. Early use of microarrays has included application to both RBC and platelet antigens. Gene chip diagnostics may prove useful for wide-scale genotyping of donors, identification of rare donor genotypes, improved matching of donor–recipient transfusions and prenatal testing.

New therapeutics

Immunology

Recent years have seen substantial growth in the application of anti-CD20 (Rituximab, IDEC Pharmaceuticals, San Diego, CA) for treatment of a wide variety of autoimmune disorders. In transfusion medicine, anti-CD20 has been used with some success for the treatment of autoimmune haemolytic anaemia, immune thrombocytopenia, thrombotic thrombocytopenic purpura, coagulation factor inhibitors and a variety of autoimmune conditions for which plasmapheresis is often tried. Despite the generally good success, there is recognition that the agent does not deplete mature immunoglobulin-producing plasma cells which limits its effect on humoral alloimmunity. Newer agents that are more specific to antibody-producing cells are needed. During the same time, there was growing use of high dose intravenous immunglobulin as an immunosuppressant. Like rituximbab, treatment with high dose immune globulin is largely done in the absence of any controlled trials.

Haemostasis

A growing number of recombinant products are available for haemostasis therapy. These include recombinant haemophilia factors, activated protein C, hirudin, tissue-type plasminogen activator and anti-platelet glycoprotein agents. Recombinant VIIa (NovoSeven, NovoNordisk, Copenhagen), licenced for treatment of bleeding in haemophilia patients with inhibitors, has been widely used off-label. Despite anecdotal evidence of benefit, several pivotal randomised controlled clinical trials failed to superiority compared with placebo. In particular, randomised trials in upper gastrointestinal bleeding, liver transplant surgery, bone marrow transplantation and trauma found no evidence of benefit. More studies are anticipated.

Transplantation

The collection and processing of haemopoietic progenitors harvested from peripheral blood or cord blood has virtually replaced bone marrow as a source of transplantation material. Stem cell processing has become a routine, established, and integral part of the transfusion medicine laboratory. The availability of increased numbers of banked cord blood cells has allowed expansion of unmatched donor transplants. Bone marrow registries worldwide continue to grow in size and have resulted in large numbers of successful marrow transplants from unrelated individuals. In addition, a growing number of tissue banks have established controlled storage of non-haemopoietic tissues.

Changes to come – what we might expect before 2015

Donor collections

Overall, the demand for blood donations is expected to rise above current levels, especially in nations where population demographics will create a large number of elderly individuals in need of surgery and medical therapies. Exclusion of plasma donated by females, failure to produce platelet concentrates from volunteer donor whole blood, and the need to exclude growing numbers of donors based on travel exposure to infectious agents may place additional strains on blood availability. The rapid economic growth in China and India would be expected to result in increased health care services in those countries and an increased demand for blood that may outstrip supply.

Product changes – infectious risk

Despite tremendous success in reducing infectious risks of transfusion, emphasis on further risk reduction will undoubtedly occur. Indeed, improved blood safety has become synonymous with reduction of infectious hazards of transfusion and has dominated the perspective of regulators, policy makers, the media and the general public. Three parallel and somewhat competing strategies for further risk reduction will likely see different degrees of implementation in the next decade: chemical pathogen reduction, nucleic acid technology and haemoglobin-based oxygen carriers.

Chemical pathogen inactivation is expected to increase. Given the formidable obstacles to develop new pathogen inactivation technology, it is likely that existing methods such as methylene blue-treatment of plasma and psoralen-light treatment of platelets will undergo further evaluation and deployment. Entirely new methodologies are unlikely to be introduced in the near term.

One might imagine initial research investigating the use of nucleic acid microarray technology – advanced by progress in genomics – applied to pathogen screening of blood donations. DNA microarrays have already been used to detect pathogens in environmental samples. Largely an engineering challenge, there are few scientific obstacles to the use of DNA array technology for blood donor testing and a single platform applied to viruses, bacteria and parasites would bring efficiencies to the screening process. High-throughput chip technology may be unexpectedly more cost-effective than current multiple platform testing systems. Microchip technology may prove fruitful for donor screening in rapidly expanding systems such as those in China or India.

Product changes, non-infectious

General policies designed to reduce the risk of TRALI should become routine and widespread during the next 7 years. Although pooling of large numbers of donor units of FFP would be expected to reduce TRALI through dilution of donor antibodies, pooling of components in the absence of a highly robust pathogen inactivation process is not likely to occur. More specific approaches to reduce the risk of TRALI may emerge. For example, screening female donors with a history of prior pregnancy for HLA antibodies, a known cause of TRALI, has already begun at some blood centres and may be more cost-effective than elimination of female donors.

Process changes – rise of information technology

Machine-readable identification of both the patient and the blood container should supplement eye-readable labels in the next decade. Because haemovigilance programmes have repeatedly documented that mis-transfusion represents one of the most common reasons for transfusion-related death or serious morbidity, there is every reason to develop, deploy and require improved methods to interrupt mis-transfusion. Two technologies – bar coding and radio-frequency chips – appear to be the most promising for this application.

Bar-coded labels have been commonplace on blood packs for decades. Bar coding is firmly established within laboratories as an important safety measure for the identification and tracking of samples and blood packs. It would be anticipated that bar coding of patient wristbands will increase and that bar code readers will be used at the bedside for several applications including the pre-transfusion safety check. Impediments to the deployment of bar code technology at the bedside may include perceived inconvenience and cost. In the US, the emphasis on proper patient identification articulated by the Joint Commission on Accreditation of Hospitals provided incentive for US hospitals to invest in proper patient identification. In the UK, the National Patient Safety Agency is promoting increased use of electronic methods for both patient identification and verification that the right blood is about to be transfused.

Radio-frequency identification (RFID) chips have undergone explosive development in the last few years. RFID carries an advantage over bar coding because direct line-of-site and alignment of the laser with the bar code is not required. Already

widely used in hospitals for security access, the declining unit cost of RFID chips makes them a practical alternative to bar codes for blood packs and patient wristbands. RFID chips on blood packs could record the pack's life history of processing steps for Good Manufacturing Practice purposes and could record environmental conditions critical to blood storage. Combined with dispensing machines, such chips could also be used for unit selection and inventory management in the laboratory. When used in combination with identification chips on the patient wristband, RFID on blood packs could be used for the bedside check prior to blood administration. Other devices, including smart infusion pumps and wireless data devices, may supplement bedside safety. For example, blood infusion pumps that 'know' the identity of the patient would alarm and refuse to infuse a blood pack labelled with an RFID chip of another patient.

Laboratory automation should increase in the near term. In the US, the Department of Labor and Statistics estimates that 120,000 new medical technologists and technicians will be needed between the year 2000 and 2010. The available workforce is not likely to meet this expected demand. The mean age of medical technologists continues to increase reflecting a decline in new graduates entering the profession and consistent with the nationwide decrease in the number of training programmes for technologists. Automation will be needed to offset this labour shortage especially during an era of increased demand for blood services by an ageing population.

Regional sharing of information about the special transfusion needs of patients can reduce the risk of haemolytic events. In Quebec province, a common database was established in which participating hospitals could record patient alloantibodies. Following implementation of this programme, the incidence of acute and delayed haemolytic transfusion reactions significantly declined. There is also every reason to believe that the explosive growth in informatics will continue to change decision-making in medicine. The trend, already begun, is for computers to migrate from repositories of data to decision support machines. For example, electronic medical libraries, such as PubMed, give practitioners rapid access to an enormous repository of medical information but make no attempt to recommend treatments. Decision support software will increasingly recommend diagnostic and therapeutic choices to guide clinical decision-making. At the very least enhanced informatics will give clinicians faster access to relevant data upon which to make clinical decisions.

Changes in diagnostics

The application of both genomics and proteomics to diagnostic medicine is expected to undergo expansive growth in the next decade leading to improved characterisation of the genotypic risk for disease, improved diagnosis and the molecular classification of diseased tissue. Blood group polymorphisms have already been explored as natural targets for genomic analysis. Continued investigation into genetic polymorphisms should redefine 'genotype and phenotype' far beyond the bounds of circulating blood cells. DNA 'chips' have already been designed to test samples for multiple RBC and platelet antigens. There is every reason to anticipate that such chip-based typing will continue to develop. It may find unique advantage for the prevention of RBC antigen sensitisation by matching blood donations for recipients who belong to minority populations.

Use of HLA testing by the transfusion service may also increase during the next decade. Three important transfusion complications result from HLA incompatibilities: febrile non-haemolytic reactions (see Chapter 8), TRALI (see Chapter 9) and platelet transfusion refractoriness (see Chapter 27). Ready access to a rapid and affordable HLA antibody screen might see wide application in the blood centre and hospital-based transfusion service. All female blood donors with a history of prior pregnancy might be tested for the presence of HLA antibodies. The routine type and screen of patients admitted for treatment of leukaemia might include an HLA type and screen. The differential diagnosis of TRALI versus volume overload or of bacterial contamination versus febrile non-haemolytic reaction may be influenced by a simple and rapid test for HLA antibodies.

Advances in diagnostic and interventional radiology and non-invasive surgery are also very likely to continue to change the use of blood components in the future. For example, the use of angiographically placed coils in vascular aneurysms, or stents in coronary arteries has already allowed many patients to avoid larger surgical procedures. Moreover, open surgical procedures of the future should become less invasive due to advances in robotics, endoscopic surgery and laparoscopic techniques. Next-generation computer processing should allow high-definition diagnostic images functional organ assessment.

New therapeutics

Complement inhibitors

Eculizimab (Alexion Pharmaceuticals) was licenced in 2007 in the US for the treatment of patients with paroxysmal nocturnal haemoglobinuria. The years to come should see initial application of this agent to a variety of transfusion-related disorders. Complement activation is central to intravascular alloimmune blood cell destruction including red cell haemolysis and platelet refractoriness. Complement activation is critical to a variety of diseases that are currently being addressed, in part, by apheresis technology. These include transplant rejection, diarrhoea-negative haemolytic uraemic syndrome, vasculitis with cryoglobulins, small vessel vasculitis and severe autoimmune haemolysis. An immediately infusable complement inhibitor may be especially valuable in situations such as ABO-mediated haemolysis or TRALI.

Growth factors

Thrombopoietin is expected to be used as a routine agent during the next 7 years especially for patients with immune thrombocytopenia. Although erythropoietin usage may decrease due to concerns of toxicity, continued development of recombinant proteins holds great promise for improved therapeutics in the coming decade (see also Chapters 31, 33 and 43). Procoagulant proteins including factors V, X, fibrinogen, prothrombin and thrombin-activated fibrinolytic inhibitor may find initial research application. Anticoagulant proteins, such as tissue factor pathway inhibitor, von Willebrand cleaving protease, protein S, thrombomodulin and plasminogen activators are equally poised for recombinant production. Newer agents, such as oral factor Xa inhibitors and oral thrombin inhibitors, will undoubtedly increase the options available to clinicians for therapeutic anticoagulation.

Haemoglobin-based oxygen carriers are likely to obtain approval for clinical use during the next 7 years although widespread implementation of these technologies may be delayed by concerns over safety and cost. Given the short intravascular half-life of most haemoglobin-based oxygen carriers, it would seem that these agents would most likely be applied to resuscitation at the point of injury, rather than as agents used to replace hospital RBC transfusions. Given the importance of the 'golden hour' (the need for adequate resuscitation during the first hour following serious injury), the effect of oxygen carriers might be especially beneficial when given to the patient on route to the hospital.

Transplantation services should continue to increase. Improved allograft survival coupled with an ageing population is expected to result in an increased demand for organ transplant services including kidney, liver, heart, lung and pancreas. These, in turn, will place ongoing demands for blood support. Progenitor cell isolation and expansion is expected to be a major focus of cancer therapy in the next decade. Research will improve the characterisation of haemopoietic pluripotent stem cells and the ex vivo processing of these cells. Research in stem cell plasticity may result in the early application of regenerative medicine whose full application is still probably in the more distant future.

Other therapeutic developments such as the advent of organ-directed gene therapy may dramatically alter the nature of transfusion support required by patients. Among the many illnesses requiring blood support, gene therapy would be expected to have most dramatic impact on inherited disorders such as haemophilia, sickle cell disease and thalassaemia. Successful gene therapy

for haemophilia, in particular, seems likely because only limited factor VIII expression is needed to ameliorate symptoms. Haemophilia gene therapy would be a natural scientific progression from decades of dependence on blood products for patients with this disorder.

Looking further ahead – 2015 and beyond

National blood donors

The widespread use of intense screening for transfusion-transmitted pathogens and the application of chemical pathogen inactivation combined with projected shortages of volunteer blood donor collections may create an environment favourable for the use of certified blood donors. Concern over emerging pathogens resulting from encroachment of humans on natural animal habitats, extreme poverty in large urban populations and global travel may fuel the rationale for certified blood donors. Drawing needed collections from a small, stable and productive group of qualified, 'card-carrying', national blood donors may prove to be the most efficient and safe means for securing an adequate blood supply.

Future product changes, infectious risk: the long road to widespread chemical pathogen reduction

While a few companies have successfully developed technology capable of providing chemically treated blood components, numerous practical hurdles lay before the widespread application of pathogen-reduced RBCs, FFP and platelets. Chemical pathogen reduction will bring the advantage of lowering not only the risk of unknown pathogens, but also reducing patient exposure to known pathogens which may not be suited to available testing strategies. As humans live in increasingly crowded conditions and continue to encroach on the habitat of wild creatures, more infectious agents are likely to 'jump' species' barriers. Continued development of pathogen reduction technology may represent a safeguard to this threat. However, the high cost of pathogen inactivation technology will surely influence its application. Ironically, the technology carries the greatest medical value when applied to poorer regions of the world where infectious agents are common among blood donors and where traditional testing is inadequate. One might hope for a future in which wealthier nations would pay a cost for the technology that would directly subsidise its application within poorer nations. A robust, safe, cost-effective and widely deployed technique for chemical sterilisation of blood would be a remarkable achievement bringing to a close the long chapter of transfusion-transmitted infections.

Future product changes, non-infectious

Given the morbidity and mortality associated with mis-transfusion of blood resulting in serious haemolytic transfusion reactions, the development of techniques designed to remove antigens from the red cell surface would represent a fundamental breakthrough. Although technology currently under development is designed to enzymatically cleave ABO antigens from the red cell surface, antigen removal is not a simple matter and will require continued refinement before application in my view. Other technical approaches include attempts to chemically 'mask' antigens ('stealth red cells') without introducing alterations that would reduce intravascular survival or microvascular function.

Future process changes

Beyond 2015, widespread application of machine-readable technology for patient identification seems nearly certain. The progress and innovation likely to occur in informatics by 2015 is almost unimaginable. Computers will continue to influence human decision-making and one would expect that computer-based informatics will move from 'passive' decision support to a more 'active' decision-making role. In passive decision support, computers respond to human decisions with approval or recommended alternatives. In active decision-making, computers will select diagnostic and therapeutic options and humans will only intervene in order to treat exceptions or to override

the computer. Computer-based simulation may eventually become the primary platform for clinical medical education. Combined with enhanced imaging, computers should be able to take control of the fine movements needed for delicate surgery, a process already begun and referred to as 'robotic surgery'.

Future diagnostics

Nanotechnology may change the trigger for transfusion

Extreme miniaturisation of mechanical devices and improved understanding of biocompatible materials may pave the way for implantable micro-devices that will provide information on tissue status. The availability of oxygen and pH sensors within a few key tissues would revolutionise the indication for RBC transfusion and oxygen support therapies. Using radio-frequency data transmission, such devices could report information by passing a 'reader' over the area of the body with an implanted chipsensor.

Genomics, proteomics, cytoplasmics and nucleonics

Beyond 2015, genomics may be advanced to analysis and understanding of genome polymorphisms for each patient. Disease susceptibility and better patient categorisation will no doubt occur as clinical outcomes are matched to detailed genotypes. Proteomics will have found a more secure foothold in medical diagnosis. Because gene analysis does not, by itself, always predict protein expression, advances in proteomics will be needed to establish genotype–phenotype correlations. In addition to proteomics, one might expect that 'cytoplasmics' and 'nucleonics' (terms not in use at this time) will be areas of organised investigation. Cytoplasmics might include analysis of cytoplasmic machinery including second messenger systems, protein chaperone activity, post-translational protein modification and endosomal and lysosomal processing. Nucleonics will explore intranuclear machinery including intranuclear messaging, DNA unfolding and gene transcription.

Future therapeutics

Haemoglobin-based therapies

Blood substitute technology will surely continue to advance in the early decades of the twenty-first century. Liposomal encapsulated haemoglobin, with a longer circulation time and improved oxygen delivery, may eventually replace free haemoglobin solutions as an oxygen carrier. Competition between these products and pathogen-inactivated blood components is expected. However, development is likely to be restricted to RBC replacement therapy. Indeed, the prospects for a functional but truly 'artificial' platelet, granulocyte, or lymphocyte appear remote.

Cellular therapies: cancer immunotherapy, tissue regeneration and immune tolerance

Three broad areas of cellular therapy are currently active and may find application during the second decade of the twenty-first century. First, immunotherapy directed against cancer and viral infections may engage transfusion medicine professionals in the harvest and manipulation of dendritic cells or other immune cells directed against unwanted pathogens. Second, exploration of the plasticity of stem cells may open new fields of tissue repair and regeneration. In nuclear transplantation therapy (also called therapeutic cloning) a nucleus from the patient's cells is transplanted into an oocyte. Culture ex vivo results in an embryonic stem cell that can then be used to differentiate under appropriate tissue-specific conditions into new autologous tissue for re-transplantation – tissue replacement therapy. While the conceptual strategy is clear-cut and while initial promising application has occurred in animal systems, numerous substantial obstacles will need to be overcome before pluripotent stem cells can be made to differentiate in vitro into useful tissue. For more information, see reviews in the cited literature. Third, the ability to induce antigen-specific immune tolerance would represent a substantial improvement from generalised non-specific immune suppression used in transplantation today. Antigen-specific tolerance would also find wide-ranging application in rheumatologic and autoimmune disorders. Adop-

tive transfer of haemopoietic progenitors, regulatory lymphocytes, or other immune cells following ex vivo modification and expansion may prove successful for the maintenance of tolerance. Ultimately, the regulation of gene transcription providing the power to turn on and off genes would represent an enormous change in medical therapeutics. Control of the human genome would unlock the potential within us for self-healing that has been a goal of medicine for centuries.

Humans, machines and biocompatibility

The development of biomechanical organs would be the natural consequence of future advances in computer technology, nanotechnology, battery–energy technology, materials research and biocompatibility. While a mechanical liver is not on the horizon, an implantable pump that could replace the human heart is foreseeable. Highly sophisticated mechanical prostheses (hands, legs, eyes, ears) may liberate victims of burns or trauma and offer new hope to those who suffer daily with severe physical disabilities. Mechanical kidneys, lungs and other vital organs await biocompatibility challenges likely to be solved through endothelial cell research.

Xenotransplantation and whole-animal cloning

The cloning of Dolly the sheep represented a landmark event in the potential use of genetically engineered whole animals for science. In principle, cloned animals in which xenoantigens have been deleted could become a new source material for xeno-transplantation freed from the substantial obstacles of acute xeno-graft rejection. Considerable guarded research has already occurred in the development of pigs whose complement protein genes have been modified towards compatibility with primates. In a general sense, whole animal cloning and xeno-transplantation is in competitive development with tissue re-growth and gene transfer therapy. Animal-to-human whole organ transplantation remains controversial bringing concerns over not only the introduction of animal pathogens into new human reservoirs, but also the ethics of whole animal cloning.

Clinical trials

Cutting across the entire timeline of technology development in transfusion medicine will be the ongoing need for intelligent clinical evaluation of new technology. All new technology should be held accountable to scrutiny regarding risk-versus-benefit to the patient and regarding cost-versus-benefit to society. All of health care, including transfusion medicine, needs to recognise that such scrutiny conducted by randomised controlled trials is well worth large investment lest we incorrectly adopt practices that later prove to be either a wasteful squandering of resources or harmful therapies misleading the public we serve (see Chapter 46). Too often in the past, technology has been imposed either through marketing pressure or through regulatory fiat. The recent application of haemovigilance programmes in the UK, France and Canada as a means to establish priorities for technical innovation has represented a breakthrough in rational strategic planning for transfusion care. In a like manner, federal funding in the US of a Clinical Trials Network in Transfusion Medicine and Hemostasis serves as an important example of national investment in the clinical investigation of new advances in our field. Similar initiatives have been established in Canada, England, Europe and Asia.

Summary

For centuries, medicine has sought to cure illness and relieve suffering through the application of improved diagnostics and therapeutics. Change has nearly always represented progress. Through the centuries, enormous human benefit derived from basic advances in hygiene, sanitation, nutrition and education. Modern science has explored the basic biologic processes that act within cells. The twentieth century witnessed an unprecedented understanding of human genetics and molecular biology coupled with advances in medical and surgical therapies that could not have been imagined in previous times. During the second half of the twentieth century, blood transfusion became an established infrastructure of modern medical and surgical practice. The last decade has seen tremendous progress in reducing the risk of transfusion-transmitted infections making blood therapies among the most spectacular life-saving remedies used in health care. The decade to come should be filled with the excitement of continued change driven by progress in both biological science and information technology. The changes that await us will bring exciting new challenges to transfusion medicine – the challenge to adopt new technology wisely and refine its use for direct patient care, to finance its application, and to remain educated to new developments. However, the greatest challenge brought by scientific discovery and its application will remain the challenge of medical ethics. Physicians and other health care professionals will need to advocate more forcefully for political and economic systems that not only promote the advance of technology in the privileged nations, but also address the greater and more pressing health care needs of impoverished nations. Looking ahead, our greatest challenge will be to balance technology with humanism, to temper the zeal for discovery with compassion for the sick, and to remember always that we are not just biological but also spiritual beings.

Acknowledgements

The author would like to thank Christine Cserti-Gazdewich (University of Toronto), Robert Makar (Harvard University) and Christopher Stowell (Harvard University) for their excellent critical reading and improvement of the manuscript. I am also indebted to the Associate Editors of the journal *Transfusion* for guidance on the topics selected for discussion and shown in Table 49.1.

Key points

1 Changing population demographics suggest that the supply of blood donors will diminish in the years ahead.

2 Some combination of chemical pathogen reduction and DNA-based testing will continue
to reduce the risk of transfusion-transmitted
injection.

3 Machine readable patient identification will represent a significant improvement in transfusion
safety.

4 Continued programme in recombinant protein
technology and cellular therapies will change the
available therapeutics in transfusion medicine.

5 Randomized clinical trials will remain the best
price of data upon which to base tranfusion
policies.

Further reading

General

Field SP & Allain JP. Transfusion in sub-Sarahan Africa:
does a Western model fit? *J Clin Pathol* 2007;60:1073–
1075.

Stowell CP & Dzik WH. (eds) *Emerging Technologies in
Transfusion Medicine*. Bethesda: AABB Press, 2003.

Zou S, Musavi F, Notari EP & Fang CT. Changing age distribution of the blood donor population in the United
States. *Transfusion* 2008;48:251–257.

Diagnostics

Alter HJ, Stramer SL & Dodd RY. Emerging infectious
diseases that threaten the blood supply. *Semin Hematol*
2007;44:32–41.

CAP Today. Positive patient identification systems and
products. *Coll Am Pathol* 2006;108–118.

Fournier-Wirth C & Coste J. Fitting new technology into
the safety paradigm: use of microarray technology in
transfusion. *Dev Biol (Basel)* 2007;127:61–70.

Goldman M, Webert KE, Arnold DM, Freedman J, Hannon J & Blajchman MA. Proceedings of a consensus
conference: towards an understanding of TRALI. *Transfus Med Rev* 2005;19:2–31.

Jain KK. Application of nanobiotechnology in clinical diagnostics. *Clin Chem* 2007;53:2002–2009.

Petrik J, de Haas M, Denomme G, Scott M & Seghatchian
J. Small world – advance of microarrays: current status
and future trends. *Transfus Apheresis Sci* 2007;36:201–
206.

Siegel DL. Recombinant monoclonal antibody technology. *Transfus Clin Biol* 2002;9:15–22.

Wu YY & Csako G. Rapid and high-throughput genotyping for human red blood cell, platelet, and leukocyte antigens and forensic applications. *Clin Chem Acta*
2006;363:165–176.

Therapeutics

Andemariam B & Bussel J. New therapies for immune thrombocytopenic purpura. *Curr Opin Hematol*
2007;14:427–431.

Cervera RP & Stojkovic M. Human embryonic stem cell
derivation and nuclear transfer: impact on regenerative
therapeutics and drug discovery. *Clin Pharmacol Ther*
2007;82:310–315.

Chang TM. Future generations of red blood cell substitutes. *J Intern Med* 2003;253:527–535.

Davies A, Stanes J, Kay J, Casbard A & Murphy M.
End-to-end electronic control of the hospital transfusion process to increase the safety of blood transfusion:
strengths and weaknesses. *Transfusion* 2006;46:352–
364.

Kunkler K. The role of medical simulation: an overview.
Int J Med Robot 2006;2:203–210.

Kuter DJ. New thrombopoietic growth factors. *Blood*
2007;109:4607–4616.

Marsh JC, Ganser A & Stadler M. Hematopoietic growth
factors in the treatment of acquired bone marrow failure states. *Semin Hematol* 2007;41:138–147.

Mimeault M, Hauke R & Batra SK. Stem cells: a revolution in therapeutics – recent advances in stem cell
biology and their therapeutic applications in regenerative medicine and cancer therapies. *Clin Pharmacol Ther*
2007;82:252–264.

Ness PM & Cushing MM. Oxygen therapeutics: pursuit of
an alternative to the donor red blood cell. *Arch Pathol
Lab Med* 2007;131:734–741.

Ponder KP. Gene therapy of hemophila. *Curr Opin Haematol* 2006;13:301–307.

Rother RP, Rollins SA, Mojcik CF, Brodsky RA &
Bell L. Discovery and development of the complement inhibitor eculizumab for the treatment of
paroxysmal nocturnal hemoglobinuria. *Nat Biotechnol*
2007;25:1256–1264.

Webert KE, Cserti CM, Hannon J *et al.* Proceedings of
a consensus conference: pathogen inactivation making decisions about new technologies. *Transfus Med Rev*
2008;22:1–34.

Index

Page numbers in **bold** represent tables, those in *italics* represent figures.

aaBB 417–18
ABO blood group system 13, 19–22
  A and B subgroups 20–1, **21**
  antibodies 20, 286
    and HDN 298
  biosynthesis and molecular genetics
    21–2, *21*, *22*
  clinical significance 19–20
  incompatibility 20, **75**, **76**
  pre-transfusion testing 246, **246**
  testing for 200–1
activated protein C 534
acute haemolytic transfusion reaction **65**
acute normovolaemic haemodilution
  375–6, 382–3
acute respiratory distress syndrome 91
acute transfusion reactions 63–71, **65–7**
  clinical presentation 63–4, **64**
  differential diagnosis 63–4, **64**
  management
    algorithm *70*, 71
    immediate action 69
    laboratory tests 69–71
  medications 64
  patient history 64
  presence of fever 68
  signs and symptoms **64**
  type of blood product 68
  volume of blood product 68
ADAMTS13 344
adaptive immunity 7
adhesion molecules *17*
adverse events
  detection/reporting 182–3, **183**
  investigation of 242
AKR-501 474
algorithms 237, 239–40
allergic transfusion reactions **65**, 86–8
  clinical presentation 86–7
  incidence 86
  management 87
  prevention 87–8
    antipyretics and/or antihistamines
    87–8
    IgA-deficient blood products 88
    leucocyte reduction 88
    washed products/plasma-reduced
    products 88

allogeneic blood transfusion 98
allogeneic mononuclear cells, TRIM effects
  100
American Association of Blood Banks *see*
  aaBB
AMG 531 474
ε-aminocaproic acid 376, **401**
aminomethyl trimethylpsoralen **108**
amotosalen **108**
anaemia 270–2, **271**
  acute 270–1
  aplastic 113
  autoimmune haemolytic *see*
    autoimmune haemolytic anaemia
  and blood conservation 370, 373, *373*,
    374
  chronic 271–2
    red cell transfusion 309
  evaluation *373*
  fetal 294, **294**
  management *373*
  neonatal 294, **294**
    management 294–5, **294**
  transfusion triggers **374**
anaphylactic transfusion reaction **66**
anaphylactoid reactions 86–7
anaphylatoxins 74
anaphylaxis 86–7
Anaplasma phagocytophilum **164**
antenatal *see* pregnancy
anti-A 73
anti-A,B 73
anti-B 73
antibodies 8, *8*, 9–10
  blood cell destruction 13
  effector functions 8, **9**
  genes encoding *10*
  HLA
    class II, restriction of response 12
    clinical relevance 38–40
    detection 37–8
    formation 36–7
  HNA 57
  humoral immune response 8, *8*
    effector functions 8, **9**
    HLA class II restriction of response 12
    T-cell-dependent 11–12
    T-cell-independent 11

  variability 8–9
  identification 247
  recombinant 348–9, **349**
    anti-HPA-1a 352
    anti-prion 351–2
    human 349–50, *350*
    human monoclonal anti-D 350–1
    'null' 352
    T-cell-dependent 11–12
    T-cell-independent 11
  testing for 201–2
  variability 8–9
  see also individual antibodies
anti-c 286, 287
anti-CD20 *see* rituximab
anticoagulants
  complications 337–8, **337**
  overdose, reversal of 404
    fresh frozen plasma 344
anti-D 24, 286, 287
  human monoclonal recombinant 350–1
  indications 289, **289**
    dose and administration, antenatal
    period 289
    postnatal period 290
    preparation 291
  pre-transfusion testing 246
antifibrinolytics 400–1, **401**
  aprotinin **269**, 270, 376, 400–1, **401**
  lysine analogues 376, 401–2
antigens
  blood group 28
  recombinant 352–3
    blood groups 352
    microbial 353
antigen presentation 16–17, *17*
antigen-presenting cells 12
anti-Gerbish 287
anti-HPA-1a, recombinant 352
anti-Jka 73
anti-K1 286
anti-K2 287
anti-Kpa 287
anti-Lea 287
anti-Leb 287
anti-Lua 73–4, 287
anti-N 287
anti-P 287